# Contents

*Foreword by Anthony Lander*                                         ix
*Foreword by Steven S Rothenberg*                                    x
*Preface*                                                            xi
*List of contributors*                                               xiii

**Section I  General**                                               **1**

1   Growth and development                                           2
    Joanne Ng

2   Fluids, electrolytes and nutritional support                    8
    Craig R Nemechek, Onyebuchi Ukabiala

3   Coagulopathies and surgical infectious diseases                 16
    Nitin Patwardhan

**Section II  Critical care**                                        **21**

4   Shock                                                            22
    Robert Baird, Pramod S Puligandla

5   Mechanical ventilation and support                              32
    Elizabeth Pilling

6   Vascular access                                                 35
    Alexander Cho, Alice Mears, Niall Jones

**Section III  Trauma**                                              **45**

7   General approach to trauma                                      46
    Marianne Beaudin, Rebeccah L Brown

8   Head and spinal injuries                                        56
    Desiderio Rodrigues

9   Thoracic trauma                                                 61
    Marianne Beaudin, Rebeccah L Brown

10  Abdominal trauma                                                71
    Marianne Beaudin, Rebeccah L Brown

# CONTENTS

11 Genitourinary trauma 84
Marianne Beaudin, Rebeccah L Brown

12 Musculoskeletal trauma and soft tissue injuries 94
Gleeson Rebello

13 Bites and burns 103
Faisal G Qureshi, Felix C Blanco, Kurt D Newman

14 Child abuse and birth injuries 116
Natasha de Vere

## Section IV  Head and neck 127

15 Cysts and sinuses in the neck 128
Ross Fisher

16 Endocrine disorders 133
Michael Skinner, Eduardo Perez

## Section V  Thorax 145

17 Breast disorders in children and adolescents 146
Marjorie J Arca

18 Chest wall deformities 156
Michael J Goretsky, Robert Obermeyer

19 Disorders of larynx, trachea and upper airway 161
Charles M Myer IV, Charles M Myer III

20 Congenital diaphragmatic hernia 170
Mary Brindle, David Sigalet

21 Congenital lung malformations 175
Matias Bruzoni, Craig T Albanese

22 Acquired lung disease 183
Matias Bruzoni, Craig T Albanese

23 Diseases of mediastinum and mediastinal masses 192
David Sigalet, Mary Brindle

24 Tracheobronchial and oesophageal foreign bodies 200
Robert Baird, Pramod S Puligandla

25 Congenital anomalies of the oesophagus 210
Ashwin Pimpalwar

# CONTENTS

26 Caustic injuries of the oesophagus 218
Brice Antao, Michael S Irish

27 Gastro-oesophageal reflux disease 226
Victoria Lane, Mark Powis

## Section VI  Cardiovascular 241

28 Congenital cardiac anomalies 242
Bassem N Mora

29 Vascular disorders 259
Alan P Sawchuk, Gary Lemmon, Raghu Motaganahalli

30 Vascular tumours and malformations 263
Cameron C Trenor III, Steven J Fishman, Arin K Greene

## Section VII  Abdomen 277

31 Congenital abdominal wall defects 278
Brice Antao, Michael S Irish

32 Hernia and hydrocele 283
Brice Antao, Michael S Irish

## Section VIII  Gastroenterology 291

33 Lesions of the stomach 292
Victoria Lane, Brice Antao, Michael S Irish

34 Intestinal atresia 300
Jason S Frischer, Richard G Azizkhan

35 Malrotation and midgut volvulus 310
Shirley Chou, Marcos Bettolli

36 Meconium ileus 317
Stephanie A Jones, Moritz M Ziegler

37 Meckel's diverticulum 330
Brice Antao, Michael S Irish

38 Alimentary tract duplications 338
Brice Antao, Shawqui Nour

39 Intussusception 344
Victoria Lane, Brice Antao, Michael S Irish

# CONTENTS

40  Necrotising enterocolitis                                              351
    Rodrigo Romao, J Ted Gerstle

41  Short bowel syndrome                                                   359
    Derek Wakeman, Jennifer A Leinicke, Brad W Warner

42  Appendicitis                                                           373
    Nitin Patwardhan

43  Inflammatory bowel disease and polypoid diseases in children          377
    A Anish, Mike Thomson

44  Gastrointestinal bleeding                                             389
    Manjula Velayudhan, Mike Thomson

45  Disorders of colonic motility                                          397
    Taiwo A Lawal, Alberto Peña, Marc A Levitt

46  Anorectal continence and constipation                                 407
    Kaveer Chatoorgoon, Alberto Peña, Marc A Levitt

47  Anorectal disorders                                                    417
    Andrea Bischoff, Alberto Peña, Marc A Levitt

**Section IX  Hepatobiliary disorders**                                   **427**

48  Biliary atresia                                                        428
    Eric Jelin, Kelly D Gonzales, Hanmin Lee

49  Choledochal cyst                                                       436
    Riccardo A Superina, Niramol Tantemsapya

50  Gallbladder disease                                                    444
    N Alexander Jones, Onyebuchi Ukabiala

51  Portal hypertension                                                    451
    Riccardo A Superina, Niramol Tantemsapya

52  Pancreatic disorders in children                                       465
    Christian J Streck Jr, Andre Hebra

53  Spleen                                                                 476
    Zachary Kastenberg, Sanjeev Dutta

**Section X  Genitourinary disorders**                                    **487**

54  Renal diseases in children                                            488
    Stephen D Marks

# CONTENTS

55 Developmental and positional anomalies of the kidney     495
Ian E Willetts

56 Cystic disease of the kidneys     502
Harish Chandran

57 Obstructive uropathies     507
Julian Roberts

58 Vesicoureteric reflux and urinary tract infection     515
Francesca Castillo, Ian E Willetts

59 Urinary incontinence     527
Ashok Rajimwale

60 Neurogenic bladder     546
Ashok Rajimwale

61 Posterior urethral valves     562
Brice Antao, George Ninan

62 Hypospadias     570
Ashok Rajimwale

63 Circumcision and disorders of penis     582
Ashok Rajimwale

64 Testicular problems and varicoceles     592
Julian Roberts

65 Disorders of sexual differentiation     600
Sarah M Lambert, Howard M Snyder III

66 Prune belly syndrome, bladder and cloacal exstrophy     607
Kate H Kraft, Howard M Snyder III

67 Gynaecological disorders in children     615
Lisa M Allen, Rachel F Spitzer

**Section XI Oncology**     **635**

68 Adjuvant therapy in childhood cancer     636
Johannes Visser

69 Renal tumours     644
Victoria Lane, Mark Powis

70 Neuroblastoma     651
Madan Samuel

71  Hepatic tumours                                                        657
    N Alexander Jones, Onyebuchi Ukabiala

72  Endocrine tumours                                                      667
    Michael Skinner, Eduardo Perez

73  Germ cell tumours                                                      679
    Roshni Dasgupta, Richard G Azizkhan

74  Lymphomas                                                              686
    Keith J August, Alan S Gamis

75  Teratoma, rhabdomyosarcoma and other tumours                           695
    Madan Samuel

**Section XII  Special areas of paediatric surgery**                       **705**

76  Paediatric radiology                                                   706
    Ashok Raghavan, Kshitij Mankad, Jeremy B Jones, Neetu Kumar

77  Paediatric anaesthesia                                                 737
    Nigel Pereira, Rob E John, Liz Storey

78  Solid organ transplantation                                            747
    Erik B Finger

79  Neonatology                                                            756
    Elizabeth Pilling

80  Paediatric orthopaedic disorders                                       761
    Gleeson Rebello

81  Paediatric neurosurgical disorders                                     775
    Desiderio Rodrigues

82  Fetal surgery                                                          779
    Ashwin Pimpalwar

83  Bariatric surgery in children                                          791
    Hariharan Thangarajah, Sanjeev Dutta

84  Medical statistics and hospital management                             801
    Madan Samuel

    *Index*                                                                806

# Foreword by Anthony Lander

I feel hugely honoured to have been asked to review these impressive multiple-choice questions that cover the depth and breadth of paediatric surgery. Questions like these are not easy to write – I know because I have tried and failed – but these many authors have achieved it and have managed to make it look so simple. The authors are all knowledgeable surgeons and are clearly skilled educators too – they tick all the boxes. If you use these works over and over again, dipping in to test yourself whenever you can, you too will soon tick all the boxes. If you are sitting an exam this could be useful!

Gaining clinical experience in the hospital and reading the textbooks and journals is not sufficient for most of us to acquire the aggregated knowledge and wisdom that underpins expert decision-making. Sadly, there are no shortcuts to this destination and, indeed, no road probably quite gets there. Nonetheless, I am sure there is no better way to revise all that underpins our practice than to test and challenge ourselves. These questions will help you do that. The answers are informative and will confirm and expand your knowledge if you are correct, and they will point you in the right direction if you are wrong. You may not always agree with the answers, but that too is a great starting point for discussion with colleagues and teachers, and it will bring you back to the evidence, science and history of this speciality that we love so much.

Brice Antao and Michael Irish have marshalled the authors and their works to produce a valuable contribution for trainees and the trained alike. These texts are something I know you will treasure – both before and, especially, *after* any examinations.

**Anthony Lander** PhD, FRCS(Paed), DCH
**Consultant Paediatric Surgeon and Clinical Director for Surgery**
**Birmingham Children's Hospital, UK**
**Clinical Lead for e-Learning in Paediatric Surgery**
**Department of Health, UK**
**Chair, Education and Training Committee**
**British Association of Paediatric Surgeons**
*October 2011*

# Foreword by
# Steven S Rothenberg

This new book, *Succeeding in Paediatric Surgery Examinations Volume 1. A complete resource for MCQs*, will be a welcome addition to the paediatric surgical literature.

It has a well-known and international panel of experts who have addressed all the major subjects within paediatric surgical practice. The format of question and then detailed answer will help not only residents and fellows who are studying for their boards but also the practising paediatric surgeon who is looking for a focused way to review current topics. All surgeons involved in the care of infants and children should benefit from reading this series.

Steven S Rothenberg MD
Clinical Professor of Surgery
Columbia University College of Physicians and Surgeons
Chief of Pediatric Surgery
Chairman, Department of Pediatrics
The Rocky Mountain Hospital for Children, Denver, CO
*October 2011*

# Preface

*Succeeding in Paediatric Surgery Examinations Volume 1. A complete resource for MCQs.*

The title of the book speaks for itself. This book is indeed a complete resource for multiple-choice questions (MCQs); all that is essential for succeeding in paediatric surgery examinations. It is also a good resource for other specialities such as paediatrics, general surgery, urology and other allied surgical specialities and also for medical students. While there are several outstanding comprehensive textbooks in paediatric surgery, it is often difficult to assimilate important and relevant information in the context of examination preparation. This book is a comprehensive yet concise review textbook, covering the entire spectrum of paediatric surgery. The questions are in a multiple-choice format, similar to most current international examinations. The questions and discussions are structured in such a way that by solving the MCQs and reading the discussions, the entire topic is covered in a systematic manner. This book is unique in that it has the advantage of covering all the important aspects of individual topics, as well as the benefit of having all MCQs under one cover. The discussions integrate various evidence-based facts and figures, practical discussion from an expert panel of authors, as well as all-important relevant information from various books, thus eliminating the need to refer to different textbooks to extract the same. Also, because all the 84 chapters are organised in a systematic manner, other specialities can easily extract information relevant to their area of interest. We hope that all prospective candidates will find it useful in preparing for the examinations, and subsequently as a reference book.

We are indebted to all the contributors, for devoting a great deal of their time and effort in preparing such top-quality material, and maintaining the high standards of this publication. We would also like to acknowledge the staff at Radcliffe Publishing, especially Gillian Nineham, Jamie Etherington, Jessica Morofke and Camille Lowe for all their expertise, help and guidance during the preparation and publication of this book. UK English spelling and editing conventions have been used throughout this book.

Brice Antao MBBS, MRCSEd, FRCSEd(Paed Surg)
Michael S Irish MD
*October 2011*

# Dedication

I would like to dedicate this book to my parents, Belarmino and Blazia, for their endless inspiration, encouragement and support throughout my life and career.

**Brice Antao**

We are appreciative and indebted to our colleague contributors in the publication of this book. I would also like to acknowledge and commend Brice Antao for his leadership, organisation and administration of this publication. Finally, to Spencer Michael Irish and Sydney Kaitlyn Irish who have contributed to the health of my patients with smiles and drawings on ward rounds since they were able to walk, I dedicate this book.

**Michael S Irish**

# List of contributors

**Chapter 1**

**Joanne Ng** MBChB, MRCPCH
Specialist Registrar in Paediatric
 Neurology
Great Ormond Street Hospital
London

**Chapter 2**

**Onyebuchi Ukabiala** MD, FRCS
Clinical Adjunct Assistant Professor of
 Surgery
The University of Iowa, Iowa City, IA
Blank Children's Hospital
Des Moines, IA

**Craig R Nemechek** MD
Chief Surgery Resident
Iowa Methodist Medical Center and
 Blank Children's Hospital
Des Moines, IA

**Chapter 3**

**Nitin Patwardhan** MS, FRCS(Paed)
Consultant Paediatric Surgeon
Leicester Royal Infirmary
Leicester

**Chapter 4**

**Pramod S Puligandla** MD, MSc, FRCSC,
 FACS
Associate Professor of Surgery and
 Pediatrics, McGill University
Attending Staff, Division of Pediatric
 Surgery
The Montreal Children's Hospital
Montreal, QC

**Robert Baird** MDCM, MSc, FRCSC
Assistant Professor of Surgery, McGill
 University
Attending Staff, Division of Pediatric
 Surgery
The Montreal Children's Hospital
Montreal, QC

**Chapter 5**

**Elizabeth Pilling** MRCPCH
Consultant Neonatologist
Jessops Neonatal Unit
Sheffield Teaching Hospitals NHS
 Foundation Trust
Sheffield

**Chapter 6**

**Niall Jones** MD, FRCSI (Paed)
Consultant Paediatric Surgeon
Barts and The London Children's
 Hospital
London

**Alexander Cho** MBBS, MSc (Hons),
 MRCS (Eng)
Specialist Registrar in Paediatric
 Surgery
Barts and The London Children's
 Hospital
London

**Alice Mears** MBChB, DTM&H,
 MRCS (Ed)
Specialist Registrar in Paediatric
 Surgery
Barts and The London Children's
 Hospital
London

*Chapter 7*
**Rebeccah L Brown** MD
Associate Director, Trauma Services
University of Cincinnati, Department
  of Pediatrics
Cincinnati Children's Hospital
Cincinnati, OH

**Marianne Beaudin** MD
Fellow in Pediatric Surgery
University of Cincinnati, Department
  of Pediatrics
Cincinnati Children's Hospital
Cincinnati, OH

*Chapter 8*
**Desiderio Rodrigues** MS, FRCS,
  FRCS(Neuro)
Consultant Paediatric Neurosurgeon
Birmingham Children's Hospital
Birmingham

*Chapter 9*
**Rebeccah L Brown** MD
Associate Director, Trauma Services
University of Cincinnati, Department
  of Pediatrics
Cincinnati Children's Hospital
Cincinnati, OH

**Marianne Beaudin** MD
Fellow in Pediatric Surgery
University of Cincinnati, Department
  of Pediatrics
Cincinnati Children's Hospital
Cincinnati, OH

*Chapter 10*
**Rebeccah L Brown** MD
Associate Director, Trauma Services
University of Cincinnati, Department
  of Pediatrics
Cincinnati Children's Hospital
Cincinnati, OH

**Marianne Beaudin** MD
Fellow in Pediatric Surgery
University of Cincinnati, Department
  of Pediatrics
Cincinnati Children's Hospital
Cincinnati, OH

*Chapter 11*
**Rebeccah L Brown** MD
Associate Director, Trauma Services
University of Cincinnati, Department
  of Pediatrics
Cincinnati Children's Hospital
Cincinnati, OH

**Marianne Beaudin** MD
Fellow in Pediatric Surgery
University of Cincinnati, Department
  of Pediatrics
Cincinnati Children's Hospital
Cincinnati, OH

*Chapter 12*
**Gleeson Rebello** MD
Instructor in Orthopedic Surgery
Harvard Medical School
Department of Pediatric Orthopedics
MassGeneral Hospital for Children
Boston, MA

*Chapter 13*
**Kurt D Newman** MD, FACS, FAAP
Professor of Surgery and Pediatrics
Surgeon-in-Chief, Children's National
  Medical Center
Washington, DC

**Faisal G Qureshi** MD, FAAP
Assistant Professor of Surgery and
  Pediatrics
Children's National Medical Center
Washington, DC

**Felix C Blanco** MD
Research Fellow, Department of
  Pediatric Surgery
Children's National Medical Center
Washington, DC

*Chapter 14*
**Natasha de Vere** MRCPCH
Specialist Registrar in Paediatrics
Sheffield Children's Hospital
Sheffield

*Chapter 15*
**Ross Fisher** MPhil, FRCS (Paed)
Consultant Paediatric Surgeon
Sheffield Children's Hospital
Sheffield

*Chapter 16*
**Michael Skinner** MD
Professor of Surgery
South Western Medical Center
Children's Medical Center
Dallas, TX

**Eduardo Perez** MD
Pediatric Surgeon
South Western Medical Center
Children's Medical Center
Dallas, TX

*Chapter 17*
**Marjorie J Arca** MD
Associate Professor of Surgery
  (Pediatric Surgery)
Children's Hospital of Wisconsin
Milwaukee, WI

*Chapter 18*
**Michael J Goretsky** MD, FACS
Associate Professor of Clinical Surgery
  and Pediatrics
Eastern Virginia Medical School
Pediatric Surgery
Children's Hospital of the King's
  Daughters
Norfolk, VA

**Robert Obermeyer** MD, FACS
Assistant Professor of Clinical Surgery
  and Pediatrics
Eastern Virginia Medical School
Pediatric Surgery
Children's Hospital of the King's
  Daughters
Norfolk, VA

*Chapter 19*
**Charles M Myer III** MD
Professor of Otolaryngology/Head and
  Neck Surgery
Department of Otolaryngology/Head
  and Neck Surgery
Cincinnati Children's Hospital
Cincinnati, OH

**Charles M Myer IV** MD
Clinical Fellow in Pediatric
  Otolaryngology-Head and Neck
  Surgery
Department of Otolaryngology/Head
  and Neck Surgery
Cincinnati Children's Hospital
Cincinnati, OH

*Chapter 20*
**David Sigalet** MD, PhD, FRCS
ACH Professor of Pediatric Surgical
  Research
Alberta Children's Hospital/University
  of Calgary
Calgary, AB

**Mary Brindle** MD, FRCSC
Assistant Professor of Surgery,
Division of Pediatric General Surgery
Alberta Children's Hospital/University
  of Calgary
Calgary, AB

*Chapter 21*
**Craig T Albanese** MD, MBA
Professor of Surgery
Department of Pediatric Surgery

Lucile Packard Children's Hospital at
  Stanford
Palo Alto, CA

**Matias Bruzoni** MD
Assistant Professor of Surgery
Department of Pediatric Surgery
Lucile Packard Children's Hospital at
  Stanford
Palo Alto, CA

*Chapter 22*
**Craig T Albanese** MD, MBA
Professor of Surgery
Department of Pediatric Surgery
Lucile Packard Children's Hospital at
  Stanford
Palo Alto, CA

**Matias Bruzoni** MD
Assistant Professor of Surgery
Department of Pediatric Surgery
Lucile Packard Children's Hospital at
  Stanford
Palo Alto, CA

*Chapter 23*
**David Sigalet** MD, PhD, FRCS
ACH Professor of Pediatric Surgical
  Research
Alberta Children's Hospital/University
  of Calgary
Calgary, AB

**Mary Brindle** MD, FRCSC
Assistant Professor of Surgery,
Division of Pediatric General Surgery
Alberta Children's Hospital/University
  of Calgary
Calgary, AB

*Chapter 24*
**Pramod S Puligandla** MD, MSc, FRCSC,
  FACS
Associate Professor of Surgery and
  Pediatrics, McGill University

Program Director, Pediatric General
  Surgery
Attending Staff, Divisions of Pediatric
  Surgery and Pediatric Critical Care
  Medicine
The Montreal Children's Hospital
Montreal, QC

**Robert Baird** MDCM, MSc, FRCSC
Assistant Professor of Surgery, McGill
  University
Attending Staff, Division of Pediatric
  Surgery
The Montreal Children's Hospital
Montreal, QC

*Chapter 25*
**Ashwin Pimpalwar** MD, FRCS(Ped Surg),
  MCh(Ped Surg), EBPS(Ped Surg), MS, DNB
Assistant Professor Pediatric Surgery
Baylor College of Medicine
DeBakey Department of Pediatric
  Surgery
Texas Children's Hospital
Houston, TX

*Chapter 26*
**Brice Antao** MBBS, MRCSEd,
  FRCSEd(Paed Surg)
Specialist Registrar in Paediatric
  Surgery
Yorkshire Deanery Training
  Programme
Leicester Royal Infirmary
Leicester

**Michael S Irish** MD
Pediatric Surgeon
Adjunct Clinical Assistant Professor of
  Surgery
The University of Iowa, Iowa City, IA
Blank Children's Hospital
Des Moines, IA

**Chapter 27**
**Mark Powis** FRCS(Paed)
Consultant Paediatric Surgeon
Department of Paediatric Surgery
Clarendon Wing
Leeds General Infirmary
Leeds

**Victoria Lane** MBChB, MRCS
Specialist Registrar in Paediatric
  Surgery
Department of Paediatric Surgery
Leeds General Infirmary
Leeds

**Chapter 28**
**Bassem N Mora** MD
Assistant Professor of Surgery
University of Chicago Medical Center
Chicago, IL

**Chapter 29**
**Alan P Sawchuk** MD
Professor of Surgery
Department of Surgery
Methodist Hospital
Indianapolis, IN

**Gary Lemmon** MD
Department of Surgery
Methodist Hospital
Indianapolis, IN

**Raghu Motaganahalli** MD
Department of Surgery
Methodist Hospital
Indianapolis, IN

**Chapter 30**
**Steven J Fishman** MD
Professor of Surgery
Harvard University Medical School
Children's Hospital Boston
Boston, MA

**Cameron C Trenor III** MD
Harvard University Medical School
Children's Hospital Boston
Boston, MA

**Arin K Greene** MD, MMSc
Harvard University Medical School
Children's Hospital Boston
Boston, MA

**Chapter 31**
**Brice Antao** MBBS, MRCSEd, FRCSEd
  (Paed Surg)
Specialist Registrar in Paediatric
  Surgery
Yorkshire Deanery Training
  Programme
Leicester Royal Infirmary
Leicester

**Michael S Irish** MD
Pediatric Surgeon
Adjunct Clinical Assistant Professor of
  Surgery
The University of Iowa, Iowa City, IA
Blank Children's Hospital
Des Moines, IA

**Chapter 32**
**Brice Antao** MBBS, MRCSEd, FRCSEd
  (Paed Surg)
Specialist Registrar in Paediatric
  Surgery
Yorkshire Deanery Training
  Programme
Leicester Royal Infirmary
Leicester

**Michael S Irish** MD
Pediatric Surgeon
Adjunct Clinical Assistant Professor of
  Surgery
The University of Iowa, Iowa City, IA
Blank Children's Hospital
Des Moines, IA

**Chapter 33**
**Brice Antao** MBBS, MRCSEd, FRCSEd
  (Paed Surg)
Specialist Registrar in Paediatric
  Surgery
Yorkshire Deanery Training
  Programme
Leicester Royal Infirmary
Leicester

**Victoria Lane** MBChB, MRCS
Specialist Registrar in Paediatric
  Surgery
Department of Paediatric Surgery
Clarendon Wing
Leeds General Infirmary
Leeds

**Michael S Irish** MD
Pediatric Surgeon
Adjunct Clinical Assistant Professor of
  Surgery
The University of Iowa, Iowa City, IA
Blank Children's Hospital
Des Moines, IA

**Chapter 34**
**Richard G Azizkhan** MD
Surgeon-in-Chief, Lester W Martin
  Chair of Pediatric Surgery
Cincinnati Children's Hospital
Cincinnati, OH

**Jason S Frischer** MD
Fellow in Pediatric Surgery
Cincinnati Children's Hospital
Cincinnati, OH

**Chapter 35**
**Shirley Chou** MD, MSc, FRCSC
Pediatric Surgeon
Division of Pediatric General Surgery
Children's Hospital of Eastern Ontario
Ottawa, ON

**Marcos Bettolli** MD
Pediatric Surgeon
Division of Pediatric General Surgery
Children's Hospital of Eastern Ontario
Ottawa, ON

**Chapter 36**
**Moritz M Ziegler** MD
The Ponzio Family Chair and Surgeon-
  in-Chief, retired
Children's Hospital Colorado
Professor of Surgery, retired
University of Colorado School of
  Medicine
Aurora, CO

**Stephanie A Jones** DO
Pediatric Surgery Fellow
Children's Hospital Colorado
Aurora, CO

**Chapter 37**
**Brice Antao** MBBS, MRCSEd, FRCSEd
  (Paed Surg)
Specialist Registrar in Paediatric
  Surgery
Yorkshire Deanery Training
  Programme
Leicester Royal Infirmary
Leicester

**Michael S Irish** MD
Pediatric Surgeon
Adjunct Clinical Assistant Professor of
  Surgery
The University of Iowa, Iowa City, IA
Blank Children's Hospital
Des Moines, IA

**Chapter 38**
**Brice Antao** MBBS, MRCSEd, FRCSEd
  (Paed Surg)
Specialist Registrar in Paediatric
  Surgery
Yorkshire Deanery Training
  Programme

Leicester Royal Infirmary
Leicester

**Shawqui Nour** MD, FRCS(Ed & Glasg), FRCS(Paed)
Consultant Paediatric Surgeon
Leicester Royal Infirmary
Leicester

*Chapter 39*
**Brice Antao** MBBS, MRCSEd, FRCSEd (Paed Surg)
Specialist Registrar in Paediatric Surgery
Yorkshire Deanery Training Programme
Leicester Royal Infirmary
Leicester

**Victoria Lane** MBChB, MRCS
Specialist Registrar in Paediatric Surgery
Department of Paediatric Surgery
Clarendon Wing
Leeds General Infirmary
Leeds

**Michael S Irish** MD
Pediatric Surgeon
Adjunct Clinical Assistant Professor of Surgery
The University of Iowa, Iowa City, IA
Blank Children's Hospital
Des Moines, IA

*Chapter 40*
**J Ted Gerstle** MD, FRCSC, FACS, FAAP
Associate Professor of Surgery
University of Toronto
The Hospital for Sick Children
Toronto, ON

**Rodrigo Romao** MD
Fellow in Pediatric Urology
University of Toronto
The Hospital for Sick Children
Toronto, ON

*Chapter 41*
**Brad W Warner** MD
Professor of Pediatric Surgery
Surgeon-in-Chief
St Louis Children's Hospital
Division of Pediatric Surgery
St Louis, MO

**Derek Wakeman** MD
Surgery Resident
St Louis Children's Hospital
Division of Pediatric Surgery
St Louis, MO

**Jennifer A Leinicke** MD
Surgery Resident
St Louis Children's Hospital
Division of Pediatric Surgery
St Louis, MO

*Chapter 42*
**Nitin Patwardhan** MS, FRCS(Paed)
Consultant Paediatric Surgeon
Leicester Royal Infirmary
Leicester

*Chapter 43*
**Mike Thomson** MBChB, DCH, FRCPCH, FRCP, MD
Consultant Paediatric Gastroenterologist
Sheffield Children's Hospital
Sheffield

**A Anish** MRCPCH
Specialist Registrar in Paediatrics
Sheffield Children's Hospital
Sheffield

*Chapter 44*
**Mike Thomson** MBChB, DCH, FRCPCH, FRCP, MD
Consultant Paediatric Gastroenterologist
Sheffield Children's Hospital
Sheffield

**Manjula Velayudhan** MBBS, MRCPCH
Specialist Registrar in Paediatrics
Sheffield Children's Hospital
Sheffield

*Chapter 45*
**Marc A Levitt** MD
Associate Director, Colorectal Center
  for Children
University of Cincinnati, Department
  of Pediatrics
Cincinnati Children's Hospital
Cincinnati, OH

**Taiwo A Lawal** MD FWACS
Colorectal Fellow, Colorectal Center
  for Children
University of Cincinnati, Department
  of Pediatrics
Cincinnati Children's Hospital
Cincinnati, OH

**Alberto Peña** MD
Director, Colorectal Center for
  Children
University of Cincinnati, Department
  of Pediatrics
Cincinnati Children's Hospital
Cincinnati, OH

*Chapter 46*
**Marc A Levitt** MD
Associate Director, Colorectal Center
  for Children
University of Cincinnati, Department
  of Pediatrics
Cincinnati Children's Hospital
Cincinnati, OH

**Kaveer Chatoorgoon** MD
Colorectal Fellow, Colorectal Center
  for Children
University of Cincinnati, Department
  of Pediatrics
Cincinnati Children's Hospital
Cincinnati, OH

**Alberto Peña** MD
Director, Colorectal Center for
  Children
University of Cincinnati, Department
  of Pediatrics
Cincinnati Children's Hospital
Cincinnati, OH

*Chapter 47*
**Marc A Levitt** MD
Associate Director, Colorectal Center
  for Children
University of Cincinnati, Department
  of Pediatrics
Cincinnati Children's Hospital
Cincinnati, OH

**Andrea Bischoff** MD
Colorectal Fellow, Colorectal Center
  for Children
University of Cincinnati, Department
  of Pediatrics
Cincinnati Children's Hospital
Cincinnati, OH

**Alberto Peña** MD
Director, Colorectal Center for
  Children
University of Cincinnati, Department
  of Pediatrics
Cincinnati Children's Hospital
Cincinnati, OH

*Chapter 48*
**Hanmin Lee** MD
Associate Professor of Surgery
Director, Fetal Treatment Center
Division of Pediatric Surgery/Fetal
  Treatment Center
University of California, San Francisco
San Francisco, CA

**Kelly D Gonzales** MD
Postdoctoral Research Fellow
Division of Pediatric Surgery/Fetal
  Treatment Center

University of California, San Francisco
San Francisco, CA

**Eric Jelin** MD
Postdoctoral Research Fellow
Division of Pediatric Surgery/Fetal
    Treatment Center
University of California, San Francisco
San Francisco, CA

*Chapter 49*
**Riccardo A Superina** MD
Professor and Head of Transplant
    Surgery
Children's Memorial Hospital
Northwestern University
Chicago, IL

**Niramol Tantemsapya** MD
Pediatric Surgery Fellow
Children's Memorial Hospital
Northwestern University
Chicago, IL

*Chapter 50*
**Onyebuchi Ukabiala** MD, FRCS
Clinical Adjunct Assistant Professor of
    Surgery
The University of Iowa, Iowa City, IA
Blank Children's Hospital
Des Moines, IA

**N Alexander Jones** MD
General Surgeon, Panama City, FL
Formally Chief Surgery Resident
Iowa Methodist Medical Center and
    Blank Children's Hospital
Des Moines, IA

*Chapter 51*
**Riccardo A Superina** MD
Professor and Head of Transplant
    Surgery
Children's Memorial Hospital
Northwestern University
Chicago, IL

**Niramol Tantemsapya** MD
Pediatric Surgery Fellow
Children's Memorial Hospital
Northwestern University
Chicago, IL

*Chapter 52*
**Andre Hebra** MD
Chief of Surgery
MUSC Children's Hospital
Charleston, SC

**Christian J Streck Jr** MD
Assistant Professor of Surgery and
    Pediatrics
MUSC Children's Hospital
Charleston, SC

*Chapter 53*
**Sanjeev Dutta** MD, MA, FACS
Associate Professor of Pediatric and
    Surgery
Division of Pediatric Surgery
Lucile Packard Children's Hospital
Stanford University
Stanford, CA

**Zachary Kastenberg** MD
Resident in General Surgery
Department of Surgery
Stanford University School of Medicine
Stanford, CA

*Chapter 54*
**Stephen D Marks** MD, MSc, MRCP(UK),
    DCH, FRCPCH
Consultant Paediatric Nephrologist
Great Ormond Street Hospital for
    Children NHS Trust
London

*Chapter 55*
**Ian E Willetts** BSc(Hons), MBChB(Hons),
    FRCS(Eng), FRCSEd, FRCS(Paed Surg)
Consultant Paediatric Urologist
John Radcliffe Hospital
Oxford

*Chapter 56*
**Harish Chandran** FRACS(Gen Surg),
  FRACS(Paed Surg), FEAPU
Consultant Paediatric Surgeon and
  Urologist
Department of Paediatric Surgery
Birmingham Children's Hospital
Birmingham

*Chapter 57*
**Julian Roberts** MS, FRCS, FRCS(Paed)
Consultant Paediatric and Urological
  Surgeon
Sheffield Children's NHS Foundation
  Hospital
Sheffield

*Chapter 58*
**Ian E Willetts** BSc(Hons), MBChB(Hons),
  FRCS(Eng), FRCSEd, FRCS(Paed Surg)
Consultant Paediatric Urologist
John Radcliffe Hospital
Oxford

**Francesca Castillo** MBChB, MRCS
Specialist Registrar in Paediatric
  Surgery
John Radcliffe Hospital
Oxford

*Chapter 59*
**Ashok Rajimwale** MS, MCh, DNB, FRCS,
  FEAPU
Consultant Paediatric and Urological
  Surgeon
Leicester Royal Infirmary
Leicester

*Chapter 60*
**Ashok Rajimwale** MS, MCh, DNB, FRCS,
  FEAPU
Consultant Paediatric and Urological
  Surgeon
Leicester Royal Infirmary
Leicester

*Chapter 61*
**George Ninan** MBBS, FRCS, FRCSG,
  FRCS(Ed), FRCSI, FRCS(Paed Surg)
Consultant Paediatric Urologist
Leicester Royal Infirmary
Leicester

**Brice Antao** MBBS, MRCSEd,
  FRCSEd(Paed Surg)
Specialist Registrar in Paediatric
  Surgery
Yorkshire Deanery Training
  Programme
Leicester Royal Infirmary
Leicester

*Chapter 62*
**Ashok Rajimwale** MS, MCh, DNB, FRCS,
  FEAPU
Consultant Paediatric and Urological
  Surgeon
Leicester Royal Infirmary
Leicester

*Chapter 63*
**Ashok Rajimwale** MS, MCh, DNB, FRCS,
  FEAPU
Consultant Paediatric and Urological
  Surgeon
Leicester Royal Infirmary
Leicester

*Chapter 64*
**Julian Roberts** MS, FRCS, FRCS(Paed)
Consultant Paediatric and Urological
  Surgeon
Sheffield Children's NHS Foundation
  Hospital
Sheffield

*Chapter 65*
**Howard M Snyder III** MD
Professor of Pediatric Urology
Children's Hospital of Philadelphia
Philadelphia, PA

**Sarah M Lambert** MD
Assistant Professor, Division of
  Urology
Children's Hospital of Philadelphia
Philadelphia, PA

*Chapter 66*
**Howard M Snyder III** MD
Professor of Pediatric Urology
Children's Hospital of Philadelphia
Philadelphia, PA

**Kate H Kraft** MD
Fellow, Division of Urology
Children's Hospital of Philadelphia
Philadelphia, PA

*Chapter 67*
**Lisa M Allen** MD, FRCSC
Section Head, Pediatric Gynecology
Associate Professor, Department of
  Obstetrics and Gynecology
Hospital for Sick Children
Mount Sinai Hospital
Toronto, ON

**Rachel F Spitzer** MD, FRCSC, MPH
Assistant Professor, Department of
  Obstetrics and Gynecology
Hospital for Sick Children
Mount Sinai Hospital
Toronto, ON

*Chapter 68*
**Johannes Visser** MD
Consultant Paediatric Oncologist
Leicester Royal Infirmary
Leicester

*Chapter 69*
**Mark Powis** FRCS(Paed)
Consultant Paediatric Surgeon
Department of Paediatric Surgery
Clarendon Wing
Leeds General Infirmary
Leeds

**Victoria Lane** MBChB, MRCS
Specialist Registrar in Paediatric
  Surgery
Department of Paediatric Surgery
Leeds General Infirmary
Leeds

*Chapter 70*
**Madan Samuel** MBBS, DM, MS, MCh,
  DPS, DCH, FRCS(Paed Surg)
Consultant Paediatric Surgeon
Addenbrooke's Hospital
Cambridge

*Chapter 71*
**Onyebuchi Ukabiala** MD, FRCS
Clinical Adjunct Assistant Professor of
  Surgery
The University of Iowa, Iowa City, IA
Blank Children's Hospital
Des Moines, IA

**N Alexander Jones** MD
General Surgeon, Panama City, FL
Formally Chief Surgery Resident
Iowa Methodist Medical Center and
  Blank Children's Hospital
Des Moines, IA

*Chapter 72*
**Michael Skinner** MD
Professor of Surgery
South Western Medical Center
Children's Medical Center
Dallas, TX

**Eduardo Perez** MD
Pediatric Surgeon
South Western Medical Center
Children's Medical Center
Dallas, TX

*Chapter 73*
**Richard G Azizkhan** MD
Surgeon-in-Chief, Lester W Martin
  Chair of Pediatric Surgery

Cincinnati Children's Hospital
Cincinnati, OH

**Roshni Dasgupta** MD, MPH
Pediatric Surgery Fellow
Division of Pediatric General and
  Thoracic Surgery
Cincinnati Children's Hospital
Cincinnati, OH

*Chapter 74*
**Alan S Gamis** MD, MPH
Professor of Pediatrics
Children's Mercy Hospital
Kansas City, MO

**Keith J August** MD, MSc
Assistant Professor of Pediatrics
Children's Mercy Hospital
Kansas City, MO

*Chapter 75*
**Madan Samuel** MBBS, DM, MS, MCh,
  DPS, DCH, FRCS(Paed Surg)
Consultant Paediatric Surgeon
Addenbrooke's Hospital
Cambridge

*Chapter 76*
**Ashok Raghavan** MD, DNB
Consultant Paediatric Radiologist
Sheffield Children's Hospital
Sheffield

**Kshitij Mankad** MRCP, FRCR
Neuroradiology Fellow
Great Ormond Street Hospital
London

**Jeremy B Jones** MBChB, MRCP
Specialist Registrar in Radiology
The Radiology Academy
Leeds General Infirmary
Leeds Teaching Hospitals NHS Trust
Leeds

**Miss Neetu Kumar** MRCS
Specialist Trainee in Paediatric Surgery
The Royal London Hospital
London

*Chapter 77*
**Nigel Pereira** MBChB, FRCA
Consultant Paediatric Anaesthetist
Sheffield Children's Hospital
Sheffield

**Rob E John** MRCP, FRCA
Consultant Paediatric Anaesthetist
Sheffield Children's Hospital
Sheffield

**Liz Storey** MBChB, FRCA
Consultant Paediatric Anaesthetist
Sheffield Children's Hospital
Sheffield

*Chapter 78*
**Erik B Finger** MD, PhD
Assistant Professor
Department of Surgery, Division of
  Transplantation
University of Minnesota
Minneapolis, MN

*Chapter 79*
**Elizabeth Pilling** MRCPCH
Consultant Neonatologist, Jessops
  Neonatal Unit
Sheffield Teaching Hospitals NHS
  Foundation Trust
Sheffield

*Chapter 80*
**Gleeson Rebello** MD
Instructor in Orthopedic Surgery
Harvard Medical School
Department of Pediatric Orthopedics
MassGeneral Hospital for Children
Boston, MA

**Chapter 81**

**Desiderio Rodrigues** MS, FRCS,
FRCS(Neuro)
Consultant Paediatric Neurosurgeon
Birmingham Children's Hospital
Birmingham

**Chapter 82**

**Ashwin Pimpalwar** MD, FRCS(Ped Surg),
MCh(Ped Surg), EBPS(Ped Surg), MS, DNB
Assistant Professor, Pediatric Surgery
Baylor College of Medicine
DeBakey Department of Pediatric
Surgery
Texas Children's Hospital
Houston, TX

**Chapter 83**

**Sanjeev Dutta** MD, MA, FRCSC, FAAP
Associate Professor of Pediatrics and
Surgery
Division of Pediatric Surgery
Lucile Packard Children's Hospital
Stanford University
Stanford, CA

**Hariharan Thangarajah** MD
Resident in General Surgery,
Department of Surgery
Stanford University School of Medicine
Stanford, CA

**Chapter 84**

**Madan Samuel** MBBS, DM, MS, MCh,
DPS, DCH, FRCS(Paed Surg)
Consultant Paediatric Surgeon
Addenbrooke's Hospital
Cambridge

# SECTION I

# General

# CHAPTER 1

# Growth and development

## JOANNE NG

**From the choices below each question, select the single best answer.**

**Q1**  Which of the following is true in relation to a newborn?
  A  Premature infants are those whose weight is below the 10th percentile for age.
  B  Premature infants are those whose height is below the 10th percentile for age.
  C  Large for gestational age (LGA) are those whose weight is above the 98th percentile.
  D  LGA are those whose weight is above the 95th percentile.
  E  Small for gestational age (SGA) are those whose birthweight is <2500 g.

**A1**  **C**  Newborns are classified based on gestational age and weight. Pre-term infants are those born before 37 weeks of gestation. Term infants are those born between 37 and 42 weeks of gestation, whereas post-term infants have a gestation that exceeds 42 weeks. Newborns with weight at or above the 90th percentile are LGA and those below the 10th percentile are SGA. Newborns whose weight falls between these extremes are appropriate for gestational age. Infants born before 37 weeks of gestation, regardless of birthweight, are considered premature. A premature infant has thin and transparent skin with an absence of plantar creases, soft malleable fingers, and ears with poorly developed cartilage. In females, the labia minora appear enlarged and the labia majora appear small. In males, the testes are usually undescended and the scrotum is underdeveloped.

**Q2** Which of the following is true for SGA?

    **A** Symmetrical SGA suggests insults late in pregnancy.

    **B** Asymmetrical SGA suggests fetus affected from early pregnancy.

    **C** Asymmetrical SGA is at a higher risk of complications.

    **D** Severe malnutrition is a cause of symmetrical SGA.

    **E** Maternal substance abuse leads to asymmetrical SGA.

**A2**   **C** SGA is defined as birthweight below the 10th percentile for gestational age. Symmetrical (proportional) SGA infants have all growth parameters symmetrically small. They usually suggest fetus affected from early pregnancy (e.g. constitutional or chromosomal disorder, intrauterine infections such as cytomegalovirus, rubella or toxoplasmosis, anaemia, maternal substance abuse). On the other hand, asymmetrical (disproportional) SGA infants have their weight centile < length and head circumference because of intrauterine growth retardation due to insult late in pregnancy (e.g. pre-eclampsia, severe malnutrition). Asymmetrical SGA infants are particularly at risk of complications. Symmetrical SGA infants often stay small, and later average intellectual ability is slightly reduced compared with appropriately grown infants. It has been suggested that these infants are at an increased risk of developing coronary vascular disease, stroke, obesity and hypertension in later life.

**Q3** Which of the following indicates normal growth for a term neonate?

    **A** Birthweight doubles by 5 months.

    **B** Birthweight doubles by 6 months.

    **C** Weight is four times birthweight by 12 months.

    **D** Body length doubles by 12 months.

    **E** Body length triples by 12 months.

**A3**   **A** A term newborn grows at a rate of 25–30 g/day over the first 6 months of life, doubling its birthweight by 5 months of age. An average infant triples his or her birthweight by 12 months, and by 3 years the weight is four times the birthweight. By the end of the first decade, the weight increases 20-fold. Body length increases 50% by the end of the first year of life and increases threefold by the end of the first decade. The pre-term infant's growth pattern is quite distinct from that of a term infant. Loss of 15% of a pre-term infant's birthweight is usual in the first 7–10 days of life, compared with a 7%–10% weight loss for a term infant. After the initial period of weight loss, a pre-term infant gains weight at a much slower rate of 10–20 g/day.

**Q4** Anaesthetists need to be concerned about the possibility of loose teeth in children until what age?

**A** 1 year

**B** 3 year

**C** 6 years

**D** 9 years

**E** 12 years

**A4** **E** Humans have two sets of teeth. The teeth that appear first are called milk teeth. These teeth are later shed and are replaced by a set of permanent teeth. Milk teeth start appearing at 6 months of age. The first milk teeth to appear are the lower central incisors. All milk teeth erupt by 3 years of age. The milk teeth are shed from 6 years onwards until about 10 years of age. The permanent teeth appear by 6 years of age. Between 6 and 9 years the child has some milk teeth as well as some permanent teeth and this period is called the mixed dentition period. By 12 years of age, all the milk teeth should be shed and be replaced by the permanent teeth.

**Q5** Which of the following is not a primitive reflex?

**A** Moro reflex

**B** grasp reflex

**C** rooting reflex

**D** stepping reflex

**E** parachute reflex

**A5** **E** Normally developing infants demonstrate a number of early or primitive reflexes that disappear by 4–6 months.

1 Moro reflex: sudden head extension causes symmetrical extension of limbs followed by flexion.

2 Grasp reflex: fingers or toes grasp an object placed on the palm or sole.

3 Rooting reflex: head turns towards a tactile stimulus placed near the mouth.

4 Stepping reflex: an infant held vertically will develop stepping motions when the sole of a foot touches a hard surface.

5 Asymmetrical neck reflex: when lying supine, if the head is turned, a 'fencing posture' is adopted with the outstretched arm on the side to which the head is turned.

The parachute reflex is a postural reflex, rather than a primitive reflex. Postural reflexes emerge later to provide the basis for the control of automatic balance, posture and voluntary movement.

**Q6**  Which of the following is true regarding gross motor development?

**A**  At 6 weeks infants should hold head upright when held sitting.

**B**  Infant should sit without support by 6 months.

**C**  Infants should be cruising round edge of furniture by 6 months.

**D**  By 2 months all children should be walking independently.

**E**  By 2 years a child can skip on both feet.

**A6**  **B**  Gross motor development shows rapid progression in the first 18 months. A newborn's head lags on pulling to a sitting position but is held in extension in ventral suspension. At 6 weeks an infant lifts its head on lying prone and moves it from side to side, and at 3 months holds head upright when held sitting. By 6 months an infant should sit without support. This relies on two reflexes, which the baby must have developed, including the parachute reflex in response to falling and the righting reflex to position head and body back to vertical on tilting. An infant becomes mobile by crawling or bottom shuffling or commando crawling. By 10 months infants tend to cruise round the edge of furniture. By 12 months, only 50% of infants are walking independently. Children tend to learn advanced motor skills after 1 year and learn to run and jump and kick a ball by 20 months. At 4 years of age, they can hop on one leg, go up and down stairs one leg at a time, and ride a bike. By 5 years of age they can skip on both feet.

**Q7**  Which of the following is true regarding fine motor development?

**A**  Infants' pincer grip develops by 6 months.

**B**  Infants' palmar grip develops by 6 weeks.

**C**  An infant at 6 weeks turns head from side to side to follow an object.

**D**  By 6 months an infant uses index finger to point to objects.

**E**  By 3 years a child can draw a triangle.

**A7**  **C**  Fine motor skills are dependent on good vision. Hence these skills should be assessed alongside visual development. A newborn can fix and follow a near face moving across the field of vision. By 6 weeks, the infant is more alert and can turn the head side to side. As the primitive grasp reflex starts to decrease, infants will start to reach for objects. At 6 months, grip is with the whole palm (palmar grasp); the infant holds objects with both hands and will bang them together and transfers objects between hands. By 10 months infants demonstrate pincer grip using thumb and first finger and by 12 months infants use index finger to point to objects. Fine motor skills can be assessed with pencil control and building bricks. At 14 months infants begin to scribble and at 3 years they can draw a circle and copy or make a bridge with building bricks. At 4 years they can draw and copy a cross. By 5 years they can draw a triangle.

**8** Which of the following is true regarding speech and language development?

  **A** By 12 weeks an infant will begin to coo and laugh.
  **B** By 6 months an infant will say 'mama' or 'dada'.
  **C** By 13 months an infant has a vocabulary of 10 words.
  **D** By 18 months an infant progresses to three-word phrases
  **E** By 2 years an infant knows its age and several colours.

**A8** **A** Speech should be assessed along with hearing. Impaired hearing will affect language development. Newborns will quieten to voices and startle to loud noises. By 6 weeks they respond to mother's voice and by 12 weeks will vocalise alone or when spoken to and begin to coo and laugh. At 6 months, infants will use consonant monosyllables and by 8 months will use non-specific two-syllable babble (e.g. 'mama' or 'dada'). By 13 months their words become more appropriate. By 18 months they have a vocabulary of 10 words and are able to demonstrate six parts of the body. Their conversation becomes increasingly complex with sentence development in the second year. At 20 months, they begin to combine two words together, progressing to three-word phrases by the age of 2 years. By 3 years they know age and several colours.

 **9** Which of the following is true regarding social and behavioural development?

  **A** An infant starts smiling by 6 weeks.
  **B** An infant drinks from a cup by 8 months.
  **C** By 12 months an infant uses a spoon to self-feed.
  **D** An infant can dress themselves by 18 months.
  **E** All of the above.

**A9** **A** At 6 weeks, the infant starts to smile and becomes socially responsive. At 8 months, they demonstrate separation anxiety when separated from parents, and begin to start to feed self using fingers. By 10 months they begin to wave 'goodbye'. At 12 months they will drink from a cup, and at 18 months use a spoon to feed self. At 2 years they can remove some clothes and will try to dress self. Some children will get potty-trained by 2 years, but others may take longer. By 24 months children start to copy actions and activities that they see around them, and progress in the second year to play on their own or alongside peers in parallel play. From 3 years they start to have interactive play, taking turns and following simple rules.

**Q10** Which of the following is true regarding developmental assessment?

  **A** Constant squints persistent beyond 8 weeks need to be referred to ophthalmologists.

  **B** A child not sitting by 9 months needs to be referred for evaluation.

  **C** A child not walking by 18 months needs to be referred for evaluation.

  **D** A cognitive function IQ test score of >70 is normal.

  **E** All of the above.

**A10** **E** Fine motor skills are dependent on good vision. Therefore fine motor skills are usually assessed alongside visual development. Some infants may demonstrate an intermittent squint. Constant squints and all those persisting beyond the 8-week check must be referred to an ophthalmologist. By 6 months an infant should sit without support. Children not sitting by 9 months should be referred for evaluation. Likewise, by 12 months 50% of infants are walking independently and children not walking by 18 months must be referred for evaluation. The Denver Developmental Screening Test is a relatively quick test of children's abilities and an assessment of whether they have achieved their age-appropriate developmental milestones. Cognitive function can be assessed by an IQ test, but this does not assess all skill areas and may be significantly affected by language problems. An IQ >70 is considered normal, 50–69 as mild learning difficulty, 35–49 as moderate learning difficulty, 20–34 as severe learning difficulty and <20 as profound learning difficulty.

## Further reading

Salt A, Sargent J. Developmental paediatrics. In: McIntosh N, Helms P, Smyth R, Logan S, editors. *Forfar and Arneil's Textbook of Paediatrics.* 7th ed. Edinburgh. Elsevier; 2008. pp. 81–110.

Tasker R, McClure R, Acerini C, editors. *Oxford Handbook of Paediatrics.* Oxford: Oxford University Press; 2008. pp. 116–20, 542–54.

# CHAPTER 2

# Fluids, electrolytes and nutritional support

## CRAIG R NEMECHEK, ONYEBUCHI UKABIALA

**From the choices below each question, select the single best answer.**

**Q1** Which of the following gives the most reliable objective measure of acute changes in nutritional status?
- **A** retinol-binding protein
- **B** weight to height index
- **C** nitrogen balance
- **D** muscle wasting
- **E** albumin and prealbumin

**A1** **A** Retinol-binding protein, prealbumin and transferrin are negative acute-phase proteins and their levels fall rapidly with acute nutritional depletion. Albumin on the other hand reflects more chronic changes. Weight to height index is a very crude way to assess chronic malnutrition.

**Q2** Which one of the following accurately approximates the protein requirements of a 28-week premature neonate?
- **A** 1.5–2.0 g/kg/day
- **B** 2.5–3 g/kg/day
- **C** extremely variable but up to 7.5 g/kg/day
- **D** 4.0–4.5 g/kg/day
- **E** 1.0–1.5 g/kg/day

**A2** **B** Protein needs often vary widely depending on age, disease and stress status as well as developmental state. Generally less is needed parenterally than enterally. Adequate protein intake is essential to maintain a positive nitrogen balance to support rapid growth. These requirements may reach 3.5 g/kg/day in premature infants or even higher in very low-birthweight infants. This level approximates intrauterine nitrogen retention rates matched for gestational age. Efficient protein utilisation requires about 200 non-protein calories/g of nitrogen – the nitrogen-sparing effect. If enough non-protein calories are not supplied, protein is wasted to provide energy instead of growth.

**Q3** Which of the following is likely to be insufficiently provided to a pre-term infant by breast milk?

  **A** essential fatty acids

  **B** phenylalanine and other aromatic amino acids

  **C** cysteine and other sulphur-containing amino acids

  **D** calcium, phosphorus and trace elements

  **E** all of the above

**A3** **D** The benefits of breast milk are universally known. Breast milk is always sufficient for protein and caloric requirements, although its caloric density can be augmented to minimise volume. It also provides useful passive immunity. However, in some infants with increased nutritional demands, breast milk may be insufficient to provide essential minerals and trace elements. For this reason it is often appropriately fortified.

**Q4** When initiating peripheral parenteral nutrition, all of the following are true *except*:

  **A** aim for minimal osmolar load with maximum caloric density

  **B** observe a maximum dextrose concentration of 12.5%, but usually start at much lower levels

  **C** eliminate lipids as a calorie source to avoid carbon dioxide retention

  **D** use filters in a closed infusion circuit to minimise microemboli and contamination

  **E** blood sugars should be monitored before and after initiation of total parenteral nutrition (TPN).

**A4** **C** Lipid emulsions in parenteral nutrition are isotonic, i.e. osmotically inert. It is essential to keep the osmolarity of TPN solutions as low as possible to minimise the incidence of peripheral vein chemical phlebitis. Glucose and amino acids on the other hand are osmotically active particles. The higher their concentration, the higher the risk of chemical phlebitis. Generally, glucose concentration starts at about 5% and should not exceed 12.5%. Blood sugars should be optimised and monitored prior to initiating TPN to prevent severe hyperglycaemia. Lipids are therefore a safe way of maximising caloric density (9 kcal/g) while minimising this complication.

**Q5** Which option below is not usually effective or recommended in the treatment of TPN-induced hyperglycaemia?

   **A** decrease in rate

   **B** add insulin to TPN

   **C** decrease dextrose concentration in TPN

   **D** insulin drip

   **E** increase the concentration of linoleic acid in TPN

**A5**   **E** All the other options will lead to improvement of hyperglycaemia; however, decreasing the rate or decreasing the concentration of glucose are frequently the most practical measures. It is seldom necessary to administer insulin in any form except in the acute situation to treat glycosuria with osmotic diuresis. Transient hyperglycaemia is common after introduction of TPN, as endogenous insulin secretion adjusts to glucose administration. The response to administered insulin can be unpredictable and unreliable. It also tends to leach into the infusion tubing.

**Q6** Which of these is true with regard to fluid management in severe burns?

   **A** Resuscitation calculations should be based on patient's weight.

   **B** Resuscitation calculations should be based on total body surface area (TBSA).

   **C** Resuscitation solution should contain ample glucose to avoid hypoglycaemia.

   **D** Target urine output should be no more than 0.25 mL/kg/hr to avoid pulmonary oedema.

   **E** Colloid is always necessary initially to maintain intravascular volume.

**A6**   **B** TBSA is the most reliable way to assess fluid requirements in serious burn injuries especially in children since the TBSA in relation to weight is greater. Because of vascular permeability the use of colloids should be discouraged, as they will leak into the tissues and defeat the aim of expanding intravascular volume. While in the interstitium, the colloids hold on to fluid thereby prolonging the oedema phase after recovery of the capillary membrane. Urine output should be kept between 1 and 2 mL/kg/hr as a good reflection of effective resuscitation. Output of 0.25 mL/kg/hr is too low and is a measure of pre-renal failure. Administration of glucose during initial resuscitation is unwise – coupled with the stress reaction, it may induce hyperglycaemia and glycosuria, which will lead to additional volume depletion. In such a case urine output will no longer be a reliable reflection of the adequacy of resuscitation.

**Q7** With respect to TPN-induced liver disease, which one of the following is *not* applicable as a risk factor?

A relative excess of any of the major substrates, particularly amino acids

B age and prematurity

C absence of enteral feedings and consequent lack of enterohepatic circulation

D recurrent septic complications

E deficiency of fat-soluble vitamins A, D, E and K.

**A7** E The fat-soluble vitamins are essential nutrients. Their deficiency, however, has not been linked to the incidence or severity of TPN-related liver disease. All the other options have been implicated in this serious long-term complication of prolonged TPN exposure, especially prematurity.

Of the exact mechanism and pathophysiology of this complication is unknown.

**Q8** Which statement below is correct with regard to fluid compartments and proportions in fetuses and neonates?

A Total body water in a 13-week fetus is approximately 95% of body weight, of which 65% is extracellular.

B Total body water and especially extracellular water volume decreases with gestational age.

C Adult levels of extracellular water (20%–25%) are reached in the neonatal period following term birth.

D A premature infant has a relatively high total body water and extracellular water.

E All of the above.

**A8** E There is a relative shift of extracellular water to the intracellular compartment during all of the transformation from fetus to neonatal life. This sequence is interrupted in the pre-term infant who at birth still has a very high total body and extracellular water. This places an additional burden on the pre-term infant for both fetal and term diuresis. A clear understanding of this is necessary for appropriate fluid management in the neonatal period. After term birth, there is a pre-diuretic phase lasting about 24–36 hours in which urine output is low – frequently less than 1 mL/kg/hr. If excessive volume is given during this period in the erroneous conclusion that the patient is oliguric from hypovolaemia, volume overload may result. The diuretic phase occurs during the second to fourth day of life, during which there is profound diuresis and natriuresis – up to 7–8 mL/kg/hr.

**Q9** Which of the following is incorrect about renal function in the neonate?
  **A** Glomerular filtration rate (GFR) increases after birth as renal vascular resistance falls and renal blood flow increases.
  **B** The GFR of neonates does not reach adult levels until about 2 years of age.
  **C** Cord blood has a very low antidiuretic hormone (ADH) level but the neonatal kidney is extremely sensitive to it.
  **D** The neonatal kidney has a limited ability to concentrate urine but is very efficient in excreting a water load.
  **E** Pre-term infants have difficulty excreting a sodium load.

**A9** **C** Cord blood has high levels of ADH but the neonatal kidney is resistant to its effects. This is thought to be because of the immaturity of the countercurrent mechanism in the loop of Henle for water reabsorption. Neonates are very efficient at excreting a water load but relatively inefficient at concentrating urine, hence the rapid and severe consequences of water deprivation. The GFR of the term infant is only 25% of the adult and does not reach adult levels for about 2 years.

**Q10** An 11-year-old white male with intestinal failure has a central venous catheter (CVC) for TPN. He has developed advanced-stage liver disease and presents with acute-onset high fevers with dehydration, lethargy and leucocytosis. The liver transaminases are higher and the patient is mildly disorientated. What is the most useful and logical next step in his management?
  **A** Immediate removal of the CVC and suspension of TPN.
  **B** Heparin-lock the CVC and start broad-spectrum antibiotics through a peripheral line.
  **C** Volume-resuscitate, draw blood cultures and start broad-spectrum antibiotics through the CVC.
  **D** Proceed to liver transplantation as soon as possible.
  **E** Repeat the blood count and liver function tests and admit to the paediatric intensive care unit for observation.

**A10** **C** This scenario is very serious and potentially life-threatening. In a patient of this description, septicaemia of some sort is the prime suspicion and will include consideration of serious line infection. Immediate removal of the catheter is not practical or necessary. These patients tend to be intravenous-access nightmares and the existing central line may be the only access available to start treatment. Certainly blood cultures should be drawn and effective antibiotics commenced. An elevation of liver transaminases may be a reflection of sepsis but can also reflect ongoing hepatocellular damage.

**Q11** In question 10, the blood culture at 48 hours is positive for *Candida parapsilosis* and the patient is still symptomatic. What is the most reasonable/effective next step?

    **A** Start appropriate antifungal antibiotics immediately through the CVC to sterilise it.

    **B** Start appropriate intravenous antifungal antibiotics and remove the CVC as soon as possible.

    **C** Sacrifice the CVC; insert a new one and use it to treat the candida septicaemia.

    **D** Stop using the CVC and start oral antifungal antibiotics.

    **E** Start appropriate intravenous antifungal antibiotics, and repeat blood cultures after another 48 hours.

**A11** **B** It is practically impossible to eradicate this organism from *in situ* catheters. Appropriate antibiotics in large enough doses, given for long enough, can lead to significant salvage rates for some infections, e.g. gram-positive cocci. While the line can be used in the meantime for treatment, plans should be made to sacrifice it as soon as possible. Unfortunately, venous access can be a very serious problem in some of these patients and while the line is now a serious hazard, it may yet constitute the only lifeline available. Certainly, placement of another long-term line should be deferred until the infection is eradicated.

**Q12** The most practical and useful method to determine the hydration and intravascular volume status of a 5-week-old baby being resuscitated for pyloric stenosis is:

    **A** urine output/kg/hr

    **B** blood pressure and heart rate

    **C** skin turgor

    **D** mental status

    **E** serum chemistry profile.

**A12** **A** The establishment of effective urine flow of 2 mL/kg/hr or more with the appropriate intravenous solution is an indication of good volume resuscitation. If this has been done with the right solution and in the right sequence the chemistry profile will improve but this is not usually a reliable measure of effective volume restoration. Skin turgor, mental status and heart rate will all improve but are less precise measurements. The author's preference is to give repeated boluses of normal saline 20 mL/kg until urine flow is established. Although potassium may have been low to begin with, it is improper to administer potassium until the patient is making urine.

    It is rarely necessary to treat the alkalosis specifically, since it invariably improves with correction of the hypochloraemia.

**Q13** A 26-week-old premature baby on a ventilator is receiving TPN through a right atrial catheter inserted through the right common facial vein. On day 10 she suddenly becomes hypotensive, tachycardic and hypoxic. The pulse pressure narrows significantly and chest X-ray confirms a widened mediastinum. What is the next best diagnostic manoeuvre?

   **A** Repeat chest X-ray to rule out barotrauma.

   **B** Check urine output to rule out fluid overload.

   **C** Echocardiogram to rule out pericardial effusion with tamponade.

   **D** Abdominal X-ray to rule out pneumatosis with pneumoperitoneum.

   **E** Arterial blood gases to determine the most appropriate ventilator changes.

**A13** **C** This scenario suggests acute cardiac tamponade. The CVC tip erodes through the superior vena cava or the thin atrial wall leading to infusion of TPN into the pericardial sac. An echocardiogram will confirm this diagnosis and ultrasound-guided catheter drainage will lead to immediate resolution. While not common, this is a well-known complication even in older children.

**Q14** All of the following are well-known risks with blood transfusions *except*:

   **A** hypokalaemia

   **B** hypocalcaemia

   **C** metabolic acidosis

   **D** hypocoagulability

   **E** non-haemolytic febrile reactions.

**A14** **A** Banked blood becomes hyperkalaemic because the sodium-potassium pump weakens over time thereby permitting potassium to leak out of the cells. Hypocalcaemia can result from the chelating activity of the anticoagulant used – citrate. There is a tendency to hypocoagulability because of dilution of clotting factors and platelets. Theses are all factors that should be borne in mind when transfusing large volumes of blood.

Q15 With regard to the otherwise stable pre-term neonate, which of these statements is invalid?

A Average daily water requirement may be in excess of 150 mL/kg.

B Excessive volume input has no association with intraventricular haemorrhage (IVH) but may lead to pulmonary oedema by reopening the ductus arteriosus.

C Calcium and phosphorus requirements are much higher than in the full-term neonate partly because of diminished reserves in the skeleton.

D Transepithelial water loss in a 27-week premature baby may be greater than 100 mL/kg/day and is associated with approximately 0.5 kcal/mL of heat loss.

E Taurine and cysteine may be essential amino acids.

A15 B Excessive volume input is clearly associated with a higher incidence of IVH as well as pulmonary flooding, which may follow reopening of the ductus. Because of the immaturity of the skin, and especially in infants under radiant warmers, massive transepithelial water loss is the rule along with associated heat loss – latent heat of evaporation. This must be accounted for in balancing the input/output equation. Taurine and cysteine are not essential in older children and adults. They are, however, considered essential amino acids in premature neonates because of their unique requirements.

## Further reading

Day AS, Abbott GD. D-lactic acidosis in short bowel syndrome. *N Z Med J.* 1999; **112**(1092): 277–8.

O'Neill JA, Rowe MI, Coran AG, *et al. Paediatric Surgery. Vol 1.* 5th ed. Philadelphia, PA: Mosby; 1998.

Wesley JR, Coran AG. Intravenous nutrition for the pediatric patient. *Semin Pediatr Surg.* 1992; 1(3): 212–20.

# CHAPTER 3

# Coagulopathies and surgical infectious diseases

## NITIN PATWARDHAN

**From the choices below each question, select the single best answer.**

**Q¹** In the absence of injury, activation of the coagulation pathway is inhibited by:

   **A** circulating plasminogen

   **B** oxygen saturation of blood

   **C** prostacyclin produced by endothelial cells

   **D** circulating heparin

   **E** none of the above.

**A¹**   **C** Prostacyclin is a vasodilator and it also inhibits platelet adhesion and aggregation. It thus provides active thromboresistance in the absence of injury. Endothelial cells have proteoglycans such as heparin sulphate that produce passive thromboresistance.

**Q²** Following a vascular injury the initial haemostatic response consists of:

   **A** vasoconstriction and platelet adhesion

   **B** platelet adhesion followed by aggregation

   **C** vasoconstriction and activation of the extrinsic pathway

   **D** platelet adhesion and activation of intrinsic pathway

   **E** activation of the intrinsic and extrinsic pathways.

**A²**   **A** Vasoconstriction leads to reduced blood flow and is due to the contraction of smooth muscle in the vessel wall. Platelet adhesion followed by aggregation are essential components of the haemostatic response. This leads to degranulation of platelets and release of important factors necessary for continuation of the haemostatic response.

**Q3** Platelets are able to release the following agents except:

    **A** serotonin

    **B** von Willebrand's factor

    **C** calcium

    **D** factor V

    **E** factor VII.

**A3**   **E** Platelets contract on adhesion to extrude storage granule contents. Dense granules release serotonin and calcium while alpha granules produce factor V and von Willebrand's factor. Factor VII is present in a circulating state and is activated by tissue factor to kick-start the extrinsic pathway.

**Q4** In the intrinsic pathway of coagulation, activation of clotting factors follows what order?

    **A** XII, XI, X, IX

    **B** XI, XII, IX, X

    **C** VII, XII, XI, IX

    **D** XII, XI, IX, X

    **E** VII, IX, V, X

**A4**  **D**

**Q5** In relation to clotting tests, which of the following statements is false?

    **A** Prothrombin time is used to screen the function of the extrinsic pathway.

    **B** Activated partial thromboplastin time is used to screen the function of the intrinsic pathway.

    **C** Specific factor assays are available for all known coagulation factors.

    **D** Normal range for platelet count in neonates is lower than adult count.

    **E** von Willebrand's disease patients may have a normal activated partial thromboplastin time.

**A5**   **D** Platelet counts are actually within normal adult range in healthy term and premature neonates. Circulating clotting factors do not cross the placenta. It is common for premature infants to have lower levels of procoagulants. Neonatal liver has very low levels of vitamin K. The main vitamin K–dependent coagulation factors are II, VII, IX and X. It is common practice to give vitamin K at birth to boost levels of vitamin K–dependent factors.

**Q6** For a patient with haemophilia, which of the following statements is true?

   **A** A mild haemophiliac can get spontaneous gum and mucosal bleeding.

   **B** A moderate haemophiliac has procoagulant factor levels between 5% and 10%.

   **C** Analgesics containing aspirin can be prescribed.

   **D** There is an increased risk of viral infections due to frequent transfusions.

   **E** None of the above.

**A6** **D** Mild haemophiliacs have procoagulant factor levels >5%. They will have bleeding problems with major trauma and surgery but not otherwise. Moderate haemophiliacs with levels between 1% and 5% can bleed with minor trauma. Viral infections related to blood transfusion remain a serious risk for these patients.

**Q7** A pre-term neonate undergoing emergency surgery generally:

   **A** requires platelet transfusion

   **B** has normal levels of coagulation factors due to placental transfer

   **C** requires intramuscular injection of vitamin K if not given at birth

   **D** has normal levels of natural anticoagulants

   **E** increased fibrinolytic activity.

**A7** **C** While neonates have low levels of some coagulation proteins, this is normally balanced by the parallel decrease in fibrinolytic activity.

**Q8** A patient with sickle-cell disease is likely to undergo:

   **A** splenectomy

   **B** cholecystectomy

   **C** orthopaedic procedures

   **D** multiple blood transfusions

   **E** all of the above.

**A8** **E** Children with sickle-cell disease can develop acute splenic sequestration resulting in hypersplenism and splenomegaly. Splenectomy is often required with repeated attacks. Because of the haemolytic nature of the disease, gallstones are common, requiring cholecystectomy. Sickle-cell crisis can result in bone infarcts and osteomyelitis.

$Q^9$ For an infection to occur, the factor *least* likely to be of importance is:
  A  size of innoculum
  B  availability of nutrient environment
  C  deficient host defence
  D  route of entry of pathogen
  E  virulence of the organism.

$A^9$  D  Different host defence mechanisms come into play depending on the route of entry. However, occurrence of infection is dependent on the other factors mentioned.

$Q10$ With regard to humoral immunity, which of the following is false?
  A  It acts against intracellular pathogens.
  B  It is mediated by B-cell lymphocytes and plasma cells.
  C  It includes the complement system.
  D  Different types of immunoglobulins have different properties.
  E  Antibodies assist phagocytosis by a process of opsonisation.

$A10$  A  Cell-mediated immunity acts against intracellular pathogens.

$Q11$ A child undergoing splenectomy is routinely vaccinated against:
  A  *Streptococcus pyogenes*
  B  *Neisseria meningitidis*
  C  *Haemophilus influenzae* type A
  D  *Mycobacterium tuberculosis*
  E  *Mycobacterium avium* complex.

$A11$  B  Levels of opsonins, splenic tuftsin and immunoglobulin M are reduced post splenectomy. This reduces the ability to clear infections by encapsulated organisms and incurs the need to routinely vaccinate against them. These include *N. meningitides*, *H. influenzae* type B and *S. pneumoniae*.

$Q12$ Which of the following antibiotics is *not* bactericidal in action?
  A  penicillin
  B  cephalexin
  C  erythromycin
  D  ciprofloxacin
  E  imipenem

$A12$  C

**Q13** Which of the following can be used effectively for intraperitoneal lavage during laparotomy for peritoneal sepsis?

   **A** antibiotic solution

   **B** normal saline

   **C** normal saline + povidone iodine

   **D** hydrogen peroxide

   **E** sterile water

**A13** **B** Various solutions have been used for peritoneal lavage. There is no evidence to suggest that addition of antibiotics or antiseptic agents has added benefits. Peritoneal lavage removes any effluent and dilutes microbial load.

## Further reading

Davidson RN, Wall RA. Prevention and management of infections in patients without a spleen. *Clin Microbiol Infect.* 2001; 7(12): 657–60.

Elhalaby EA, Teitelbaum DH, Coran AG, *et al.* Enterocolitis associated with Hirschsprung's disease: a clinical histopathological correlative study. *J Pediatr Surg.* 1995; 30(7): 1023–6, discussion 1026–7.

Kimber CP, Hutson JM. Primary peritonitis in children. *Aust N Z J Surg.* 1996; 66(3): 169–70.

Luong A, McClay JE, Jafri HS, *et al.* Antibiotic therapy for nontuberculous mycobacterial cervicofacial lymphadenitis. *Laryngoscope.* 2005; 115(10): 1746–51.

Połubinska A, Winckiewicz M, Staniszewski R, *et al.* Time to reconsider saline as the ideal rinsing solution during abdominal surgery. *Am J Surg.* 2006: 192(3): 281–5.

# SECTION II

# Critical care

# CHAPTER 4

# Shock

## ROBERT BAIRD, PRAMOD S PULIGANDLA

**From the choices below each question, select the single best answer.**

**Q1** Hypovolaemic shock in the paediatric population, as compared with adults, includes all of the following *except*:

**A** Children have a tendency towards delayed hypotension, followed quickly by complete cardiovascular collapse.

**B** Blood products should only be administered after two boluses of 5–10 mL/kg of crystalloid solution.

**C** Children are at increased risk of heat loss, due to an increased body surface area.

**D** The first-choice fluid for volume resuscitation in infants should be a crystalloid solution.

**E** Resuscitation may necessitate the placement of an intraosseous intravenous in children <6 years of age.

**A1** **D** Several differences exist in the manifestation of hypovolaemic shock in the paediatric population when compared with adults. Children have an increased physiologic reserve and show signs of hypovolaemic shock much later, with hypotension followed quickly by complete cardiovascular collapse. Less obvious signs of hypovolaemia such as decreased pulse pressure (<20 mmHg), mottled skin, cool extremities, capillary refill and lethargy can be the clues to a shock state in the eyes of the experienced clinician. Thermoregulation is an important consideration in the treatment of paediatric patients, as their increased body surface area places them at increased risk of heat loss and hypothermia. The total estimated blood volume of a child is approximately 80 mL/kg, indicating that a 1-year-old child weighing 10 kg who has lost 200 mL of blood will actually have a 25% blood volume deficit.

Intravenous access may prove challenging during a paediatric resuscitation; an intraosseus intravenous is a simple technique applicable to children less than 6 years of age. As in the adult, the fluid of choice for resuscitation of hypovolaemia remains crystalloid, but Advanced Trauma Life Support (ATLS) guidelines suggest two boluses of **10–20 mL/kg** before the administration of blood products.

**Q2** The most common aetiology of shock in the paediatric population is:

    **A** cardiogenic

    **B** hypovolaemic

    **C** septic

    **D** distributive

    **E** obstructive.

**A2**  **B**  Hypovolaemic shock is by far the most common aetiology of shock in the paediatric population. Causes include hypovolaemia from GI losses (diarrhoea), renal losses (diabetes) or haemorrhage. Other less common mechanisms of shock include the following:

- **Cardiogenic:** a primary pump failure. Causes include myocarditis or a congenital heart defect.
- **Septic:** a physiologic response (systemic inflammatory response syndrome) in the presence of suspected or confirmed infection. Most commonly due to bacteraemia.
- **Distributive:** consists of pathological and inappropriate vasodilatation, endothelial dysfunction with capillary leak, loss of vascular tone or a combination of these factors. Causes include anaphylaxis and spinal shock.
- **Obstructive:** produced by the impairment of venous return to the heart. Causes include cardiac tamponade or tension pneumothorax.

**Q3** Which of following statements is *false*?

    **A** Cardiac output is the product of stroke volume and heart rate.

    **B** Stroke volume is dependent upon ventricular filling (preload), myocardial contractility and systemic vascular resistance (afterload).

    **C** Oxygen delivery is the product of cardiac output and oxygen content.

    **D** Oxygen content is determined by the total oxygen in whole blood available to tissues.

    **E** Mixed venous oxygen tension $(S_vO_2)$ is an accurate reflection of oxygen delivery.

**A3**  **E**  *See* Figure 4.1. The statements in options A, B, C and D are correct. $S_vO_2$ reflects the oxygen content in blood returning to the heart after delivery. It is dependent upon oxygen delivery, but importantly also on oxygen consumption at the tissue level.

oxygen delivery $(DO_2)$ = oxygen content × cardiac output

$(1.36 × Hb × O_2sat) + (P_aO_2 × 0.003)$     heart rate × stroke volume

**FIGURE 4.1** The equation describing tissue oxygen delivery

Hb = haemoglobin
$P_aO_2$ = partial pressure of $O_2$ in blood

 **Q4** Which of the following associations is *incorrect*?
  A  Hypovolaemic shock:    ↓ Preload, ↑ HR, ↑↑ SVR
  B  Neurogenic shock:      − Preload, ↑ HR, ↓ SVR
  C  Cardiogenic shock:     − Preload, ↑ HR, ↑ SVR
  D  Obstructive shock:     ↓ Preload, ↑ HR, ↑ SVR
  E  Septic shock:          − Preload, ↑ HR, ↑ SVR

**A4**  **B**  Hypovolaemic shock results in a decrease in circulating blood volume and a drop in left ventricular volume (preload). Compensatory mechanisms include tachycardia and an increase in systolic vascular resistance to maintain cardiac output. Neurogenic (or spinal) shock is a form of distributive shock, whose primary event is loss of vascular tone. While circulatory volume (preload) remains unchanged, neurogenic shock is characterised by an inappropriate **absence of tachycardia**. Cardiogenic shock is characterised by a primary failure of myocardial activity. There is no change in preload, and tachycardia and vascular constriction are compensatory mechanisms. Obstructive shock results from a primary decrease in venous return to the heart (preload) secondary to an 'obstruction'. Tachycardia and ↑ SVR are compensatory. Septic shock is often described as either a 'warm' and 'cold' phase. Answer 'E' accurately portrays the more commonly observed 'cold' phase of septic shock with primary myocardial dysfunction followed by tachycardia and increased vascular tone.

**Q5** Which of the receptor/action associations is *incorrect* regarding medications useful in the treatment of shock?

| Drug | Receptor | Action |
| --- | --- | --- |
| A. dopamine | dopamine, ß, α | chronotropy, inotropy, vasoconstriction |
| B. dobutamine | α | chronotropy, inotropy, vasoconstriction |
| C. epinephrine | ß, α | chronotropy, inotropy, vasoconstriction |
| D. milrinone | PDE inhibitor | inotropy, lusitropy, vasodilatation |
| E. vasopressin | V1 vascular receptors | vasoconstriction |

**TABLE 4.1** Mechanism of action of vasopressors and inotropes

**A5** **D** *See* Table 4.2. Dobutamine preferentially affects the ß receptor, resulting in chronotropy, inotropy and **vasodilatation**.

| Drug | Receptor | Action |
| --- | --- | --- |
| dopamine | dopamine, ß, α | chronotropy, inotropy, vasoconstriction |
| dobutamine | ß | chronotropy, inotropy, vasodilatation |
| epinephrine | ß, α | chronotropy, inotropy, vasoconstriction |
| norepinephrine | α, ß | vasoconstriction, chronotropy, inotropy |
| milrinone | PDE inhibitor | inotropy, lusitropy, vasodilatation |
| nitroprusside | NO donor, smooth muscle relaxation | vasodilatation |
| vasopressin | V1 vascular receptors | vasoconstriction |

**TABLE 4.2 Mechanism of action of vasopressors and inotropes**

**Q6** Which of the following is true regarding the outcomes of shock?

**A** Colloid resuscitation has been demonstrated to be superior to crystalloid in the management of shock in the neonate.

**B** A superior outcome is associated with early resuscitation in the paediatric patient with shock, regardless of aetiology.

**C** Volume restriction in paediatric septic shock has been associated with decreased mortality.

**D** Shock-related mortality is dependent on normalising and maintaining blood pressure.

**E** Liberal fluid resuscitation has resulted in increasing rates of acute respiratory distress syndrome (ARDS).

**A6** **B** No difference in outcome has been demonstrated when comparing crystalloids with colloids in paediatric shock, including the neonate. A possible indication for colloid is in the context of a congenital heart anomaly and the concern of fluid overload.

Multiple studies in the adult and paediatric literature have demonstrated improved mortality rates with early, goal-directed therapy. This is the single greatest parameter that can be modified by healthcare providers – including emergency room physicians.

Mortality is significantly decreased when children with septic shock receive early, liberal fluid resuscitation when compared with those who are volume restricted. Shock-related mortality is independent of maintaining or normalising the blood pressure alone, but is directly related to low cardiac index and low mixed venous oxygen saturations. Furthermore, Carcillo and Fields (2002) did not find a difference in the occurrence of ARDS between groups with restricted fluid resuscitation compared with those who received liberal fluid resuscitation.

**Q7** Which of the following is not a well-demonstrated surrogate marker of tissue perfusion?

  **A** serum bicarbonate

  **B** serum pH

  **C** serum glucose

  **D** serum lactate

  **E** base deficit

**A7**  **C**  Serum pH, lactate, base deficit and bicarbonate are accepted surrogate markers of tissue perfusion that correlate with the severity of shock and the adequacy of resuscitation. Normalisation of serum bicarbonate and lactate are associated with patient recovery in paediatric septic shock. Successful resuscitation should be accompanied by a decreasing anion gap, decreasing lactate and improving base excess. While increases in serum glucose have been associated with an increased risk of death, hyperglycaemia indicates excessive circulating counter-regulatory hormones (like catecholamine) that result in the failure of insulin to suppress hepatic gluconeogenesis. Glucose is not a surrogate marker for tissue perfusion.

**Q8** Which of the following is true regarding relative adrenal insufficiency?

  **A** It occurs in nearly 25% of all paediatric intensive care unit (PICU) admissions for septic shock.

  **B** Routine administration of steroid replacement therapy is warranted in cases of hypovolaemic shock.

  **C** Patients who increase serum cortisol levels in response to test-dose corticotropin have a 60% mortality compared with patients who do not.

  **D** Steroid therapy should be given in septic shock if hypotension is refractory to vasopressor therapy.

  **E** Steroids should be administered only in children with suspected or proven adrenal insufficiency.

**A8**  **E**  Relative adrenal insufficiency is common in the PICU, occurring in over 75% of patients in septic shock. Steroid replacement has no direct role in the care of hypovolaemic shock, unless an underlying steroid dependence exists. Adrenal suppression is diagnosed by a failure to increase cortisol levels after the administration of a test dose of corticotropin. Non-responders who fail to increase serum cortisol levels after this test dose have a 60% mortality compared with responders (normal adrenal function). Routine treatment of paediatric patients with stress-dose steroids cannot be recommended, as stated by the Surviving Sepsis Campaign. This publication recommends administering steroid therapy to **adults** in septic shock who respond poorly to vasopressors. However, evidence in the paediatric population is lacking. Nonetheless, in children with catecholamine-refractory shock or in whom the presence of risk factors (such as history of chronic or recent high-dose steroid treatment) is present, steroid administration should be considered.

**Q⁹** Changes in a child's cardiac output is most dependent upon which of the following variables?

**A** end-diastolic volume

**B** blood pressure

**C** heart rate

**D** stroke volume

**E** myocardial contractility

**A⁹** **C** Cardiac output = heart rate × stroke volume

Children are mostly dependent on their heart rate to increase cardiac output. Stroke volume (the volume of blood pumped from one ventricle of the heart with each beat) cannot be altered in children to the same degree as in adults. Factors that affect stroke volume include blood pressure (afterload), end-diastolic volume (preload) and myocardial contractility. Blood pressure and end-diastolic volume have limited ranges while the ability to increase contractility in response to catecholamine stimulation is limited because of insufficient muscle mass and 'stiffness' of the young myocardium as compared with the adult heart.

**Q10** Which of the following is essential in the definition of shock?

**A** inadequate systemic oxygen and nutrient supply to meet metabolic demands

**B** the delivery of oxygen ($DO_2$) is less than oxygen consumption ($VO_2$)

**C** hypotension refractory to volume and vasopressors

**D** A and B

**E** all of the above

**A10** **D** Shock ensues when systemic oxygen and nutrient supply become acutely inadequate to meet the metabolic demands of the body's organ systems. This can be expressed in mathematical terms, where:

$DO_2$ (oxygen delivery) < $VO_2$ (oxygen consumption).

Hypotension is often associated with shock states, but it is **not** necessary. Indeed, fatal shock can ensue in spite of a normal arterial blood pressure if metabolic demands are not being met.

Q11 Shock in the neonatal period has several unique characteristics. These include:
A the development of pulmonary hypertension
B may benefit from prostaglandin infusion
C may result from maternal factors
D shock is less likely, given the increased heart rate of the newborn
E may benefit from indomethacin.

A11 **D** Several important differences exist in neonates as they transition from fetal to extrauterine physiology. A patent ductus arteriosus (PDA) may contribute to or cause shock through the failure of a compensatory increase in the cardiac output. This may be secondary to myocardial immaturity or a ductal steal phenomenon, which accounts for a uniform reduction in systolic and diastolic blood pressure. This is particularly true of extremely premature infants, who benefit from efforts to close this shunt. A PDA may close after a dose of indomethacin or ibuprofen. Alternatively, surgical closure is sometimes required. On the other hand, several duct-dependent cardiac lesions present in shock that is refractory to fluid therapy. These neonates benefit from early prostaglandin infusion to maintain duct patency, and require a cardiac echocardiogram to confirm the diagnosis.

Neonates are also at risk for the development of pulmonary hypertension. This results in increased afterload for the right ventricle and reduced pulmonary blood flow that ultimately compromises oxygen exchange and worsens oxygen delivery. Other causes of neonatal shock include hypovolaemia (GI losses, haemorrhage), obstructive shock (tension pneumothorax) and cardiogenic shock (arrhythmias). Neonates are uniquely at risk for developing sepsis as a consequence of maternal infection, most commonly Group B Streptococcus. This should be considered in any newborn manifesting evidence of unexplained shock.

Neonates are less able to vary their heart rate to meet metabolic demands, placing them at an **increased** risk of developing shock.

Q12 Regarding vasopressin in the treatment of paediatric septic shock, which of the following is *incorrect*?
A It significantly reduces 28-day mortality when compared with placebo for paediatric patients in septic shock.
B It may be useful in cases of hypotension unresponsive to conventional vasopressor therapy.
C It acts via a catecholamine-independent V1 vascular receptor.
D It has a direct antidiuretic effect on the distal renal tubule and collecting duct.
E It may reduce cardiac output by increasing afterload.

A12 **A** Vasopressin, otherwise know as antidiuretic hormone, is a peptide hormone with multiple effects, mediated by different receptors. It acts through a second messenger system to increase water absorption in the distal renal tubule and collecting duct. It also acts through a catecholamine–independent V1 receptor on vascular endothelium to promote vasoconstriction. This increases afterload, which can lower cardiac output in the absence of compensatory changes in heart rate or contractility. While vasopressin has been demonstrated to increase mean arterial pressure and improve urine output in patients with catecholamine-unresponsive hypotension, a recent randomised, multicentre trial (Choong *et al.*, 2009) investigating low-dose vasopressin in the treatment of paediatric vasodilatory shock did not demonstrate any beneficial effects. Although not statistically significant, there was a concerning trend towards increased mortality.

Q13 A 16-year-old presents to the trauma bay after sustaining a gunshot wound to the abdomen. His pulse is 130 beats per minute, and his blood pressure is 80/50. He is anxious but *conscious and orientated*. A Foley catheter drains a small amount of urine output. His estimated blood loss is:

**A** <15%

**B** 15%–25%

**C** 25%–40%

**D** >40%

**E** not estimable given above information.

A13 **C** While paediatric patients tend to maintain normal vital signs in the face of hypovolaemia, this adolescent is manifesting evidence of significant blood loss. His tachycardia and hypotension suggest blood loss greater than 25% of his circulating blood volume, but the maintenance of end-organ function (mental activity, renal function) suggests that the blood loss does not exceed 40% – see Table 4.3.

| % Blood loss | Clinical signs | | | | | |
|---|---|---|---|---|---|---|
| | Heart rate | Blood pressure | Capillary refill | Respiratory rate | Urine output | Mental status |
| <15 | Normal to slightly increased | Normal or increased | Normal | Normal | Normal | Anxious |
| 15–25 | Slightly increased | Might be decreased | Prolonged | Mildly tachypnoeic | Normal to slightly decreased | Anxious, might be agitated |
| 25–40 | Increased | Decreased | Prolonged | Moderately tachypnoeic | Decreased (<0.5 mL/ kg/hr) | Anxious, confused |
| >40 | Increased | Decreased | Prolonged | Severely tachypnoeic | Absent | Confused, lethargic, unresponsive |

**TABLE 4.3 Estimated blood loss percentages based on clinical signs**

Q14 A 6-year-old child who weighs 30 kg presents to the hospital with fever, tachycardia (pulse = 140) and mental status changes. She has a history of urinary tract infections. Intravenous access is obtained and three successive boluses of 600 mL normal saline are administered. She is started on antibiotic therapy but continues to have delayed capillary refill and remains lethargic. After transfer to the intensive care unit, the next step in her care is:

   A  transfuse with 10 mL/kg of packed red blood cells

   B  administer hydrocortisone

   C  begin a milrinone infusion at 0.25 mcg/kg/min

   D  begin a dopamine infusion at 10 mcg/kg/min

   E  consider initiating extracorporeal life support (ECLS).

A14 **D** This child presents with fluid refractory septic shock. The next appropriate step is to begin a dopamine infusion. The dosage should be adequate to activate adrenergic receptors and thereby provide chronotropy, inotropy and peripheral vasoconstriction. There is no reason to suspect acute blood loss; a transfusion is not indicated at this time. Milrinone may be useful if there is evidence of myocardial hypocontractility, but it is also not indicated at this time. Hydrocortisone is important if the child has documented or suspected adrenal insufficiency. While ECLS has been shown to be of value in the treatment of septic shock, it should be instituted only after other treatment options (catecholamines) have been exhausted and a shock state persists.

Q15 As compared with crystalloid resuscitation, which of the following is a documented advantage of colloid fluid resuscitation?

   A  decreased cost

   B  decreased risk of allergic reaction

   C  decreased volume of fluid required

   D  decreased risk of disease transmission

   E  decreased overall mortality rates

A15 **C** Colloid solutions effectively restore blood pressure, especially in young neonates. However, there is a concern over the potential adverse effects of using natural and synthetic colloids, which include infectious disease transmission/exposure and the potential for allergic reactions. In a recent paediatric open-label trial, children with septic shock were randomised to receive either normal saline or gelatin polymer in saline. Both groups achieved haemodynamic stability, and mortality and organ failure rates were similar in both groups. The colloid-resuscitated group required 40% less volume than the saline-resuscitated group. For this reason, the use of colloids and/or hypertonic solutions may be of particular benefit in postoperative cardiac surgery patients where volume load is a concern.

**Q16** Signs of compensated shock include all of the following *except*:

    **A** tachycardia

    **B** cool extremities

    **C** prolonged capillary refill (despite warm ambient temperature)

    **D** weak peripheral pulses compared with central pulses

    **E** low blood pressure.

**A16** **E** Shock progresses over a continuum of severity, from a compensated to a decompensated state. Physiologic attempts to compensate include tachycardia and increased systemic vascular resistance (vasoconstriction) to maintain cardiac output and blood pressure. As compensatory mechanisms fail, signs of inadequate end-organ perfusion develop. In addition to the above, these signs include hypotension and evidence of end-organ dysfunction (mental status changes, decreased urine output, metabolic acidosis). Hypotension is defined based on systolic blood pressure and the patient's age:

- <60 mmHg in term neonates (0–28 days)
- <70 mmHg in infants (1 month to 12 months)
- <70 mmHg + (2 × age in years) in children 1–10 years
- <90 mmHg in children ≥10 years of age.

## Further reading

American College of Surgeons, Committee on Trauma. *Advanced Trauma Life Support for Doctors (ATLS).* 8th ed. Chicago, IL: 2008.

Boluyt N, Bollen CW, Bos AP, *et al.* Fluid resuscitation in neonatal and pediatric hypovolemic shock: a Dutch Pediatric Society evidence-based clinical practice guideline. *Intensive Care Med.* 2006; **32**(7): 995–1003.

Carcillo JA, Fields AI. Clinical practice parameters for hemodynamic support of pediatric and neonatal patients in septic shock. *Crit Care Med.* 2002; **30**(6): 1365–78.

Choong K, Bohn D, Fraser D. Vasopressin in pediatric vasodilatory shock: a multicenter randomized controlled trial. *Am J Respir Crit Care Med.* 2009; **180**(7): 632–9.

DeRoss AL, Vane DW. Early evaluation and resuscitation of the pediatric trauma patient. *Semin Pediatr Surg.* 2004; **13**(2): 74–9.

Zaritsky AL, Nadkarni VM, Hickey RW, *et al.*, editors. *Pediatric Advanced Life Support Provider Manual.* Dallas, TX: American Heart Association; 2002.

# CHAPTER 5

# Mechanical ventilation and support

## ELIZABETH PILLING

From the choices below each question, select the single best answer.

**Q1** From Figure 5.1, which of the following is true?

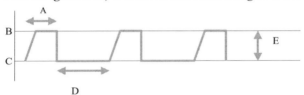

**FIGURE 5.1** Standard spirometer trace showing the various lung function tests

    **A** A indicates inspiratory time.
    **B** D indicates tidal volume.
    **C** E indicates expiratory time.
    **D** All of the above.
    **E** None of the above.

**A1**   **A**

**Q2** To increase $CO_2$ clearance for a baby ventilated using pressure-limited time-cycled ventilation:
    **A** increase the positive end-expiratory pressure (PEEP)
    **B** increase the inspiratory time
    **C** increase the positive inspiratory pressure (PIP)
    **D** increase the fraction of inspired oxygen ($F_iO_2$)
    **E** decrease the respiratory rate.

**A2**   **C**  $CO_2$ is controlled by the minute ventilation, which is a product of tidal volume (the size of breath) and the ventilatory rate. In these examples, to increase $CO_2$

clearance, the tidal volume needs to be increased. This can be done by increasing the PIP, or reducing the PEEP. To reduce the $CO_2$ the opposite is needed. Note, a reduction of PEEP will also result in a reduction in the mean airway pressure and therefore oxygenation.

**Q3** To improve oxygenation for a patient ventilated using pressure-limited time-cycled ventilation:

**A** increase the PEEP

**B** decrease the tidal volume

**C** decrease the PIP

**D** decrease the inspiratory time

**E** decrease the respiratory rate.

**A3** **A** Oxygenation is controlled by the mean airway pressure. This is a function of the inspiratory time, PIP and PEEP. To improve oxygenation, the PIP or PEEP can be increased. Note, increasing the PEEP will reduce the tidal volume and therefore reduce $CO_2$ clearance.

**Q4** Common complications of extracorporeal membrane oxygenation (ECMO) do not include:

**A** barotrauma to lungs

**B** intracranial haemorrhage

**C** pulmonary haemorrhage

**D** carotid artery ligation

**E** need for renal haemofiltration.

**A4** **A** ECMO is used to 'rest' the lungs while the underlying pathology recovers. Patients are placed on a cardiopulmonary bypass circuit to provide oxygenation and $CO_2$ removal. Pulmonary barotrauma therefore does not occur as minimal pressure is used to ventilate. Haemorrhage is a complication due to the need for anticoagulation to maintain patency of the ECMO circuit, with 15% of neonates suffering an intracranial haemorrhage and 12% pulmonary haemorrhage in one study. In the same study, 25% of infants required haemofiltration.

**Q5** The highest neonatal ECMO survival rate is in infants with:

**A** persistent pulmonary hypertension

**B** congenital diaphragmatic hernia

**C** meconium aspiration syndrome

**D** sepsis

**E** pulmonary hypoplasia.

**A5**    **C**   Ninety-four per cent of infants with meconium aspiration syndrome survive to discharge. This compares with 79% with PPHN, 75% with sepsis and 54% with congenital diaphragmatic hernia. Pulmonary hypoplasia alone is not an indication for ECMO as it is a non-reversible condition.

**Q6**   Contraindications to ECMO include:

     **A**   respiratory distress syndrome (RDS)

     **B**   gestational age below term (37 weeks)

     **C**   ventilation for less than 7 days

     **D**   ventilation more than 14 days

     **E**   cardiac abnormality.

**A6**    **D**   ECMO can be used for infants with reversible disease, therefore RDS can be an indication if other selection criteria are met. Pre-term infants below 35 weeks are not considered candidates for ECMO because of the risk of intraventricular haemorrhage, which is increased because of their gestation and need for anticoagulation on ECMO. Ventilation for over 14 days is considered a contraindication because of the irreversible lung damage that will have occurred, whatever the underlying pathology. There is no minimum time of ventilation before ECMO is considered, and early referral is considered best practice to minimise barotraumas. Cardiac abnormality per se is not a contraindication, and ECMO can be used occasionally as a bridge to cardiac transplantation.

**Q7**   Contraindications for continuous positive airway pressure (CPAP) include:

     **A**   gastroschisis (postoperative)

     **B**   oesophageal atresia (preoperative)

     **C**   congenital diaphragmatic hernia (preoperative)

     **D**   cardiac malformation

     **E**   laryngomalacia.

**A7**    **C**   CPAP provides a continuous distending pressure to the lungs. It is most commonly used in infants with RDS to minimise the work of breathing and reduce atelectasis. For infants with repaired gastroschisis, it may help with the respiratory complications of increased intra-abdominal pressure. Preoperatively CPAP should be avoided in infants with gastroschisis, exomphalos and congenital diaphragmatic hernia, as it will cause intestinal distension. It is safe to deliver CPAP to infants with pure oesophageal atresia provided a Replogle tube is in place or frequent aspiration of the upper pouch is performed. CPAP can be used as supportive therapy for infants with laryngomalacia, because of the airway support provided.

# CHAPTER 6

# Vascular access

## ALEXANDER CHO, ALICE MEARS, NIALL JONES

**From the choices below each question, select the single best answer.**

**Q1** Which of the following is true regarding the rate of flow through vascular access catheters?

  A  The rate of flow is governed by the Poisson–Hagen formula.

  B  The rate of flow through a rigid tube $= \dfrac{8\eta \cdot L}{P \cdot r^4 \cdot \prod}$

  C  The greatest flow is achieved with long, wide catheters.

  D  The length of the catheter has the greatest impact on flow rate.

  E  Central lines are not the most effective means of rapid fluid administration.

**A1**  E  Flow rate through a tube is described by the Hagen–Poiseuille formula:

$$\frac{P \cdot r^4 \cdot \prod}{8\eta \cdot L}$$

where $P$ is driving pressure, $r$ is radius of the tube, $\eta$ is viscosity of the liquid and $L$ is length of the tube. Thus the fastest flow can be achieved through a *short*, wide catheter. However, the width, not the length, of the catheter will have the greatest impact, as the flow is proportional to the fourth power of the catheter's radius. Central lines are long and slim and therefore are not the most effective means of rapid fluid administration.

**Q2** Which of the following is true regarding umbilical arteries?

  A  A single umbilical artery is found in approximately 5% of neonates.

  B  They are a continuation of the external iliac arteries.

  C  They twist around the umbilical vein.

  D  When fetal circulation ceases, the pelvic portion remains patent as the inferior vesical artery.

  E  The non-patent obliterated part of the artery becomes the lateral umbilical ligament.

$A^2$    **C**   A single umbilical artery is a rare abnormality, present in only around 0.3% of neonates. It is associated with an increased incidence of chromosomal and congenital abnormalities. In fetal circulation, the internal iliac artery is twice the size of the external iliac artery and is a direct continuation of the common iliac artery. On each side of the body the umbilical artery, arising from the internal iliac artery, ascends along the side of the bladder, then runs along the underside of the anterior abdominal wall to enter the umbilical cord. Within the umbilical cord the two arteries twist around the umbilical vein, ending in the placenta.

     After birth, the main length of the umbilical arteries becomes obliterated into a fibrous cord called the medial umbilical ligament. The pelvic portion of the artery remains patent as the superior vesical artery.

$Q^3$   Which of the following correctly states the infection rate of central venous catheters?

   **A**   1 episode per 1000 catheter days

   **B**   1 episode per 100 catheter days

   **C**   5 episodes per 100 catheter days

   **D**   5 episodes per 1000 catheter days

   **E**   1 episode per 500 catheter days

$A^3$    **D**   The infection rate of central lines is 5 episodes per 1000 catheter days. Up to 60% of central lines become infected, half of which require removal. The commonest infecting organisms are *Staphylococcus aureus* and *Staphylococcus epidermidis*, with gram-negative infections being more prevalent in immunocompromised patients.

$Q^4$   Which of the following veins is *not* suitable for an open technique of central line insertion?

   **A**   cephalic

   **B**   saphenous

   **C**   internal jugular

   **D**   subclavian

   **E**   femoral

$A^4$    **D**   Open ('cutdown') techniques can be used to insert peripherally inserted central catheters (PICCs) into the cephalic and saphenous veins and central lines into internal jugular and femoral veins. In addition to these veins, percutaneous insertion techniques can be used on scalp veins and subclavian veins.

**Q5** Which of the following is *not* a contraindication to using the intraosseous route?

**A** bone fracture

**B** neonate

**C** older child

**D** use as long-term access

**E** previous failed attempt

 **A5** **B** Intraosseous needles are useful for emergency access in neonates and young children. With the intraosseous route, fluid is infused into the non-collapsible venous network of sinusoids within the medullary cavity of the bone. The most reliable and safe site is 2–3 cm distal to the tibial tuberosity on the flat anteromedial surface of the tibia, as the surface of the bone is close to the skin and there are no nearby vital nerves or vessels to damage. The tibia cannot be used if there is a fracture in that limb. An alternative site is the iliac crest.

Intraosseous needles have a high success rate of insertion – 98% – but should not be attempted multiple times in the event of a failed insertion because of the increased risk of complications such as epiphyseal damage and osteomyelitis. They should not be used for long-term access or non-emergency access, as the risks include fat embolus, osteomyelitis and needle displacement resulting in subperiosteal infiltration or subcutaneous extravasation. In older children the bone cortex is too thick to be easily penetrated with an intraosseous needle, unless a powered device is used.

 **Q6** Validated techniques to improve the success rate of peripheral intravenous cannulation in the children over the age of one, include all except:

**A** local warming

**B** transillumination with fibre-optic 'cold light'

**C** transillumination with an otoscope

**D** Lidocaine with prilocaine topical cream (EMLA)

**E** topical nitroglycerine (GTN)

 **A6** **D** Local warming dilates the arterioles and decreases alpha-2-adrenergic vasoconstriction, improving the success of cannulation. Transillumination with cold-light fibre optics is commonly used to good effect but the user should be aware of the rare complication of burns. Transillumination using an otoscope has been shown in the emergency department setting to increase the success rate of venous access with a reduction in number of events. EMLA cream causes local reaction in up to 50% of patients including erythema or oedema and irritation. It may improve patient compliance, but has no direct effect on the vasculature. GTN positively affected venous dilatation, choice of cannulation site and ease of cannulation, in a double-blinded trial of 104 children aged between 1 and 11 years.

**Q7** With reference to pericardial effusion and cardiac tamponade associated with central venous catheters, the following are true *except*:

A present chiefly in neonates and infants

B peripherally inserted central catheters are associated with a decreased risk

C managed with prompt withdrawal of the central venous catheter

D managed with pericardiocentesis

E can present with hypotension.

**A7** **B** There is evidence that peripherally inserted central catheters are associated with an increased risk of cardiac tamponade and pericardial effusion, particularly soon after birth. A 10-year review demonstrated no occurrence in patients over 3 weeks of age. Prematurity is a risk factor with reported mean gestational age of 30–33 weeks at birth. This is thought to be due to thin cardiac tissue associated with small premature infants. A study in 2005 identified five occurrences in patients less than 1500 g due to the peripherally inserted central catheter. Prompt recognition of signs, which include cardiac arrest, increased respiratory rate or oxygen requirements, tachycardia or hypotension, followed by line removal and pericardiocentesis is a highly effective therapy.

**Q8** When inserting a percutaneous central venous catheter the following are true *except*:

A The right side is preferable due to avoidance of the thoracic duct.

B The patient should be placed in reverse Trendelenburg's position for the subclavian or internal jugular veins.

C It should be noted that the subclavian vein position is more cephalad in younger children.

D Gentle negative pressure should be applied during needle insertion.

E Accessing the femoral vein is aided by inguinal compression over the femoral vein.

**A8** **B** The thoracic duct enters at the junction of the left subclavian and left jugular veins. In the infant population, placing the patient in reverse Trendelenburg's position (head up) increases the cross-sectional area of the femoral vein by 15%. When combined with inguinal pressure over the femoral vein, this increases by 30%. Trendelenburg's position (head down) for subclavian and internal jugular veins similarly increases the cross-sectional area and also minimises risk of cerebral air embolism. Gentle negative pressure is recommended during needle insertion so that the vein does not collapse during venepuncture. In infants, the subclavian vein was found to have a significant superior arch as it coursed centrally, that was more apparent on the right. The horizontal position of the subclavian vein that is seen in adults does not become evident until over 12 months of age.

**Q9** In a haemophilia patient undergoing central vascular access, which of the following is false?

A Factor VIII levels should be optimised preoperatively.

B Most catheters tend to be removed, as they are no longer needed.

C Complications requiring catheter removal include infection, blockage, line fracture, inability to access the port and pain.

D Factor VIII inhibitors are associated with more catheter complications.

E Even when the device has to be removed for complications, most patients and carers opt for the insertion of a further device.

**A9** B Catheter-related complications are the most common reason for removal of central venous catheters in patients with haemophilia. These include (in reducing incidence): infection, blockage, catheter fracture, inability to access port and pain. Optimisation of factor VIII levels (above 100%) preoperatively with a bolus and subsequent infusion maximises success of the insertion procedure. This can prevent even the slightest bruising around the wounds, a suspected nidus of infection particularly in inhibitor-positive children. Inhibitors are associated with a 67% increase in infections, and most infected devices need to be removed for successful treatment. The formation of antibodies against factor VIII inhibits replacement therapy and is the most serious treatment-related complication faced by patients with haemophilia. The majority of patients and carers will opt for reinsertion of another implantable device after removal because of complication. This is very likely related to the trauma of repeated peripheral access procedures, and the overall satisfaction with implantable devices. Overall, the salient features of successful outcome when inserting an implantable venous access device in children with haemophilia are (a) a robust protocol for catheter insertion, (b) the management of the catheter and (c) the timing of administration of factor VIII.

**Q10** With reference to central venous catheter–related complications, the following are true *except*:

A Passing the guide wire while monitoring the electrocardiogram rhythm strip (to observe for rhythm disturbances to indicate that the guide wire is in the heart) is a safe practice.

B Air embolism should be suspected in severe hypotension with a normal electrocardiogram tracing.

C Phrenic nerve paresis has a worse prognosis in neonates.

D Too medial insertion of subclavian lines should be avoided.

E Pneumothorax should not be a fatal complication.

$A$10 **A** There are several reports of dysrhythmias in children, secondary to guide wire placement, requiring medications and/or cardioversion for correction. Guide wires can also be associated with direct cardiac injury and perforation despite their relatively soft tip. The typical finding in air embolism is severe hypotension with a normal electrocardiogram tracing. The classic 'millwheel' murmur, a loud churning sound as the air mixes with the blood in the right ventricle in the setting of an air embolism, may be heard but is transient. In larger children, phrenic nerve paresis is much better tolerated and typically resolves within 1–3 years. In pre-term infants with phrenic nerve paresis, weaning from ventilation can be problematic and respiratory function can dramatically worsen with inadequate diaphragm function. Too medial insertion of subclavian lines may lead to 'pinching' between the clavicle and first rib. Pneumothorax should not be a fatal complication because it is a well-known complication and is easily controlled with a tube thoracostomy. There has been only one reported death.

$Q$11 Which of the following statements is incorrect with regard to Hickman and Broviac catheters?

**A** The internal diameter of a 6.6Fr single lumen catheter is twice that of a 2.7Fr single lumen catheter.

**B** They have a tissue ingrowth cuff that takes 2–4 weeks to take effect.

**C** They are radio-opaque.

**D** They can be placed in the right atrium.

**E** They can be removed by simple traction alone.

$A$11 **D** The internal diameter of a 6.6Fr single lumen catheter is 10 mm. The internal diameter of a 2.7Fr single lumen catheter is 5 mm. Tissue grows into the Dacron cuff after 2–4 weeks. These catheters are radio-opaque but the small-sized catheters may require water-soluble contrast during radiological screening to determine the current position. These catheters are *not* right atrium catheters. The preferred position is at the junction of the superior vena cava and the right atrium. There are several documented methods of catheter removal, dependent on whether the catheter is sutured internally at the cuff site or at the vessel insertion site. Catheters may be removed by simple traction without dissecting the cuff unless it is retained post removal.

**Q12** In children with difficult peripheral access, which of the following is *not* correct?

  A Clinical studies show that only 53%–76% of children are successfully cannulated on the first attempt

  B Blood products can be given via the intraosseous route.

  C Subcutaneous absorption of isotonic fluids can be accelerated by the concomitant administration of hyaluronidase.

  D Fluid given via the subcutaneous route can be used in emergency situations.

  E Similar serum drug levels are achieved with both intravenous and intraosseous routes.

**A12** **D** Studies have demonstrated that only 53%–76% of children are successfully cannulated on the first attempt. Approximately 5%–33% require more than two attempts to achieve intravenous access. The intraosseous route allows for the rapid delivery of a variety of drugs, crystalloid solutions and blood products. Human recombinant formulation of hyaluronidase has been approved for use as an adjunct to accelerate subcutaneous fluid and drug administration. It is an enzymatic spreading agent and early evidence indicates that it is safe and effective in children with mild and moderate dehydration. Subcutaneous administration of fluid is not recommended in emergency situations, as systemic absorption is significantly reduced by compromised peripheral perfusion. Similar serum drug levels are achieved with intraosseous and intravenous routes. There is evidence that drug delivery may be faster than via an intravenous route.

**Q13** Which of the following statements is *incorrect* with regard to positioning of central venous catheters?

  A A left femoral venous catheter should cross the midline.

  B Common malpositions include the contralateral subclavian vein and the ipsilateral internal jugular vein.

  C Catheter tip position can be elicited with fluoroscopy, ultrasound scan or a lateral cross-table radiograph.

  D Risk of severe allergic reaction to intravenous contrast injection should not be a barrier to performing contrast injection for determining central line placement.

  E A postoperative chest X-ray can help prevent complications.

**A13** **E** A femoral venous catheter placed in the left side should be demonstrated to cross the midline to sure that it is in the inferior vena cava rather than a lumbar or other non-central vein. A retrospective review of 11 306 paediatric patients demonstrated an incidence of 0.18% of acute allergic reaction. Only three patients had a severe reaction. Many institutions routinely use fluoroscopy intraoperatively to ascertain catheter tip position. A limitation of anterior–posterior radio-graphs/fluoroscopy is that only a two-dimensional view is obtained. This may be addressed with a lateral cross-table radiograph. Sonography has been used to used determine catheter position, especially in the context of trapped central lines. Although routine chest radiographs immediately post-insertion can be used to verify the position of the catheter, there is no evidence that they can help prevent complications.

**Q14** Which of the following advanced paediatric life support statements with regard to venous access is *incorrect*?

  **A** Surface anatomy of the saphenous vein of an infant is half a finger's breadth superior and anterior to the medial malleolus.

  **B** Surface anatomy for tibial intraosseous infusion is the anterior surface, 2–3 cm below the tibial tuberosity.

  **C** Surface anatomy for femoral intraosseous infusion is the antero-medial aspect, 3 cm above the medial condyle.

  **D** The femoral vein lies medial to the femoral artery.

  **E** The external jugular vein can be seen passing over the sternoclei-domastoid muscle at the junction of its middle and lower thirds.

**A14** **C** The saphenous vein of an infant is half a finger's breadth superior and anterior to the medial malleolus. In small children, this is found one finger's breadth away. Surface anatomy for tibial intraosseous insertion is as stated. For femoral inser-tion, the landmark is the anterolateral aspect, 3 cm above the lateral condyle. The femoral vein lies medial to the femoral artery ('VAN' – from medial to lateral: vein, artery, nerve). The external jugular vein passes over the sternocleidomastoid at its middle and lower thirds. Digital pressure over the lower end above the clavicle stabilises and distends this vein.

**Q15** Which of the following is true regarding the tip position of peripherally inserted central venous catheters (PICCs) in neonates?

  **A** Catheter tip angulation or looping is strongly associated with cardiac tamponade.

  **B** The ideal tip position is in the right atrium.

  **C** Cardiac tamponade is generally well tolerated.

  **D** Migration of the catheter tip occurs in 1% of all PICCs.

  **E** All of the above.

**A15** **A** Approximately 25% of neonatal unit admissions will undergo PICC placement. Distal catheter angulation, curvature or looping as well as right atrial tip place-ment are all strongly associated with cardiac tamponade. Cardiac tamponade leads to death in 44% of such cases unless pericardiocentesis is performed.

Migration of line tips after initial placement and securing occurs in approximately 10% of cases and is usually distal in nature. Recommendations for PICC placement in neonates include the following:

- Use PICCs only when there is a clear indication.
- Do not place tips in the right atrium; tips should be in either the superior or inferior vena cava.
- Perform regular radiographs to identify migration.
- Withdraw any migrated lines from the right atrium.
- Train staff to perform pericardiocentesis for acute collapse when initial resuscitation fails.

**Q16** When deciding which vascular access device to insert, the following should be taken into account *except*:

A the child and carer's wishes

B the length of treatment required

C the need for regular blood tests

D a history of previous vascular access procedures

E the child's age.

**A16** **D** Most children admitted for surgery will have some form of vascular access during their admission. This ranges from peripheral venous cannulation to emergency intraosseous cannulation in a resuscitation setting. Working together with the child and parents and keeping them informed during the process of vascular access will ensure more success. When given all the options, the older child who enjoys swimming may choose an implantable vascular access device (VAD) rather than an external tunnelled line, for instance. The duration of treatment is important and generally PICCs will suffice when therapy extends from 7 days to several months. Peripheral access will suffice for shorter durations and either tunnelled or implanted, subcutaneous VADs should be considered for therapy beyond 6 months. Double-lumen tunnelled lines will be appropriate if frequent blood tests are required, whereas an implantable device is ideal when access is less frequent, e.g. once a week. A history of previous vascular access is important in choosing which site to use, and which technique to use in the event of thrombosed veins. It should not have any bearing on the choice of which device to use. The child's age is important, e.g. when choosing implantable ports. A smaller child with little or no subcutaneous tissue would be at risk of port erosion. Equally a larger teenager with thick subcutaneous tissue would not be suitable for a port as needle access would be difficult or impossible.

## Further reading

Askegard-Giesmann JR, Caniano DA, Kenney BD. Rare but serious complications of central line insertion. *Semin Pediatr Surg.* 2009; **18**(2): 73–83.

Chokshi NK, Nguyen N, Cinat M. Access in the neonatal and paediatric patient. In Wilson SE. *Vascular Access: principles and practice.* 5th ed. Philadelphia, PA: Lippincott Williams & Wilkins; 2009. pp. 139–49.

Milbrandt K, Beaudry P, Anderson R, *et al.* A multiinstitutional review of central venous line complications: retained intravascular fragments. *J Pediatr Surg.* 2009; **44**(5): 972–6.

Rauch D, Dowd D, Eldridge D, *et al.*, Peripheral difficult venous access in children. *Clin Pediatr (Phila).* 2009; **48**(9): 895–901.

Suk EH, Kim DH, Kil HK, *et al.* Effects of reverse Trendelenburg position and inguinal compression on femoral vein cross-sectional area in infants and young children. *Anaesthesia.* 2009; **64**(4): 399–402.

Upadhyaya M, Richards M, Buckham S, *et al.* Long-term results of central venous access devices in children with haemophilia. *Pediatr Surg Int.* 2009; **25**(6): 503–6.

Weil BR, Ladd AP, Yoder K. Pericardial effusion and cardiac tamponade associated with central venous catheters in children: an uncommon but serious and treatable condition. *J Pediatr Surg.* 2010; **45**(8): 1687–92.

# SECTION III

# Trauma

# CHAPTER 7

# General approach to trauma

## MARIANNE BEAUDIN, REBECCAH L BROWN

**From the choices below each question, select the single best answer.**

**Q1** What is the most frequent cause of death in children between 1 and 14 years old?
 A  cancer
 B  congenital malformation
 C  trauma
 D  infectious diseases
 E  heart disease

**A1** C  Trauma is the leading cause of death in children between ages 1 and 14 years, accounting for more than 5000 deaths per year. The second most common cause of death varies according to the age group. For children between 1 and 4 years of age, congenital anomalies are the second leading cause of death, whereas for children between 5 and 14 years of age, it is cancer. For children between 0 and 1 year of age, the leading causes of death are congenital anomalies, short gestation and sudden infant death syndrome. Trauma is the fifth leading cause of death in that age group.

**Q2** What is the most frequent cause of paediatric trauma death?
 A  head trauma
 B  thoracic trauma
 C  abdominal trauma
 D  spinal trauma
 E  drowning

**A2** A  The leading cause by far of traumatic death in children is head trauma. It accounts for more than 80% of paediatric trauma mortality. Overall, the incidence of traumatic brain injuries in the United States is 200 per 100 000 children. About 5% of all these brain injuries are fatal. It is estimated that around 3000 children die of head injury each year in the United States.

Q3 Which trauma mechanism is the leading cause of death in children?
  A  fall
  B  motor vehicle collision – occupant
  C  motor vehicle collision – pedestrian
  D  bicycle
  E  drowning

A3  B  Motor vehicle–related injuries account for approximately 50% of all traumatic
deaths in children. According to the Center for Disease Control and Prevention
(CDC) in 2007, the most frequent mechanism of unintentional death for children
aged between 1 and 14 years is motor vehicle collisions in which children are
occupants. The other leading causes of unintentional death in this age group, in
order of frequency, are drowning and pedestrians hit by motor vehicles. However,
in children aged between 1 and 4 years, drowning is the leading cause of death,
accounting for 28% of all unintentional injuries. The proportion of traffic-related
death increases as the age of the child increases. Although falls remain the most
common mechanism of injury in children, they are less commonly fatal.

Q4 Which one of the following is not classically associated with non-
accidental trauma?
  A  subdural haematoma
  B  posterior rib fractures
  C  retinal haemorrhages
  D  spiral fracture of humerus
  E  pelvic fracture

A4  E  There are four reported types of child abuse: neglect, physical abuse, sexual
abuse and emotional abuse. In 2008, the CDC estimated that 772 000 children
were victims of maltreatment. It was also estimated that 1740 children died from
abuse, with 80% of these deaths being in children under 4 years of age. Factors
that should increase the suspicion of child abuse include delay in seeking medical
care, vague or inconsistent history reported by caregivers, as well as specific patterns of injuries. For example, the presence of subdural haematoma and retinal
haemorrhages is essentially pathognomonic of shaken baby syndrome. Because
the chest wall of a child is very compliant, the presence of rib fractures, especially
posterior rib fractures, implies significant force was exerted, more so than can
be explained by simple falls. Likewise, spiral fractures of long bones and bucket-
handle fractures are classically associated with non-accidental trauma. Although
pelvic fractures may occur, they are not classically associated with non-accidental
trauma, except in extreme cases.

**Q5** Waddell's triad is a pattern of injuries that occur when pedestrian children are struck by motor vehicles. What are the injuries that comprise this triad?

    **A** head, neck and torso (chest/abdomen)

    **B** head, torso (chest/abdomen) and lower extremities

    **C** head, neck and upper extremities

    **D** neck, torso (chest/abdomen) and upper extremities

    **E** neck, torso (chest/abdomen) and lower extremities

**A5**   **B** Waddell's triad of injuries refers to injuries to head, torso (chest/abdomen) and lower extremities. This is a pattern of injury that is seen among pedestrians hit by cars. The first point of impact is to the lower extremities as the bumper of the car strikes the child; the second point of impact is to the torso (chest/abdomen) from the front of the car (bumper or bonnet); and the third point of impact is to the head as the child is thrown to the windscreen or the ground. Commonly, the injuries to the torso (chest/abdomen) or lower extremity are on the same side and the injury to the head is on the opposite side. Although this triad of injuries is not always present, it emphasises the importance of mechanism of injury in predicting specific injury patterns useful in the assessment of the injured child.

**Q6** Which of the following is the most frequent cause of airway obstruction in the injured child?

    **A** vomit

    **B** foreign body

    **C** tongue

    **D** laryngospasm

    **E** adenoid tissue and tonsils

**A6**   **C** The most frequent cause of airway obstruction in the injured child occurs when the tongue falls back and obstructs the glottis. This can be prevented by using a simple chin-lift or jaw-thrust manoeuvre, always taking care to maintain in-line cervical traction in case of cervical spine injury in the setting of trauma. Children with airway obstruction may also benefit from insertion of an oropharyngeal or nasopharyngeal airway. However, if a child can tolerate such an airway adjunct, there is a need for respiratory assistance because it indicates an altered level of consciousness such that the child can no longer protect his or her airway. Other causes of upper airway obstruction in the trauma patient include foreign bodies (i.e. broken teeth), secretions (i.e. blood) and vomit.

**Q7** Which of the following is *not* true regarding differences in the paediatric airway?

  **A** A straight laryngeal blade may be preferred for intubation of young children because of an omega-shaped epiglottis.

  **B** Intubation of the right mainstem bronchus is more frequent than in adults.

  **C** The narrowest part of the airway is the thyroid cartilage.

  **D** The larynx is more cephalad and anterior in children.

  **E** The infant must be placed in a different position in order to avoid airway obstruction.

**A7**  **C**  There are many differences between children and adults that must be considered during evaluation of the paediatric airway. The tongue is a major cause of upper airway obstruction. A straight laryngeal blade is generally preferred for endotracheal intubation because of the omega-shaped, floppy epiglottis in children, although there are those who prefer a curved blade. The trachea is shorter, which results in more frequent right mainstem bronchus intubation. The correct position of the endotracheal tube must be confirmed by both auscultation and chest X-ray. During intubation, it is also important to remember that the larynx is more cephalad and anterior in children, making it more difficult to visualise the vocal cords. Finally, the narrowest part of the airway in children is the cricoid cartilage. Because of this, uncuffed endotracheal tubes are generally preferred in children up to the age of 8 years. A cuffed endotracheal tube can be used, but one needs to be careful to avoid overinflation of the balloon, as it can lead to tracheal injury, necrosis and subglottic stenosis. Because the head of an infant or young child is much larger proportional to the body, and the neck is shorter, there is a propensity for the posterior pharynx to buckle anteriorly, thereby obstructing the airway and causing passive flexion of the cervical spine. The child must be positioned such that the plane of the face is parallel to the backboard. This may be accomplished by placing a 1-inch layer of padding beneath a child's torso to preserve the neutral alignment of the spine.

 **Q8** In children under 1 year of age, what drug is generally administered in combination with succinylcholine as part of rapid-sequence intubation?

  **A** epinephrine

  **B** atropine

  **C** rocuronium

  **D** fentanyl

  **E** lidocaine

**A8**    **B** Rapid-sequence intubation is recommended for children who need to be intubated urgently unless they are already in cardiac arrest. Following pre-oxygenation, a sedative and paralytic are administered. Cricoid pressure is maintained to prevent aspiration of gastric contents. The sedative agent of choice is often etomidate, which can be safely used in haemodynamically unstable and brain-injured patients. In children, the paralytic agent of choice is often succinylcholine unless contraindicated (i.e. burns, crush injury). For children in whom elevated intracranial pressure is suspected, premedication with lidocaine is recommended. Furthermore, in children under 1 year of age, children younger than 5 years of age receiving succinylcholine, and in all children receiving a second dose of succinylcholine, atropine should be given to prevent bradycardia. Atropine may decrease the incidence of bradycardia associated with direct laryngoscopy (stimulation of parasympathetic receptors in the laryngopharynx) and administration of succinylcholine (direct stimulation of cardiac muscarinic receptors).

**Q9**  A 5-year-old child presents to the emergency department after being hit by a car. During the initial assessment, auscultation of the chest reveals decreased breath sounds on the right side. The trachea is also deviated to the left side. What should be done first?
   **A** Administer 100% oxygen by a non-rebreather mask.
   **B** Perform a needle decompression of the right chest in the second intercostal space in the mid-clavicular line.
   **C** Insert a chest tube in the right chest at the fourth intercostal space in the anterior axillary line.
   **D** Perform a chest X-ray immediately.
   **E** Perform a computed tomography (CT) scan of the chest immediately.

**A9**    **B** A tension pneumothorax is a clinical diagnosis and should be addressed as soon as suspected. The correct management is to perform a needle decompression (usually with a 14-gauge needle) in the second intercostal space in the mid-clavicular line, just above the third rib. This can be achieved in a few seconds and the primary survey can then proceed. After a needle decompression is done, a chest tube should be inserted in the fourth intercostal space along the anterior axillary line, above the rib to avoid the intercostal vessels. This is usually at the level of the nipple. There is no place for a chest CT or chest X-ray in the immediate management of a suspected tension pneumothorax.

**Q10** A child presents to the emergency department after a motor vehicle collision. He has an obvious open femur fracture that is bleeding. What is the first step in fluid resuscitation?

    **A** transfuse 10 mL/kg of packed red blood cells (PRBCs)

    **B** transfuse 20 mL/kg of PRBCs

    **C** bolus 10 mL/kg of normal saline (NS)

    **D** bolus 20 mL/kg of NS

    **E** bolus 20 mL/kg of colloid

**A10** **D** In the paediatric trauma patient, fluid resuscitation is begun by bolus administration of 20 mL/kg of NS or lactated Ringer's solution (LR). As soon as hypovolaemic shock is suspected, a type and cross-match should be sent. If the child needs further fluid resuscitation, a second bolus of 20 mL/kg of NS or LR should be given. If the child does not respond appropriately to crystalloid infusion, blood transfusion is begun with 10 mL/kg of PRBCs. If cross-matched blood is available, it should be given. If not, O-negative blood should be given until cross-matched blood becomes available. There is no place for colloid administration in the acute trauma setting.

**Q11** Which of the following is not a potential site of haemorrhage leading to hypotensive shock in children?

    **A** intracranial

    **B** thorax

    **C** abdomen

    **D** pelvis

    **E** femur

**A11** **A** Haemorrhagic shock is classified in four categories based on the estimated blood loss (EBL). Class I shock is less than 15% EBL, class II is 15%–30% EBL, class III is 30%–40% EBL, and class IV is more than 40% EBL. Patients in class I shock usually show minimal findings; patients in class II shock are mildly anxious with tachycardia, have normal blood pressure (BP) with narrow pulse pressure, and prolonged capillary refill; patients in class III shock may have marked tachycardia, hypotension with narrowed pulse pressure, altered mental status with marked anxiety and confusion, and cool, mottled extremities; patients in class IV shock show severe signs of hypoperfusion with loss of central and peripheral pulses, wide pulse pressure, loss of consciousness, and cold, cyanotic extremities. Children have a unique ability to compensate for major blood loss. Decompensation tends to be abrupt. Tachycardia precedes hypotension which is a late, ominous sign. Except for infants with fontanelles that can bulge, intracranial bleeding alone can never account for haemorrhagic shock. Other sources of haemorrhage should be sought.

**Q12** A 1-year-old child presents to the emergency department after sustaining a fall from the arms of his parent. His vital signs are the following: respiratory rate 35/min, heart rate 150/min, BP 80/40. What is the correct diagnosis?

    **A** This child is in respiratory distress and needs emergency intubation.

    **B** This child is hypotensive and needs emergency fluid resuscitation.

    **C** This child shows signs of intracranial bleeding and needs a head CT immediately.

    **D** This child needs to be monitored in an intensive care unit because of his unstable condition.

    **E** This child has normal vital signs for his age.

**A12 E** It is important for the trauma care provider to be familiar with normal vital signs for each paediatric age group. In children 1–10 years of age, a formula that can be used to approximate the normal systolic BP is 70 + 2 × (age in years). Normal vital signs values for different age groups are provided in Table 7.1.

| Age | Breaths/min | Heart rate | Systolic BP | Diastolic BP |
| --- | --- | --- | --- | --- |
| Infant | 30–60 | 120–60 | 60–90 | 30–55 |
| Toddler | 24–40 | 80–130 | 70–100 | 45–65 |
| School age | 20–34 | 70–110 | 90–110 | 50–70 |
| Adolescent | 12–16 | 60–100 | 95–130 | 60–80 |

TABLE 7.1 Normal vital sign values for paediatric age groups

**Q13** A 5-year-old child presents to the emergency department after being involved in a high-speed motor vehicle collision. He is hypotensive and needs immediate fluid resuscitation. Nurses are unable to insert a peripheral intravenous (IV) catheter after several attempts. What should be done next?

    **A** Try to insert a small-bore peripheral IV catheter yourself.

    **B** Insert a central venous catheter in the femoral vein.

    **C** Insert a peripheral venous catheter in the external jugular vein.

    **D** Perform a saphenous vein cutdown.

    **E** Insert an intraosseous (IO) cannula.

**A13 E** Placement of peripheral IVs can be difficult in young children, especially in the presence of shock. After unsuccessful attempts at inserting a peripheral IV catheter, the next step should be to obtain IO access. The preferred sites are the proximal tibia and distal femur. IO access should not be obtained distal to a fracture. If there is a lower extremity or pelvis fracture, it is possible to insert an IO cannula in the proximal humerus. IO access can be obtained in children who are conscious or unconscious. IO access is generally safe, efficacious and expeditious. Complications of IO infusion include osteomyelitis, compartment syndrome and iatrogenic fracture. Other options for venous access are to insert a femoral central line (unless there is a suspicion of pelvis fracture) or perform a venous cutdown at the antecubital or saphenous sites. If a central line is placed, it should be a large-bore introducer rather than a standard central line.

**Q14** A toddler is being evaluated in the emergency department after a motor vehicle collision. He is haemodynamically stable but his abdomen is markedly distended on physical exam. What should be done next?

  **A** Perform an abdominal CT immediately.

  **B** Take the patient to the operating room for an emergency exploratory laparotomy.

  **C** Perform a diagnostic peritoneal lavage.

  **D** Transfuse 10 mL/kg PRBCs.

  **E** Insert a naso- or orogastric tube and re-evaluate clinically.

**A14** **E** Infants and young children commonly develop a distended abdomen because of a stomach filled with air or gastric contents, often due to crying and screaming. This can be erroneously mistaken for a sign of an intra-abdominal injury. Inserting a naso- or orogastric tube should be done rapidly in the paediatric trauma management algorithm. FAST exam (Focused Assessment with Sonography for Trauma) can also aid in the diagnosis of intra-abdominal injury that would cause abdominal distension. Diagnostic peritoneal lavage is rarely performed in children.

**Q15** A child presents to the emergency department after being involved in a high-speed motor vehicle collision. He initially presents with a Glasgow Coma Scale (GCS) score of 12 and gradually improves to a score of 15. He is now complaining of weakness and paraesthesias in both upper extremities, although his sensory and motor exam are otherwise normal. He is still wearing a cervical collar. As part of his initial evaluation, a head and cervical spine CT were obtained, both of which were normal. What should you do?

  **A** Discontinue the cervical collar since there is no cervical spine fracture on CT.

  **B** Discontinue the cervical collar and perform flexion-extension X-rays.

  **C** Repeat the cervical spine CT.

  **D** Discontinue the cervical collar and ask for a neurology consult.

  **E** Leave the cervical collar in place and ask for a neurosurgery consult.

**A15** **E** Spinal cord injury without radiographic abnormality (SCIWORA) is a phenomenon that is more commonly seen in children than in adults because of the laxity of the cervical ligaments in children. In children younger than 8 years of age, SCIWORA accounts for 30%–40% of all spinal cord injuries. A thorough neurologic evaluation and examination of the cervical spine is crucial to exclude spinal injury in a child with a suspicious mechanism of injury, and to determine the need for further radiological imaging studies. In children without a distracting injury, neurologic deficit, and who are not intoxicated, the sensitivity and negative predictive value of the clinical exam approaches 100%. Children younger than 2 years of age may constitute an exception. For children with midline tenderness or deformity on exam, a standard three-view X-ray of the cervical spine (cross-table lateral, anteroposterior and odontoid) should be done. If the cervical spine is incompletely visualised on the X-ray and there are symptoms that suggest a cervical spine injury, a cervical spine CT can be done. If this exam does not show a fracture and the child has either midline tenderness or neurologic symptoms, a cervical spine magnetic resonance imaging scan can be done to evaluate for ligamentous and spinal cord injuries. A cervical collar should never be removed in the face of neurologic symptoms without consulting a neurosurgeon.

**Q16** What is the GCS score of a child who opens his eyes to pain, moans in response to pain, and has abnormal flexion in response to pain?
  **A** 4
  **B** 5
  **C** 6
  **D** 7
  **E** 8

**A16** **D** There is a modified GCS to evaluate infants and children. Table 7.2 summarises the adult, child and infant GCS.

| Response | Adult | Child | Infant | Score |
|---|---|---|---|---|
| **Eye opening** | Spontaneous | Spontaneous | Spontaneous | 4 |
| | To speech | To speech | To speech | 3 |
| | To pain | To pain | To pain | 2 |
| | None | None | None | 1 |
| **Best verbal response** | Orientated | Orientated | Coos and babbles | 5 |
| | Confused | Confused | Irritable, cries | 4 |
| | Inappropriate words | Inappropriate words | Cries in response to pain | 3 |
| | Incomprehensible words | Incomprehensible words or non-specific sounds | Moans in response to pain | 2 |
| | None | None | None | 1 |

| Response | Adult | Child | Infant | Score |
|----------|-------|-------|--------|-------|
| Best motor response | Obeys | Obeys | Moves spontaneously and purposely | 6 |
| | Localises pain | Localises pain | Withdraws to touch | 5 |
| | Withdraws to pain | Withdraws to pain | Withdraws to pain | 4 |
| | Abnormal flexion to pain | Abnormal flexion to pain | Abnormal flexion to pain | 3 |
| | Abnormal extension to pain | Abnormal extension to pain | Abnormal extension to pain | 2 |
| | None | None | None | 1 |
| Total score | | | | 3–15 |

**TABLE 7.2 Glasgow Coma Scale and Modified Glasgow Coma Scale for Infants and Children**

**Q17** Contraindications to insertion of a nasogastric tube include all of the following *except*:

 **A** Battle's sign (retroauricular ecchymosis)

 **B** raccoon eyes (periorbital ecchymosis)

 **C** cerebrospinal fluid (CSF) leakage from nose

 **D** CSF leakage from ear

 **E** epistaxis.

**A17** **E** Basal skull fracture is a contraindication to insertion of a nasogastric tube and is suspected if there is a Battle's sign (retroauricular ecchymosis), raccoon eyes (periorbital ecchymosis), CSF rhinorrhoea or otorrhoea, and haemotympanum. The patients should be evaluated with a head CT. Epistaxis alone is not a contraindication to insertion of a nasogastric tube, but severe midface fracture is.

## Further reading

Avarello JT, Cantor RM. Pediatric major trauma: an approach to evaluation and management. *Emerg Med Clin North Am.* 2007; **25**(3): 803–36.

Cooper A. Early assessment and management of trauma. In: Ashcraft KW, Holcomb GW, Murphy JP, editors. *Pediatric Surgery.* 4th ed. Philadelphia, PA: Elsevier; 2005. pp. 167–81.

Lukish JR, Eichelberger MR. Accident victims and their emergency management. In: Grosfeld JL, O'Neill JA, Fonkalsrud EW, *et al.*, editors. *Pediatric Surgery. Vol. 1.* 6th ed. Philadelphia, PA: Mosby; 2006. pp. 265–74.

Mendelson KG, Fallat ME. Pediatric injuries: prevention to resolution. *Surg Clin North Am.* 2007; **87**(1): 207–28.

Ralston M, Hazinski MF, Zaritsky A, *et al.* Pediatric assessment. In: *Pediatric Advanced Life Support, Provider Manual.* American Heart Association; 2006. pp. 1–32.

# CHAPTER 8

# Head and spinal injuries

## DESIDERIO RODRIGUES

**From the choices below each question, select the single best answer.**

**Q1** Which one of the following statements is true regarding skull fractures?
  A  Skull fractures are uncommon in young children.
  B  Linear fractures are less likely to be associated with underlying brain injury or haemorrhage than complex fractures.
  C  The vast majority of linear skull fractures in young children are caused by road traffic accidents.
  D  CT scan is the best imaging modality to demonstrate a linear fracture of the skull.
  E  Growing skull fracture is a well-recognised complication, occurring in 10% of children.

**A1**  **B**  Skull fractures are common in young children and represent the most common abnormal radiographic finding. Linear fractures in children may be associated with haemorrhage or significant underlying brain injury, but usually are not. Multiple fractures, and complex fractures crossing venous sinuses, are usually associated with underlying brain injury or haemorrhage. The vast majority of linear fractures in young children are caused by falls. Plain radiograph is the best modality to identify a linear fracture; an axial slice of CT scan may occasionally miss an axially orientated fracture. Growing skull fracture is a well-recognised complication occurring in 1% of children with skull fractures. They occur because of underlying dural laceration.

**Q2** Which one of the following statements is true with regard to infantile acute subdural haematoma?
  A  It is usually due to falling from a height.
  B  It results in coma from the onset of the fall.
  C  It usually occurs in babies <6 months old.
  D  It usually presents with a generalised seizure.
  E  It is due to a tear in the branch of the middle meningeal artery.

A2  **D** Infantile acute subdural haematoma is due to a minor head injury, without initial loss of consciousness, and is usually due to a rupture of a bridging vein. The most common trauma is a fall backwards from a sitting or standing position. Patients are usually <2 years old – the age when they first begin to pull themselves up or begin to walk. They often present with generalised seizures within minutes to an hour following the injury.

Q3  Which one of the following statements is true with regard to cephalhaematoma?

  **A** Its extent is limited by sutures and hence remains localised to region.
  **B** Bleeding occurs in the loose connective tissue above the periosteum.
  **C** Eighty per cent will need evacuation as can result in calcification if not treated.
  **D** It should be treated with aspiration rather than open drainage.
  **E** It is most commonly seen in newborns delivered by caesarean section.

A3  **A** Cephalhaematoma is most commonly seen in newborns associated with parturition. Bleeding elevates the periosteum and hence extent is limited by the sutures while a subgaleal haematoma is between the periosteum and the galea in the loose connective tissue and crosses the sutures. Eighty per cent of cephalhaematomas reabsorb over 2–3 weeks and may occasionally calcify. They should never be aspirated because the risk of infection exceeds the risk following them up expectantly, and in the newborn removal of the blood may make them anaemic.

Q4  Which one of the following is not a characteristic finding in shaken baby syndrome?

  **A** retinal haemorrhages
  **B** bilateral subdural haematomas in 80% of cases
  **C** multiple fractures of ribs
  **D** significant brain injury
  **E** extensive external signs of trauma

A4  **E** All the statements are correct except that there may be few or no external signs of trauma. In some cases there may be finger marks on the chest.

**Q5** Which of one the following statements is true with regard to the outcome following head injury?

**A** The outcome of epidural haematomas overall is unfavourable.

**B** For children needing a craniotomy for subdural haematoma, a mortality as well as morbidity of about 30% has been described.

**C** Less than 10% of severely head-injured children with mass lesion die or remain severely disabled.

**D** Previously head-injured children who arrest or regress in their recovery are likely to have hydrocephalus.

**E** Post-traumatic seizures occur more frequently in younger adults than in children.

**A5** **D** The overall outcome of extradural haematomas is favourable. In children needing craniotomy for subdural haematoma a mortality as well as morbidity of 8% has been described. In severely head-injured children with mass lesions, 50% either died or remained severely disabled. If a patient arrests or regresses in their recovery following a head injury they should be scanned to rule out post-traumatic hydrocephalus, which can develop as late as 2–3 years following the initial injury. Post-traumatic seizures are a well-recognised complication of head injury. They are more common in children and older adults.

**Q6** Which one of the following statements is true with regard to atlantoaxial rotatory subluxation?

**A** A history of trauma is always present.

**B** Cock robin head position is the characteristic deformity.

**C** Antibiotics along with anti-inflammatory medications will result in spontaneous correction of the deformity.

**D** Reduction and internal fixation as early as possible is the gold standard in its management.

**E** MRI scan should be done as a priority in its management.

**A6** **B** Atlantoaxial rotatory subluxation can occur spontaneously – with rheumatoid arthritis, following minor or major trauma, or even with infection of the head or neck including upper respiratory tract infection (**known as Grisel's syndrome**). Patients are usually young and neurologic deficit is rare. The characteristic finding is a 'Cock robin' head position with torticollis. Manual reduction, either with traction or under anaesthesia, and immobilising external bracing (with a well-fitting Minerva jacket or a halo ring vest) for 6 weeks to 3 months, will usually be sufficient. In cases with upper respiratory tract infection a course of antibiotics will be necessary in addition to reduction and immobilisation. X-ray and dynamic CT scan of the spine is usually diagnostic. MRI may be undertaken only to assess competency of the transverse ligament.

Q7  Which of one the following statements is true with regard to thoracic spine injuries in children?

    A  They are relatively common compared with cervical spine injuries.

    B  They are commonly avulsion-type fractures of the superior spinous processes.

    C  In the young child, every effort should be to treat them with closed reduction and external immobilisation.

    D  The majority will have purely thoracic spine injury.

    E  They never cause neurological deficits.

A7  C  Injuries to the thoracic spine are relatively uncommon compared with cervical injuries in children (13% cases). Hadley *et al.* reported only 11 out of 122 children with purely thoracic spine injuries. These injuries are usually due to axial load, or high-velocity injuries where the flexion force is transmitted into the thoracic spine. They are usually seen as wedge fractures or a three-column injury. Every effort should be made, especially in the young child, to treat these with closed reduction and external bracing because operative fixation, which may need multiple segment fixation, can result in growth restriction. If there is canal compromise there can be cord compression and a partial neurological deficit, in which case surgery is warranted.

Q8  Which of one the following statements is true with regard to the epidemiology of spinal cord injury?

    A  About 12% of all paediatric trauma patients suffer some form of either spinal column or spinal cord injury.

    B  Cervical and lumbar spinal cord injury tends to be complete while the thoracic spinal cord injury tends to be incomplete.

    C  The mortality rate associated with paediatric spinal cord injury is estimated to be 2.5 times higher than that for spinal cord injury in adults.

    D  Survivors of spinal cord injury have improved outcome and recovery in adults than in children.

    E  In the paediatric group, the risk of spinal cord injury increases with younger age.

A8  C  Approximately 3.4% of all paediatric trauma patients suffer some form of either spinal column or spinal cord injury. The risk of spinal cord injury is increased with older age, more severe overall trauma, and other systemic injury like chest and abdomen. Cervical and lumbar spinal cord injuries tend to be incomplete; thoracic spinal cord injury is more often complete. Compared with adults the mortality associated with spinal cord injury is 2.5 times higher in children; whereas children have a better recovery and improved outcome among the survivors than adults.

**Q9** All the following are indications for elevating a depressed skull fracture in a child *except*:

    **A** to reduce post-traumatic epilepsy

    **B** to correct cranial deformity and help cosmesis

    **C** to repair dural laceration

    **D** to treat compound depressed fractures

    **E** to reduce any mass effect.

**A9**   **A** Elevation of the depressed fracture neither decreases the incidence of post-traumatic epilepsy nor substantially improves associated neurologic deficits.

**Q10** Which of the following statements is *not* true for children with severe traumatic brain injury?

    **A** All children with a Glasgow Coma Scale (GCS) score of 8 or less should be electively intubated and ventilated.

    **B** They should have an urgent CT scan of the head once stabilised.

    **C** Malignant intracranial hypertension is a common complication of severe traumatic brain injury.

    **D** Intracranial pressure monitoring is indicated.

    **E** Pupillary size and light reaction are the early indicators of intracranial hypertension.

**A10**  **E** All children with a GCS score of 8 or less following traumatic brain injury should be electively intubated and ventilated to prevent hypoxia and secondary brain injury. They should be stabilised and then a CT scan of the head should be performed to look for any surgical lesion. Malignant intracranial hypertension is a common complication of severe traumatic brain injury. It has long been recognised that clinical signs like pupillary size and light response fail as early indicators of intracranial hypertension. Intracranial pressure monitoring is indicated as it provides a window into the global pressure status of the brain and helps manage the cerebral perfusion pressure.

## Further reading

Albright AL, Pollack IF, Adelson PD. *Operative Techniques in Pediatric Neurosurgery.* New York, NY: Thieme; 2001.

Albright AL, Pollack IF, Adelson PD, editors. *Principles and Practice of Pediatric Neurosurgery.* 2nd ed. New York, NY: Thieme; 2008.

Greenberg MS. *Handbook of Neurosurgery*, 6th ed. New York, NY: Thieme; 2006.

Hadley MN, Zabramski JM, Browner CM, *et al.* Pediatric spinal trauma. *J Neurosurg.* 1988; **68**: 18–24.

# CHAPTER 9

# Thoracic trauma

## MARIANNE BEAUDIN, REBECCAH L BROWN

**From the choices below each question, select the single best answer.**

**Q1** What type of thoracic traumatic injury is the most frequent in children?
  **A** rib fractures
  **B** flail chest
  **C** lung contusion
  **D** pneumothorax
  **E** haemothorax

**A1** **C** Overall, traumatic thoracic injuries account for only 5%–12% of trauma admissions in children. Most thoracic injuries are the result of blunt trauma. Rib fractures are not as frequent in children as in adults because of the greater flexibility of the thoracic cage in children. Therefore, energy transmitted to the thorax can cause a significant lung contusion without any rib fractures. For the same reason, flail chest is also very rare in children. Pneumothorax and haemothorax are usually associated with rib fractures.

**Q2** What type of injury is not associated with first-rib fracture?
  **A** clavicular fracture
  **B** spinal cord injury
  **C** aortic injury
  **D** subclavian vein injury
  **E** liver laceration

**A2** **E** A first-rib fracture implies a significant mechanism of injury and should prompt a search for other associated injuries, including aortic injury, clavicular injury, thoracic spine and spinal cord injury, and neurovascular injury (i.e. subclavian vessels, brachial plexus). There is currently controversy in the trauma literature as to whether or not all patients with first-rib fractures should undergo chest CT-angiography. However, a chest CT should be done, and if there is any suggestion of aortic injury (i.e. widened mediastinum), a completion CT angiography should be done. Liver lacerations are more often associated with lower rib fractures.

 A child is seen in the emergency department after a motor vehicle colli-sion. He has a Glasgow Coma Scale score of 6 and is rapidly intubated in the trauma bay. The intubation is difficult and the patient vomited prior to intubation. An initial chest X-ray showed no intrathoracic injury. Twenty-four hours later, in the intensive care unit, a chest X-ray shows a unilateral basal alveolar infiltrate. What is the most plausible cause?

  **A** lung contusion

  **B** aspiration pneumonia

  **C** ventilator-associated pneumonia

  **D** acute respiratory distress sydrome (ARDS)

  **E** haemothorax

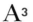 **B** Lung contusions are usually present on the initial chest X-ray. Aspiration pneumonia usually becomes visible on chest X-ray within 24–48 hours. Alveolar infiltrates may be unilateral (most commonly on the right side) or bilateral but are often in the lower lobes. Ventilator-associated pneumonia is a bacterial pneumo-nia that develops at least 48 hours after intubation. Aspiration is also a risk factor for bacterial pneumonia although there are currently no recommendations for prophylactic administration of antibiotics to prevent this complication. ARDS is a clinical diagnosis that presents with bilateral patchy infiltrates on chest X-ray and requires a $PO_2/F_iO_2$ ratio under 200 mmHg for diagnosis. Haemothorax does not present with alveolar infiltrates on chest X-ray.

 Which of the following is not a sign of tension pneumothorax?

  **A** deviation of the trachea to the contralateral side

  **B** decreased breath sounds on the ipsilateral side

  **C** distended jugular veins

  **D** tachycardia

  **E** hypertension

**A4** **E** Tension pneumothorax is a clinical, not radiological, diagnosis that should be suspected with any of these findings: deviation of the trachea to the contralateral side, decreased breath sounds on the ipsilateral side, distended jugular veins, tachycardia and hypotension. Entrapment of air in the pleural cavity leads to a collapse of the ipsilateral lung and a shift of the mediastinum to the contralateral side that subsequently causes decrease in venous return and cardiac output. This condition needs to be addressed immediately since cardiorespiratory collapse can ensue rapidly. A tension pneumothorax needs to be decompressed by inserting a 14-gauge needle into the second intercostal space at the mid-clavicular line. A chest tube must then be inserted.

**Q5** A patient comes to the emergency department after a penetrating injury to the right chest. He presents with a large open wound on the lateral aspect of the chest and has difficulty breathing. What should be done initially?

   **A** Insert a needle in the second intercostal space.

   **B** Insert a chest tube in the fourth intercostal space.

   **C** Apply a completely occlusive dressing over the wound.

   **D** Apply an occlusive dressing taped on three sides.

   **E** Intubate the patient as soon as possible.

**A5** **D** An open pneumothorax seriously compromises ventilation if its diameter is larger than ¾ the diameter of the trachea. In that case, air preferentially enters the thorax through the chest wound rather than the trachea. During inspiration, negative intrathoracic pressure is created, and air will enter the pleural cavity through this wound. If air is allowed to enter and cannot escape because of a tissue flap, a tension pneumothorax can develop. The initial treatment (even in the field), should be to apply an occlusive dressing taped on three sides to create a flutter-valve effect. As the patient inhales, the dressing occludes the wound, preventing air entry, but with exhalation, the open end of the dressing allows air to escape. The definitive treatment is to insert a chest tube and then change the dressing to a completely occlusive dressing. Applying an occlusive dressing if one is not ready to insert a chest tube may convert an open pneumothorax to a tension pneumothorax. Intubation needs to be considered but should not delay placement of a chest tube. Decompressing the chest with a needle should be done only if a tension pneumothorax is suspected.

**Q6** Which finding is not suspicious for cardiac tamponade?

   **A** decreased heart sounds

   **B** jugular venous distension

   **C** widened mediastinum

   **D** decreased bilateral breath sounds

   **E** hypotension

**A6** **D** The classic findings of cardiac tamponade are described in Beck's triad: decreased heart sounds, jugular venous distension and hypotension. This is a clinical triad, but all three elements are not always present. Moreover, it is often difficult, if not impossible, to accurately assess heart sounds in a noisy emergency department environment, especially in children. However, tamponade should be suspected in presence of any of these findings. Cardiac tamponade is most commonly due to a penetrating injury. As blood fills the pericardium, venous return and cardiac output are decreased, leading to the clinical triad of symptoms. A widened mediastinum on chest X-ray should arouse suspicion, especially in the presence of a penetrating chest injury. It can, however, be difficult to assess the size of the mediastinum on a supine anteroposterior chest X-ray. Decreased bilateral breath sounds are more often associated with bilateral pneumothoraces, although cardiac tamponade could coexist.

 **Q7** A child presents to the emergency department after sustaining a penetrating chest injury just to the left side of the sternum, at the nipple level. He is hypotensive, has decreased heart sounds, and a widened mediastinum on chest X-ray. What should be done immediately?

**A** Intubate the patient as soon as possible.

**B** Insert a needle in the second intercostal space.

**c** Insert a chest tube in the fourth intercostal space.

**D** Perform a pericardiocentesis.

**E** Do a chest CT urgently.

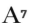 **A7** **D** Cardiac tamponade should be a clinical diagnosis based on findings of decreased heart sounds, distended jugular veins and hypotension. A chest X-ray may reveal a widened mediastinum but management should not be delayed to obtain a chest X-ray. Another diagnostic tool that is being used more frequently in the emergency department is the FAST (Focused Assessment Sonography in Trauma) exam. It takes only a few seconds and can confirm the diagnosis of haemopericardium. As soon as tamponade is either strongly suspected or diagnosed, a pericardiocentesis should be performed by inserting a large-bore angiocatheter connected to a syringe beneath the xyphoid process at a 45° angle angulated towards the left shoulder. Negative pressure should be applied to the syringe as the needle is inserted, all the while monitoring for signs of ventricular arrhythmias. If ventricular arrhythmias are seen on the monitor, the needle should be slightly retracted. Usually, blood that is withdrawn from the cardiac chambers will clot whereas blood from the pericardium will not. As little as 15 mL of blood withdrawn from the pericardium can relieve the tamponade. The needle is then removed, and the catheter is left in place, attached to the syringe. Immediate surgical consultation is warranted. Another technique for evacuation of pericardial tamponade is creation of a pericardial window, a procedure that is performed by experienced surgeons in the operating room.

**Q8** Which diagnostic study is now considered the study of choice for aortic dissection?

  **A** chest CT
  **B** chest CT angiography
  **C** aortography
  **D** transthoracic echocardiography
  **E** transoesophageal echocardiography

 **A8** **B** Traumatic aortic dissection is rare in children but can occur with a rapid acceleration–deceleration mechanism such as in a high-speed motor vehicle collision or in a fall from great height. The tear in the intima is usually distal to the left subclavian artery at the level of the ligamentum arteriosum. Although aortography has been the gold standard for many years, the diagnostic study of choice for blunt aortic injury is now chest CT angiography. The use of aortography is limited because it is a very invasive study that requires a specialised team and is also associated with complications of its own. Chest CT angiography has excellent sensitivity and negative predictive value. Transoesophageal echocardiography is a diagnostic test of lesser value as it can miss injuries of the ascending aorta and its branches.

 **Q9** Which of the following is a finding commonly seen with *commotio cordis*?

  **A** cardiac contusion
  **B** coronary abnormality
  **C** pre-existing arrhythmia
  **D** valvular abnormality
  **E** normal heart

 **A9** **E** *Commotio cordis* is a traumatic condition that results from sudden impact to the chest causing cessation of cardiac activity. It is most frequently associated with sports such as baseball or hockey. The sudden impact leads to a recalcitrant arrhythmia, usually ventricular fibrillation, that rapidly evolves into cardiovascular collapse. This phenomenon is characterised by a sudden arrhythmia in a normal heart with no cardiac contusion or coronary injury and no underlying structural or conduction defect. It is thought to occur more often in children because of the more compliant chest wall that allows direct transmission of energy to the heart. Survival from *commotio cordis* is reported to be around 25%, mainly because the arrhythmias are often resistant to resuscitative efforts and also because the mechanism is often not initially recognised, causing delays in treatment. Recognition of this phenomenon has led to more frequent use of mid-chest protective gear in baseball and hockey players as well as increased availability of automatic external defibrillators at organised athletic events.

**Q10** After chest tube placement, a patient has persistent, large air leak noted in the Pleurovac. He also has extensive crepitus in the neck. What is the most likely cause?

**A** bilateral pneumothorax

**B** tracheobronchial tree injury

**C** Pleurovac malfunction

**D** oesophageal perforation

**E** diaphragmatic rupture

**A10** **B** Tracheobronchial tree injuries are rare both in children and in adults. They occur more commonly with penetrating than with blunt chest trauma. Most injuries resulting from blunt trauma occur in the distal trachea or proximal bronchi. They should be suspected in the context of bilateral or unilateral pneumothorax with persistent air leak after chest tube placement. Hoarseness, respiratory distress, and extensive cervical or thoracic subcutaneous emphysema may be seen. A pneumomediastinum can also be seen on chest X-ray or CT of the chest. These injuries are highly lethal if not addressed immediately. These children require intubation assisted with fibre-optic guidance. Bronchoscopy should be performed to assess the airway when a tracheobronchial injury is suspected. Occasionally, in a stable patient, a CT of the chest can help delineate the anatomy. Treatment usually requires operative intervention.

**Q11** After chest tube placement for a suspected haemothorax in a 10 kg child, 300 mL of blood is returned immediately. What should be the next step?

**A** insertion of another chest tube on the ipsilateral side

**B** insertion of a chest tube on the contralateral side

**C** clamping of the chest tube

**D** intubation

**E** prepare for surgical intervention.

**A11** **E** Massive haemothorax should increase suspicion of a serious intrathoracic injury that needs to be addressed surgically. Some volumetric guidelines for surgical intervention described in the paediatric literature include more than 15 mL/kg of initial drainage or more than 2–3 mL/kg/hr of continuous drainage. Possible aetiologies for massive haemothorax include lacerations to intercostal vessels, lung parenchyma, heart or great vessels. These children need to be resuscitated aggressively and brought to the operating room as soon as possible. Patients that are haemodynamically unstable should undergo thoracotomy rather than thoracoscopy. The approach chosen depends on the clinical suspicion of the injury. Most authors would agree that the correct approach in an unstable child would be a left anterolateral thoracotomy.

Q12 A child has been on mechanical ventilation in an intensive care unit for 1 week following a multiple trauma. He now has a $P_aO_2$ of 65 mmHg with a $F_iO_2$ of 60%, a pulmonary capillary wedge pressure of 10 mmHg, and bilateral alveolar infiltrates on chest X-ray. What is the diagnosis?

   A  bilateral pneumonia
   B  acute pulmonary oedema
   C  acute lung injury (ALI)
   D  ARDS
   E  bilateral pleural effusions

A12  **D**  ARDS can occur in children with multiple trauma with or without associated thoracic trauma. It is the result of widespread inflammation with endothelial cell damage. Ventilation/perfusion impairment ensues with secondary hypoxaemia. By definition, the pulmonary capillary wedge pressure is <18 mmHg, whereas it is elevated in pulmonary oedema. The difference between ARDS and ALI is the level of hypoxaemia: $P_aO_2/F_iO_2$ is <300 mmHg in ALI and is <200 mmHg in ARDS. Both can present with bilateral patchy alveolar infiltrates. The treatment of ARDS relies on supportive measures such as high-frequency oscillatory ventilation. Although ARDS occurs infrequently in children, mortality is very high, reflecting the severity of the trauma.

Q13 All the following can be appropriate treatment of an empyema secondary to a haemothorax *except*:

   A  IV antibiotics only
   B  chest tube placement if not done initially
   C  fibrinolytic therapy through a pre-existing chest tube
   D  decortication with video-assisted thoracoscopy (VATS)
   E  decortication with thoracotomy.

A13  **A**  Empyema is a collection of pus in the pleural space. Undrained haemothorax predisposes to empyema. Therefore, in the setting of trauma, even small haemothoraces require drainage to prevent the formation of empyema. Although empyemas may vary from simple to complex, it may be adequate to start with less invasive measures such as placement of a chest tube to drain the empyema. The child can then be reassessed and followed with serial chest X-rays. Fibrinolytic therapy instilled through the chest tube has also been described as an effective treatment for empyema. If fever persists and the lung doesn't re-expand adequately despite chest tube drainage and fibrinolytic therapy, surgery must be considered. Surgery is also the appropriate treatment if the chest CT or ultrasound shows multiple loculations unlikely to be adequately drained with a chest tube. The procedure can be done either by VATS or mini-thoracotomy, although most paediatric surgeons would prefer VATS as it is a less invasive procedure. Removal of pus and fibrinous exudate that prevents the lung from re-expanding is achieved during the procedure. A chest tube is left in place after the procedure and antibiotics are continued. The use of antibiotics alone is not an effective treatment for a proven post-traumatic empyema.

**Q14** After a child sustained a penetrating injury to the chest, unexplained fever is noted the following day. The only findings are fever and pneumomediastinum. What diagnosis should be suspected?

  A  necrotising pneumonia

  B  empyema

  C  lung abscess

  D  oesophageal perforation

  E  tracheobronchial injury

**A14**  **D**  Oesophageal injury is rare after blunt trauma since the oesophagus is a well-protected, posteriorly located intrathoracic organ. Oesophageal injury is more likely after penetrating chest trauma. It is a type of injury that can be missed initially if not thoroughly searched for. Clinical findings suggestive of oesophageal injury include unexplained fever, pleural effusion, empyema or pneumomediastinum. When suspected, an oesophageal injury should be evaluated with a contrast study and oesophagoscopy. The combination of a contrast study and endoscopy increases the likelihood of identifying an injury. The treatment will depend on the extent of the injury as well as the time since injury and may involve primary closure, debridement and drainage, or even diversion.

**Q15** What would be the appropriate management in the trauma bay of a child with a suspicion of thoracic spine fracture after a motor vehicle collision?

  A  Leave the patient on the backboard.

  B  Maintain spine precautions, log-roll patient off the backboard, and keep the cervical collar in place until imaging is completed.

  C  Maintain spine precautions, log-roll patient off the backboard, and remove the cervical collar since there is no suspicion of cervical spine fracture.

  D  No spine precautions needed for the thoracic vertebrae fracture but the cervical collar needs to be kept in place until imaging is completed.

  E  No spine precautions are needed.

A15  **B**  Thoracic spine injuries are rare compared with cervical spine injuries which account for 60%–80% of spine injuries. The primary mechanisms of injury for thoracic and thoracolumbar vertebral fractures are motor vehicle collisions and falls from great heights. Spine precautions, both for the cervical and thoracolumbar spine, need to be maintained until appropriate imaging can be done. This includes a cervical collar for potential cervical spine injury and keeping the patient in a supine position with log-roll only for potential thoracolumbar spine injury. Although total spine precautions must be maintained, the patient can be log-rolled off the backboard since it can rapidly lead to pressure-related complications. Plain X-rays should be done first, but if a plausible mechanism of injury and midline focal tenderness are present, further imaging with CT scan should be done.

Q16  Which of the following is the most appropriate diagnostic study to screen for cardiac contusion after blunt chest trauma in a haemodynamically stable child?

　　**A**  electrocardiogram (ECG)

　　**B**  CK-MB

　　**C**  troponins

　　**D**  echocardiography

　　**E**  all of the above

A16  **A**  Cardiac contusion occurs as a result of blunt trauma to the chest (i.e. impact against the steering wheel in motor vehicle collisions, direct blows to the chest or crush injuries). Initial screening includes an ECG. The patient can then be placed on a cardiac monitor for 8 hours. There is no need to routinely obtain labs or imaging tests. If cardiac contusion is suspected because of arrhythmia, a FAST should be performed immediately to exclude a haemopericardium. A formal cardiology consultation should be requested and a transthoracic echocardiography performed. If only cardiac contusion is found, treatment is supportive and requires cardiac monitoring for approximately 24 hours if the patient remains stable. Cardiac biomarkers (CK-MB and troponins) have no proven prognostic value, and their use is controversial.

**Q17** A child sustained a penetrating injury with a knife in the seventh inter-costal space on the left side of the chest along the anterior axillary line. What would be the correct management to exclude a diaphragmatic injury in a stable patient?

**A** CT of the chest

**B** CT of the chest and abdomen

**C** CT of the abdomen

**D** diagnostic laparoscopy

**E** none of the above

**A17** **D** Thoracoabdominal penetrating injuries often result in diaphragmatic injuries which are difficult to diagnose. Patients may be asymptomatic in the absence of herniation. With a penetrating injury to the chest beneath the nipple line, diaphragmatic and intra-abdominal injury must be suspected. CT scan of the chest or abdomen is not sensitive for detection of diaphragmatic injuries in the absence of herniation. Similarly, FAST or diagnostic peritoneal lavage are not sensitive for detection of diaphragmatic injuries. Diagnostic laparoscopy is the most sensitive study to exclude diaphragmatic and intra-abdominal injury as a result of penetrating thoracoabdominal trauma.

## Further reading

Bliss D, Silen M. Pediatric thoracic trauma. *Crit Care Med.* 2002; **30**(11 Suppl.): S409–15.

Lofland GK, O'Brien JE. Thoracic trauma in children. In: Ashcraft KW, Holcomb GW, Murphy JP, editors. *Pediatric Surgery.* 4th ed. Philadelphia, PA: Elsevier; 2005. pp. 185–200.

Mendelson KG, Fallat ME. Pediatric injuries: prevention to resolution. *Surg Clin North Am.* 2007; **87**(1): 207–28.

Tovar JA. The lung and pediatric trauma. *Semin Pediatr Surg.* 2008; **17**(1): 53–9.

Wesson DE. Thoracic injuries. In: Grosfeld JL, O'Neill JA, Fonkalsrud EW, *et al.*, editors. *Pediatric Surgery. Vol. 1.* 6th ed. Philadelphia, PA: Mosby; 2006. pp. 275–95.

# CHAPTER 10

# Abdominal trauma

## MARIANNE BEAUDIN, REBECCAH L BROWN

From the choices below each question, select the single best answer.

**Q1** Which intra-abdominal organ is the most frequently injured in children due to blunt abdominal trauma?

   **A** liver
   **B** spleen
   **C** kidney
   **D** pancreas
   **E** duodenum

**A1**  **B** Among the solid organs, the spleen is the most frequently injured in blunt abdominal trauma, followed by the liver and kidney. The pancreas is injured in approximately 3% of the cases of paediatric blunt abdominal trauma. Children are more susceptible to solid organ injury after sustaining blunt abdominal trauma because of distinct anatomical differences compared with adults. The abdominal wall is thinner with less fat and muscular padding, resulting in more intense energy transmission and closer proximity to vital organs. The ratio between the size of the intra-abdominal organs and the torso is higher than in adults, also making them more vulnerable to injury. Because of smaller body mass, children are more likely to incur multiple organ injuries. Children also have a higher incidence of upper abdominal injuries (i.e. liver and spleen) because of more flexible ribs.

Hollow viscus injury following blunt abdominal trauma is rare, occurring in only 1%–15% of patients. The most common injury is intestinal perforation, with jejunum and ileum being most frequently injured, followed by duodenum.

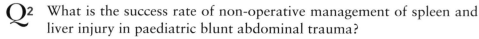

**Q2** What is the success rate of non-operative management of spleen and liver injury in paediatric blunt abdominal trauma?

A 20%

B 30%

c 50%

D 70%

E 90%

**A2** **E** The success rate for non-operative management of spleen and liver injuries in paediatric blunt abdominal trauma has been reported to be as high as 90%–95%. This differs significantly from the success rate reported in the adult literature, which is approximately 75% for blunt splenic injury. This needs to be taken into account when caring for the injured child. Children treated for blunt splenic trauma at adult trauma centres are nearly twice as likely to undergo splenectomy. Non-operative management of solid organ injury in children is predicated on physiologic rather that radiological parameters. The only absolute contraindication to non-operative management of the child with solid organ injury is haemodynamic instability unresponsive to fluid and blood resuscitation (usually >40 mL/kg of packed red blood cells) or the presence of associated injuries requiring laparotomy. Although CT grade of injury and degree of haemoperitoneum correlate with severity of injury, they do not necessarily correlate with the need for immediate operative intervention or failure of non-operative management. The child should be monitored closely in a setting that allows for immediate intervention should non-operative management fail.

**Q3** A child sustained a blunt abdominal trauma and CT scan of the abdomen demonstrates a 4 cm parenchymal laceration with devascularisation of less than 25% of the spleen. No other injuries are identified. The child is haemodynamically stable and haemoglobin is 13. What is the most appropriate management?

A exploratory laparotomy and splenectomy

B exploratory laparotomy and partial splenectomy

c exploratory laparoscopy and splenectomy

D admission to intensive care unit (ICU) for monitoring

E admission to the floor for monitoring

**A3** **E** In 2000, evidence-based guidelines were proposed by the American Paediatric Surgical Association Trauma Committee for the non-operative management of blunt splenic or liver injuries. These recommendations were made based on a thorough review of the medical literature as well the retrospective analysis of more than 800 children who sustained blunt abdominal trauma and were treated conservatively. Guidelines were proposed to address need for ICU monitoring, length of hospital stay, need for pre-discharge or post-discharge imaging, and appropriate activity restrictions. The level of activity implied in these guidelines is normal activity for the age of the child. Return to full-contact activities is left to the discretion of the physician. Grade V injuries were excluded from this study, and patients had to meet the criteria for non-operative management. Table 10.1 summarises the proposed guidelines.

|  | CT grade | | | |
| --- | --- | --- | --- | --- |
|  | I | II | III | IV |
| ICU stay (d) | None | None | None | 1 |
| Hospital stay (d) | 2 | 3 | 4 | 5 |
| Pre-discharge imaging | None | None | None | None |
| Post-discharge imaging | None | None | None | None |
| Activity restriction (wk) | 3 | 4 | 5 | 6 |

TABLE 10.1 Evidence-based guidelines for resource utilisation in children with isolated spleen or liver injury (Stylianos, 2000)

The patient described is haemodynamically stable with an isolated grade III splenic injury according to the American Association for the Surgery of Trauma organ injury grading scale and thus can be managed non-operatively. According to the proposed guidelines, he does not require ICU admission and can be safely admitted to the floor for monitoring.

 **Q4** All the following are complications of the non-operative management of blunt splenic trauma *except*:

 **A** bleeding
 **B** splenic pseudocyst
 **C** splenic pseudoaneurysm
 **D** overwhelming post-splenectomy sepsis (OPSI)
 **E** missed intra-abdominal injury.

 **A4** **D** Bleeding is the most common complication of non-operative management of blunt splenic trauma. The need for an operation in children with grade I–III splenic injuries is less than 3%. Bleeding is more likely with higher-grade injuries and tends to occur early after injury. Close monitoring of these children with serial abdominal exams and serial haemoglobin levels identify those patients with early bleeding. Late bleeding can be because of the formation of a splenic pseudoaneurysm. The rate of formation of pseudoaneurysms and natural history if left untreated is unclear. Although routine follow-up imaging is not currently recommended for non-operative management of splenic trauma, if a splenic pseudoaneurysm is identified on subsequent imaging because of symptoms, it can usually be successfully embolised. Splenic pseudocysts are asymptomatic most of the time, and for this reason, their incidence is unknown. However, symptoms including pain and vomiting may occur with enlargement of the cyst and compression of the stomach. If symptomatic, treatment may include simple fenestration of the cyst or partial splenectomy. Splenic abscess is a rare complication of splenic trauma and is generally managed with antibiotics and percutaneous drainage. Pleuropulmonary complications, including development of pleural effusions, atelectasis, pneumonia and empyema may occur in up to 50% of patients with splenic trauma. The risk of missing an intra-abdominal injury is fairly low but does exist. For this reason, non-operative management is contraindicated in children with diffuse peritonitis. Accordingly, a child who develops increasing abdominal tenderness with peritonitis during the observation period should undergo exploration. OPSI is a complication that occurs after splenectomy.

 **Q5** Following splenectomy in children, vaccines need to be administered to prevent OPSI by which of the following organisms?

**A** *Streptococcus pneumoniae*

**B** *Neisseria meningitidis*

**C** *Haemophilus influenzae*

**D** all of the above

**E** none of the above

**A5** **D** The risk of OPSI is higher for children than adults. The incidence is 0.23%–0.42% per year with a lifetime risk of 5% in children, compared with a 2% lifetime risk in adults. Although the risk is low, mortality may exceed 50% when this complication occurs. Splenectomised children are most susceptible to sepsis due to encapsulated microorganisms, including *S. pneumoniae*, *N. meningitidis* and *H. influenzae*. The exact timing of vaccinations in this situation is controversial, however, it is generally recommended that children receive vaccines against these pathogens prior to discharge from the hospital to avoid problems with non-compliance. Another area of controversy is the use of prophylactic antibiotics in asplenic children. It is generally recommended that children under the age of 5 years receive penicillin for prophylaxis.

**Q⁶** A child involved in a motor vehicle collision is haemodynamically unstable on presentation to the emergency department and has diffuse peritonitis on abdominal exam. He is rapidly taken to the operating room for an exploratory laparotomy. An isolated, large, actively bleeding right liver laceration is found. The child remains haemodynamically unstable despite aggressive fluid and blood resuscitation. What is the appropriate management at this point?

   **A** right hepatectomy

   **B** hepatorrhaphy

   **C** right hepatic artery ligation

   **D** packing of the liver with laparotomy pads and temporary closure of the abdomen

   **E** none of the above

**A⁶** **D** The armamentarium for operative management of liver injuries is vast. Hepatorrhaphy can be safely done for smaller lacerations. Adjuncts to hepatorrhaphy include application of sealants such as Tisseel or BioGlue and packing of the laceration with omentum. For extensive injuries, bleeding can initially be controlled by packing the involved area with laparotomy pads. The Pringle manoeuvre is a useful technique to temporarily occlude the hepatic hilum when there is extensive haemorrhage not controlled by other means. A large haemostat is used to clamp the hepatoduodenal ligament thereby interrupting the flow of blood through the hepatic artery and the portal vein and thus helping to control bleeding from the liver.

Complicated procedures such as hepatic resection are generally not recommended but may be considered in experienced hands if it can be accomplished safely and expeditiously and the patient is haemodynamically stable. Another option for uncontrollable bleeding is right or left hepatic artery ligation. This technique is fraught with complications and should be considered only when other options fail. In the context of extensive bleeding and shock, the safest option is to expeditiously pack the abdomen to control the bleeding, perform a temporary abdominal wall closure, and continue aggressive fluid resuscitation and rewarming of the patient in the ICU. This technique can also be combined with the postoperative angiographic embolisation prior to returning to the operating room for reassessment.

**Q7** All of the following findings are associated with abdominal compartment syndrome *except*:

  **A** decreased urine output

  **B** increased respiratory peak pressures

  **C** increased cardiac output

  **D** decreased venous return

  **E** splanchnic hypoperfusion.

**A7**  **C** Abdominal compartment syndrome occurs when there is increased abdominal pressure causing decreased perfusion to the body wall and intra-abdominal organs. It has become an increasingly recognised clinical entity associated with multiple trauma, massive intra-abdominal haemorrrhage, and aggressive fluid and blood resuscitation. Abdominal compartment syndrome has been described not only in postoperative patients but also in patients managed non-operatively. Increased intra-abdominal pressure leads to decreased renal and splanchnic perfusion, decreased venous return and cardiac output, and respiratory failure with increased peak respiratory pressures and ventilation/perfusion mismatch. Increased ventilator pressures, oliguria and a 'tight' abdomen in the multiple trauma patient should arouse suspicion for abdominal compartment syndrome. Once suspected, it must be diagnosed and treated immediately to prevent progression to intestinal ischaemia/infarction, multiple system organ failure and death. Indirect measurement of intra-abdominal pressure can be accomplished by measuring bladder pressures using a Foley catheter and a pressure transducer. Decompression of the abdomen should be considered when intra-abdominal pressures exceed 15–20 mmHg. Abdominal compartment syndrome may be prevented by leaving the abdomen open in the severely injured child undergoing laparotomy and avoiding overaggressive fluid resuscitation. Several devices can be used for temporary closure of the abdomen in children: Bogota bag, vacuum-assisted closure dressing, and Silastic sheeting among others.

**Q8** All these injuries should be suspected in a child presenting with the seat-belt sign *except*:

  **A** splenic laceration

  **B** intestinal injury

  **C** mesenteric injury

  **D** thoracic spine fracture

  **E** lumbar spine fracture.

**A8**  **A** The seat-belt syndrome is a pattern of injuries attributed to use of the lap seat belt in children involved in motor vehicle collisions. It consists of the triad of abdominal wall contusion (seat-belt sign), intestinal and/or mesenteric injury and thoracic and/or lumbar spine fracture. It has been commonly associated with a Chance fracture, which is a fracture that occurs after hyperflexion of the back over a fixed object and most commonly involves T12, L1 and L2. Intestinal and mesenteric injuries result from deceleration, shearing and compressive forces, and present with intestinal perforation, intestinal bruising, mesenteric haematoma and/or mesenteric laceration with active bleeding. The presence of a seat-belt sign (abdominal wall contusion caused by a seat belt) should raise suspicion for underlying intestinal injury as well as thoracolumbar spine fractures (i.e. Chance fractures), which may be accompanied by paraplegia. CT scan may reveal bowel thickening or free fluid without solid organ injury, findings that should heighten suspicion for bowel injury. A low threshold for surgical exploration should be maintained in this setting. A thorough clinical and radiological evaluation for lumbar or thoracic trauma should also be pursued in these patients. Although solid organ injury such as splenic laceration can occur with the same mechanism of injury (high-impact motor vehicle collision), it is not classically associated with the seat-belt syndrome.

 A child presents to the emergency department after a bicycle crash. His abdominal exam reveals an abrasion with contusion over the epigastrium and he complains of localised epigastric pain. A CT scan was done and does not show any injuries. Which injuries should be included in the differential diagnosis?

  **A** duodenal injury

  **B** pancreatic injury

  **C** small-bowel injury

  **D** all of the above

  **E** none of the above

 **D** This abdominal wall contusion is most likely the result of the bicycle handle bar impaling the upper abdomen as the child falls from the bicycle. Handlebar injuries are classically associated with duodenal, pancreatic, and small-bowel injuries. In up to two-thirds of cases, duodenal injury and pancreatic injury coexist. Duodenal, pancreatic and small-bowel injuries are not infrequently missed on the initial CT scan. One must maintain a high index of suspicion for these injuries. Adding oral contrast to the intravenous contrast when performing the CT scan may increase the sensitivity to detect these injuries. Patients with localised tenderness and a normal CT scan should be monitored with serial exams.

Although clinical examination is usually reliable, repeating a CT scan at 24–48 hours in the setting of persistent symptoms may reveal evolving injuries. Although amylase levels may initially be normal, they are usually elevated at 24 hours after the injury if a pancreatic injury is present. These children may therefore benefit from serial blood tests.

**Q10** A 10-year-old child is kicked in the upper abdomen while playing soccer. He presents to the emergency department 4 days after the injury because of persistent pain and vomiting. A CT scan of the abdomen reveals a duodenal haematoma. What is the appropriate management of this patient?

   **A** exploratory laparoscopy and drainage of haematoma

   **B** exploratory laparotomy and drainage of the haematoma

   **C** exploratory laparotomy and duodenal resection

   **D** nasogastric decompression and parenteral or enteral nutrition

   **E** none of the above

**A10** **D** Most duodenal haematomas can be managed non-operativey in the absence of peritoneal signs on physical examination. Children with duodenal haematomas usually present with gastric distension, vomiting and intolerance to feeds. Conservative management consists of decompressing the stomach with a nasogastric tube and either total parenteral nutrition or enteral nutrition with nasojejunal feedings. It may take up to 3–4 weeks for complete resolution of obstructive symptoms. Rarely, patients develop a stricture at the site of the haematoma.

When an intramural duodenal haematoma is found intraoperatively while exploring for another injury, the serosa of the duodenum overlying the haematoma can be incised to evacuate the haematoma. This should be done carefully so as not to disrupt the submucosa. Alternatively, the haematoma can also be left in place as long as it is not a full-thickness haematoma. It can be beneficial to pass a nasojejunal tube under direct vision to provide enteral feedings in the postoperative period. A nasogastric tube should also be left in place.

**Q11** What is the appropriate management for a child brought to the operating room 24 hours after an injury who is found to have a complex, stellate 4 cm perforation on the lateral aspect of the second part of the duodenum with massive intra-abdominal contamination?

   **A** primary repair

   **B** primary repair with drain left near the repair

   **C** tube duodenostomy, pyloric exclusion, feeding jejunostomy, nasogastric tube

   **D** Whipple's procedure (pancreaticoduodenectomy)

   **E** none of the above

**A11** **C** Management of duodenal injury varies depending on type of injury (haematoma vs. laceration), location of injury, and complexity of injury. Most duodenal haematomas can be managed non-operatively with nasogastric tube decompression and total parenteral nutrition or nasojejunal feedings. Perforations should be managed operatively. If the perforation is small, primary closure should be performed. Because of the often-tenuous status of duodenal repairs, a closed suction drain is often left near the repair. However, if the perforation is more complex such that primary closure is not feasible, or there is significant intra-abdominal contamination (in cases of delayed exploration), other options must be considered. One option is primary repair, if this can be done without significantly narrowing the duodenal lumen, with pyloric exclusion to protect the repair. If the perforation cannot be closed primarily, a tube duodenostomy may be left in place, and a pyloric exclusion and/or gastrojejunostomy performed. For both procedures, a drain should be left near the duodenum, a nasogastric tube used to decompress the stomach, and a feeding jejunostomy created to provide postoperative enteral nutritional support. A Whipple's procedure is not generally recommended in the acute trauma setting unless there is significant vascular injury in the pancreaticoduodenal area that precludes repair.

**Q12** What is the appropriate management of a laceration involving 50% of the circumference of the descending colon in an otherwise stable child?

  **A** primary repair

  **B** primary repair with proximal loop colostomy

  **C** primary repair with proximal loop ileostomy

  **D** exteriorisation of proximal and distal ends of the colon as stomas

  **E** Hartmann's procedure (exteriorisation of proximal end of the colon as a stoma while leaving the distal end as a stump in the abdomen)

**A12  A** Both small-bowel and colon injuries are managed by debridement and primary repair for smaller, less complex lacerations vs. resection and primary anastomosis for larger, more complex lacerations or complete transections. Factors that may alter this approach include haemodynamic instability, extensive gross contamination, severe burden of injuries, or extensive blood loss with hypothermia and coagulopathy. In such cases, a damage-control procedure is a wiser option. The stomach is decompressed with a nasogastric tube, all injured bowel is stapled off to prevent further contamination, a temporary abdominal wall closure is performed, and the patient is taken to the ICU for further resuscitation and warming, with re-exploration in 24–48 hours once the patient is stable. At the time of re-exploration, a decision can be made regarding primary repair, resection and reanastomosis, or resection and ostomy depending upon the clinical status of the child and the degree of contamination. Rectal injuries are repaired primarily with or without a colostomy depending on the extent and location (intraperitoneal vs. extraperitoneal) of the injury.

**Q13** What is the appropriate diagnostic study in a child who was involved in a motor vehicle collision and presents to the emergency department with a seat-belt sign and localised abdominal pain?
  **A** FAST (Focused Assessment with Sonography for Trauma) exam
  **B** diagnostic peritoneal lavage (DPL)
  **C** ultrasound of the abdomen
  **D** CT scan of the abdomen and pelvis
  **E** diagnostic laparoscopy

**A13** **D** CT scan of the abdomen and pelvis with intravenous contrast is the gold standard for evaluation of blunt abdominal trauma in children. Adding oral contrast may increase the sensitivity for detection of duodenal and proximal small-bowel injuries; however, this benefit should be weighed against the risk of aspiration. The role of the FAST exam and DPL is limited to children who are too unstable to undergo CT scan. A FAST exam that demonstrates a large amount of free intraperitoneal fluid in a child who is haemodynamically unstable mandates operative exploration. DPL can be useful in the case of an equivocal FAST exam in a haemodynamically unstable child. If the DPL is positive, the child requires exploration, whereas if it is negative, other causes of bleeding should be sought, such as a pelvic fracture.

**Q14** All the following are criteria for a positive DPL in blunt trauma *except*:
  **A** aspiration of 1 mL of gross blood
  **B** >100 000 red blood cells per mL
  **C** >500 white blood cells per mL
  **D** aspiration of bile or gastrointestinal contents
  **E** Gram stain positive for bacteria.

**A14** **A** DPL is rarely indicated in children; however, DPL can be helpful in situations where the patient is too unstable to undergo a CT scan of the abdomen and a FAST exam is not available or is equivocal. It can be performed either percutaneously or using an open technique with a small incision above or below the umbilicus. A supraumbilical approach is preferred in cases where a pelvic fracture is suspected. The percutaneous technique is done in a Seldinger fashion, using a needle, a guide wire, a dilator, and a catheter. For both techniques, the first step is to aspirate. If more than 10 mL of gross blood is returned upon aspiration, the exam is positive and the patient needs to go to the operating room. The exam is also positive if bile, vegetable fibres, or gastrointestinal contents are aspirated. If less than 10 mL of gross blood is aspirated, 10 mL/kg of normal saline should be infused in the peritoneal cavity and then aspirated and sent to the lab. The criteria for a positive DPL are >100 000 RBC/mL, >500 WBC/mL and positive Gram stain. DPL is a diagnostic study with excellent sensitivity, but diaphragmatic and retroperitoneal injuries may be missed.

**Q15** What is the appropriate management in a child who is haemodynami- cally unstable after 40 mL/kg of packed red blood cells, has a Glasgow Coma Scale score of 3, and a distended abdomen with a positive FAST exam?

A emergency head CT

B emergency abdominal CT

C emergency craniotomy

D emergency laparoscopy

E emergency laparotomy with placement of an intracranial pressure monitor perioperatively

**A15** **E** Whenever an intra-abdominal injury leading to haemorrhagic shock coex- ists with a traumatic brain injury (TBI), the intra-abdominal bleeding should be addressed first since secondary brain hypoperfusion can have devastating consequences on the outcome of the TBI. A child that is haemodynamically unstable due to major intra-abdominal haemorrhage and is in a state of shock not responsive to fluid and blood resuscitation is too unstable to undergo CT scan- ning and needs to be transported immediately to the operating room to undergo exploratory laparotomy. The cause of the bleeding has to be addressed as quickly as possible, and a damage control procedure may be indicated. Neurosurgeons should be consulted while the patient is still in the emergency department so that a neurologic evaluation can be completed. Depending on the clinical context and available resources, further management can vary from perioperative intracranial pressure monitor placement, emergency burr holes, portable head CT in the operating room, or immediate transport to CT scan after the procedure.

**Q16** Which of the following is the most frequent complication of non- operative management of blunt liver trauma?

A bile leak

B haemobilia

C abscess

D abdominal compartment syndrome

E necrotising cholecystitis

**A16** **A** The most frequent complication of non-operative management of blunt trauma of the liver, other than bleeding, is a bile leak. The development of fever, ileus, right upper quadrant pain, and persistently elevated liver function tests after liver trauma should arouse suspicion for liver-related complications. An ultrasound or CT scan should be performed to evaluate for a possible biloma or abscess. If a fluid collection is found, it can usually be drained percutaneously under ultrasound guidance. The nature of the fluid retrieved determines the diagnosis, i.e. bile with biliary leak; gross pus with abscess. Hepatobiliary imino-diacetic acid scan is also a useful adjunct for detection of biliary leaks. Endoscopic pancreatography (ERCP) may be both diagnostic and therapeutic. If a bile leak is identified by ERCP, a sphincterotomy may be performed to facilitate ampullary drainage, and an endoscopic stent may be placed. Abscess may occur due to an infected biloma but can also be secondary to infected necrosis of the liver when the liver is devitalised by trauma. Some patients will ultimately require hepatic resection to remove the necrotic part of the liver. Gangrenous cholecystitis may occur secondary to injury to the right hepatic artery or cystic artery. Acalculous cholecystitis may also occur in multiply-injured patients who have a prolonged length of stay in the intensive care unit, although this is not usually attributed to liver trauma. Haemobilia is acute gastrointestinal bleeding arising from the biliary tract that may occur after major liver injury. Patients classically present with right upper quadrant pain, jaundice, and acute gastrointestinal bleeding. Diagnosis is made by either angiography or upper endoscopy.

These complications tend to occur in higher-grade liver injuries, such as grades IV and V.

**Q17** For evaluation of a stab wound to the anterior abdominal wall of a child who has localised abdominal tenderness but is haemodynamically stable, all of the following are useful *except*:

**A** local wound exploration

**B** DPL

**C** diagnostic laparoscopy

**D** observation and serial physical exams

**E** angiography.

**A17** **E** There are several ways to approach a stab wound to the anterior abdomen. Emergency exploration is mandated in children with diffuse peritonitis who are haemodynamically unstable. In those who are stable with only localised pain, the stab wound may be locally explored to exclude peritoneal violation. If there is no peritoneal violation on local exploration, an intra-abdominal injury is excluded. In patients with violation of the peritoneum, further evaluation may include DPL, CT scan or diagnostic laparoscopy. Observation and serial abdominal examination alone is also an option for the haemodynamically stable patient with minimal abdominal tenderness. The overall accuracy rate for serial examination for detection of intra-abdominal injury approaches 94% but is labour intensive and requires a thorough, experienced examiner. Angiography is not typically utilised in the assessment of anterior abdominal wall stab wounds.

## Further reading

Brown RL. Abdominal trauma. In: Wheeler DS, Wong HR, Shanley TP, editors. *Paediatric Critical Care Medicine: basic science and clinical evidence*. New York, NY: Springer-Verlag; 2007. pp. 1572–8.

Gaines, BA. Intra-abdominal solid organ injury in children: diagnosis and treatment. *J Trauma*. 2009; **67**(2 Suppl.): S135–9.

Stylianos S. Evidence-based guidelines for resource utilisation in children with isolated spleen or liver injury. *J Pediatr Surg*. 2000; **35**(2): 164–7.

Stylianos S, Hicks BA. Abdominal and renal trauma. In: Ashcraft KW, Holcomb GW, Murphy JP, editors. *Pediatric Surgery*. 4th ed. Philadelphia, PA: Elsevier; 2005. pp. 201–16.

Stylianos S, Pearl RH. Abdominal trauma. In: Grosfeld JL, O'Neill JA, Fonkalsrud EW, *et al.*, editors. *Pediatric Surgery*. Vol. 1. 6th ed. Philadelphia, PA: Mosby; 2006. pp. 295–316.

Sutherland I, Ledder O, Crameri J, *et al.* Pancreatic trauma in children. *Pediatr Surg Int*. 2010; **26**(12): 1201–6. Epub 2010 Aug 28.

# CHAPTER 11

# Genitourinary trauma

### MARIANNE BEAUDIN, REBECCAH L BROWN

**From the choices below each question, select the single best answer.**

Q1 Which genitourinary organ is the most frequently injured?
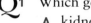
    **A** kidney
    **B** ureter
    **C** bladder
    **D** urethra
    **E** testis

A1   **A**  The kidney is the genitourinary organ most frequently involved in both blunt and penetrating trauma, accounting for more than 50% of the genitourinary traumas. It is thought that the kidney is involved in 10%–20% of all the paediatric blunt abdominal traumas. More than 90% of all kidney injuries are secondary to blunt trauma. Blunt renal injuries are associated with other intra-abdominal injuries in 42%–74% of patients. When isolated kidney injuries occur, they are usually minor injuries. The bladder is the second most commonly injured genitourinary organ, and injury occurs as a result of blunt abdominal trauma in up to 80% of patients. Bladder injuries are associated with pelvic fractures in 75%–95% of blunt abdominal trauma. Ureteral injuries are rare and occur in less than 1% of blunt abdominal trauma and 4% of penetrating abdominal trauma. Urethral injuries are different in children than in adults because of the fact that the prostate is less developed and does not protect the posterior urethra in children. Posterior urethral trauma is associated with pelvic fractures whereas anterior urethral trauma is associated with straddle injuries. Testicular injuries are rare in children although scrotal haematoma is more frequent.

**Q2** Children are more vulnerable to renal trauma for all of the following reasons *except*:

   **A** kidneys are proportionally smaller in children

   **B** kidneys are positioned lower in the abdomen in children

   **C** Gerota's fascia is less developed in children

   **D** children have weaker abdominal wall musculature

   **E** children can have persistent fetal lobulations

**A2** **A** There are many anatomical differences between children and adults that render the kidney more susceptible to injury in children. Kidneys are proportionally larger in children relative to the size of the body and are positioned lower in the abdomen and therefore not as protected by the rib cage. Furthermore, since the rib cage is not completely ossified, it does not offer as much protection as in adults. Because children have weaker abdominal wall musculature, there is less perirenal fat to offer additional protection. Likewise, Gerota's fascia and the renal capsule are also not as thick as in adults and make the kidney more vulnerable to lacerations, non-confined bleeding and urinary extravasation. Since many paediatric kidneys retain their fetal lobulations, lower pole amputation is more likely. Renal trauma is also more prevalent in children with underlying congenital anomalies. The reported incidence of pre-existing renal disease in children sustaining renal trauma varies between 1% and 23%. Associated anomalies may include hydronephrosis (commonly secondary to ureteropelvic junction obstruction), abnormal kidney position (horseshoe kidney), abnormal kidney consistency (polycystic kidney disease, urinary reflux), and tumour (Wilms's tumour).

**Q3** Which sports-related injury has been most commonly associated with renal trauma in children?

   **A** hockey

   **B** football

   **C** baseball

   **D** martial arts

   **E** bicycle collisions

**A3** **E** Although the most common mechanism of blunt renal trauma in children is motor vehicle collisions, the most common sports-related injuries are from bicycle crashes. Bicycle crashes are four times as frequent as contact sports in paediatric blunt renal trauma. All-terrain vehicles have also been recognised as an important mechanism of injury for paediatric kidneys. This has led to some questioning of the advice about safe activities that should be provided to children with kidney abnormalities or after renal trauma.

**Q4** What should be done when blood is seen at the urethral meatus in a child who sustained blunt trauma?

 **A** Insert a Foley catheter with caution.

 **B** Insert a suprapubic cystostomy tube.

 **C** Insert a nephrostomy tube.

 **D** Perform a retrograde urethrography.

 **E** Perform a CT of the abdomen and pelvis with intravenous (IV) contrast.

**A4** **D** Signs and symptoms suggestive of urethral injury include blood at the meatus, gross haematuria, scrotal haematoma, and inability to void or the sensation of voiding without passing urine. Another commonly reported sign in the adult literature is the presence of a high-riding prostate, which can be difficult to assess in children. If any of these signs and symptoms are present, urethral trauma should be suspected and investigated. Insertion of a urinary catheter should not be attempted because of the risk of creating a false passage with the catheter and aggravating the injury. Insertion of a suprapubic cystostomy or nephrostomy tube is not recommended in the acute setting prior to any other studies. The imaging modality of choice is retrograde urethrography. If a urethral injury is confirmed, a urologist should be consulted to insert a Foley catheter. A cystogram is then completed to exclude an associated bladder injury. Although most patients with blunt abdominal trauma will require a CT scan to exclude intra-abdominal injury, CT is not a very sensitive study for detection of urethral injuries.

**Q5** What is the diagnostic study of choice for investigation of haematuria in children?

 **A** intravenous pyelogram (IVP)

 **B** cystogram

 **C** ultrasound

 **D** CT of the abdomen and pelvis with IV contrast

 **E** CT of the abdomen and pelvis without IV contrast

**A5** **D** The management of haematuria in children is an area of controversy. All agree that children with gross haematuria require further investigation. However, the degree of microscopic haematuria that mandates further investigation has not been clearly defined in the literature. Some recommend further investigation for microscopic haematuria >5 red blood cells (RBCs) per high-power field (HPF), while others recommend further investigation for >20 RBCs/HPF, >50 RBCs/HPF, or >100 RBCs/HPF. In the presence of any signs of shock, any degree of microscopic haematuria should be investigated. One of the reasons why some experts recommend performing diagnostic studies for any level of haematuria in children is the fact that it may be associated with an underlying renal abnormality such as ureteropelvic junction obstruction or Wilms's tumour. Historically, IVP has been the diagnostic study of choice. This has now been replaced by CT of the abdomen and pelvis with IV contrast. An early-phase contrast bolus will detect arterial injuries to kidneys, a delayed phase (>80 seconds) will detect venous and renal parenchymal injuries, while an excretory phase (2–10 minutes) will detect injuries to ureters and bladder. CT is not sensitive for diagnosis of bladder injury if the bladder is not fully distended. If a bladder injury is strongly suspected, a CT or conventional cystogram should be performed. Ultrasound has decreased sensitivity compared with CT, especially for renal parenchymal injuries.

 Which one of the following is the appropriate initial management of urinary extravasation?

**A** observation

**B** ureteral stent

**C** percutaneous drainage

**D** all of the above

**E** none of the above

 **D** Urinary extravasation can occur with grade IV and V renal injuries according to the organ injury grading scale of the American Association for the Surgery of Trauma (AAST). In the past, urinary extravasation was an indication for surgical exploration whereas now most of these injuries are managed non-operatively. Most urinomas will resolve spontaneously without any intervention. An enlarging or infected urinoma can manifest itself with an expanding flank mass, pain, fever, or ileus. If an enlarging urinoma is suspected, an ultrasound or CT of the abdomen and pelvis with IV contrast should be performed. This can still be managed non-operatively with percutaneous drainage and/or ureteral stenting by cystoscopy. The use of routine antibiotics for urinary extravasation is controversial with some authors recommending its use only when ureteral stents are used. If an infected urinoma is suspected, it should be treated with antibiotics and percutaneous drainage, with or without ureteral stents.

**Q7** What is the most important criterion to consider when deciding on operative vs. non-operative management of renal trauma?

**A** large perirenal haematoma

**B** extensive urinary extravasation

**C** parenchymal laceration extending through the renal cortex, medulla and collecting system

**D** renal artery thrombosis

**E** haemodynamic instability

**7** **E** The only absolute indication for operative intervention for renal trauma is haemodynamic instability unresponsive to fluid and/or blood resuscitation.

Even complex grade IV and V renal injuries may be successfully managed non-operatively as long as the patient remains haemodynamically stable. Ongoing bleeding and increasing transfusion requirements are indications for operative management. Radiographic signs on CT indicative of ongoing renal bleeding include an expanding or uncontained retroperitoneal haematoma or complete avulsion of the main renal artery or vein with extravasation. Whereas some of these radiographic findings may be managed non-operatively with angiography and selective embolisation in the stable paediatric patient, surgery is mandated in the unstable paediatric patient. During surgical exploration, if the kidney appears salvageable, a conservative approach should be attempted with renorraphy or partial nephrectomy. If the kidney appears unsalvageable or the patient is too unstable to undergo conservative management, a nephrectomy should be performed.

**Q8** What is the most common complication after non-operative management of renal trauma?

**A** bleeding

**B** urinoma

**C** perinephric abscess

**D** hydronephrosis

**E** hypertension

**A8** **B** The most common complication of non-operative management of renal injuries is development of urinoma secondary to urine extravasation. It has been reported that approximately two-thirds of urinomas in children will resolve spontaneously. Accordingly, it is appropriate to observe a small non-infected urinoma. Percutaneous drainage and/or ureteral stents are indicated for enlarging and/or infected urinomas. Delayed bleeding is rare in renal trauma. Perinephric abscesses can be associated with infected urinomas or perinephric haematomas. Most can be treated by CT-guided percutaneous drainage and antibiotics while some loculated abscesses will eventually require operative drainage. Hypertension is thought to occur in less than 5% of the renal traumas managed non-operatively. Blood pressure should be monitored annually after renal trauma. Late complications of renal trauma are rare and include hydronephrosis, arteriovenous fistula, arterial pseudoaneurysm, pyelonephritis and calculus formation.

**Q9** What is the appropriate management of a renovascular injury diagnosed in a stable patient who presents to the emergency room 2 hours after a blunt abdominal trauma?

**A** observation

**B** surgical exploration with attempted revascularisation if the kidney appears salvageable

**C** surgical exploration and nephrectomy

**D** angiography and endovascular stent

**E** none of the above

**A9** **B** Renovascular injuries are rare in children. The most frequent mechanism of renovascular injury in blunt trauma is rapid deceleration that results in stretching of the renal vasculature with disruption of the arterial intima and subsequent arterial thrombosis. The proposed treatment algorithm is based on the duration of warm ischaemia. The time of warm ischaemia for which surgical revascularisation is more likely to be successful in blunt renal trauma is less than 4–6 hours. The chances of successful revascularisation are greater with penetrating trauma than with blunt trauma. In blunt trauma, renovascular injuries are associated with severe disruption of the renal parenchyma that can make the kidney unsalvageable. If there is significant parenchymal disruption, nephrectomy would be more appropriate than attempts at revascularisation. When the diagnosis is made more than 4–6 hours after injury, observation may be an appropriate treatment if the patient is haemodynamically stable. Others recommend angiography and endovascular stenting in this setting. Revascularisation should always be attempted in patients with bilateral kidney injuries or a solitary kidney.

**Q10** Which one of these is the most appropriate for the management of a distal ureteral injury?

**A** observation

**B** ureteral stent

**C** psoas hitch and/or Boari flap

**D** transureteroureterostomy

**E** ureteral ligation

**A10** **C** The management of ureteral trauma depends on the location of injury and the haemodynamic stability of the patient. In a haemodynamically unstable patient, it can be appropriate to ligate the ureter, insert a tube nephrostomy, and plan a delayed intervention. All devitalised tissue must be debrided and this sometimes results in a length deficit in the ureter. In distal ureteral injury, primary repair can usually be achieved using a psoas hitch and/or a Boari flap. The psoas hitch consists of fixing the bladder on the psoas muscle to allow a tension-free anastomosis. The Boari flap uses a tubularised flap of the bladder to increase the length of the distal ureter. These primary repairs are often done over ureteral stents. Another option to increase ureteral length is to mobilise the kidney to add up to 3–5 cm of length. For more proximal injuries, a spatulated end-to-end anastomosis can be performed or a transureteroureterostomy if a large deficit is present. Other more complicated options include renal auto-transplantation and ileal interposition.

**Q11** What is the most appropriate management of extraperitoneal bladder rupture?

    **A** observation

    **B** Foley catheter insertion

    **C** suprapubic cystostomy

    **D** nephrostomy tube

    **E** operative repair

**A11** **B** The most appropriate management of extraperitoneal rupture noted on cystogram is bladder drainage with a Foley catheter. Surgical repair of these injuries entails manipulation of an extraperitoneal haematoma which increases the risk of bleeding as well as converting a closed pelvic fracture into an open fracture thereby increasing the risk of infection. According to the literature, approximately 90% of bladder injuries will heal in 10 days and the remainder within 3 weeks with only transurethral catheter drainage. The literature doesn't support the routine use of a contrast study before removing the urinary catheter, although it is commonly performed.

**Q12** What is the most appropriate management of intraperitoneal bladder rupture?

    **A** observation

    **B** Foley catheter

    **C** suprapubic cystostomy

    **D** nephrostomy tube

    **E** operative repair

**A12** **E** Intraperitoneal bladder rupture requires surgical exploration. Transurethral drainage of the bladder alone is not sufficient since protracted extravasation of urine into the peritoneal cavity can lead to serious metabolic and septic complications. Furthermore, many of these injuries are associated with other intra-abdominal injuries that require exploration. The bladder is more likely to be injured if it is distended at the time of injury. The most common area of injury is at the dome of the bladder. At the time of repair, the ureteral orifices inside the bladder must be visualised through the defect to ensure their patency. The defect can then be repaired with absorbable sutures in two layers. A closed-suction drain can be left in place over the repair. A Foley catheter is generally left in place for 5–10 days. Some authors recommend performing a contrast study prior to removal of the closed-suction drain and Foley catheter. Antibiotics are not required.

**Q13** What is the most appropriate management of partial disruption of the posterior urethra following blunt trauma?

  **A** observation

  **B** Foley catheter

  **C** suprapubic cystotomy

  **D** nephrostomy tube

  **E** operative repair

**A13** **B** Urethral injuries are classified into five categories according to the AAST: contusion, stretching, partial disruption, complete disruption of less and more than 2 cm. Urethral injuries are most commonly due to pelvic fractures. The posterior urethra is more prone to injuries in children as it is not protected by the prostate. Urethral injuries are diagnosed by retrograde urethrography. Low-grade injuries can be treated with observation alone. If the child is unable to void, a urinary catheter can be inserted carefully by a urologist. Most children with partial disruption of the urethra can be managed with a urinary catheter only. Higher grade injuries can be managed with early surgical repair or delayed surgical repair after insertion of a suprapubic cystostomy tube. The advantage of delayed repair is avoiding entering a pelvic haematoma with increased risk of bleeding.

**Q14** All of these are complications of urethral trauma *except*:

  **A** impotence

  **B** retrograde ejaculation

  **C** incontinence

  **D** stricture

  **E** Peyronie's disease.

**A14** **E** The long-term sequelae of urethral trauma can be devastating and may include incontinence and urethral strictures, as well as impotence and retrograde ejaculation in boys, and urethrovaginal fistula and vaginal stenosis in girls. Some of these complications may be a direct consequence of the trauma itself or may be related to surgical attempts at repair. Delays in diagnosis of urethral injuries in girls occur frequently and can lead to other complications such as sepsis and necrotising fasciitis. Peyronie's disease is a curvature in the penis that is secondary to an area of fibrosis in the tunica albuginea. The cause of this disease is uncertain but it is thought to be due to vascular trauma or injury to the penis. It is not secondary to urethral injury.

Q15 What is the most common mechanism of injury to the penis in children?

  A straddle injuries

  B zipper injuries

  C blunt injuries

  D penetrating injuries

  E iatrogenic injuries

A15 E The most common mechanism of injury to the penis is iatrogenic and most often occurs during circumcision. Complications of circumcision include penile amputation, urethral fistulisation, laceration of the glans, and inaccurate removal of the foreskin that can later lead to phimosis. Penile injuries from penetrating and blunt trauma are rare in children. Zipper entrapment of the penis is a well-described mechanism of injury in children. It can often be managed in the emergency room with sedation, but general anaesthesia may be necessary.

Q16 What is the most appropriate management of haematocele in children?

  A observation

  B anti-inflammatory medication

  C percutaneous drainage

  D surgical exploration

  E none of the above

A16 D Ultrasound is very useful for evaluation of scrotal and testicular injuries. It can differentiate between scrotal haematoma, hydroceles, haematoceles, testicular rupture and infarction. Patients with haematoceles should be considered for surgical exploration to evacuate blood from the tunica vaginalis because this approach reduces morbidity and hastens recovery. Testicular rupture and infraction are surgical emergencies. Testicular rupture should be managed with debridement and primary closure.

Q17 What is the most appropriate management in a 4-year-old girl who was found to have a vaginal laceration after a motor vehicle collision?

  A observation

  B antibiotics

  C repair of laceration in the emergency room

  D exam under general anaesthesia

  E none of the above

A17 D Vaginal lacerations associated with blunt trauma are particularly worrisome for associated injuries. Attempts at exam and repair should not be attempted in the emergency department. These patients should be brought to the operating room in order to perform a thorough exam under general anaesthesia. Speculum examination and vaginoscopy can then be performed, as well as urethroscopy and proctoscopy to exclude associated injuries that can have devastating consequences if diagnosis is delayed. Depending on the extent, vaginal lacerations can be simply observed or repaired in a single layer with absorbable sutures. There is no need for antibiotics. Vaginal lacerations are usually associated with straddle injuries and pelvic fractures when found after blunt trauma. The possibility of abuse has to be kept in mind if the mechanism of injury is not consistent with the findings.

## Further reading

Brown RL, Garcia VF. Genitourinary tract trauma. In: Grosfeld JL, O'Neill JA, Fonkalsrud EW, *et al.*, editors. *Paediatric Surgery*. Vol. 1. 6th ed. Philadelphia, PA. Mosby; 2006.

Buckley JC, McAninch JW. The diagnosis, management and outcomes of pediatric renal injuries. *Urol Clin North Am.* 2006; **33**(1): 33–40.

Fraser JD, Aguayo P, Ostlie DJ, *et al.* Review of the evidence on the management of blunt renal trauma in pediatric patients. *Pediatr Surg Int.* 2009; **25**(2): 125–32.

McAleer IM, Kaplan GW. Pediatric genitourinary trauma. *Urol Clin North Am.* 1995; **22**(1): 177–88.

Stylianos S, Hicks BA. Abdominal and renal trauma. In: Ashcraft KW, Holcomb GW, Murphy JP, editors. *Pediatric Surgery*. 4th ed. Philadelphia, PA: Elsevier; 2005.

# CHAPTER 12

# Musculoskeletal trauma and soft tissue injuries

**GLEESON REBELLO**

**From the choices below each question, select the best single answer.**

1 Children's fractures differ from adults because the musculoskeletal system in a child differs from that of an adult in all the following ways *except*:

- **A** presence of growth plate
- **B** higher collagen-to-bone ratio in children
- **C** thicker and stronger periosteal sleeve
- **D** ligaments in children are relatively stronger than bone as compared with adult
- **E** decreased ratio of cartilage to bone.

1 **E** The increased ratio of cartilage to bone in children improves resilience but makes evaluation by radiography more difficult, as the size of the articular fragment is often underestimated. The most obvious difference between the bones of a child and an adult is the presence of a growth plate. The growth plate facilitates remodelling that corrects residual angulation over time but when injured can lead to asymmetrical growth causing angular deformity. The higher collagen-to-bone ratio reduces the tensile strength of bone thus reducing the tendency of fractures to propagate with less fracture comminution. Thick periosteum permits less fracture displacement and also when intact, aids in fracture reduction during manipulation. It is also more metabolically active which explains the exuberant callus formation, quicker healing and increased potential for remodelling. Avulsion injury patterns in childhood are more common because ligaments are relatively stronger than bone.

**Q2** Fracture remodelling in children depends on:
  A the number of years of growth remaining
  B the proximity of fracture to a rapidly growing growth plate
  C the magnitude of original angular deformity
  D the plane of angulation relative to adjacent joints
  E all of the above.

**A2** E Remodelling at the fracture site occurs by reorientation of the growth plate with improvement in overall alignment of the limb as well as bone resorption on the convexity and deposition on the concavity of the fracture. It may continue for 5–6 years after fracture as long as growth occurs during the process of remodelling. Fractures in the plane of joint motion and near rapidly growing physes have the greatest capacity to remodel. For instance remodelling in a fracture of the proximal humerus is far superior than a fracture of the distal humerus, as the proximal humeral growth plate contributes to 80% of the growth of the humerus. Fractures with the smallest degrees of malunion are more likely to remodel completely. Remodelling of rotational deformity is less predictable than angular remodelling.

**Q3** Regarding physeal (growth plate) injury, which of the following is *not* true?
  A Physeal bridging and altered growth occurs in 1% of physeal injuries.
  B It occurs more commonly in Salter–Harris type 3, 4 and 5 injuries.
  C For best results anatomical reduction is essential in Salter–Harris type 3 and 4 injuries.
  D Growth need not be monitored when physeal injury is suspected.
  E Imaging physeal bars may be done best with CT or MRI scans.

**A3** D Growth needs to be monitored to detect physeal bridges that develop following injury and lead to either angular deformity or limb length discrepancy or both, all of which occur over time. They happen most commonly following Salter–Harris type 3, 4 and 5 injuries. These bony bridges are best imaged using coronal and sagittal reformats of 1 mm CT scans or MRI studies. MRI scans provide more soft tissue information but may be difficult to interpret. Anatomical reduction of Salter–Harris type 3 and 4 injuries is essential for improving outcomes. Open reduction and internal fixation that does not traverse the physis is best. If fixation is necessary across growth plates then a small, smooth K wire must be used.

Q4 The principles of fracture fixation in children include all *except*:
   A supplementation with cast using minimal fixation techniques
   B external fixation in open fractures
   C avoid crossing the physis (growth plate)
   D use of 'flexible fixation' options in long bones
   E rigid intramedullary fixation.

A4 E Cast immobilisation is used to supplement minimal internal fixation in most instances. Growth plates can be crossed with smooth K wires only. Flexible intramedullary fixation is ideal for transverse long-bone fractures with lack of comminution or obliquity. External fixation is used in long-bone fractures with severe soft tissue injuries. Rigid intramuscular fixation exposes child to risk of physeal damage or avascular necrosis (especially in the proximal femur) and is not used in children with open physes.

Q5 Open fractures in children differ from open fractures in adults in all the following ways *except*:
   A soft tissue healing is much more rapid and complete
   B devitalised bone that is not contaminated can be left in place and will incorporate
   C periosteum will generate new bone when lost
   D delayed or non-union is more common in children
   E external fixators may be left in place till union.

A5 D Delayed or non-union is uncommon in paediatric fractures because of the overall enhanced healing potential. The soft tissue healing potential is far superior to adults and limb salvage is usually feasible in the large majority of cases. External fixation may result in being the only form of treatment utilised to achieve union and bone loss is not as big a problem as it would be in an adult with a similar injury. The management of open fractures otherwise is similar to an adult in terms of using antibiotic prophylaxis, doing a thorough debridement and fracture stabilisation in order to promote soft tissue healing.

Q6 Fractures that have a high complication rate if inadequately treated include all *except*:
   A supracondylar fractures
   B lateral condylar fractures
   C distal radial buckle fractures
   D femoral neck fractures
   E distal femoral physeal fractures.

**A⁶**    **C**   Buckle fractures of the distal radius are easily treated with immobilisation in a short arm cast or splint for 3 weeks. Improperly treated supracondylar fractures can develop malunion (cubitus varus) and ischaemic contracture secondary to undiagnosed compartment syndrome. Lateral condylar fractures have the potential for displacement and non-union. Distal femoral metaphyseal fractures often develop growth arrest and angular deformity. Femoral neck fractures can develop avascular necrosis of the femoral head.

**Q⁷**   Which of the following statements is untrue about proximal femoral fractures in the paediatric age group?

   **A**   As in the elderly, paediatric proximal femoral fractures occur following low energy trauma.

   **B**   On presentation a child has a typically flexed, abducted and externally rotated posture.

   **C**   They have a high complication rate due to unique vascular anatomy of the femoral head.

   **D**   In cases of intracapsular femoral neck fracture, urgent anatomical reduction is critical to restore blood flow to the femoral head.

   **E**   The most frequent and devastating complication of hip fractures is osteonecrosis of the femoral head.

**A⁷**    **A**   Hip fractures in children occur nearly always as a result of high-energy trauma, such as motor vehicle accident or a fall from height, placing children with these injuries at risk for multiple injuries. In the elderly population with osteoporotic bone, most proximal femoral fractures occur following low energy trauma.

Clinical presentation of affected extremity is typically that of flexion, abduction and external rotation at the hip. The femoral head is essentially an end organ supplied exclusively by branches from the medial circumflex femoral artery, which puts it at risk of osteonecrosis if blood supply is disrupted by the trauma. Urgent, anatomical reduction is critical to restore/maintain blood supply to the femoral head in intracapsular fractures in order to warrant a good outcome. Extracapsular fractures have a more favourable prognosis because the blood supply is usually preserved but can have complications like varus malunion.

Q8   Paediatric femoral shaft fracture:

A   that occurs in children younger than 1 year should be viewed with suspicion for non-accidental injury.

B   is usually treated with a Pavlik harness in infants and spica casting in toddlers.

C   when casted, is usually immobilised at 90 degrees flexion at the hip and knee with approximately 30 degrees of abduction and 20 degrees of external rotation and may be preceded by a few days of traction.

D   plating and external fixation are never used as a method of fixation.

E   is usually treated by flexible femoral nailing in preschool children.

A8   D   External fixation is usually used to manage open femoral fractures, or in patients with head or vascular injuries. The benefits of external fixation include avoidance of long incisions, exposure of the fracture site and significant blood loss. Plate fixation, though done less frequently, is used in atypical fracture patterns. A technique called submuscular bridge plating is being utilised in some centres to treat extensively comminuted, length unstable fractures. Infants with femoral fractures can be managed in a Pavlik harness and spica casting is the method of choice in preschoolers 1–5 years of age. Flexible nailing is a form of fixation utilised in average-build school-going children with greatest success in transverse fracture patterns. Bigger adolescents with femoral fractures are treated with lateral entry femoral nails. These nails avoid the piriform fossa and reduce the chance of disrupting the blood supply of the femoral head, which can lead to avascular necrosis.

Q9   Regarding injuries in and around the paediatric knee, which of the following statements is false?

A   Physeal injuries of the distal femur do not carry much risk of growth disturbance.

B   Proximal tibial physeal disruptions should be carefully evaluated for neurovascular injuries and compartment syndrome.

C   Tibial tubercle avulsion can lead to genu recurvatum.

D   Conservative treatment is the mainstay of patellar dislocations.

E   Surgical reconstruction provides superior results if the child desires to continue an active lifestyle following anterior cruciate ligament (ACL) injury.

A9   A   Physeal injuries of the distal femur carry a significant risk of growth disturbance because of its complex undulating shape, which decreases the odds of a clean cleavage plane when injured thus increasing the risk of focal damage to the physis. The neurovascular structures about the knee are at some risk with any injury in that region but this risk is greatest for injury to the proximal tibia because of tethering of the popliteal artery at its trifurcation, to the peroneal nerve around the proximal fibula and to the tibial nerve at the proximal interosseous membrane. Genu recurvatum can develop rarely in tibial tubercle fractures that occur in patients younger than 11 years because of disruption of the anterior aspect of the proximal tibial growth plate. Conservative treatment is the mainstay of patellar dislocations and includes strengthening of the vastus medialis obliquus, hamstring stretching, proprioceptive training and patellar bracing or taping. Intra-articular reconstruction using bone tunnels may be performed on boys that have achieved skeletal maturity or on girls that are at least 14 years of age. In younger children with ACL injuries controversy exists regarding treatment for fear of disrupting adjacent growth plates during surgery.

Q10 Which of the following is *not* true regarding paediatric ankle fractures?
   A  Most commonly occur in patients 8–15 years of age.
   B  The non-uniform closure of the distal tibial physis results in transitional fracture patterns like the triplane fracture and Tillaux's fracture.
   C  Diagnostic imaging should only include CT scans.
   D  If the fracture does not involve the joint surface it can usually be treated with closed reduction and casting ± minimal fixation.
   E  One of the most common ankle injuries in children is the isolated Salter–Harris 1 fracture of the distal fibula, which is often misdiagnosed as an ankle sprain.

A10  C  Initial diagnostic imaging should always consist of antereoposterior, lateral and mortise radiographs of the affected ankle. Accessory ossification centres should not be confused with fractures. CT scanning is recommended when plain radiographs show intra-articular fractures with questionable displacement, as CT allows for more accurate estimation of articular displacement and surgical planning.

   The closure of the distal tibial physis starts centrally and then proceeds in a medial to posterior direction with the anterolateral portion of the physis being last to close. The unfused areas of this physis represent areas of relative weakness and are prone to fracture. Salter–Harris 1 fractures of the distal fibula can be misdiagnosed with ankle sprains and are treated with 3–4 weeks of cast immobilisation.

**Q11** Which of the following statements about a humerus fracture is not true?

    **A** The proximal humerus fracture has tremendous potential for remodelling and malunions are rare.

    **B** The proximal humerus fracture can be treated with a sling and a swathe.

    **C** An entrapped biceps tendon in the fracture site is an indication for open reduction and internal fixation of the proximal humerus.

    **D** Humeral shaft fractures in children are always treated with open reduction and internal fixation.

    **E** Almost all associated radial nerve injuries in a paediatric patient can be treated conservatively with observation.

**A11**   **D**  Humeral shaft fractures in children are rarely treated with open reduction. Almost all associated radial nerve injuries in paediatric patients can be treated conservatively with observation, and full recovery should be expected. In the event of non-recovery within 3–4 months, electrodiagnostic tests and surgical exploration are warranted.

    The proximal humeral physis contributes 80% of the growth of the humerus as a result of which there is good remodelling and malunions are rare. Most fractures of the proximal humerus are treated conservatively with a sling and swathe, which serves to provide comfort. Interposition of an entrapped biceps tendon is a clear indication for open reduction and internal fixation.

**Q12** Regarding fractures of the paediatric elbow which of the following statements is untrue?

    **A** Knowledge of the sequence, timing and appearance of secondary ossification centres around the elbow is essential for making the correct diagnosis.

    **B** Most displaced fractures of the lateral condyle can be treated conservatively.

    **C** A high incidence of medial epicondylar fractures (60%) has been reported in association with elbow dislocations.

    **D** Radial neck fractures with malalignment of greater than 30 degrees should be reduced.

    **E** The most common nerve injured in paediatric supracondylar fractures is the anterior interosseous branch of the median nerve.

A12  B  All displaced lateral condyle fractures require open reduction and internal fixation as they involve an articular surface. Care is taken to avoid disruption of the blood supply of the trochlea by avoiding posterior dissection. Careful anterior exposure is performed of the joint and fracture to ensure adequate reduction of articular surface. Knowledge of the sequence, timing and appearance of secondary ossification centres around the elbow is essential in making the correct diagnosis. The order of appearance may be abbreviated by CRITOE, which stands for capitellum, radial head, medial (internal) epicondyle, trochlea, olecranon and lateral (external) epicondyle. A high incidence of medial epicondylar fractures (60%) has been reported in association with elbow dislocations. A major concern following this injury is incarceration of the medial epicondyle in the joint. Radial neck fractures with a malalignment of greater than 30 degrees should be reduced using closed or percutaneous means. Open reduction in these situations has a high rate of osteonecrosis and non-union.

The anterior interosseous branch of the median nerve is the most common nerve injured in paediatric supracondylar fractures. Median nerve function is assessed by testing thenar opposition for intrinsic innervation, and the anterior interosseous nerve is evaluated by assessing flexor pollicis longus and flexor digitorum profundus to the index finger. Most displaced paediatric supracondylar fractures are treated by closed reduction under radiographic control followed by stabilisation with two to three lateral-entry divergent K wires and long arm casting. Medial pins are avoided for fear of iatrogenic ulnar nerve injury.

Q13  Which of the following is untrue for paediatric forearm fractures?

A  Diaphyseal fractures of the forearm can be divided into three categories according to pattern of injury: plastic deformation, incomplete or greenstick, and bicortical or complete fractures.

B  Reducing and stabilising the ulnar fracture is the key to maintaining radial head reduction in Monteggia's fractures.

C  Indications for surgical treatment in bicortical forearm fractures include irreducible or unstable fractures, floating elbow injuries.

D  Distal radial fractures are rare in children.

E  Most distal radial physeal fractures are Salter–Harris type 2 fractures that are treated with closed reduction and above-elbow cast mobilisation.

A13  D  Between 75% and 84% of all forearm fractures in children involve the distal radius, of which 15%–20% involve the distal radial physis. Diaphyseal fractures of the forearm can be divided into three categories based on pattern of injury. Clinical and radiographic manifestations of plastic deformation may be subtle and at times, if left uncorrected, may result in limitation of forearm rotation. Greenstick fractures account for approximately 50% of diaphyseal fractures and typically occur in younger children. Greenstick fractures are treated with closed reduction followed by a well-moulded cast. Bicortical fractures occur in older children and have a higher predisposition for instability. Indications for surgical treatment in bicortical forearm fractures include irreducible or unstable fractures and floating elbow injuries. Stabilisation may be achieved with a plate and screw construct or intramedullary fixation. Intramedullary fixation usually requires additional postoperative cast immobilisation as it does not provide rotational stability.

**Q14** Which of the following is true regarding injuries of the paediatric spine?

    **A** Special care needs to be during immobilisation and transport of the paediatric patient, keeping in mind certain anatomical differences in the paediatric upper body from adult patients.

    **B** SCIWORA (spinal cord injury without radiological abnormality) is more common in the paediatric population than the adult population.

    **C** MRI is the test of choice for determining and defining spinal cord injury.

    **D** Spondylolysis is believed to be related to repetitive microtrauma.

    **E** All of the above.

**A14** **E** Compared with adults, the head of a child is proportionately larger. As a result, immobilisation on a standard adult backboard will lead to flexion of a child's neck and potentially worsen a cervical spine injury. Hence an infant or toddler with possible neck injury should be transported with a pad under the shoulders in order to maintain the neck in a neutral position. SCIWORA is characterised by presence of a spinal cord injury in a patient with normal radiographic studies. The cervical spine is most commonly involved and neurologic injuries may be complete or incomplete. MRI can usually delineate cord changes such as swelling, contusion or infarction. Spondylolysis, which is a stress fracture of the pars interarticularis, is not caused by a single traumatic event but believed to be related to repetitive microtrauma. It usually occurs in adolescents who are highly active. Bracing, physical therapy focused on hamstring stretching and abdominal strengthening are the mainstays of treatment.

## Further reading

Anglen JO, Choi L. Treatment options in pediatric femoral shaft fractures. *J Orthop Trauma.* 2005; **19**(10): 724–33.

Dormans JP, Squillante R, Sharf H. Acute neurovascular complications with supracondylar humerus fractures in children. *J Hand Surg Am.* 1995; **20**(1): 1–4.

Pang D. Spinal cord Injury without radiographic abnormality in children, 2 decades later. *Neurosurgery.* 2004; **55**(6): 1325–42, discussion 1342–3.

# CHAPTER 13

# Bites and burns

## FAISAL G QURESHI, FELIX C BLANCO, KURT D NEWMAN

**From the choices below each question, select the single best answer.**

**Q1** The treatment of severe snakebite envenomation includes all *except which one of the following?*

**A** The initial dose of snake antivenin in children is half the required dose for adults.

**B** Aggressive intravenous hydration should follow the administration of antivenin.

**C** Extremity fasciotomy is rarely necessary.

**D** The polyvalent form of antivenin is more allergenic than the ovine Fab antivenin.

**E** Alkalinise the urine with bicarbonate and administer mannitol.

**A1** **A** Mild snakebite envenomation manifests with localised oedema and absence of systemic symptoms. These patients can be discharged from the hospital after an observation period of 24 hours. The oedema in moderate envenomation is more pronounced; there may be localised blisters and the patient experiences non-specific systemic effects such as nausea, vomiting or tachycardia. Signs of severe envenomation include rapid progression of local and systemic signs, hypotension, petechiae, abnormal laboratory values, coagulopathy, seizures and death. It is important to transport the victim immediately to a specialised centre where the antivenin is administered without delay. Snake antivenin should be administered in cases of moderate or severe envenomation, not mild. Because the blood volume in children is small in relation to the venom concentration, the dose of antivenin in paediatric patients is usually double the required dose for adults, not half. Immediately after the administration of antivenin, aggressive resuscitation with intravenous fluids should be instituted. Rarely wound debridement and limb fasciotomy are needed, but the affected limb should be examined constantly in search of signs of compartment syndrome.

Crotalide polyvalent antivenin is frequently associated with allergic reactions compared with the new ovine Fab antivenin, which is safer in children.

In cases of moderate envenomation, an abnormal coagulation value without bleeding is common. Coagulopathy after severe snake envenomation usually presents with active bleeding. In this case, ICU admission and aggressive management of coagulopathy should be implemented.

Similarly, extensive rhabdomyolysis puts the patient at risk for renal failure. In this case, the urine should be alkalinised with intravenous bicarbonate and mannitol.

 **Q2** Which one of the following statements regarding spider bites is *correct*?

   **A** The brown recluse spider is identified by its eight paired eyes and a violin-shaped cephalothorax.
   **B** The management of mild spider envenomation requires the use of antivenin.
   **C** Systemic signs after black widow and funnel web spider bites include autonomic and neuromuscular hyperactivity.
   **D** The neurotoxin released by *Loxosceles reclusa* (brown recluse spider) causes severe cutaneous necrosis.
   **E** Dapsone is the first-line treatment for brown recluse bite.

**A2** **C** The two most common species of spider responsible for arachnidism in the United States are the black widow (*Lactrodectus* spp.) and brown recluse (*Loxosceles reclusa*) spiders. Characteristically, the brown recluse spider has six paired eyes (most spiders have eight). The funnel web (*Atrax* spp.) spider is a common venomous spider in Australia. Mild to moderate symptoms of arachnidism are treated with supportive measures only. Systemic signs indicate severe envenomation and require prompt use of antivenin in children; black widow and funnel web spiders produce a potent neurotoxin responsible for autonomic hyperactivity, muscle rigidity, spasms and occasionally respiratory arrest.

Localised cutaneous necrosis is often found after brown recluse spider bite and is caused by local enzymatic destruction secondary to cytotoxic venom, not a neurotoxin. This should be treated with limb elevation, ice compresses and local wound care. Healing takes several weeks and rarely requires extensive debridement. There is no strong evidence to support the use of Dapsone in humans although it is frequently administered.

Rarely, loxoscelism presents with systemic toxicity such as hypotension, renal failure, seizures or even coma.

**Q3** Which one of the following statements is *not* true regarding scorpion sting?

**A** Severe scorpion envenomation is more common in children than adults.

**B** Scorpion antivenin is contraindicated in children.

**C** The syndrome of severe envenomation includes neuromotor hyperactivity, cardiorespiratory compromise and visual abnormalities.

**D** Neuromotor hyperactivity may be treated in the ICU with high doses of benzodiazepines.

**E** The administration of scorpion antivenin can successfully reduce the symptoms of severe envenomation.

 **A3** **B** *Centruroides* is the only species of scorpion responsible for severe envenomation in the United States. Mild envenomation causes only local burning pain and resolves spontaneously within a few hours. However, this is not the case in children who usually have a serious clinical syndrome consisting of neuromotor hyperactivity, visual abnormalities, and respiratory compromise due to excessive secretions, bronchospasm and pulmonary oedema. Traditionally, and before the availability of the antivenin, these patients were treated in the ICU with high doses of benzodiazepines and ventilatory support. The prompt administration of scorpion antivenin obviates the need for such extreme measures. This is not contraindicated in children.

**Q4** Which one of the following statements is *true* regarding dog bites?

**A** The majority of dog bites in children occur in the upper extremity.

**B** Routine use of systemic antibiotics is recommended to treat any type of dog bite.

**C** Primary closure of bite wounds should only be attempted in deep lacerations involving the face.

**D** Staphylococcus is the most common pathogen responsible for delayed wound infection after dog bites.

**E** Prophylaxis against rabies should be started within the first week if the dog's vaccination certificate cannot be obtained.

**A4** **D** Dog bites are common in children under 10 years of age. The head and neck area is affected almost 50% of the time, followed by the upper and lower extremities with 28% and 18%, respectively. Superficial bite wounds should be treated with local care and the patient discharged from the emergency department with no antibiotics. For deep lacerations, admission to the surgical floor, administration of systemic antibiotics and early surgical intervention is recommended. Copious irrigation, debridement of devitalised tissue and closure of all deep lacerations is the standard treatment. Although *Pasteurella multocida* is found in the oral flora of dogs and is associated with very early infections, *Staphylococcus* spp. is for the most part responsible for wound infections occurring 24 hours after the bite.

If the dog's certificate of vaccination against rabies cannot be obtained within 24 hours, the patient should be placed on a rabies vaccine schedule. Tetanus status should be investigated.

 **Q5** Which one of the following statements is not true regarding the epidemiology of paediatric?

**A** Burn injuries constitute the second leading cause of accidental death of children in the United States.

**B** Most scald burn injuries occur in children younger than 4 years of age.

**C** Areas commonly affected by scald burns include the face and hands.

**D** A stocking-glove distribution of a burn indicates possible child abuse.

**E** Contact with hot liquids at temperatures of 100°F for more than 3 seconds can cause severe thermal burns in children

**A5** **E** Thermal injuries can be caused by flame, by contact with hot surfaces or by scalding due to hot fluids. Over 500 children per year die from severe burns in the United States making it the second leading cause of accidental death.

Spillage of hot food or beverages is the commonest cause of scald burns in children under 4 years of age. The areas usually affected are the hands and face. Child abuse should be suspected when the burn is localised in the perineum, has a stocking-glove distribution or when burn care has been neglected.

For a thermal burn to occur, the contact with the offending agent should be for at least for 3 seconds at a temperature greater than 120°F (49°C). Therefore most homes in the United States have the hot water temperature set at less than 110°F (43°C).

 **Q6** Which one of the following statements is *correct* regarding skin and burn physiology?

**A** The total surface area of skin in a newborn is approximately $0.5 \, m^2$.

**B** According to the Lund and Browder chart, the surface area of skin represented by the head and neck in infants is approximately 25%.

**C** A neurovascular plexus separates the epidermis from the papillary dermis.

**D** Full thickness burns re-epithelialise from retained appendages in the reticular dermis.

**E** The zone of stasis in burned tissue has impaired blood flow secondary to an increase in local inflammatory mediators.

A6   **E**   The skin exerts an essential role in body thermoregulation and fluid homeostasis, and is the main barrier against opportunistic organisms. The total surface area of skin in a newborn is 0.25 m². Unlike adults, the head represents approximately 18% of the body surface area in children under 4 years of age according to the Lund and Browder chart. This chart estimates the surface area in children more precisely than the classic Rule of Nines.

The depth of the burn is classified according to the affected skin layer. Superficial or first-degree burns affect only the epidermis, are erythematous, oedematous and resolve in about a week without scarring. Partial thickness or second-degree burns are divided into superficial and deep if the papillary or reticular dermis respectively, is affected. Because a rich neurovascular plexus separates the papillary from the reticular dermis, a superficial partial-thickness burn is exquisitely painful, with blanching erythema and often with blisters (Figure 13.1). It re-epithelialises in 2 weeks from residual epidermal appendages without scarring. A deep partial-thickness burn penetrates into the reticular dermis, clinically presents with non-blanching erythema and is often insensate (Figure 13.2). It usually requires skin grafting. A full-thickness burn involves all layers of the skin into the subcutaneous tissue. Its clinical appearance is dry and leathery and is insensate because of the complete destruction of all nerve terminals (Figure 13.3). This burn will not re-epithelialise and will require a skin graft.

Some recognise a fourth category in which the burn penetrates into the muscle, tendon or bone.

The centre of the burn is called the zone of coagulation and represents the necrotic eschar. Immediately around this area, the zone of stasis represents all the borderline viable tissue that can be rescued with appropriate management. Intense local release of inflammatory mediators decreases the blood flow to this area. Finally, the hyperaemic zone is the viable tissue surrounding the burn.

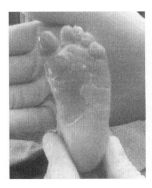
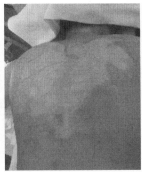
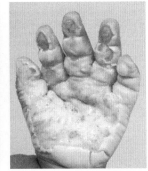

FIGURE 13.1 Superficial partial-thickness burn

FIGURE 13.2 Deep partial-thickness burn

FIGURE 13.3 Full-thickness burn

**Q7** Which one of the following statements regarding initial resuscitation after burn injuries is *not* correct?

**A** Intubation and ventilator support should be instituted in cases of extensive burns and burns in closed spaces.

**B** The preferred initial resuscitation fluid in children is 0.9% normal saline solution.

**C** The estimation of fluid requirements should consider partial- and full-thickness burns only.

**D** The fluid requirement in children with burns equals the sum of the fluid estimated by the Parkland formula plus the maintenance requirement.

**E** Urine output of 1 mL/kg/hr accurately reflects appropriate fluid resuscitation.

 **A7** **B** The ABC of resuscitation should be applied to all victims of burns, and endotracheal intubation should be considered not only in patients subjected to inhalation injury but also in those with extensive burns. Signs of inhalation injury include singed nasal hair and carbonaceous sputum. Following the management of the airway, large-bore IV lines should be obtained, preferably but not necessarily away from the area burned. Anticipate the need for central lines to avoid displacement of short IV catheters when massive oedema is expected. Lactated Ringer's solution (LR) is perhaps the best initial resuscitation fluid, not only because of its low sodium concentration but also because of its buffering effect on metabolic acidosis.

Estimates of resuscitation fluid may be achieved by various methods and are based on the affected body surface (TBSA), weight and only begun for partial- and full-thickness burns, not superficial. In addition, most clinicians agree that resuscitation should be started only when the TBSA burned is more than 15% in children. The Parkland formula is the most used and is applied for the first 24 hours as follows:

$$4\,mL \times TBSA(\%) \times weight(kg).$$

Half the estimated amount should be administered within the first 8 hours after the event (not the first time seen in the ER) and the other half in the remaining 16 hours. For children under 4 years old, the maintenance fluid requirement and dextrose should be added to the calculated amount, as D5 LR. After the first 24 hours, when capillary permeability has stabilised, the addition of albumin may be beneficial.

The end point of resuscitation is the appropriate perfusion of end organs. A good indicator of a good resuscitation is a urine output of at least 1 mL/kg/hr.

| Age (y) | 0 | 1 | 5 | 10 | 15 | Adult |
|---|---|---|---|---|---|---|
| A = Half of head | 9.5 | 8.5 | 6.5 | 5.5 | 4.5 | 3.5 |
| B = Half of thigh | 2.75 | 3.25 | 4 | 4.25 | 4.25 | 4.75 |
| C = Half of leg | 2.5 | 2.5 | 2.75 | 3 | 3.25 | 3.5 |

**TABLE 13.1 Lund and Browder chart**

 **Q**8 Which one of the following statements is *true* regarding topical agents for burns?

**A** Silver sulfadiazine penetrates the burn eschar efficiently but causes hyponatraemia.

**B** Silver sulfadiazide is effective against Pseudomonas.

**C** The main side effect of Sulfamylon is leucopenia.

**D** Silver nitrate is an alternative topical agent for facial burns.

**E** Antibiotic ointments are recommended for facial burns and small partial-thickness burns.

 **A**8 **E** The initial management of most partial- and full-thickness burns consists of topical preparations. These agents prevent, or at least minimise, the bacterial colonisation of the wound and provide a favourable environment for wound healing or in preparation for skin grafting. Superficial or first-degree burns do not require any special treatment. Aloe vera ointments and protection from the sun are sufficient measures to promote healing. For partial-thickness burns, excision of large blisters and debridement of the eschar under sedation is necessary for proper burn care. Small blisters are left alone because they act as a natural barrier against microbial invasion. Once exposed, the dermis or deeper tissues should be covered with various preparations.

Silver sulfadiazide is an excellent agent, but does not penetrate the eschar and sometimes produces reversible leucopenia. It has poor coverage against Pseudomonas. Mafenide acetate or Sulfamylon penetrates the eschar and protects against Pseudomonas, but its administration is painful and causes metabolic acidosis due to carbonic anhydrase inhibition. Silver nitrate has a broad coverage and its application is painless. Its major side effects are electrolyte abnormalities such as hyponatraemia and silver staining of the skin. This side effect limits its use on the face.

For small partial-thickness burns or burns on the face, antibiotic ointment is recommended.

**9** Which one of the following statements concerning burn dressings is *not* correct?

A The ideal wound dressing promotes spontaneous epithelialisation, acts as a scaffold, provides moisture and is durable.

B Site, extent and depth of the wound determines the type of dressing selection.

C Membrane dressings are biological films that promote epithelialisation after adherence to the burn bed.

D Decellularised dermis serves as a scaffold for epithelial cell migration in full-thickness burns.

E Porcine skin can be used as a temporary skin substitute when large burned surfaces need coverage.

 **C** The first step in the management of partial- or full-thickness burns is the application of an appropriate dressing. This should not only provide coverage and prevent fluid losses but also act as a barrier against infection, serve as a scaffold for re-epithelialisation, and provide moisture and durability, thus avoiding frequent and painful dressing changes. The type of dressing depends largely on the depth and extent of the burn.

For most superficial partial-thickness burns, topical creams such as silver sulfadiazide followed by the application of membrane dressings is enough. Membrane dressings are synthetic films that adhere to the burned skin, serving as a scaffold. Silver-impregnated films are an example and they do not have to be changed at all because they separate off after complete epithelialisation has occurred. Silver components should be avoided on the face because they cause staining. Decellularised dermis is a biologic agent that serves the same purpose and its use is appropriate in cases of full-thickness burns.

Often, large burns require extensive coverage that can only be achieved through the use of temporary substitutes such as porcine skin. Meshing the skin graft is a simple method to expand the graft and accomplish coverage, but should be avoided on the face, neck or hands because of poor cosmetic results.

**Q10** Which of the following statements is *true* regarding skin grafting?

A Excision and skin grafting should be delayed for at least 2 weeks after the inflammatory response has subsided.

B Blood loss from excision of the eschar is prominent during the first 48 hours.

C Partial thickness autografts are less prone to wound contraction and their 'take' is always 100%.

D Full-thickness allografts are prone to excessive contraction.

E The donor site of full-thickness grafts may be closed primarily.

A10  **E**  It is important to remove burned devitalised tissue to cease the immunosuppressive and inflammatory response. Several studies demonstrated that delayed excision and grafting expose the patient to risk of wound infection, sepsis and multiorgan failure. After the first 48 hours, the burn has already started the process of angiogenesis, this may be responsible for substantial bleeding during the delayed excision of the eschar.

The most common technique of excision is the tangential method, using a sharp blade or dermatome. The excision should be continued until viable tissue is observed or sometimes to the fascial plane.

Skin grafts are named according to their origin. A graft from the same patient is an autograft; it as an isograft if it comes from a twin, an allograft if it comes from another human and a xenograft if it comes from another species. According to the layers of skin included in the graft, it is classified as split-thickness skin graft (STSG) if it includes the epidermis and dermis, and full-thickness skin graft (FTSG) if it includes all layers of the skin. The STSG donor sites should be covered with a temporary dressing such as petroleum gauze. These dressings will slough off the wound after epithelialisation occurs.

FTSG take is excellent and it undergoes less contraction than STSG, which is paramount when a graft is used in hands or joints. Even more, the colour matching is optimal in cosmetic areas like the face. For FTSG, primary closure or STSG should be done.

Q11  Which one of the following statements is *incorrect* regarding the hypermetabolic response to burns?

  **A**  Between 20% and 40% of the total caloric intake should be derived from proteins.

  **B**  Intravenous hyperalimentation is currently recommended to boost the immune system.

  **C**  Enteral feeding prevents intestinal mucosal atrophy and decreases the level of catabolic hormones

  **D**  Formulas to calculate the caloric requirements in burned children are based on burned body surface.

  **E**  Hyperglycaemia in burn patients is caused by hepatic insulin resistance.

A11  **B**  The paediatric patient is extremely vulnerable to malnutrition after burns. The small proportion of fat and muscle in children compared with adults makes them prone to protein-caloric malnutrition. Hence it is important to provide a balanced nutrition consisting of protein-derived calories of about 20%–40% and carbohydrate-derived calories of 40%–70%. Several catabolic hormones such as catecholamines and cortisol are released as a primary response and their action can persist for months. These, along with the potent inflammatory response cause physiologic stress and increased metabolic demands.

Intravenous hyperalimentation, once thought to be useful in burned patients, is now avoided because of its deleterious effects on the immune system and the gut. The enteral route is preferred because it not only achieves the nutritional goals but also prevents intestinal mucosal atrophy, translocation and indirectly decreases the levels of catabolic hormones.

The estimation of the caloric requirements can be obtained from the Curreri formula as follows:

25 kcal/kg + 40 kcal/% TBSA.

Appropriate enteral nutrition should be instituted as soon as possible either by the oral route or through feeding tubes. Delays can result in malnutrition, organ dysfunction and delayed wound healing.

Hyperglycaemia in the burned patient results from hepatic insulin resistance and the persistent effect of catabolic hormones.

**Q12** Which one of the following statements is *correct* regarding inhalation injury?

**A** Severe symptoms of inhalation injury include cough, wheezing and shortness of breath.

**B** Pulmonary injury can be ruled out if the initial chest X-ray (CXR) and arterial blood gas (ABG) are normal.

**C** Oxygen therapy should be started when carboxyhaemoglobin levels exceed 20%.

**D** The half-life of carboxyhaemoglobin is approximately 2 hours.

**E** Lactic acidosis, high mixed-venous saturations and unresponsiveness to oxygen therapy are indicators of cyanide toxicity

**A12** **E** The clinical presentation of inhalation injury ranges from mild respiratory symptoms such as cough, shortness of breath and wheezing to a more-severe clinical picture with confusion, coma and cardiopulmonary arrest.

Smoke inhalation injury affects four different levels: (1) upper airway, causing swelling and ulceration of the mucosa; (2) tracheobronchial, causing oedema and formation of 'airway casts' leading to bronchial obstruction; (3) alveolar, causing alveolar oedema, loss of surfactant and excessive inflammatory infiltrate; and (4) systemic, due to hypoxaemia and the absorption of toxins such as carbon monoxide (CO) and cyanide.

A baseline CXR and ABG should always be obtained and repeated in 12–24 hours because pulmonary injury is often underestimated by initial radiographs.

Supplemental oxygen at 100% by non-rebreather mask should be instituted early in the management of smoke inhalation injury and not delayed by waiting on

CO levels. If appropriate, intubate the patient in anticipation of worsening airway oedema. Perform an early bronchoscopy to determine the extent of injury and to clear the bronchi from soot, accumulated mucus and airway casts. Administer bronchodilators and institute aggressive pulmonary toilet. The role of steroids in the management of inhalation injury is controversial.

CO has 200-fold affinity for haemoglobin compared with oxygen and shifts the dissociation curve left, making oxygen less available. Symptoms secondary to elevated carboxyhaemoglobin are usually present when the level is above 10%. The administration of 100% oxygen decreases the half-life from 6 hours to 60 minutes. Hyperbaric oxygen at 2–3 atm reduces even more the half-life of CO to 15 minutes, but its availability is limited.

Cyanide blocks oxidative phosphorylation by inhibition of the cytochrome oxidase, resulting in increased lactic acid levels, metabolic acidosis and high mixed-venous saturation. It is released from the partial combustion of plastics. Treatment of cyanide toxicity should include a combination of oxygen with sodium thiosulfate or amyl nitrite. Hydroxycobalamin (vitamin $B_{12}$) creates cyanide compounds that facilitate its excretion by the kidneys.

**Q13** Which one of the following statements regarding caustic dermal injuries is *not correct*?

  **A**  Irrigation of alkali burns should be performed for at least 12 hours.
  **B**  High-pressure burn irrigation is preferred to low-pressure irrigation.
  **C**  Exothermic acid–base reactions limit the use of neutralising agents.
  **D**  The corneal pH after irrigation should be at least 7.3 to prevent permanent damage.
  **E**  Intravenous magnesium is as effective as intra-arterial calcium infusion for hydrofluoric acid burns.

**A13**  **B**  Caustic agents include acids and alkalis. They are found in multiple detergents, housecleaning and plumbing agents. Acids produce coagulation necrosis and their penetration is limited by the formation of a thick eschar. Sulphuric acid is the most common acid associated with chemical burns and typically produces a black eschar. Once identified, an acid burn should be irrigated for at least 2–3 hours. Alkalis produce liquefaction necrosis that may persist for several hours, so it is important to irrigate the affected tissues for at least 12 hours.

After the contaminated clothing is removed, low-pressure irrigation should be started. Tap water is preferable to neutralising agents because the latter could generate an exothermic acid–base reaction that would produce further tissue damage.

Ocular chemical burns should be irrigated from 30 to 60 minutes and the pH of the cornea measured. Any level below pH 7.3 requires that the irrigation should be continued. Ophthalmology consultation should be obtained immediately.

Fluoride ions released by hydrofluoric acid avidly penetrate tissues and cause severe burns with uncontrollable pain. For small and superficial burns with hydrofluoric acid, the application of 2.5% calcium gluconate gel is sufficient. For deep burns or burns on the hand, it is necessary to inject calcium gluconate either subcutaneously or intra-arterially. Calcium sequesters fluoride ions. Recent studies have shown that intravenous administration of magnesium is as effective as, and less complicated than, the administration of intra-arterial calcium.

**Q14** Which one of the statements below is *not correct* regarding electrical injuries?

A  High voltage is defined as greater than 1000 V.

B  The entry and exit wounds caused by alternating current are usually full thickness.

C  Breaks in the skin lower its resistance to electrical current.

D  The electrical path in the direction of one hand to another can be associated with ventricular fibrillation.

E  An asymptomatic patient with a normal initial ECG does not require continuous monitoring.

**A14**  **B**  Electrical injuries are common in children. The *current* and *voltage* are directly related to the degree of injury caused by electricity. Alternating current of low voltage (< 1000 V), commonly found in homes, deliver an electrical current that generates a prolonged muscle tetany and cardiac conduction abnormalities. Ventricular fibrillation is the most common arrhythmia.

The entry and exit electrical injury wounds are usually small and full thickness. They are not usually associated with alternating current, rather, are the result of direct-current or high-voltage electricity and may indicate serious injury to internal organs.

*Impedance* is defined as resistance to electrical current flow. The resistance is low in tissues such as muscles, nerves and vessels and high in the skin, bone and fat. So, the skin offers significant protection against electrical injuries. This resistance decreases when the skin is wet or damaged.

An electric current path from a hand to a hand or hand to foot, travels through the chest and may cause cardiac arrhythmias such as ventricular fibrillation.

All patients with electrical burns should have a workup that includes an ECG, complete blood cell count, electrolytes, creatine phosphokinase level and urinalysis. A normal initial ECG in a patient with a low-voltage electrical injury, no history of seizures or loss of consciousness and a normal urinalysis can be discharged after a few hours of observation in the emergency room.

Patients with severe injuries, ECG abnormalities, loss of consciousness during the event, myoglobinuria or high-voltage injuries must be hospitalised.

## Further reading

Boyer LV, Theodorou AA, Berg RA, *et al.* Antivenom for critically ill children with neurotoxicity from scorpion stings. *N Engl J Med.* 2009; **360**(20): 2090–8.

Corneille MG, Larson S, Stewart RM, *et al.* A large single-center experience with treatment of patients with crotalid envenomations: outcomes with and evolution of antivenin therapy. *Am J Surg.* 2006; **192**(6): 848–52.

Grosfeld JL, O'Neill JA, Fonkalsrud EW, *et al.*, editors. *Pediatric Surgery. Vol. 1.* 6th ed. Philadelphia, PA: Mosby; 2006.

Koumbourlis AC. Electrical injuries. *Crit Care Med.* 2002; **30**(11 Suppl.): S424–30.

Monstrey S, Hoeksema H, Verbelen J, *et al.* Assessment of burn depth and burn wound healing potential. *Burns.* 2008; **34**(6): 761–9.

Palao R, Monge I, Ruiz M, *et al.* Chemical burns: pathophysiology and treatment. *Burns.* 2010; **36**(3): 295–304.

Rehberg S, Maybauer MO, Enkhbaatar P, *et al.* Pathophysiology, management and treatment of smoke inhalation injury. *Expert Rev Respir Med.* 2009; **3**(3): 283–97.

Saucier JR. Arachnid envenomation. *Emerg Med Clin North Am.* 2004; **22**(2): 405–22.

# CHAPTER 14

# Child abuse and birth injuries

## NATASHA DE VERE

**From the choices below each question, select the single best answer.**

**Q1** Which of the following are *not* at increased risk of child abuse or neglect?

   **A** families living in areas of community violence

   **B** children born prematurely

   **C** children with learning disability

   **D** families with religious faith participation

   **E** children exposed to domestic violence

**A1** **D** Several risk factors have been identified for child abuse and neglect. These risk factors fall into the categories of child factors, parental factors and environmental factors. More recently researchers and policy makers have identified protective factors against abuse. The most significant risk factors are having a parent aged younger than 21 years, having a history of mental illness or depression, or living with a violent adult. Religious faith participation has been found to be one of several social/environmental protective factors.

**Q2** Which of the following is not true?

   **A** Parental responsibility may be acquired through the court by a residence order.

   **B** Both parents have parental responsibility if they were married at the time of the child's birth.

   **C** Both parents have parental responsibility if they were cohabiting at the time of the child's birth.

   **D** A father may acquire parental responsibility by marrying the mother.

   **E** Parental responsibility can be exercised by one person independently.

**A2** **C** Parental responsibility – the Children Act 1989 introduced the concept of parental responsibility. Parental responsibility can be held by one or more people at a time. It is important in cases of abuse or for consenting to medical treatment. Fathers have responsibility only if they were married to the mother at the time of birth, they marry the mother later, they obtain a court order, they have a formal agreement with the mother, or are present at the registration of the birth and are recorded as such.

**Q3** Bruising to which of the following areas is likely to be accidental?

 **A** neck

 **B** ear

 **C** buttocks

 **D** hip

 **E** genitalia

**A3** **D** Bruising is a common injury from physical child abuse and from accidental causes. Bruises in certain areas are predictive of abuse. Any bruise in an area that is protected should be given a high index of suspicion (neck, ears, torso, genitalia), areas over bones are more likely to be accidental (limbs, spine, hips).

**Q4** In a mobile child who is currently well, with multiple bruises to her legs and buttocks and a slightly swollen left ankle, which of the following is most likely?

 **A** meningococcal sepsis

 **B** von Willebrand's deficiency

 **C** idiopathic thrombocytopenic purpura (ITP)

 **D** Henoch–Schönlein's purpura (HSP)

 **E** Ehlers–Danlos's syndrome

**A4** **A** Meningococcal sepsis causing multiple bruises is usually seen in a child who is very unwell, peripherally shut down, drowsy and who may be pyrexial. Von Willebrand's deficiency usually presents with prolonged bleeding after a surgical/dental procedure or because of a family history. This picture could be seen in ITP but the bruising is usually all over the body rather than confined to the lower limbs. HSP commonly presents with petechiae and purpura and often with inflamed joints. Ehlers–Danlos's can present with easy bruising but this is rarely seen, and would not normally be seen acutely.

**Q5** Which of the following is least likely to be mistaken for child abuse?

 **A** capillary haemangioma

 **B** Mongolian blue spot

 **C** café au lait macules

 **D** varicella zoster infection

 **E** sucking blisters

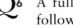**5** **D** Capillary haemangiomas, though often present at birth, tend to darken and become more visible after a few weeks/months and can therefore be mistaken for new unexplained bruises. Mongolian blue spots look very similar to bruises over the spine and therefore if not known about could cause confusion. Café au lait macules also develop over time and are often on the buttocks and thighs. Varicella zoster is usually easily recognised because it is so common. Sucking blisters are small blisters that can be mistaken for burns but are always in an area that a baby can get into their mouth to be able to suck.

**Q6** A full blood count and coagulation screen will miss which of the following?

 **A** haemophilia

 **B** platelet function defect

 **C** idiopathic thrombocytopenic purpura

 **D** warfarin ingestion

 **E** disseminated intravascular coagulation

**6** **B** Haemophilia can be diagnosed with a very raised activated partial thrombo-plastin time (aPTT). Blood count in ITP will show very low platelet count. Warfarin ingestion will show a raised prothrombin time (PT) and INR (interenational nor-malised ratio). Disseminated intravascular coagulation will show raised aPTT, PT and fibrinogen is likely to be low. In a platelet function defect the platelet count will be normal and therefore platelet function testing is needed if suspected.

**Q7** Which of these investigations would not usually be required in a 9-month-old with unexplained bruising to the abdomen?

 **A** skeletal survey

 **B** vitamin D levels

 **C** CT head

 **D** CT abdomen

 **E** ophthalmological examination

**7** **B** Bruising to the cheek in a non-mobile child would be indicative of non-accidental injury. In a child under 2 years a skeletal survey, CT head and ophthalmology examination are indicated. With bruising to the abdomen a CT abdomen is important to look for internal injuries. Vitamin D levels would not be required unless these investigations show fractures or bony abnormalities.

Q8 Which of the following fractures has a high specificity for child abuse?
 A long bone diaphyseal
 B rib
 C long bone metaphyseal
 D scapula
 E spine

A8 **A** Diaphyseal fractures are four times more common than metaphyseal fractures. Metaphyseal fractures can be caused by gripping, twisting, pulling and possibly shaking. They are often not accompanied by swelling and bruising, and may not develop callus.

Q9 Rib fractures are best detected:
 A by chest X-ray (CXR) following acute presentation of injury
 B as part of skeletal survey
 C by delayed CXR
 D clinically with bruising
 E following detection of visceral injuries.

A9 **C** Rib fractures may not be easy to see on an acute CXR, or on skeletal survey if the injury has been recent, therefore a delayed CXR (2 weeks later) is advised.

Q10 Indicators of sexual abuse include:
 A recurrent UTIs in a toddler
 B constipation in a 10-year-old requiring regular laxatives to ensure regular bowel movements
 C a 7-year-old girl wanting to dress like her mum
 D rectal prolapse in a toddler
 E wrist-cutting in a 14-year-old girl.

A10 **E** Recurrent UTIs are common in children who aren't yet potty-trained, particularly if there is constipation. Constipation itself is very common in all ages of children but if it is intractable or more often there is encopresis then all forms of abuse should be considered. Young girls commonly wish to mimic their mother's behaviour and appearance. Rectal prolapse is common in children under 5 and is usually secondary to constipation but can be associated with cystic fibrosis and Hirschprung's disease. Self-harm is an important presentation of sexual abuse but may be hard to elucidate.

Q11 A 13-year-old girl is referred with abdominal pain and is found to be pregnant. She discloses that her Mum's partner is likely to be the father of the child. She states she doesn't want her mother to know. What should you do?

A Tell her that what she tells you is confidential.

B Refer to the obstetric unit and expect that they will look into the relationship.

C Contact social services without telling her.

D Advise her that her safety is a concern and in this case you must break her confidence to inform social services.

E Talk to her mother and mother's partner about these allegations.

A11 **D** Confidentiality is the responsibility of any doctor who suspects abuse. Although the patient's relationship may be consensual, there is a high likelihood the girl has been manipulated and the age difference is likely to be big. As she is only 13, a sexual relationship is illegal.

Q12 A 3-year-old boy with quadriplegic cerebral palsy is brought to your outpatient clinic. He had a percutaneous endoscopic gastrostomy (PEG) tube inserted by you last year because of unsafe swallowing. He has gained very little weight over the last year and appears very quiet. His PEG site is very inflamed and excoriated. When you examine him his nappy is soiled and he has an extensive excoriated nappy rash. There is also an area of skin breakdown over his back. Mum tells you she saw the GP recently but he did not do anything. When you check the notes he has failed to attend his neurodisability clinic appointments. The best course of action would be:

A referral to social services

B ask Mum to take him back to the GP about the areas of skin breakdown

C discuss his case with other professionals involved

D admit him for observation of his feeding

E copy a clinic letter to the neurodisability consultant he sees.

A12 **A** This child is showing many signs of neglect. He is at increased risk of abuse because of his disability. A referral to social services is indicated as a child in need. It would also be useful to follow this up with discussions with other professionals involved in his case. A multi-agency assessment would be indicated. Options C and E would also be important but not the most important.

**Q13** An 18-month-old boy was transferred to a neurosurgical unit with severe head trauma. The history given was that he had climbed onto a chest of drawers and fallen onto a wooden floor. Initial investigations at the referring hospital showed a mildly reduced haemoglobin, normal urea and electrolytes and raised transaminases (AST 250, ALT 458). Bilirubin level was normal. What should your next step be?

   **A** exclude abdominal injury on clinical examination

   **B** repeat transaminases and if falling, observe

   **C** CT abdomen

   **D** laparotomy

   **E** clinical observation

**A13** **C** Occult liver injuries occur as a result of physical abuse. Raised transaminases are a good indicator of abdominal injury. The result should be followed up by CT abdomen. The history given is unlikely to have caused such severe head trauma, therefore abuse is likely.

**Q14** Which of the following should be treated urgently with vitamin K and fresh frozen plasma?

   **A** a large subaponeurotic haemorrhage

   **B** a chignon

   **C** a cephalhaematoma

   **D** a caput succedaneum

   **E** a laceration to the scalp from forcep use

**A14** **A** A subaponeurotic haemorrhage is a haemorrhage between the aponeurosis and periosteum and is therefore not limited by the suture lines. It is rare but is associated with vacuum and instrumental deliveries. A chignon is the area where the vacuum was applied in a vacuum delivery. A cephalhaematoma may follow an instrumental or normal delivery but is differentiated from the subaponeurotic haemorrhage because the haemorrhage does not cross suture lines. A caput is a serosanguineous subcutaneous effusion over the presenting part in a vaginal delivery. It does cross the suture lines but resolves quickly. Lacerations are not uncommon and may require a Steri-Strip, but extremely rarely any further treatment.

**Q15** Which of the following is not suggestive of an Erb's palsy?

   **A** weak hand movements

   **B** biceps paralysis

   **C** grasp reflex present

   **D** Moro reflex is asymmetric

   **E** over 70% recover completely without intervention

A**15** **A** In an Erb's palsy (C5, C6) the arm is limp from paralysis of deltoid, biceps, brachioradialis and long wrist extensors but finger movements and grasp reflex are preserved.

Q**16** In hypoxic ischaemic encephalopathy, which is the most appropriate intervention?
- **A** controlled hypothermia
- **B** anti-epileptic medication
- **C** hyperventilation to reduce $PCO_2$
- **D** fluid resuscitation
- **E** nasogastric feeding

A**16** **A** Controlled hypothermia has been shown to improve outcome in the mild to moderate encephalopathy groups. It is now used in tertiary neonatal units under strict criteria.

Q**17** A 6-month-old is referred to your outpatient clinic with undescended testes. When you examine him you notice he has dirt under his nails and a severe nappy rash. What should you do?
- **A** Treat him the same as any other referral.
- **B** Contact his health visitor.
- **C** Ask Mum why he is dirty.
- **D** Contact the local safeguarding board to find out if they have information on the child.
- **E** Record in your notes that he appears dirty.

A**17** **B** Dirt under the nails of a non-mobile child could signify neglect. Nappy rash is common but a caring parent would have sought advice for it. Contacting the health visitor would enable further monitoring and then lead onto social services referral if necessary.

Q**18** A 7-year-old boy is brought into the emergency department with a supracondylar fracture of his right arm. This is his third fracture over 2 years. He says he jumped off a wall and slipped. What should you do?
- **A** Contact social services.
- **B** Contact local safeguarding board.
- **C** Ask a paediatrician to see him.
- **D** Treat his fracture and then allow home.
- **E** Treat his fracture and then ask a paediatrician to see him.

A18  **D**  It is not uncommon for mobile normal children aged 4–7 years to have several fractures. The sites are commonly radius/ulna and tibia.

Q19  A 3-year-old child is referred to the child development centre for a developmental assessment. He is found to be microcephalic and an MRI shows an underdeveloped brain. Which of the following could not be the cause?

**A**  antenatal infection

**B**  lack of stimulation during early life

**C**  neonatal stroke

**D**  meningitis at age 2½

**E**  a chromosomal disorder

A19  **D**  Antenatal 'TORCH' infections are well-known causes of microcephaly and developmental delay. They include toxoplasmosis, rubella, cytomegalovirus and herpes. Lack of stimulation is a well-recognised cause of developmental delay and microcephaly. The orphans in Romanian orphanages (Rutter, 1998) are a clear example of this. Neonatal stroke if severe could cause profound long-term problems, and many chromosomal disorders may be found at investigation for microcephaly. A more recent meningitis may well cause arrest of development and brain growth but would be unlikely to cause an underdeveloped brain.

Q20  The United Nations convention on the Rights of the Child does not state that:

**A**  governments must do all they can to fulfil the rights of every child

**B**  a child with a disability has a right to live a full and decent life

**C**  every child has the right to privacy

**D**  every child has the right to relax, play, and join in a wide range of cultural and artistic activities

**E**  everyone under the age of 16 has all the rights in the convention.

A20  **E**  Article 4 of the Convention on the Rights of the Child states that governments must do all they can to fulfil the rights of every child. Article 23 states that a child with a disability has a right to live a full and decent life. Article 16 states that every child has the right to privacy. Article 31 states that every child has the right to relax, play and join in a wide range of cultural and artistic activities, and Article 1 states that everyone under the age of **18** has all the rights in the convention.

**Q21** A 33-month-old girl is brought to clinic for follow-up. These are her growth charts. Which of the options is most likely?

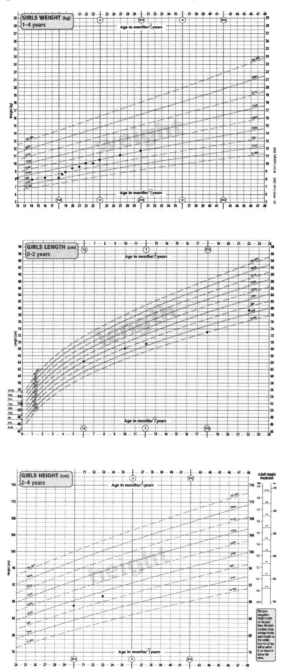

**FIGURE 14.1** Growth charts of this 33-month-old girl

A The child is PEG fed.

B She has been in foster care from age 18 months to 2½ years.

C She suffers from a malabsorption syndrome.

D She is fed by parenteral nutrition.

E She is on long-term steroid treatment.

A21 **B** The child's growth charts show the 'saw-tooth' appearance of non-organic faltering growth. The height was on the 50th centile at birth but then steadily dropped down. She went into foster care at 18 months and her weight quickly improved. Her height then caught up. As she went back to the care of her parents she stopped gaining weight as well.

## Further reading

Barnes PM, Norton CM, Dunstan FD, *et al*. Abdominal injury due to child abuse. *Lancet*. 2005; **366**(9481): 234–5.

Coant DN, Kornberg AE, Brody AS, *et al*. Markers for occult liver injury in cases of physical abuse in children. *Pediatrics*. 1992; **89**(2): 274–8.

Pierce MC, Kaczor K, Aldridge S, *et al*. Bruising characteristics discriminating physical child abuse from accidental trauma. *Pediatrics*. 2010; **125**(1): 67–74.

Royal College of Radiologists, Royal College of Paediatrics and Child Health. *Standards for Radiological Investigations of Suspected Non-Accidental Injury*. London: RCPCH and RCR; 2008.

Rutter M. Developmental catch-up, and deficit, following adoption after severe global early privation. English and Romanian Adoptees (ERA) Study Team. *J Child Psychol Psychiatry*. 1998; **39**(4): 465–76.

Vallone R, Addona F, D'Elia L, *et al*. Child abuse: a multidisciplinary approach. *Paediatr Child Health*. 2009; **19**(Suppl. 2): S207–10.

# SECTION IV

# Head and neck

# CHAPTER 15

# Cysts and sinuses in the neck

## ROSS FISHER

From the choices below each question, select the single best answer.

**Q1** Which of the following is true regarding thyroglossal cyst?
- **A** It is due to entrapment of epithelial tissue during the descent of the thyroid gland.
- **B** The gland passes inferiorly through the midsection of the cricoid.
- **C** Less than 5% of cysts are found lateral to the midline.
- **D** The primordial thyroid forms from the third branchial arches.
- **E** The most common presentation is with a discharging sinus.

**A1** **A** The thyroid gland develops as an out-pouching of the floor of the embryonic pharynx at the foramen caecum and descends through the hyoid bone to its final position in the anterior neck. Entrapped epithelial tissue left behind during this descent gives rise, in later life, to a thyroglossal cyst. More than 75% of cysts are diagnosed during childhood. The most common presentation is with an asymptomatic midline lump rather than the less common discharging sinus. At least 25% of cysts are found lateral to the midline and may be intrathyroid, intralingual, suprahyoidal or suprasternal.

**Q2** Which of the following is true regarding a preauricular sinus?
- **A** Routine renal ultrasound is indicated because of high incidence of associated anomalies.
- **B** It is more common in Caucasians than African Americans.
- **C** The risk of recurrence after excision surgery is less than 5%.
- **D** It is not found in patients with Treacher Collins's syndrome.
- **E** There is a male predominance.

**A2** **C** The incidence of associated renal anomalies in patients with preauricular sinuses is very low and most authorities would not require ultrasound in such children. The anomaly is more common in African Americans than Caucasians and occurs with no sex preponderance. It is common in various syndromes, not the least the Treacher Collins's and branchio-oto-renal syndromes. Surgical excision is indicated for frequent infection and is associated with a recurrence rate in major studies approaching 10%.

**Q3** Which of the following is *not* true regarding piriform sinus fistula?
- **A** It occurs on the left in over 90% of cases.
- **B** It may lead to acute thyroiditis.
- **C** The piriform sinus fistula develops from the second branchial pouch.
- **D** It may be effectively treated with trichloracetic acid.
- **E** It should be considered in the differential diagnosis of acute deep neck infection.

**A3** **C** Piriform sinus fistulas are a very rare, but important cause of acute deep neck infection. There is debate regarding the exact embryological origin, whether due to third or fourth branchial pouch problems. The condition occurs almost uniformly on the left side. The anatomical connection to the thyroid gland leads to marked inflammation of the gland, infection probably being reduced in severity because of the high iodine content of the tissue and the protective effect of the capsule. Surgical excision is recommended but because of the associated risks of surgery, some fistulas are effectively treated using injection of 40% trichloracetic acid into the mouth of the sinus.

**Q4** Which of the following is a true statement regarding branchial arch embryology?
- **A** Third cleft anomalies are the most common.
- **B** Anomalies of first pouch typically have their external orifice inferior to the ramus of the mandible.
- **C** Overall, cleft anomalies are more commonly right-sided.
- **D** Sinuses of third arch anomalies common pass anterior to the carotid bifurcation up to the piriform fossa.
- **E** Fourth cleft anomalies, although rare, occur more frequently than first cleft anomalies.

**A4** **B** Branchial arch anomalies most frequently occur on the left and most commonly in those derived from the second arch. The uncommon third arch sinus passes posterior to the carotid bifurcation to its drainage in the piriform fossa of the pharynx. First arch anomalies, although very rare do drain inferior to the ramus of the mandible. There is debate as to whether fourth arch anomalies actually exist at all.

**Q5** Which of the following is true of atypical mycobacterial sinus formation in the neck?

    **A** The intestinal tract is the primary route for *Mycobacterium avium* infection.

    **B** *Mycobacterium scrofulaceum* is associated with lymphadenitis in immunocompetent children.

    **C** Disseminated atypical mycobacterial disease is the second most common opportunistic infection in children with HIV infection.

    **D** All of the above.

    **E** None of the above.

**A5**   **E** Atypical mycobacteria are a problematic cause of recurrently infected and discharging lymph node abscesses in the neck often leading to chronic sinus formation. The common organisms encountered are *M. avium* and *M. scrofulaceum*, which most frequently enter the body via the enteral route. Such infections present significant risk for immune compromised children, in particular those with HIV.

**Q6** Which one of the following statements about cystic lymphatic obstruction is *not* true?

    **A** It may be because of abnormalities of *VEGF-C* and its receptors.

    **B** It is strongly associated with genetic abnormalities.

    **C** It is most commonly seen on the right side of the neck.

    **D** If occurring only in the third trimester of pregnancy, genetic abnormalities are rare.

    **E** It may be effectively treated using intralesional bleomycin.

**A6**   **C** Cystic lymphatic malformations are variously described as lymphangioma, cystic hygroma and lymphatic obstruction sequence and occur because of a combination of lymphatic obstruction, failure of connection to the venous circulation and abnormalities of the VEGF-C endothelial growth factor and its receptors. It is most commonly related to the lymphatic duct on the left side of the neck and has a strong association with genetic abnormalities, particularly trisomy 13, 18 and 21 if noted early in pregnancy. Interestingly, cystic hygroma occurring only in the third trimester virtually never shows this genetic anomaly. Surgical treatment is fraught with difficulty and conservative approaches have been tried, with varying success using sclerosants such as OK432, bleomycin, alcohol and even fibrin sealant.

**Q7** The preoperative workup for a child with a midline cyst should include:
- **A** ultrasound scan of the thyroid gland
- **B** fine needle aspiration
- **C** methylene-diphosphonate isotope scan
- **D** serum thyroid antibody-level measurement
- **E** all of the above.

**A7** **A** There is debate in the literature regarding the value of any investigation of a clinically euthyroid child with a suspected thyroglossal cyst. It would be reasonable to include at the very least ultrasound examination of the thyroid gland. Some practitioners persist in assessing thyroid function with serum thyroid-stimulating hormone (TSH) levels and even radioactive [123]I scans. Fine needle aspiration is contraindicated in children and antibody levels have no place in the assessment of such lesions.

**Q8** Which of the following is *not* true regarding bronchogenic neck cysts?
- **A** They are congenital malformations of ventral foregut development.
- **B** They may be directly connected to the tracheobronchial airway.
- **C** They usually present with sinus tract formation and external drainage of purulent material.
- **D** They have a 4 : 1 male-to-female ratio.
- **E** They are lined by ciliated pseudostratified columnar epithelium.

**A8** **C** Bronchogenic cysts form as a result of abnormal budding of the bronchial tree during embryogenesis. The connection with the tracheobronchial tree is usually lost but the cellular lining directly reflects their respiratory origin: ciliated pseudostratified columnar epithelium. There is a significant male predominance (4 : 1) The majority of cervical lesions are asymptomatic and present not with discharge but due to coincidental factors including size. Sinuses are uncommon in bronchogenic cysts.

**Q9** Which of the following statements is true with respect to surgical removal of a branchial arch remnant?
- **A** The recurrent laryngeal nerve is at risk as it crosses through the carotid bifurcation with the fistula.
- **B** The midsection of the hyoid bone must be excised to ensure low recurrence rates.
- **C** The facial nerve must be formally identified when excising first arch anomalies.
- **D** The piriform fossa must be explored to facilitate complete excision of second pouch anomalies.
- **E** The accessory nerve is encountered at the medial border of sternocleidomastoid with the fistulous opening of second arch.

A⁹  **C** Intimate knowledge of the anatomy of this region is required before undertaking surgery. The facial, hypoglossal, recurrent laryngeal and spinal accessory nerves are at most risk and should be formally identified. The facial nerve lies close to the auditory canal and is at risk during first arch surgery. The recurrent laryngeal nerve lies principally in the tracheo-oesophageal groove and the accessory nerve is at risk if surgery extends to the posterior border of sternocleidomastoid. The internal opening of the second arch sinus is commonly in the posterior tonsillar fossa. The hyoid bone is excised during the Sistrunk procedure for excision of thyroglossal cysts.

Q10 The differential diagnosis of an isolated midline neck cyst does not include:

    **A** branchial arch cyst

    **B** dermoid cyst

    **C** lymph node

    **D** thyroglossal cyst

    **E** cervical cleft.

A10  **A** Because of the laterality of embryological origin, branchial cysts are never midline. An isolated prehyoid lymph node and a dermoid cyst must be included as part of the differential, the diagnosis often being made only during surgery. Both may be firmly adherent to the hyoid bone, due to inflammation, and thus move with tongue protrusion. The sticky, honey-like contents of a thyroglossal cyst are pathognomonic. Congenital midline cervical cleft is a rare condition usually presenting as a cleft of pink tissue in the anterior midline neck, often with an associated protuberance of skin superiorly and a blind sinus tract inferiorly.

## Further reading

Brewis C, Mahadevan M, Bailey CM, *et al.* Investigation and treatment of thyroglossal cysts in children. *J R Soc Med.* 2000; **93**(1): 18–21.

Schroeder JW Jr, Mohyuddin N, Maddalozzo J. Branchial anomalies in the pediatric population. *Otolaryngol Head Neck Surg.* 2007; **137**(2): 289–95.

Tan T, Constantinides H, Mitchell TE. The preauricular sinus: a review of its aetiology, clinical presentation and management. *Int J Pediatr Otorhinolaryngol.* 2005; **69**(11): 1469–74.

# CHAPTER 16

# Endocrine disorders

## MICHAEL SKINNER, EDUARDO PEREZ

**From the choices below each question, select the single best answer.**

**Q1** Which one of these genes is involved in the pathogenesis of multiple endocrine neoplasia type II?

A *APC*

B *p53*

C *RET*

D *VLH*

E none of the above

**A1** C Multiple endocrine neoplasia syndromes are inherited in an autosomal dominant pattern with very high penetrance. The genetic defect in these disorders involves the *RET* proto-oncogene, a tyrosine kinase receptor, on chromosome 10q11.2. All clinical manifestations of the multiple endocrine neoplasia type 2 (MEN2) syndromes relate to a defect in transduction of growth and differentiation signals in several developing tissues that express *RET*. So far, mutation analysis in MEN2 families has identified over 50 different mutations related to the disease.

**Q2** Which of the following is *not* true regarding hypothyroidism in children?

A Thyroid-stimulating hormone (TSH) is elevated.

B Patients are usually symptomatic at birth.

C It can present as a sublingual mass.

D It is congenital in 90% of cases.

E Surgical treatment is rarely required.

**A2** B Children may be rarely afflicted with acquired or congenital diseases of thyroid hormone production, resulting in either increased or decreased hormone production and secretion. Thyroid gland dysgenesis is the most common cause of hypothyroidism diagnosed in neonatal screening programmes, accounting for approximately 90% of these patients. In about one-third of these babies, no thyroid tissue is seen on radionuclide scanning. In the rest of the patients, a rudimentary gland may be found in an ectopic location, usually the base of the tongue. Often, there has been enough transplacental thyroid hormone present throughout development so even children with complete thyroid agenesis are asymptomatic at birth. In some cases, ectopically located thyroid tissue may supply a sufficient amount of thyroxin for many years or may fail in childhood. This condition can be identified with the development of a sublingual or midline neck mass. When evaluating neck masses in children, attention should be paid to this fact and a radionuclide thyroid scan should be considered, prior to removing any unusual neck mass. This will ensure that functioning thyroid tissue is not accidentally resected. Because of its sensitivity, TSH is the best screening method for this condition. Disorders of hypothyroidism are rarely treated surgically, and may result from a defect anywhere in the hypothalamic–pituitary–thyroid axis.

 **Q3** Which of the following is *not* true about Graves's disease?

   **A** It is the most common cause of hyperthyroidism in childhood.
   **B** Infection may elicit the production of autoantibodies against the TSH receptor.
   **C** The condition is seen in girls about five times more than in boys.
   **D** The condition is more frequent in the adolescent years.
   **E** The congenital form occurs in 20% of infants born to mothers with active Graves's disease.

**A3**   **E**   Graves's disease is the most common cause of hyperthyroidism in childhood. It is characterised by autoimmunity by thyroid-stimulating antibodies that result in activation of thyrotropin receptors leading to unregulated hyperthyroidism. This is mediated by immunoglobulins of the IgG class, and is present in 95% of the patients. The event that initiates the production of these antibodies is unknown, but it has been postulated that it could be related to infection. This is suggested by the presence of TSH-binding sites in gram-negative and gram-positive bacteria and also by epidemiologic reports of disease clustering. The disease is seen in girls 5 times more than boys, and is higher in the adolescent population. Congenital Graves's disease occurs in 1% of infants born to women with active disease.

**Q4** While evaluating an infant on rounds, you notice that his mother looks anxious, complains of fatigue and heat intolerance, and admits to some weight loss despite having an increased appetite. You examine her carefully and discover that she is tachycardic, with a tremor. Furthermore she has fullness in her neck and in her eyes. She denies prenatal care. The infant is most likely at risk for development of:

- **A** constipation
- **B** heart failure
- **C** macrocephaly
- **D** third-degree heart block
- **E** thrombocytosis.

**A4** **B** The infant is likely at risk for neonatal thyrotoxicosis. Neonatal thyrotoxicosis usually disappears within 2–4 months as the concentration of thyroid-stimulating immunoglobulin (TSI) diminishes. Unlike TSI, TSH does not cross the placenta. All forms of thyrotoxicosis are more common in females, with the exception of neonatal thyrotoxicosis, which has an equal sex distribution. Symptoms include tachycardia and tachypnoea, irritability and hyperactivity, low birthweight with microcephaly, severe vomiting and diarrhoea, thrombocytopenia, jaundice, hepatosplenomegaly and heart failure. In severely affected infants, the disease could be fatal if not treated vigorously and promptly. Third-degree heart block is not a feature of this disease, but is sometimes seen in infants born to mothers with systemic lupus erythematosis.

**Q5** A 16-year-old female has had elevated serum calcium levels since birth. During her workup she is found to have a normal parathormone (PTH) level and hypocalciuria. She denies any symptoms. What would be the most appropriate treatment?

- **A** 3½ parathyroidectomy
- **B** technetium-99m sestamibi scintigraphy
- **C** bisphosphonate
- **D** observation
- **E** single adenoma parathyroidectomy

**A5** **D** The case describes a patient with familial hypocalciuric hypercalcaemic disease. It is an autosomal dominant disease that expresses itself as an error in the calcium-sensing receptor. This results in higher-than-normal serum calcium levels. These patients are usually asymptomatic and laboratory findings include hypercalcaemia, hypocalciuria and normal or slightly elevated PTH levels. The diagnosis of familial hypocalciuric hypercalcaemia can be made by measuring urine calcium levels, which are lowered in these patients. It is important to exclude this diagnosis in all patients with high serum calcium. The treatment of this disease is strictly observational. Patients do not require surgery or further workup.

 **Q6** What is the most common cause of primary hyperaldosteronism in children?

**A** Conn's syndrome

**B** adrenocortical hyperplasia

**C** adrenocortical carcinoma

**D** Bartter's syndrome

**E** none of the above

 **A6** **B** Overproduction of aldosterone is known as primary hyperaldosteronism when the cause is related to adrenal dysfunction. This hypersecretion may be the result of bilateral nodular hyperplasia, or from an adrenocortical tumour (adenoma or carcinoma). Adrenocortical hyperplasia is the most common cause in the paediatric population. Children present with hypertension, hypokalaemia, elevated plasma aldosterone levels, and low plasma renin activity. Children with hyperplasia are treated medically with spironolactone, an inhibitor of aldosterone biosynthesis, which is usually quite effective in managing the hypertension. Bilateral adrenalectomy has not always been effective in curing the hypertension associated with this condition. Bartter's syndrome is a renal tubular defect that is characterised by hypochloraemic metabolic alkalosis, hypokalaemia, elevated urinary chloride, potassium and prostaglandin levels. Patients have normal blood pressure, but hyperreninaemia and hyperaldosteronism are present.

 **Q7** A 5-year-old male is referred to your clinic after presenting with a few months of muscle weakness, polydipsia and polyuria. His BP is 150/80. What is the next step in management?

**A** head CT scan

**B** aldosterone level

**C** potassium level

**D** check a renin level

**E** arterial blood gas

 **A7** **C** Signs and symptoms of primary hyperaldosteronism are non-specific. Children usually present with hypertension, muscle weakness, polydipsia and polyuria. Constant high levels of aldosterone causes the total body sodium level to increase, thus increasing the total fluid volume. This also suppresses renin and angiotensin. When a child presents with hypertension and hypokalaemia, one should consider a diagnosis of primary hyperaldosteronism. This is the reason why potassium levels are the initial screening test in children with hypertension.

**Q8** In the previous scenario, CT scan shows no discrete masses. What is the next step in management?

**A** exploratory laparotomy

**B** selective adrenal vein sampling

**C** MRI scan

**D** abdominal ultrasonography

**E** none of the above

**A8** **B** Once the diagnosis of hyperaldosteronism is confirmed, one has to distinguish between an adenoma and bilateral adrenal hyperplasia. If a mass greater than 1 cm is identified by a CT scan or an MRI, the diagnosis of adenoma is entertained. If no masses are visualised, a selective adrenal vein sampling can differentiate unilateral vs. bilateral adrenocortical hypersecretion.

**Q9** Which of the following is true about goitres in children?

**A** Most are euthyroid, and surgery is rarely indicated.

**B** With simple colloid goitre, the patient is hyperthyroid.

**C** Exogenous thyroid hormone is the treatment of choice for simple goitres

**D** Graves's disease is the most common cause.

**E** None of the above.

**A9** **A** Diffuse thyroid enlargement can be due to a defect in hormone production, autoimmune disease or a response to an inflammatory condition. Most children with goitres are euthyroid and surgical indication is rarely indicated. The most common diagnosis of enlarged thyroid is simple goitre. Other diagnoses include chronic lymphocytic thyroiditis, Graves's disease, benign adenomas, and cysts. Exogenous thyroid hormone does not enhance resolution of the goitre.

**Q10** Which of the following is not a manifestation or associated condition of Graves's hyperthyroidism in children?

**A** Addison's disease

**B** diffuse goitre

**C** ophthalmopathy

**D** diffuse arthropathy

**E** localised dermopathy

**A10** **D** Graves's disease is characterised by autoimmunity by thyroid-stimulating anti-bodies that results in activation of thyrotropin receptors leading to unregulated hyperthyroidism. It is the most common cause of hyperthyroidism in children. The clinical manifestations specific to Graves's disease include diffuse goitre, exophthalmos, dermopathy and lymphoid hyperplasia. Common diseases associated with Graves's are diabetes mellitus, Addison's disease, vitiligo, pernicious anaemia, myasthenia gravis, alopecia areata and other autoimmune diseases. Patients will often present with signs and symptoms of hyperthyroidism. Most children with Graves's disease have a family history of some type of autoimmune thyroid disease.

**Q11** A 7-year-old obese female presents to your clinic with growth failure. Which is the most sensitive test to order in this patient to screen for Cushing's syndrome?

**A** high-dose dexamethasone suppression test

**B** 24-hour urine free cortisol

**C** adrenocorticotropic hormone (ACTH) stimulation test

**D** corticotropin-releasing hormone (CRH) test

**E** plasma cortisol level

**A11** **B** The most sensitive and specific test to determine hypercortisolism is the 24-hour urine free cortisol test. This avoids the episodic nature of cortisol secretion. ACTH level can be elevated, suppressed or normal in hypercortisolism. The CRH test is used to differentiate between a pituitary cause for hypercortisolism and other causes. The high-dose dexamethasone test separates a pituitary source of hypercortisolism from an ectopic source of ACTH.

The ACTH stimulation test is used to determine the function of the adrenal gland(s) and is the test of choice to diagnose adrenal insufficiency. The low-dose dexamethasone suppression test is used to diagnose hypercortisolism. Although plasma ACTH level will most likely be elevated in adrenal insufficiency, this test is not specific for this condition. Random serum cortisol levels are quite variable because of the episodic nature of cortisol secretion, and thus this test is not sensitive enough for diagnosing adrenal insufficiency.

**Q12** Non-endocrine manifestations of MEN2B include all the following *except*:

**A** megacolon

**B** lichen amyloidosis

**C** mucosal neuromas

**D** hypertrophied corneal nerves

**E** pectus excavatum.

**A12** **B** MEN syndromes are a group of endocrine disturbances that affect hormone-secreting glands. These are rare autosomal dominant conditions that predispose affected individuals to benign and malignant tumours of the pituitary, thyroid, parathyroids, adrenals, endocrine pancreas, paraganglia or non-endocrine organs. The classic MEN syndromes include MEN type 1 (MEN1) and MEN type 2 (MEN2). MEN2 syndrome is often first suspected when a patient is found to have one or more of the tumours described in the syndrome, usually medullary thyroid cancer, or a family history. These syndromes are accompanied by a series of non-endocrine manifestations that help in the diagnosis, especially in children with no known family history of the disease. Cutaneous lichen amyloidosis is a component of the MEN2A syndrome that has been described in families with the disease. It can be present before the onset of medullary thyroid carcinoma , and the identification of this skin lesion should prompt an evaluation for MEN2A. The skin lesion is usually described as as intensely pruritic, red-brown hyperkeratotic papules most commonly seen in the interscapular region or on the extensor sur-faces of the extremities. The first early symptom is usually pruritus; the amyloid deposition is seen later and is thought to be secondary to repeated scratching. Amyloid deposition has been documented histologically. MEN2B presents with mucosal neuromas, intestinal ganglioneuromas and marfanoid habitus. Clinically the neuromas present in the tongue, lips and eyelids, with characteristic facial features including enlarged lips, a 'bumpy' tongue, and eversion of the eyelids. The marfanoid body habitus physic is accompanied by increased joint mobility and decreased subcutaneous fat. Ganglioneuromatosis presents with thickening of the corneal nerves or in the gastrointestinal tract, resulting in abdominal disten-sion, megacolon, constipation, or diarrhoea. All these physical traits are usually evident in early childhood, and are sometimes already present at birth.

**Q13** You are evaluating an 8-year-old female who complains of short stat-ure. She is in the 10th percentile for her age. On further questioning, you notice that she had vaginal spotting for the last couple of months and she is also constipated. Her school performance has changed. On examination, she seems overweight and has a puffy face; no obvious masses are palpated on her neck, and she has muffled heart sounds. Which of the following conditions is most likely to present with these findings?

**A** rickets

**B** scurvy

**C** hypothyroidism

**D** microcytic anaemia

**E** adrenocortical insufficiency

**A13** **C** Acquired hypothyroidism is the most common disturbance of thyroid function in childhood. Most cases of acquired hypothyroidism in children are the result of autoimmune thyroid disease. The most common manifestation is a decrease in growth rate resulting in short stature. If hypothyroidism occurs in adolescence, it is also associated with delayed puberty. Another common presentation is altered school performance. Other common symptoms are sluggishness, lethargy, cold intolerance, constipation, dry skin, brittle hair, facial puffiness and muscle aches and pains. On physical examination, findings include short stature and increased weight for height. A goitre may or may not be present. Children with long-standing hypothyroidism have puffy myxoedematous facies. Cardiovascular examination may show bradycardia, low systolic blood pressure, and muffled heart tones if a pericardial effusion is present. On neurologic examination, deep tendon reflexes tend to have a delayed return phase. A minority of children may actually present with pseudoprecocious puberty. Rickets results from a deficiency of vitamin D. This condition predominantly affects the long bones and skull. Vitamin C deficiency results in scurvy, a condition with impaired collagen formation. The clinical manifestations may include changes in the gums, loosening of teeth, brittle bones and swollen joints. Pallor is the most important sign of iron-deficiency anaemia. Children may also have the desire to ingest unusual substances such as ice or dirt. Finally, hyponatraemia and hypoglycaemia are the prominent presenting signs of adrenal insufficiency in infants.

**Q14** A 10-year-old boy has recently been diagnosed with sporadic hyperparathyroidism (HPT). Compared with MEN1 associated HPT, this patient's disease is most likely to involve:

**A** a single parathyroid gland

**B** all four parathyroid glands

**C** the thyroid gland

**D** the pituitary gland

**E** none of the above.

**A14** **A** Sporadic primary hyperparathyroidism (HPT) is genetically distinct from its MEN-associated disease. Whereas MEN-associated disease tends to produce diffuse multiglandular parathyroid involvement, sporadic primary HPT tends to involve only a single gland. The difference in number of glands involved in sporadic vs. MEN-associated disease has important implications for surgical management of patients with primary HPT. In MEN-associated HPT, most surgeons advocate exploration with identification of all four glands. The specifics of which procedure to perform in MEN-associated disease, however, are controversial. Some surgeons advocate total parathyroidectomy with autotransplantation while others prefer subtotal or 3½ gland parathyroidectomy. In contrast, surgical therapy for sporadic adenomas may be directed at removal of the single adenomatous gland – especially with the use of localisation imaging and intraoperative parathyroid hormone testing.

Q15 A 12-year-old male with known diagnosis of HPT and awaiting surgical resection, presents with hypercalcaemia. Which of the following is not an acceptable treatment for hypercalcaemia?

  **A** intravenous hydration

  **B** furosemide

  **C** thiazide

  **D** bisphosphonate

  **E** calcitonin

A15 **C** The treatment for symptomatic hypercalcaemia begins with inpatient admission for continuous cardiac monitoring. Any medication that may increase calcium levels should be discontinued. This includes vitamin D supplements and thiazide diuretics. Any dietary calcium (dairy products) should also be stopped. Intravenous hydration and furosemide will generally correct symptoms and bring calcium levels to normal in those patients with hyperparathyroidism as the cause of their hypercalcaemia. Malignant hypercalcaemia may be more difficult to manage and may require the use of disodium etidronate or other bisphosphonates. These agents work by inhibiting the action of osteoclast activity. Calcitonin is another agent that can be used to lower calcium levels. It is a comparatively poor hypercalcaemia treatment agent, but has a short time to action and minimal adverse effect profile. Mithramycin is also effective and high-dose steroids work well for sarcoid patients with hypercalcaemic symptoms.

Q16 You are evaluating a female newborn with tonic–clonic seizures. Patient and mother did not have any prenatal significant history. On her initial workup she is found to have glucose of 10 mg/dL. After correcting her hypoglycaemia, which of these tests is not indicated in the workup of this patient?

  **A** TSH

  **B** insulin level

  **C** cortisol level

  **D** growth hormone level

  **E** PTH level

A16 **E** Hypoglycaemia is the most common metabolic disorder in the first year of life. It is potentially a devastating cause of severe brain damage, mental retardation and even death if not recognised and treated early. The differential diagnosis for hypoglycaemia in the newborn includes persistent hyperinsulinaemic hypoglycaemia of infancy (PHHI), also called nesidioblastosis; lack of substrate for gluconeogenesis (e.g. glycogen-storage disease); and inadequate gluconeogenic hormones (e.g. hypothyroidism, adrenal insufficiency or growth-hormone deficiency). When working up a neonate with hypoglycaemia, all these causes should be ruled out. PTH is useful in the screening for parathyroid disease and is not indicated in this patient.

**Q17** Laboratory studies show a serum insulin of 9.0 mcU/mL when her plasma glucose was 24 mg/dL (insulin : glucose = 0.35) (normal <0.3), along with negative findings for serum acetone; cortisol, 17.2 ug/dL (normal = 6–23 mcg/dL) and growth hormone, 18.8 ng/mL (normal = 10–40 ng/mL). What is the most likely diagnosis?

**A** nesidioblastosis

**B** Addison's disease

**C** Cushing's disease

**D** thyroid dysgenesis

**E** none of the above

**A17** **A** Nesidioblastosis or PHHI is the most common cause of persistent hypoglycaemia in infants. It is characterised by inadequate suppression of insulin secretion in the presence of severe, recurrent, fasting hypoglycaemia. There are two forms of PHHI, a focal and a diffuse type. Both forms have similar clinical presentation, and pathological analysis is required for proper distinction between the two. Neonates with PHHI present with hypoglycaemic symptoms, which include lethargy, hypotonia and seizures shortly after birth. Serum glucose, ketone and insulin levels should be obtained while the patient is hypoglycaemic. The finding of nonketotic hypoglycaemia in association with elevated insulin levels (>10 μU/mL) and normal levels of free fatty acid supports the diagnosis of hyperinsulinism. The insulin-to-glucose ratio may range from 0.4 to 2.7 (normal <0.3). Cortisol and growth hormone levels are usually elevated in specimens taken during an episode of hypoglycaemia (appropriate and normal response to hypoglycaemia) and are usually within the reference range during periods of normoglycaemia. Serum metabolic screens, pH, lactate and ammonia studies may be obtained to exclude other metabolic diseases.

**Q18** If medical management fails, what is the most appropriate surgical management?

**A** pancreatoduodenectomy

**B** near-total pancreatectomy

**C** trans-sphenoidal microadenoma

**D** liver transplant

**E** pancreatic transplant

A18  B  The initial therapy is directed towards correcting the hypoglycaemia. This should consist of intravenous glucose, frequent feedings if possible, and drug administration to control insulin secretion. Diazoxide and octreotide are the first-line medications. They act by inhibiting insulin secretion. Other medical therapy may consist of glucocorticoids to promote insulin resistance and streptozotocin to decrease the number of insulin-secreting cells. In cases where medical therapy fails, pancreatic resection has been the mainstay of surgical therapy for patients with PHHI. The clinical distinction between the two forms of PHHI is important because patients with focal PHHI may respond to a topographically guided partial pancreatic resection, whereas patients with diffuse PHHI may require a near-total pancreatectomy to alleviate symptoms of hypoglycaemia. However, long-term follow-up has reported a significant incidence of diabetes after such a resection.

Q19  A 5-day-old girl is admitted to a hospital for evaluation of vomiting and dehydration. Physical examination is otherwise normal except for a small urethral phallus, apparent hypertrophy of a clitoris and near fusion of the labioscrotal folds. Serum sodium and potassium concentrations are 121 mEq/L and 8.5 mEq/L, respectively; serum glucose is 122 mg/dL. The most likely diagnosis is:

A  panhypopituitarism
B  congenital adrenal hyperplasia
C  secondary hypothyroidism
D  pyloric stenosis
E  hyperaldosteronism.

A19  B  This infant most likely has congenital adrenal hyperplasia, usually manifested during the first 5–15 days of life as anorexia, vomiting, diarrhoea and dehydration. Hypoglycaemia can also occur. Affected infants can have increased pigmentation, and female infants show evidence of virilisation (ambiguous external genitalia). Hyponatraemia, hyperkalaemia and urinary sodium wasting are the usual laboratory findings. Pyloric stenosis seems unlikely in this infant in that the vomiting with this disease usually begins after the third week of life. Hypothyroidism would present as a lethargic, poor-feeding infant with delayed reflexes, persistent jaundice and hypotonia. Hyperaldosteronism would be expected to cause decreased potassium, not increased levels. Panhypopituitarism usually presents with apnoea, cyanosis or severe hypoglycaemia.

Q20 Which of the following is the best test to confirm the diagnosis in this patient?

   A  abdominal ultrasonography

   B  measurement of 17-hydroxyprogesterone

   C  somatomedin C measurement

   D  measurement of T3, T4 and TSH

   E  measurement of serum renin levels

A20  B  The enzymatic defect in the steroidogenesis pathway causes a decrease in cortisol secretion, with consequent increased ACTH production, which acts in a vicious cycle to further drive the production of other steroids in the pathway (other than cortisol). The excess adrenal androgens are converted peripherally to testosterone. The most common enzymatic deficiency is 21-hydroxylase deficiency, responsible for more than 90% of the congenital adrenal hyperplasia. It is manifested by elevation of serum levels of 17-hydroxyprogesterone beyond 3 days of life (in the first 3 days of life they can normally be high). Treatment of this disorder consists of glucocorticoid and mineralocorticoid replacement and in the case of the female pseudohermaphrodite, the external genitalia are surgically modified to be female. Death can occur if the diagnosis is missed and appropriate treatment is not instituted.

## Further reading

Holcomb GW, Murphy JP. *Ashcraft's Pediatric Surgery*. 5th ed. Philadelphia, PA: Saunders; 2010.

Kappy MS, Allen DB, Geffner ME, editors. *Principles and Practice of Pediatric Endocrinology*. 1st ed. Springfield, IL: Charles Thomas Publishers Ltd; 2005.

Oldham KT, Colombani PM, Foglia RP, *et al.*, editors. *Principles and Practice of Pediatric Surgery*. 4th ed. Philadelphia, PA: Lippincott Williams & Wilkins; 2005.

# SECTION V

# Thorax

# CHAPTER 17

# Breast disorders in children and adolescents

## MARJORIE J ARCA

**From the choices below each question, select the single best answer.**

**Q1** A 2-day-old baby presents with unilateral breast discharge. On examination, milky thin fluid can be expressed from the right nipple. What is the appropriate management?

  **A** check oestrogen level, prolactin level, progesterone level

  **B** pelvic ultrasound

  **C** breast ultrasound

  **D** reassurance and observation

  **E** trauma workup

**A1**  **D**  By birth neonatal mammary tissue may be functional and may secrete colostrum for the first week of life. The fluid, termed 'witch's milk', consists of cellular debris. This is not a pathological finding. Parents should be advised that this condition is self-limiting.

**Q2** Which of the following is *not* true regarding the anatomy and embryology of the breast?

  **A** The internal mammary artery and lateral thoracic artery supply the majority of blood to the breast.

  **B** Breast tissue is derived from ectoderm.

  **C** The tail of Spence is the portion of the breast that projects towards the clavicle.

  **D** Breasts begin to form at 5–7 weeks' fetal development from the base of the forelimbs to the hind limbs.

  **E** Sensory innervation of the anterolateral and anteromedial breast is from T3 to T5 nerve roots.

**A2**   **C**   The tail of Spence is the part of the breast that extends towards the axilla. Careful palpation of this part is essential for a complete breast exam.

**Q3**   Which of the following statements is *not* true regarding the anatomy of the breast?

   **A**   Cooper's ligaments support the nipple–areola complex.

   **B**   Breast tissue is composed of skin, subcutaneous tissue, parenchyma and stroma.

   **C**   Collecting ducts of breast drain each segment, converging into lactiferous sinuses that drain into milk ducts.

   **D**   Breast parenchyma overlies the deep pectoral fascia and is enveloped by superficial pectoral fascia.

   **E**   Lymphatic drainage is to the axillary nodes and the mammary nodes.

**A3**   **A**   Cooper's ligaments are bands of fibrous tissue that span the superficial and deep pectoral fascia, supporting the whole breast. Alveoli make up lobules, and 20–40 lobules make up a lobe. Lobes are grouped into segments. Segments are located radially around the nipple with 15–20 segments present in each breast. There are up to 10 milk ducts per breast.

**Q4**   All of the following statements are true regarding congenital breast deformities *except*:

   **A**   Ectopic breast tissue may be subject to the same pathology as normally located breast.

   **B**   Patients with polythelia should have a renal ultrasound.

   **C**   Athelia is always bilateral.

   **D**   Athelia is highly associated with a syndrome or cluster of other abnormalities.

   **E**   Amastia may or may not be associated with athelia.

**A4**   **C**   Deficiency in parathyroid-related hormone is thought to lead to lack of proliferation of the mesenchyme that forms the nipple–areola complex.

   Polythelia, the presence of supernumerary nipple(s) should prompt a workup for renal abnormalities such as duplication, obstruction and agenesis. Polythelia is treated by excision of the supernumerary nipple in a healthy child.

   Athelia, the absence of nipple–areola complex, is not addressed until puberty.

   Athelia may be unilateral or bilateral and is almost always associated with syndromes such as Poland's syndrome, ectodermal dysplasia, choanal atresia and athelia syndrome.

   Polymastia is the presence of ectopic breast tissue within the breast line. Complete resection is recommended for patients with polymastia for reasons of cosmesis and symptoms. Risks and outcomes of supernumerary mastectomies have not been analysed.

Amastia may or may not be associated with athelia.

**Q5** A 2-month-old baby girl presents with a tender, inflamed left breast abscess. The following are true regarding the treatment course of the disease *except*:

**A** Treatment may include IV or oral antibiotics.

**B** Drainage of the infected fluid may be performed by needle aspiration.

**C** If surgical drainage is necessary, care must be exercised in order to avoid damage to the breast bud.

**D** All breast abscesses should be drained surgically since the infection would damage the developing breast tissue.

**E** Staphylococcus and streptococcus are the most common organisms that have been implicated in breast abscesses in infants.

**A5** **D** Breast infection usually presents as a tender, fluctuant mass. Antibiotic administration is the initial course of therapy. The most common organisms causing breast infections include *Staphylococcus aureus*, beta haemolytic streptococcus, *Escherichia coli* and *Pseudomonas aeruginosa*. Because of the widespread distribution of the methicillin-resistant *S. aureus*, this organism should be covered pending definitive identification of the causative organism. Aspiration or incision and drainage may be required. Care must be exercised in procedures performed to the prepubertal breast as damage to the breast bud may occur with injudicious procedures.

**Q6** An 11-year-old female presents with Tanner stage II breast development on the right side and Tanner stage I development on the left side. What is the most appropriate course of action?

**A** Advise the child and her parents that asymmetric development is common and that most asymmetry will not have discernible size discrepancy at adulthood.

**B** Check follicle-stimulating hormone and luteinising hormone levels.

**C** Perform a careful family history evaluation, paying close attention to a history of early breast carcinoma and male breast carcinoma.

**D** Obtain serum oestrogen, progesterone and prolactin levels.

**E** Ultrasonography of the breast.

**A6**  **A** Thelarche marks the onset of puberty and is the first sign of puberty. It should occur by age 13. In the early stages, it is very common for the breast development to be asymmetrical. A careful examination in the office is necessary to rule out masses or infections. Thereafter, the child and the family should be reassured that asymmetrical development is common in the early stages of puberty.

There are five Tanner stages of breast development.

I  Elevation of breast papilla only.

II  Elevation of breast bud and papilla as a small round enlargement of the areola diameter. Areola becomes pinker.

III  Further enlargement of the breast and areola show no separation of their contours. Appearance of Montgomery's tubercles.

IV  Further enlargement with projection of the areola and papilla to form a secondary mound above the level of the breast.

V  Projection of the papilla only resulting from the recession of the areola to the general contour of the breast.

**Q7**  A 14-year-old female with Tanner V breast development presents with a 2 cm well-rounded mass in the upper inner quadrant of the right breast. There is no nipple discharge or erythema around the breast. She states that the mass becomes slightly larger and more tender a few days before her menstrual period. On exam, the mass is easily palpable with regular edges and is freely moveable. There is no adenopathy in the bilateral axillae, supraclavicular or infraclavicular areas. Each of the following is a reasonable course of action except:

**A** ultrasound of the mass

**B** excisional biopsy of the mass

**C** bilateral mammography

**D** observation

**E** serial examination.

**A7**  **C** A fibroadenoma is the most commonly encountered breast mass in the female adolescent population. On examination, these are discrete, rubbery, moveable and nontender. They may be bilateral (10% of the time) and multiple (10%–15% of the time). The average size of a lesion is 2–3 cm. On ultrasound fibroadenomas are hypoechoic and well circumscribed.

Two histological types of fibroadenomas have been described: simple and complex. Simple fibroadenomas have both epithelial and connective elements. There is no increased risk of breast carcinoma in these patients with any family history of breast carcinoma or proliferative breast disease. Complex fibroadenomas show foci of cysts, sclerosing adenomas, epithelial calcifications and papillary apocrine metaplasia. The future risk of breast cancer in patients with complex fibroadenomas is higher. Overall, malignant transformations of fibroadenomas are considered to be rare, in the order of 0.002%–0.00125%. Complete resolution of fibroadenomas is reported in 16%–59% of longitudinal studies. Of those that did not regress, half become smaller and the other half enlarged.

Solitary discrete fibroadenomas may be excised or observed. Observation requires serial examinations and ultrasound every 6 months to a year to monitor size. Operative indications include rapid size, enlargement, symptoms, desire by the patient and her family or radiological findings that differ from a typical fibroadenoma. Excision does not require a margin of normal breast.

**Q8** A 14-year-old female presents with a 7 cm rapidly growing mass of the left breast. On examination, there is significant left breast distortion, overlying warmth with dilatation of superficial breast veins. Differential diagnoses include all of the following *except*:

**A** breast cancer

**B** giant fibroadenoma

**C** infection

**D** cystosarcoma phyllodes

**E** prolactinoma.

**A8** **E** Giant fibroadenoma (also known as juvenile cellular fibroadenoma) is an uncommon variant of fibroadenoma characterised by rapid growth. The lesions are generally over 5 cm, encapsulated, benign and may have dilated veins on the overlying skin.

Cystosarcoma tumours present as bulky breast masses, which may reach up to 20 cm in size. These masses are firm and mobile. The overlying skin may be thin and shiny with increased vascularity. Typically, skin dimpling, nipple retraction or nipple discharge is not seen. Patients usually present with a rapidly growing, non-tender breast mass or with accelerated growth of a previously stable mass. Ultrasonography and MRI cannot distinguish between a fibroadenoma and a phyllodes tumour. Microscopically, benign phyllodes tumours have a hyperplastic and cellular stromal component. Cellular atypia and increased mitotic figures are seen more commonly in the malignant variant. Not fully encapsulated, the abnormal phyllodes tissue often extends projections into the surrounding normal breast tissue.

Breast abscess and cellulitis present with a rapidly growing isolated tender mass. Although uncommon in this age group, inflammatory breast lesions have a similar presentation to the one described. Prolactin-secreting tumours typically present with galactorrhoea and not a unilateral mass.

**Q9** The following agents have been implicated in problems associated with nipple piercing *except*:

A platinum

B *Mycobacterium fortuitum*

C *S. aureus*

D nickel

E anaerobic bacteria.

**A9** A *M. fortuitum* and *Prevotella melaninogenica* (anaerobic organism) have been implicated in breast abscesses. Other organisms that have been reported to be associated with nipple piercing include coagulase-negative staphylococcus, streptococcus and gordonea. Nickel allergies have also been well described as the cause of post-piercing inflammation. Platinum has not been implicated in piercing-associated inflammation.

**Q10** To investigate nipple discharge in a 16-year-old female the following may be useful *except*:

A complete history and physical examination

B list of current medications including illicit drugs

C cytology of discharge fluid

D thyroid function tests

E serum prolactin level.

**A10** C Brown episodic discharge may occur from Montgomery's tubercles, areolar tubercles involved in lactation. Causes of milky discharge or galactorrhoea include prolactin-seeding tumours, pregnancy, hypothyroidism, hyperthyroidism, papillary duct ectasia, papillary duct hyperplasia and the postpartum state. Hyperprolactinaemia has been associated with thoracotomy, nipple irritation and chest trauma. Nipple discharge may be associated with primary or secondary amenorrhoea, interrupted puberty and medication such as oral contraceptives, tricyclic antidepressants, H2 antagonists, cannabis, phenothiazines and hypertensive agents. Exfoliative cytological examination of nipple discharge and scrape smears has a low sensitivity for diagnosis.

Q11 Which one of the following statements about juvenile papillomatosis is *not* true?

  A It occurs as a localised mass.

  B Microscopically it is characterised by cysts in combination with epithelial hyperplasia, marked papillomatosis, papillary apocrine metaplasia and mild cytologic atypia.

  C Treatment is simple mastectomy.

  D Ultrasound features include poor mass definition with internal echoes of variable strength and one or more small, rounded, echo-free areas at the border of the lesion.

  E It is a marker for families with a high frequency of breast carcinoma.

A11 C Juvenile papillomatosis is a distinct entity seen at a young age. It presents as a localised mass. It occurs in women <30 years of age, but has been described in men. Treatment is total resection with preservation of normal breast. There is an increased risk of breast cancer in patients with juvenile papillomatosis and therefore close follow-up is needed.

Q12 Which of the following is *not* true regarding the clinical course of phyllodes tumours of the breast?

  A Phyllodes tumours may metastasise or locally recur.

  B The lymphatic route is the primary means of spread for malignant cystosarcoma phyllodes.

  C Clinically positive nodes are present about 20% of the time.

  D If local recurrence is present, re-excision or mastectomy may be necessary.

  E Phylloides tumours in children and adolescents have a more favourable prognosis than their adult counterparts.

A12 B Cystosarcoma phyllodes or phyllodes tumours are stromal tumours. They are histologically classified as benign, intermediate or malignant. They occur more commonly on the left breast. Benign tumours should be surgically excised with at least a 1 cm margin. Benign phylloides tumours are often difficult to differentiate from fibroadenomas on ultrasonography and MRI. On cytopathology, several properties are seen in phyllodes tumours that are not seen in fibroadenoma, such as fibromyxoid stromal fragments with spindle nuclei, fibroblastic pavements, and appreciable numbers of spindle cells of fibroblastic nature among dispersed cell population. Malignant tumours should be treated with simple mastectomy. Recurrent tumours may be treated by re-excision or mastectomy. The haematogenous route is the primary route of spread and metastases to lung, pleura, soft tissue, bone, pancreas and CNS has been described. Radiation therapy should be considered if an adequate margin cannot be achieved on the chest wall. Prognosis for phylloides tumours in adolescents is more favourable than in adults.

**Q13** Which of the following is *not* true regarding primary breast tumours in adolescents?

  **A** Chest wall radiation for Hodgkin's disease has been implicated as a risk factor in primary breast cancer.

  **B** The usual presentation is an enlarging, non-tender, firm, immobile lesion in the lateral breast quadrants.

  **C** Nipple discharge and nipple retraction are less common in adolescents with primary breast cancer than in adults with primary breast cancer.

  **D** Secretory carcinoma is a type of invasive ductal carcinoma with favourable prognosis that may spread beyond the breast to regional lymph nodes or may metastasise by the haematological route.

  **E** Secretory carcinoma almost always requires adjuvant chemotherapy and radiation therapy.

**A13**   **E**   Primary breast cancer has been reported in 39 children as of the year 2000. The average age is 11 (range 3–19). Histological subtypes of breast carcinoma seen in adolescents include the secretory subtype which has a thick-walled capsule. For the secretory subtype, surgical excision is the primary treatment and adjuvant therapy is rarely needed. Other subtypes described in children and adolescents include inflammatory breast cancer and medullary carcinoma. Surgical options for infiltrating lobular or intraductal carcinoma in adolescents include breast-sparing surgery (lumpectomy with axillary node dissection and irradiation) or modified radical mastectomy. Younger women tend to have more-aggressive disease. Systemic adjuvant chemotherapy is strongly advised in all young women with breast carcinoma.

**Q14** Regarding the inherited predisposition to breast cancer, the following are true *except*:

  **A** *BRCA1* is located on chromosome 17 and *BRCA2* is located on chromosome 13.

  **B** Recommendations for girls with predisposition to breast cancer include monthly breast examination between 18 and 21 years of age and mammography at age 23–35 years.

  **C** Annual bilateral breast MRI is recommended beginning at age 16.

  **D** *BRCA1* and *BRCA2* are felt to be responsible for 7%–9% of breast cancers.

  **E** Not all women with the *BRCA* genes will develop breast cancer.

**A14** **C** There are two genes responsible for 5%–9% of all breast cancers, *BRCA1* located on chromosome 17 and *BRCA2*, located on chromosome 13. Studies imply that carriers for *BRCA1* have a 65%–80% lifetime risk of breast cancer and *BRCA2* carriers have a 45%–85% lifetime risk of breast cancer. Adolescent genetic testing has been deemed ethically unacceptable by most professional organisations because of the current absence of beneficial medical interventions in children that would affect the course of disease. In adults, surveillance of *BRCA* carriers includes monthly breast examinations, clinical breast examinations once or twice yearly, yearly mammograms, and MRI of breast starting at age 25–30.

**Q15** The most common malignant breast tumour in the adolescent female is:

**A** a metastasis

**B** secretory breast carcinoma

**C** malignant cystosarcoma phyllodes

**D** infiltrating ductal carcinoma

**E** rhabdomyosarcoma.

**A15** **A** Metastatic lesions are more common than primary lesions in children and adolescents. Hodgkin's and non-Hodgkin's lymphoma, rhabdomyosarcoma, melanoma and neuroblastoma have been described to metastasise in the breast.

**Q16** A 12-year-old male presents with bilateral 2 cm tender masses just underneath the areola complex. There is no nipple discharge bilaterally. The rest of physical examination is normal. The patient has Tanner II intrascrotal testes and Tanner II hair development in the axilla and pubic areas. There were no palpable masses on abdominal examination. The next best course of action is:

**A** bilateral breast biopsies

**B** bilateral testicular biopsies

**C** abdomen and pelvic CT scan

**D** detailed history of current medications used by the patient

**E** genetic workup.

**A16** **D** Pubertal gynaecomastia is a benign, usually self-limited condition noted in 50%–60% of boys during early adolescence. Breast findings vary from a discrete 1–3 cm round, mobile and usually tender mass, just underneath the areola, to diffusely enlarged breasts. Changes may be unilateral or bilateral. Often, these young men may be followed in the clinic and reassured that the condition is self-limiting. If the breast enlargement is such that it causes pain, discomfort or psychological trauma, subcutaneous mastectomies may be performed.

Further workup may be necessary if the mass is large or fixed, if a discharge is present, or if it occurs between the neonatal period and adolescence. Causes for pathological gynaecomastia include Klinefelter's syndrome, testicular feminisation, hormone-secreting tumours, hyperthyroidism, hypothyroidism, cirrhosis, drugs (cimetidine, marijuana) and familial predisposition. Obese patients may have pseudogynaecomastia, where the preponderance of subcutaneous tissue in the chest wall may give the appearance of enlarged breasts.

## Further reading

Bengaulid V, Singh V, Singh H, *et al.* Myobacterium fortuitum and anaerobic breast abscess following nipple piercing: case presentation and review of the literature. *J Adolesc Health.* 2008; **42**(5): 530–2.

Diehl T, Kaplan W. Breast masses in adolescent females. *J Adolesc Health Care.* 1985; **6**(5): 353–7.

Fallat ME, Ignacio RC Jr. Breast disorders in children and adolescents. *J Pediatr Adolesc Gynecol.* 2008; **21**(6): 311–16.

Greydanus ME, Matytsina L, Gains M. Breast disorders in children and adolescents. *Prim Care.* 2006; **33**(2): 455–502.

Latham K, Fernandez S, Held L, *et al.* Pediatric breast deformity. *J Craniofac Surg.* 2006; **17**(3): 454–67.

Santen SJ, Mansel R. Benign breast disorders. *N Engl J Med.* 2005; **353**(3): 275–85.

Templeman C, Hertwick SP. Breast disorders in the pediatric and adolescent patient. *Obstet Gynecol Clin North Am.* 2000; **27**(1): 19–34.

# CHAPTER 18

# Chest wall deformities

## MICHAEL J GORETSKY, ROBERT OBERMEYER

**From the choices below each question, select the single best answer.**

**Q1** Thoracoscopy should be used:
 **A** from the right side only
 **B** from the left side only
 **C** from both sides
 **D** never
 **E** any of the above, at the discretion of the surgeon.

**A1** **E** The use of the thoracoscope has decreased the incidence of intraoperative collateral structure injury. The decision to use the thoracoscope on the left or right side is up to the surgeon. Even bilateral thoracoscopy is reasonable and actually recommended in cases of severe pectus excavatum, redo Nuss's procedure, or if visualisation from one side is inadequate. Although some advocate not using thoracoscopy, we have found it very helpful and it definitely makes the dissection safer.

**Q2** The best age to repair pectus excavatum using the minimally invasive technique is:
 **A** 3–6 years
 **B** 7–10 years
 **C** 11–14 years
 **D** 15–20 years
 **E** 21 and over.

**A2** **C** Repair of pectus excavatum prior to pubescence is not ideal because of the fact that most patients will outgrow the bar as they go through puberty. Repair of pectus excavatum after puberty is not ideal because the patient's chest begins to develop less compliance. Watching the patient's growth trajectory during the ages 11–14 years will typically allow for a time frame that is more optimal for pectus repair via the minimally invasive technique.

**Q3** It is easier to correct pectus excavatum before the child reaches puberty because:

  A  the psychological effects of the chest wall deformity will be prevented

  B  the patient will require only one bar

  C  the rib and cartilage structures are more pliable

  D  the pectus bar is smaller and easier to bend into position

  E  the patient has no physiologic benefit until after puberty.

**A3**  C  Prior to puberty the cartilage of the anterior rib cage as well as the bone of the lateral and posterior rib cage is more pliable. Changes in the density of the bony rib cage and ossification of the cartilaginous rib cage result in a much stiffer chest after puberty and into adulthood.

**Q4** Additional equipment kept immediately available in the cardiothoracic OR includes all *except*:

  A  sternoscopy tray

  B  sternal saw

  C  sternal retractors

  D  vascular clamps

  E  suction.

**A4**  A  Although the risk of cardiac injury is low, preparation for the steps that follow are of vital importance to improve the chances of patient survival. If a cardiac injury is recognised during introduction of the stabiliser, the first step is to leave the introducer in place and then call for assistance. Having the sternoscopy tray in the room will prevent this from being a source of delayed treatment.

**Q5** The pectus bar may be removed as an outpatient procedure after a minimum of _____ years?

  A  1

  B  2

  C  3

  D  4

  E  5

**A5**  B  Long-term assessment of pectus excavatum repair has been classified into four categories: excellent, good, fair or failed. An excellent repair is defined as a patient with no evidence of recurrence and resolution of associated symptoms. More patients fall into the excellent and good categories when the bar is left in place 24 months or longer.

**Q6** Pad placement for defibrillation in patients with a pectus bar should be:

   **A** posterior/mid-axillary

   **B** bilateral anterior

   **C** anterior/mid-axillary

   **D** anterior/posterior

   **E** bilateral axillary.

**A6**   **D**  Placement of the defibrillator in the typical recommended sites of the chest wall may result in ineffective delivery of energy to the heart because of the energy taking the path of least resistance along the bar. For this reason, in order to optimise delivery of energy to the myocardium, pad placement should be such that one pad is placed on the anterior thorax and one on the posterior thorax.

**Q7** Bar removal is facilitated by:

   **A** palpating the ends of the bar

   **B** reviewing chest X-ray preoperatively if bar cannot be palpated

   **C** fluoroscopy during surgery if needed

   **D** opening both incisions if needed

   **E** all of the above.

**A7**   **E**  Bar removal can be a complicated matter with significant complications if not done correctly. Knowing exactly where the bar is, is critical and imaging may be necessary if significant calcifications have developed. Counterbending the bar to straighten, by opening both incisions, is the safest method, to minimise the bar pulling on any tissue or organ on removal.

**Q8** Bar infection *may* require:

   **A** short-term high-dose antibiotic therapy

   **B** long-term preventive maintenance antibiotic therapy

   **C** incision drainage and packing of the wound

   **D** bar removal after failed conservative therapy

   **E** all of the above.

**A8**   **E**  Bar infection should be rare and occurs <2.5% of the time. Appropriate sterile technique and use of antibiotics minimises the risk of infection. When an infection occurs aggressive treatment can often save the bar. This includes long-term antibiotics, incision and drainage and use of wound-closure devices. Complete blood count, erythrocyte sedimentation, and C-reactive protein are useful inflammatory markers to use in determining duration of therapy. Repeat course of antibiotics has been able to preserve the bar when repeat infection occurs. Testing for metal allergy is also warranted for any 'atypical' wound issue.

**Q9** Stabilisers and polydioxanone (PDS) sutures placed around the ribs and the bar have reduced the incidence of bar displacement from 15% to:

   **A** 12%

   **B** 10%

   **C** 5%

   **D** <2%

   **E** 0%.

**A9** **D** Bar displacement is the most common complication associated with Nuss's procedure. Various modifications over the last 20 years have significantly decreased the incidence. Generally one stabiliser per bar is recommended since bilateral stabilisers did not change the incidence and can lead to rib compression in those patients who are actively growing. The use of PDS around the ribs and the liberal use of two bars have greatly decreased the incidence of bar displacement. If the bar rotates less than 10–15 degrees and still provides the same support it can be observed without reoperating. Slight rotation within 1 month of surgery may be best treated by adding a second bar or resecuring.

**Q10** Patients with known metal allergies should have:

   **A** a custom titanium bar

   **B** a TRUE patch (Thin-layer Rapid-Use Epicutaneous test)

   **C** no antibiotics pre-op

   **D** referral to an allergy specialist

   **E** no umbilical piercings.

**A10** **A** Metal allergies can occur in up to 3% of pectus patients. Any patient with a history of a metal or jewellery allergy or atopic history should be tested with a TRUE patch. This tests for multiple allergens including nickel and cobalt specific for the Nuss bar. Anyone who tests positive should have titanium bars made. It is important to remember to also use a titanium stabiliser and not use wire to secure the bar to stabiliser. Anyone with a bar that has atypical symptoms should be tested for nickel allergy.

**Q11** When planning to place two bars, do all *except*:

   **A** place introducer in easiest location first

   **B** elevate sternum while passing second introducer through deepest defect

   **C** make sure at least one bar is under the sternum

   **D** make sure both bars are under the sternum

   **E** put stabilisers on opposite sides.

A11  **D**  The use of 2 bars has significantly increased in the last 10 years. Their use is increased in older patients >16 years with stiff chests, saucer-shaped defects, asymmetrical pectus patients, sterna torsion, recurrent pectus excavatum patients, and those patients with Marfan's syndrome or similar phenotype. When placing two bars it is easier to place the more superior bar first since this will be an easier dissection. It is frequently helpful to leave the first introducer in place to facilitate dissecting the second tunnel. It is imperative that at least one bar is fully under the sternum, but the second bar does not necessarily need to be under the sternum if the defect is low.

Q12  Techniques to avoid pericardial injury include all *except*:
  **A**  maintaining dissection immediately adjacent to the posterior sternum
  **B**  turning up pulse oximeter volume while passing the introducer
  **C**  use of a thoracoscope
  **D**  dissection predominantly in an anterior to posterior direction
  **E**  reviewing pre-op CT scan for sternal torsion/anatomy.

A12  **B**  Any hole in the pericardium may lead to post-pericardiotomy syndrome. This can easily be treated with non-steroidal anti-inflammatory drugs. Although a hole should be avoided it is sometimes impossible not to have it occur if there are a lot of adhesions. The bar should NEVER be allowed to go through the pericardium since this may lead to cardiac rupture at time of removal. Thoracoscopy is invaluable in avoiding this injury and more importantly recognising it if it occurs and allowing repositioning of the bar outside the pericardium.

## Further reading

Goretsky MJ, Kelly RE Jr, Croitoru DP, *et al*. Chest wall anomalies: pectus excavatum and pectus carinatum. *Adolesc Med Clin*. 2004; **15**(3): 455–71.

Redlinger RE Jr, Rushing GD, Moskowitz AD, *et al*. Minimally invasive repair of pectus excavatum in patients with Marfan syndrome and marfanoid features. *J Pediatr Surg*. 2010; **45**(1): 193–9.

Rushing GD, Goretsky MJ, Gustin T, *et al*. When it is not an infection: metal allergy after the Nuss procedure for repair of pectus excavatum. *J Pediatr Surg*. 2007; **42**(1): 93–7.

Shin S, Goretsky MJ, Kelly RE Jr, *et al*. Infectious complications after the Nuss repair in a series of 863 patients. *J Pediatr Surg*. 2007; **42**(1): 87–92.

# CHAPTER 19

# Disorders of larynx, trachea and upper airway

## CHARLES M MYER IV, CHARLES M MYER III

**From the choices below each question, select the single best answer.**

**Q1** The most serious complication of closure of a tracheocutaneous fistula is:

- **A** bleeding
- **B** wound infection
- **C** wound breakdown
- **D** scar
- **E** pneumothorax.

**A1** **E** Tracheocutaneous fistula is a result of epithelialisation of the skin tract from the anterior neck to the trachea that fails to close following decannulation. While all answers are complications of tracheocutaneous fistula, pneumothorax following fistula closure can result in rapid airway compromise and death. Traditional primary closure, a multilayered technique, can result in air that extravasates from the trachea becoming trapped under the reapproximated cutaneous and deeper layers. This air can track into the chest, resulting in a pneumothorax or pneumomediastinum. Drain placement and observation may decrease this risk, as will the use of a secondary intention closure, in which the skin tract to the level of the trachea is excised and no dermal or epidermal closure is performed.

**Q2** Which of the following symptoms occurs most frequently with either congenital or acquired?

- **A** inspiratory stridor
- **B** cough
- **C** dysphagia
- **D** hoarseness
- **E** cyclical cyanosis

A2    **A** Subglottic stenosis is defined as a narrowing of the airway located in the area directly below the vocal cords. Independent of the aetiology, this narrowing produces turbulent inspiratory flow which creates stridor, a high-pitched noise. Stridor may be created from narrowing anywhere in the airway and the characteristics may help to predict location of the lesion. The gold standard for diagnosis of subglottic stenosis remains airway endoscopy with examination of the supraglottis, glottis and trachea.

Q3    In epiglottitis, patients frequently assume what characteristic position to facilitate breathing?

**A** supine

**B** prone

**C** tripod

**D** open-mouth

**E** lateral-decubitus

A3    **C** Although relatively uncommon since the introduction of the *Haemophilus influenzae* type b immunisation policy, epiglottitis is still seen secondary to both infectious and non-infectious causes. Inflammation of the epiglottis and associated supraglottic structures results in narrowing of the airway above the glottis. To maximise airflow through the oedematous tissues, the child often leans forward with hands on the bed or chair and the head tilted in the sniffing position. This manoeuvre functions to open the upper airway and improve dynamics of respiratory muscle use.

Q4    A patient with a type IV laryngeal cleft has a defect at the level of the:

**A** tip of arytenoid

**B** supraglottis

**C** vocal cords

**D** mid-trachea

**E** carina.

A4    **E** A laryngeal cleft is a congenital defect that results from incomplete fusion of the cricoid cartilage or incomplete tracheo-oesophageal septum formation. The most widely utilised classification system was described by Benjamin and Inglis in 1989. In this system, clefts are divided into four categories based upon the extension of the defect. A type I cleft extends between the arytenoids of the posterior glottis to the level of the vocal folds. Type II clefts involve the posterior cricoid cartilage but lack complete involvement of the cartilage. Extension through the cricoid cartilage, with or without extension into the cervical trachea defines a type III cleft. A type IV cleft extends to the thoracic trachea and may include the carina. In general, the severity of the symptomatology correlates to the severity of the cleft present.

**Q5** Expiratory stridor is commonly associated with abnormalities of the:

A nasopharynx

B oropharynx

C glottis

D subglottis

E tracheobronchial tree.

**A5** E Stridor, a noise created by turbulent flow through a narrowed portion of the airway, can be classified by phase of respiration. Inspiratory stridor generally corresponds to blockage of the supraglottic or glottic airway. Expiratory stridor is often a symptom of tracheal or bronchial obstruction and may be associated with a prolonged expiratory phase. Biphasic stridor is traditionally described in subglottic or high tracheal lesions. Obstruction of the nasopharynx and oropharynx will produce stertor, a snore-like respiratory noise. While symptomatology may suggest a site of lesion, airway endoscopy is required to definitively diagnose the obstruction.

**Q6** Patients with type I laryngeal cleft commonly present with all of the following *except*:

A aspiration

B choking

C cough

D recurrent pneumonia

E expiratory stridor.

**A6** E In the Benjamin and Inglis classification, a type I laryngeal cleft is described as a supraglottic cleft involving the interarytenoid region extending to, but not involving, the tissues inferior to the level of the true vocal cords. As complete separation of the oesophagus and airway is not achieved, patients typically present with symptoms of difficulty feeding as well as recurrent pulmonary insults, including aspiration and associated pneumonias. Stridor is a frequent associated symptom, especially in patients with a co-diagnosis of laryngomalacia. It is primarily inspiratory in nature.

**Q7** An 8-year-old patient presents with a 1-day history of inspiratory stridor and radiographic evidence of tracheal wall irregularities and tracheal membranes. Flexible endoscopy reveals crusting in the subglottis. The most likely diagnosis is:

A croup

B epiglottitis

C retropharyngeal abscess

D subglottic haemangioma

E bacterial tracheitis.

**A7** **E** Infectious diseases of the airway, including croup, epiglottitis and bacterial tracheitis, all produce an acute obstructive insult resulting in stridor and difficulty breathing. Bacterial tracheitis differs from croup and epiglottitis in the presence of exudates lining the tracheal lumen causing the airway obstruction rather than primarily tissue oedema. Identification of the child with bacterial tracheitis is key as treatment involves endoscopic removal of the exudate and crusts to prevent complete airway obstruction. While suspicion may be based upon a failure of response to traditional treatment of viral laryngotracheitis, primarily inhaled epinephrine and steroids, definitive diagnosis is made with flexible endoscopic evaluation showing tracheal crusts or secretions that do not clear with cough. Radiographs in bacterial tracheitis show tracheal wall irregularities, different from the findings of subglottic oedema (steeple sign) in croup, and epiglottic smudging (thumbprint sign) in epiglottitis.

**Q8** A 3-year-old male presents with a 3-day history of fever, sore throat and lethargy. The parents noted a recent upper respiratory infection prior to his acute illness. Examination reveals marked torticollis with fullness in the right neck. The most likely diagnosis is:

A peritonsillar abscess

B oesophageal foreign body

C tonsillitis

D retropharyngeal abscess

E epiglottitis.

**A8** **D** The retropharyngeal space houses the retropharyngeal lymph nodes which involute at approximately 5 years of age. Suppurative lymphadenitis, often following an antecedent head or neck infection, is the primary aetiology in children, although direct extension from adjacent infection as well as direct inoculation secondary to trauma may also be causative. Symptoms include fever, lethargy, torticollis, odynophagia and decreased oral intake. Physical examination may include cervical lymphadenopathy or an appreciable bulge or mass in posterior pharynx, although these are frequently absent. Classic teaching describes airway compromise and diagnostic confusion with epiglottitis. Recent studies, however, show a low incidence of airway symptoms with retropharyngeal abscess and postulate its absence until progression of disease has occurred. High-voltage airway radiography and CT scanning are useful clinical adjuncts to diagnosis. Treatment includes parenteral antibiotics and surgical drainage dependent on response to conservative measures and overall condition of the child.

**Q⁹** Evaluation of an infant with expiratory stridor demonstrated no remarkable findings other than noisy breathing. Airway radiographs were obtained and showed no obvious lesions. Bronchoscopy was performed, demonstrating asymmetrical narrowing of the distal trachea with compression of the right anterior tracheal wall. The most likely diagnosis is:

**A** complete tracheal rings

**B** double aortic arch

**C** innominate artery compression of the trachea

**D** aberrant subclavian artery

**E** pulmonary sling.

**A⁹** **C** Narrowing of the trachea, tracheomalacia, can produce airway obstruction and result in stridor, often in the expiratory phase of respiration, in association with a prolonged expiratory phase as well as dying spells or apnoea. Tracheomalacia can be due to defects of the tracheal wall or secondary to an external compression, often a result of anomalies of the mediastinal vasculature. Double aortic arch and aberrant subclavian artery will produce a distal tracheal collapse, primarily posterior in nature. Right-sided anterior tracheal wall compression may be secondary to either a pulmonary sling or innominate artery compression with the latter being the more common aetiology. Not all patients with an anomalous innominate artery course will be symptomatic. Airway fluoroscopy may show an anterior narrowing approximately 1–2 cm above the carina and endoscopy reveals an often pulsatile compression over the distal right trachea. Compression of the pulsatile area with the bronchoscope can diminish the pulse in the right upper extremity. Diagnosis is based on evaluation of the surrounding vasculature with MRI or an equivalent study.

**Q10** A 6-year-old female child presents to your office with chronic hoarseness. She has no symptoms of airway obstruction. Her parents state that she is a 'loud' child and screams often. What is the most likely diagnosis?

    **A** subglottic stenosis

    **B** recurrent respiratory papillomatosis

    **C** unilateral vocal fold paralysis

    **D** vocal fold nodules

    **E** unilateral vocal fold cyst

**A10** **D** Vocal fold nodules are the most common cause of hoarseness in children. Voice overuse or abuse are often cited as the primary causes(s) of the lesions. Diagnosis is made by flexible laryngoscopy/stroboscopy. Management usually consists of behavioural modifications and voice therapy.

**Q11** A 2-year-old child undergoes microlaryngoscopy and rigid bronchoscopy for acute airway obstruction. The examination demonstrates wart-like lesions obstructing the airway. What is the organism associated with this lesion?

    **A** *Haemophilus influenzae*

    **B** Respiratory syncytial virus

    **C** Human papilloma virus

    **D** Human immunodeficiency virus

    **E** Herpes simplex virus 1

**A11** **C** Human papilloma virus is the causative agent in recurrent respiratory papillomatosis (RRP). RRP is most commonly diagnosed between ages 2 and 5 years in children. The disease is characterised by wart-like lesions that cause airway obstruction and hoarseness. Management is airway stabilisation and surgical debridement of the obstructing papillomas.

**Q12** Injury to what structure during a patent ductus arteriosus (PDA) ligation would cause a weak, breathy cry and aspiration in a neonate?

    **A** sympathetic chain

    **B** recurrent laryngeal nerve

    **C** phrenic nerve

    **D** superior laryngeal nerve

    **E** ansa cervicalis

**A12** **B** The recurrent laryngeal nerve is at risk during PDA ligation. Injury can present as either a weak cry or aspiration. Diagnosis is made by flexible fibre-optic laryngoscopy. Neonates less than 28 weeks and below 1250 g weight are at higher risk of injury to the nerve. Treatment involves management of the feeding disorder. The acute paralysis can be managed with a unilateral temporary vocal fold injection. Long-term management involves observation to determine the ultimate outcome of the paralysis.

Q13 A 3-month-old previously healthy baby girl presents to your clinic (*see* Figure 19.1). Mum reports that over the last several weeks her child has had noisy breathing. The respiratory sounds are described as being especially pronounced during crying and feeding.

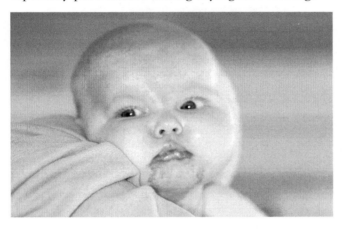

FIGURE 19.1 A 3-month-old child with breathing difficulty

The most likely diagnosis for this child's breathing difficulties is:
A  subglottic stenosis
B  laryngomalacia
C  laryngotracheomalacia
D  nasal airway obstruction
E  subglottic haemangioma.

A13  E  Segmental facial haemangiomas in a beard distribution are commonly associated with airway haemangiomas. Segmental haemangiomas in the submental area especially are highly associated with airway haemangiomas. Airway haemangiomas can occur in the oral cavity, nasopharynx, hypopharynx, glottis or subglottis. In contrast to the other sites, haemangiomas of the subglottis are typically bulky and can significantly narrow the upper respiratory tract leading to respiratory insufficiency. Children with obstructive airway haemangiomas typically present at 2–3 months of age. Important to remember is that only 50% of children with a subglottic haemangioma have a cutaneous haemangioma.

Q14 A 5-month-old child is referred to you by her paediatrician for evaluation of a possible subglottic haemangioma since the child is noted to have a large segmental facial haemangioma (*see* Figure 19.2). However, after eliciting a history from the parents, you note that the child has no feeding or airway symptoms. Furthermore, a flexible laryngoscopy, and soft tissue airway films demonstrate no obvious subglottic lesions.

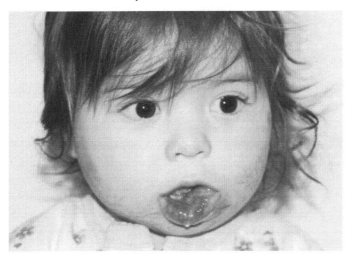

FIGURE 19.2 A 5-month-old child with segmental facial haemangioma

At this point the next reasonable step in management is:

A Assure the parents that given there is no subglottic haemangioma at the moment, there is unlikely to be one later.

B Since the airway is normal, send the patient to a facial plastic surgeon for treatment of the lip deformity.

C Refer the patient to an ophthalmologist, cardiologist and neurologist for evaluation of PHACES.

D Tell the parents that there is no airway haemangioma present on initial exam, and advise that the patient should undergo serial airway evaluations in the operating room for the next 4 months.

E Discharge the patient home with no follow-up.

A14 C Segmental facial haemangiomas can be associated with PHACES syndrome, especially when the haemangioma occurs in a V1 distribution. However, some children have facial haemangiomas that cross all three dermatomes and thus cannot be classified easily into those that are at high risk for airway haemangiomas and those that are at high risk for PHACES syndrome. PHACES is an acronym that stands for **P**osterior cranial fossa malformations, **H**aemangioma, **A**rterial anomalies, **C**ardiac defects, **E**ye anomalies, and **S**ternal clefts or **S**upraumbilical raphe.

**Q15** Medical treatment options for subglottic haemangiomas include all of the following *except*:

   **A**  systemic propranolol

   **B**  systemic steroids

   **C**  intralesional steroids

   **D**  systemic vincristine

   **E**  intralesional vincristine.

**A15**  **E**  Medical treatment options for the management of subglottic haemangioma include all of the above except for intralesional vincristine injections. Currently, the most efficacious medical treatment option for subglottic haemangioma appears to be systemic propranolol. However, in the recent past both systemic and intralesional steroids have been fairly effective. Some have even advocated a combination treatment with both systemic propranolol and steroids (intralesional or systemic).

## Further reading

Haggstrom AN, Garzon MC, Baselga E, *et al*. Risk for PHACE syndrome in infants with large facial hemangiomas. *Paediatrics*. 2010; **126**(2): e418–26. Epub 2010 Jul 19.

Metry DW, Haggstrom AN, Drolet BA, *et al*. A prospective study of PHACE syndrome in infantile hemangiomas: demographic features, clinical findings, and complications. *Am J Med Genet A*. 2006; **140**(9): 975–86.

O TM, Alexander RE, Lando T, *et al*. Segmental hemangiomas of the upper airway. *Laryngoscope*. 2009; **119**(11): 2242–7.

Orlow SJ, Isakoff MS, Blei F. Increased risk of symptomatic hemangiomas of the airway in association with cutaneous hemangiomas in a 'beard' distribution. *J Pediatr*. 1997; **131**(4): 643–6.

Perkins JA, Duke W, Chen E, *et al*. Emerging concepts in airway infantile hemangioma assessment and management. *Otolaryngol Head Neck Surg*. 2009; **141**(2): 207–12.

Rosbe KW, Suh KY, Meyer AK, *et al*. Propranolol in the management of airway infantile hemangiomas. *Arch Otolaryngol Head Neck Surg*. 2010; **136**(7): 658–65.

# CHAPTER 20

# Congenital diaphragmatic hernia

## MARY BRINDLE, DAVID SIGALET

**From the choices below each question, select the single best answer.**

**Q1** Which aspect of fetal pulmonary development is most significantly affected by congenital diaphragmatic hernia (CDH)?
  **A** embryonal
  **B** pseudoglandular
  **C** canalicular
  **D** saccular
  **E** alveolar

**A1** **C** Lung development proceeds from initial lung bud formation through a series of branchings and alveolarisation. Embryonal phase is associated with lung bud formation, while pseudoglandular represents formation of the large bronchi. The canalicular phase of lung development generally occurs from week 16 to week 24 and it is this stage at which the terminal bronchioles are formed. Disruption at this stage results in 'pruning' of the pulmonary airways with large branching points but missing the small branches crucial for optimal gas exchange. Alveoli start forming in the fetal saccular stage and progress during the alveolar stage which continues postnatally.

**Q2** What is the most common presentation of CDH?
  **A** prenatal diagnosis on ultrasound
  **B** fetal distress preceding delivery
  **C** respiratory deterioration within hours of delivery
  **D** incidental finding on chest radiograph
  **E** late diagnosis after 1 year of age

**A2** **A** Prenatal diagnosis on ultrasound is the most common presentation of CDH in North America and in most developed nations. As routine antenatal sonography is generally performed between 18 and 20 weeks, the defect itself will be present at this time. Occasionally the diagnosis of CDH is missed on this early ultrasound.

Liver and lung have similar echogenicity early on and liver herniated into the chest may be mistaken for lung. Bowel within the chest is less likely to be missed; however, occasionally when the defect is present the intestinal contents do not herniate into the chest. If prenatal ultrasound is not performed or the diagnosis is missed, the most common presentation of CDH is shortly after birth. Delivery itself is rarely complicated by the condition as the fetus is untroubled by pulmonary hypoplasia. Late diagnoses and incidental findings of CDH are less common.

**Q3** The best time to repair CDH is:

  **A** prior to birth
  **B** as shortly after delivery as is feasible
  **C** electively after extubation
  **D** when infant is on minimal ventilator settings
  **E** if hypoxia is worsening despite maximal support.

**A3**  **D** At the present time, prenatal intervention for CDH is an experimental therapy undertaken on a small subset of high-risk patients. Repair itself is not pursued in fetal interventions but the trachea itself is plugged causing lung growth. The goal of the surgery is to salvage the small proportion of very high-risk infants. These infants will still require formal repair postnatally. Timing of surgical repair has shifted from its early conception as a surgical emergency to a repair that is undertaken once stability is achieved. Infants who die prior to surgical repair generally represent a subset for whom surgery does not change outcome. Ideally surgery is performed prior to extubation once the patient is stable on conventional ventilation and pulmonary arterial pressures are sub-systemic (ideally normalised).

**Q4** Measures used by clinicians in the first days of life to provide an estimation of severity of pulmonary hypertension in CDH include all *except*:

  **A** right-to-left flow on patent ductus arteriosus
  **B** flattening of the intraventricular septum
  **C** tricuspid regurgitation velocity of flow
  **D** right ventricular hypertrophy
  **E** difference in pre- and post-ductal saturation measurement.

**A4**  **D** During development of pulmonary hypertension, pressures build up within the pulmonary arteries. There is increasing resistance to flow which results in shunting of blood from the pulmonary circulation to the systemic circulation via the ductus arteriosus. With worsening hypertension, pressure backs up into the ventricle causing the interventricular septum, which naturally curves into the right ventricle, to flatten and then bow into the left ventricle. The ventricular muscle also becomes hypertrophied and pressure may even force blood to regurgitate through the tricuspid valve. The velocity of this flow provides an indirect estimation of the degree of pulmonary hypertension. Ventricular hypertrophy is a late development in pulmonary hypertension and is not often seen in the first few days of life.

 **Q5** Which prenatal ultrasound finding is most predictive of poor outcome for an infant with CDH?

A lung-to-head ratio <1.0

B MRI findings of lung volume <50% of predicted.

C presence of liver in the chest

D double-outlet right ventricle

E right-sided CDH

 **A5** **D** The presence of a significant cardiac anomaly has grave repercussions for the fetus. Survival for infants with CDH complicated by complex heart disease has been estimated at 20%. Other features that can be examined to help determine prognosis are often related to factors that provide some estimation of lung volume. Liver within the chest is a strong predictor of poor lung volume and complications related to pulmonary hypoplasia. There is controversy as to the most sensitive predictor of pulmonary hypoplasia. Presence of liver in the chest (and the volume of liver as based on MRI) represents one measure that is predictive in most studies. There is less consistency in terms of direct measures of lung volumes. On ultrasound, this usually involves a two-dimensional measure of the contralateral lung at the level of the four-chamber view of the heart. The measurement of the lung is compared with some normal measure, often the fetal head. The lung-to-head ratio can be further normalised by comparing the lung-to-head ratio of the fetus with that of a fetus at similar gestational age without CDH (an observed-to-expected ratio). This is commonly performed in European centres to predict the most severely affected fetus. Lung-to-head ratio less than 1.0 has been associated with worse outcomes in many but not all centres. MRI provides further information to enable a more precise estimate of lung volume. Right-sided CDH has poor outcome compared with left-sided CDH. One reason for this may be that small defects on the right side are not clinically apparent and it is only with large defects and liver herniation that right-sided CDH is diagnosed. MRI lung volumes currently show that survivors with CDH have lung volumes about 30% of expected, while fetuses that do not survive have lung volumes around 19%–20% of expected.

**Q6** Common long-term complications of CDH include all *except*:
  A  gastro-oesophageal reflux
  B  reactive airway disease
  C  pectus excavatum
  D  tracheomalacia
  E  impairment of lung function on pulmonary function testing.

**A6**  **D**  Tracheomalacia is a complication typically associated with tracheo-oesophageal fistula and does not commonly present in CDH. Chest wall deformities are relatively common with CDH. Long-term respiratory compromise has been demonstrated quantitatively with both obstructive and restrictive impairment in pulmonary function testing and is likewise clinically apparent with increase in bronchodilator use in this patient population. Gastro-oesophageal reflux is a common issue with these infants due to disruption of the anatomical relationship between the diaphragm and the distal oesophagus.

**Q7** A small, rubbery piece of tissue is identified at the margin of the diaphragm at the time of surgical repair. This most likely represents:
  A  pulmonary sequestration
  B  splenule
  C  accessory hepatic tissue
  D  neuroblastoma
  E  benign adrenal tumour.

**A7**  **A**  Small extralobar pulmonary sequestrations are relatively common occurrences in conjunction with large diaphragmatic hernia and often are present at the border between the chest and the abdomen.

**Q8** Which of the following treatment strategies would *not* be used for a term infant with severe pulmonary hypertension and worsening ventilatory impairment associated with diaphragmatic hernia?
  A  administration of surfactant
  B  allowing persistent elevation of $PCO_2$ beyond the normal limits
  C  inhaled nitric oxide
  D  high-frequency oscillation
  E  extracorporeal membrane oxygenation (ECMO)

**A8**  **A**  Surfactant has not been associated with improved survival for infants with CDH. One of the crucial strategies for improving neonatal outcomes was the development of 'gentle ventilation' allowing for the accumulation of carbon dioxide or 'permissive hypercapnia' to minimise barotrauma. In infants with poor oxygenation, this strategy may involve using a high-frequency oscillator to delivery very small volume breaths. Although the indications for ECMO vary from centre to centre, it is a therapy that has a recognised role in the management of some high-risk patients with congenital diaphragmatic hernia. Inhaled nitric oxide may have some benefit in diminishing pulmonary hypertension in infants with diaphragmatic hernia.

 For a mother who has a child with an isolated CDH with a normal karyotype, the likelihood of having a second child with CDH is:

**A** 1 : 5000

**B** 2%

**C** 10%

**D** 50%

**E** 1 : 1000.

 **B** The frequency of diaphragmatic hernia in the general population is between 1 : 2500 and 1 : 5000 live births. Although uncommon, a future sibling will have between a 1% and a 2% chance of having a diaphragmatic hernia.

## Further reading

Ba'ath ME, Jesudason EC, Losty PD. How useful is the lung-to-head ratio in predicting outcome in the fetus with congenital diaphragmatic hernia? A systematic review and meta-analysis. *Ultrasound Obstet Gynecol.* 2007; **30**(6): 897–906.

Bagolan P, Morini F. Long-term follow up of infants with congenital diaphragmatic hernia. *Semin Pediatr Surg.* 2007; **16**(2): 134–44.

Bootstaylor BS, Filly RA, Harrison MR, *et al.* Prenatal sonographic predictors of liver herniation in congenital diaphragmatic hernia. *J Ultrasound Med.* 1995; **14**(7): 515–20.

Downard CD. Congenital diaphragmatic hernia: an ongoing clinical challenge. *Curr Opin Pediatr.* 2008; **20**(3): 300–4.

Javid PJ, Jaksic T, Skarsgard ED, *et al.* Survival rate in congenital diaphragmatic hernia: the experience of the Canadian Neonatal Network. *J Pediatr Surg.* 2004; **39**(5): 657–60.

Smith NP, Jesudason EC, Featherstone NC, *et al.* Recent advances in congenital diaphragmatic hernia. *Arch Dis Child.* 2005; **90**(4): 426–8.

Van den Hout L, Sluiter I, Gischler S, *et al.* Can we improve outcome of congenital diaphragmatic hernia? *Pediatr Surg Int.* 2009; **25**(9): 733–43.

# CHAPTER 21

# Congenital lung malformations

## MATIAS BRUZONI, CRAIG T ALBANESE

**From the choices below each question, select the single best answer.**

**Q1** The most common site for congenital lobar emphysema is the:
 **A** right upper lobe
 **B** left lower lobe
 **C** left upper lobe
 **D** right lower lobe
 **E** right middle lobe.

**A1** **C** Congenital lobar emphysema is a congenital cystic lung lesion in which the fundamental abnormality consists of an abnormal bronchus that allows passage of air on inspiration but only limited expulsion of air on expiration leading to lobar overexpansion. These lesions do not always cause symptoms. In severe cases, prenatal hydrops or postnatal fatal respiratory distress can occur. The most common site of involvement for congenital lobar emphysema is the left upper lobe (40%–50%), followed by the right middle lobe (30%–40%), right upper lobe (20%), lower lobes (1%) and multiple sites for the remainder.

**Q2** The most common location for a congenital pulmonary adenomatoid malformation (CPAM) is in the:
 **A** right upper lobe
 **B** lingula
 **C** left upper lobe
 **D** either lower lobe
 **E** right middle lobe.

**A2** **D** CPAMs represent about 30%–40% of developmental lung bud anomalies and are diagnosed both antenatally and postnatally. Evidence suggests that lesions arise from insults that may occur from 5 to 22 weeks of gestation. CPAMs are characterised by an adenomatoid increase of terminal respiratory bronchioles that form cysts of various sizes. It consists of a discrete, intrapulmonary mass that contains cysts ranging in diameter from less than 1.0 mm to over 10.0 cm. CPAMs usually arise from one lobe of the lung, with the lower lobes being the most common site. Bilateral lung involvement is rare. Congenital cystic adenomatoid malformation lesions have an equal left- and right-sided incidence.

Q3 The systemic perfusion and venous drainage of an extralobar pulmonary sequestration (ELS) consists of:

A systemic artery and mostly systemic venous drainage

B systemic artery and mostly pulmonary venous drainage

C pulmonary artery and pulmonary venous drainage

D pulmonary artery and systemic venous drainage

E variable inflow and systemic pulmonary drainage.

A3 A Bronchopulmonary sequestrations (BPSs) are microscopic cystic masses of non-functioning pulmonary tissue that lack an obvious communication with the tracheobronchial tree. An accepted embryologic theory is that a supernumerary lung bud arises caudal to the normal lung bud and continues to migrate distally with the oesophagus. If this lung bud arises prior to the development of the pleura, it is invested with adjacent lung and becomes an intralobar sequestration (ILS). If supernumerary lung development occurs subsequent to pleura formation, the bud will grow separately and acquire its own pleural covering, forming an ELS. All the ELSs have a systemic arterial blood supply. In most ELSs, there are systemic venous connections, which include the superior vena cava, the azygous and hemiazygous veins. ILSs are supplied by systemic vessels and drain into the pulmonary circulation.

Q4 The microscopic features that distinguish a CPAM from other pulmonary lesions are all of the following *except*:

A polypoid projections of the mucosa

B increased smooth muscle and elastic fibres within the cyst wall

C increased cartilage within the mass

D mucus-secreting cells

E absence of inflammation.

A4 C Macroscopically, CPAMs can be very difficult to differentiate from pulmonary sequestrations or congenital lobar emphysema. Microscopically, a CPAM is distinguished from other lesions and normal lung by several features. These include polypoid projections of the mucosa, an increase in smooth muscle and elastic tissue within cyst walls, an absence of cartilage, the presence of mucus-secreting cells and the absence of inflammation.

**Q5** CPAMs that consist of large cysts surrounded by smaller cysts and account for 50%–65% of all CPAMs are classified as:

A  type I

B  type II

C  type I and II

D  type III

E  type IV.

**A5**  **A**  The type 0 CPAM, also known as acinar dysplasia or agenesis, is a rarely occurring malformation that is incompatible with life. Affected infants survive for only a few hours. Type I CPAM is the predominant cystic type, comprising 50%–65% of postnatal cases. They consist of single or multiple large cysts (3–10 cm in diameter) surrounded by smaller cysts and compressed normal parenchyma. Type II lesions account for 10%–40% of postnatal CPAMs and consist of more numerous smaller cysts (0.5–2.0 cm in diameter) that are lined by cuboidal-to-columnar epithelial cells with a thin, underlying, fibromuscular layer. Type III lesions account for only 5%–10% of postnatal cases and have a male predominance. These lesions consist of small cystic lesions that appear solid on gross examination. Microscopically, lesions resemble an immature lung devoid of bronchi. These cells are surrounded by alveolar ductules and saccules also lined by epithelial cells. Finally, type IV CPAM (10%–15% of cases) consists of a hamartomatous malformation of the distal acinus. Macroscopically, large thin-walled cysts are located at the periphery of the lobe and are lined by a smooth membrane. Microscopically, type IV cysts are lined by flattened type I and II epithelial cells over most of the cyst wall.

**Q6** The *most* accurate prognostic factor for prenatally diagnosed CPAMs is:

A  presence or absence of hydrops

B  type IV CPAM

C  size

D  location

E  gestational age at diagnosis.

**A6**  **A**  The classification described above may correlate with a favourable or unfavourable prognosis depending on the subtype; however, it does not affect treatment decisions and is not sufficient to provide an accurate prognosis. Rather, prognosis for prenatally diagnosed lesions largely depends on the presence or absence of hydrops. Additionally, prognosis for both prenatally and postnatally diagnosed lesions depends on the size of the lesion and the extent of pulmonary hypoplasia, as well as the presence of other significant anomalies.

**Q7** A 28-year-old female is 27 weeks pregnant with a fetus whose prenatal ultrasound reveals a 3.5 cm cystic mass in the left lower lobe. There is mediastinal shift and no hydrops. The next step in management should be:

**A** counselling for termination of pregnancy

**B** intrauterine drainage of the mass

**C** observation with serial ultrasounds

**D** placement of thoracoamniotic shunt

**E** *in utero* excision of the mass.

 **A7** **C** The size of the CPAM can cause mediastinal shift and low-output cardiac failure from caval and cardiac compression. This results in polyhydramnios and hydrops. Hydrops manifests as skin/scalp oedema, ascites, pleural or pericardial effusions and placentomegaly. The single characteristic most commonly noted with fetal demise or perinatal death is hydrops. In the absence of hydrops, the survival of fetuses with CPAMs is excellent. Ultrasound-guided interventions or prenatal surgery are not indicated for fetuses who are not hydropic. Termination of pregnancy would not be recommended since there is a high chance that this fetus will probably have a good outcome. Symptomatic patients may require surgery or drainage of the cyst soon after birth for adequate ventilation. Observation with serial ultrasounds is the appropriate management in this case.

 **Q8** An otherwise healthy newborn has a prenatal diagnosis of a cystic lesion in the right lung. His chest radiograph is unremarkable and he is on room air. Appropriate management at this point includes:

**A** elective radiographic (e.g. CT scan) localisation

**B** operative resection as soon as possible

**C** emergency CT of the chest

**D** follow up with observation and chest X-rays until the patient becomes symptomatic

**E** serial chest ultrasounds.

 **A8** **C** Occasionally, CPAMs or sequestrations will decrease in size or even disappear by the time of delivery. If not seen on chest X-ray, a chest CT with intravenous contrast is still recommended since small lesions are not well seen on plain radiographs. In addition, it is important to recognise a systemic arterial blood supply, which may help during resection. Asymptomatic masses do not require urgent surgery and can be watched over the first several months. Most authors suggest that the child with a persistent lung mass undergoes resection before the first year of life to avoid infectious complications. While the incidence of malignancy is unknown, undiagnosed lesions have been reported to experience malignant transformation several decades after birth.

**Q9** Even though infrequent, case reports show that CPAMs can have malignant transformation into all of the following tumour types *except*:

A rhabdomyosarcoma

B squamous cell carcinoma

C adenocarcinoma

D bronchioalveolar carcinoma

E pleuropulmonary blastoma.

**A9** **B** The management of asymptomatic CPAMs continues to be controversial, with some authors advocating observation and others recommending elective resection. However, most agree that there is substantial evidence against a 'wait and see' approach. A growing number of reports document malignancies such as myxosarcoma, embryonal rhabdomyosarcoma, pleuropulmonary blastoma and bronchioalveolar carcinoma arising in CPAMs. Although primary lung tumours are rare during the first 2 decades of life, up to 8% of these tumours are associated with congenital cystic lesions of the lung, including CPAMs. The youngest reported patient with a malignancy arising within a CPAM was only 13 months of age. Squamous cell carcinomas have not yet been described in the literature in this setting.

**Q10** The operation recommended for a 3 cm microcystic lesion located in the left lower lobe of the lung is:

A wedge resection

B drainage of the cyst

C marsupialisation of the cyst

D lobectomy

E lobectomy and local lymph node dissection.

**A10** **D** Most authors recommend elective resection either at birth or at about 1 month of age after allowing some time for family bonding at home. Most CPAMs can be treated with single lobectomy. The rationale behind lobectomy is that visually, it is very difficult to predict how much of the lobe can be preserved without leaving cystic disease unresected. In cases where two lobes are affected, bi-lobectomy is the preferred treatment of choice. There have been several series reported describing thoracoscopic lobectomy for cystic lung lesions, and in many institutions it is now the preferred approach.

Q11 Which of the following statements about BPSs is true?

   **A** They are macrocystic lesions located mostly in the pulmonary parenchyma.

   **B** They are microcystic lesions that lack an obvious communication with the airway.

   **C** They are macrocystic lesions that communicate at the level of segmental bronchi.

   **D** They are usually symptomatic at birth.

   **E** Most of their blood supply arises from a branch of the pulmonary artery.

A11 **B** A BPS is a microcystic mass of non-functioning lung tissue that is supplied by an anomalous systemic artery and does not have a bronchial connection to the native tracheobronchial tree. Typically, the lung tissue in BPS receives all or most of its blood supply from an anomalous systemic artery of variable origin. Two forms of sequestration are recognised: ILS and ELS. Although rare, both forms can occur simultaneously. ILSs are incorporated into the normal surrounding lung, whereas ELSs are completely discrete from the normal lung and are enveloped by a separate pleura. The most widely accepted embryologic theory is that a supernumerary lung bud arises caudal to the normal lung bud and continues to migrate caudally with the oesophagus. If this lung bud arises prior to the development of the pleura, it is invested with adjacent lung and becomes an ILS. If supernumerary lung development occurs subsequent to pleura formation, the bud will grow separately and acquire its own pleural covering, forming an ELS.

Q12 The following features distinguish congenital lobar emphysema from sequestrations and CPAMs except:

   **A** endobronchial obstruction from inspissated mucus

   **B** absence of systemic blood supply

   **C** decreased echogenicity on ultrasound

   **D** presence of dysplastic bronchial cartilages which cause a valve effect

   **E** lobar hyperexpansion.

A12 **C** Air trapping in the emphysematous lobe may be due to (1) dysplastic bronchial cartilages creating a ball-valve effect or complete bronchial atresia; (2) endobronchial obstruction from inspissated mucus or extensive mucosal proliferation and infolding; (3) extrinsic compression of the bronchi from aberrant cardiopulmonary vasculature or enlarged cardiac chambers; and (4) diffuse bronchial abnormalities that may or may not be related to infection. Congenital lobar emphysema can be distinguished prenatally from other cystic lung lesions on ultrasonography by increased echogenicity and reflectivity compared with a microcystic CPAM, and the absence of systemic arterial blood supply compared with a BPS. At the time of birth, the affected lobe may be radio-opaque on chest radiography because of delayed clearance of fetal lung fluid.

**Q13** The following have proven to be effective treatments of hydrops due to a congenital cystic lesion of the lung *except*:
  A thoracoamniotic shunt
  B maternal steroid administration
  C resection using the *ex utero* intrapartum treatment (EXIT) strategy
  D percutaneous, *in utero* drainage of the cyst
  E maternal prostaglandin administration.

**A13** **E** The development of hydrops usually mandates emergency intervention. Centres with high fetal surgery volume have reported their experience in the management of these lesions. Surgical interventions such as thoracoamniotic shunting, ultrasound-guided drainage and fetal resection have shown to be effective in some cases. In patients who show signs of severe mediastinal shift and cardiac compression, EXIT-to-resection may be indicated. The EXIT-to-resection procedure is a thoracotomy and resection of the CPAM performed on placental support. Although surgical intervention remains the best treatment option for CPAMs associated with hydrops, some patients may not be appropriate candidates because of either medical or psychosocial contraindications. These contraindications include chromosomal abnormality, multiple gestation, the presence of other significant anatomical abnormalities, and the presence of other maternal medical or psychosocial risk factors. In these cases, a course of maternal steroids (betamethasone or dexamethasone) may be effective in limiting CPAM growth and resolving hydrops. Prostaglandins have not shown to be effective in treating this condition.

**Q14** Which one of the following statements is *true* regarding the CPAM volume: head-circumference ratio (CVR)?
  A A CVR lower than 1.6 is predictive of increased risk for hydrops.
  B Serial measurements of the CVR showed that the growth of a CPAM often reaches a plateau by 28 weeks' gestation.
  C The CVR is most helpful in CPAMs that consist of a dominant cyst.
  D If the CVR measured at 26 weeks' gestation suggests an increased risk for hydrops, the recommendation is to perform ultrasounds every 3 weeks.
  E The CVR is of no value in predicting hydrops.

**A14** **B** In 2002, Cromblehome *et al.* developed an ultrasound-derived CPAM volume: CVR, which allows a gestational age-corrected volume ratio to be used to predict the risk of hydrops within the setting of a CPAM. The CVR is obtained by dividing the CPAM volume by the head circumference to correct for differences in gestational age. The authors found that a CVR >1.6 was predictive of an increased risk of hydrops, with 80% of these CPAM fetuses developing hydrops. Those fetuses with CVR <1.6 have only a 2% risk of hydrops. The major exception to this rule is that CPAMs with a dominant cyst may be unpredictable in their growth and expansion. If the CVR is >1.6 at presentation, the authors suggest following the pregnancy with ultrasounds twice a week to help detect early signs of hydrops. The development of marked hydrops may indicate the need to consider open fetal surgery, especially if there is a large microcystic CPAM. By performing serial CVR measurements, it has been shown that CPAM growth generally reaches a plateau by week 28 of gestation.

**Q15** Which one of the following statements is *true* regarding the features of an ELS?

**A** They are more common in females.

**B** They share the same pleural lining as the rest of the lung.

**C** Twenty per cent of ELSs have an infradiaphragmatic systemic feeding vessel.

**D** The venous drainage consists of a branch of the pulmonary vein.

**E** Associated anomalies are not common.

**A15** **C** Extralobar BPS has predominance in males (3 : 1), is more common on the left side, and can be associated with conditions such as congenital diaphragmatic hernia, vertebral deformities and congenital heart disease in about 40% of the cases. Approximately 5% of neonates with a congenital diaphragmatic hernia will have an extralobar BPS, which is usually an incidental intraoperative finding. All the ELSs have a systemic arterial blood supply. In 20% of patients, the feeding artery originates from the infradiaphragmatic aorta. In most ELSs, there are systemic venous connections, which include the superior vena cava and the azygous and hemiazygous veins.

## Further reading

Adzick NS, Farmer, DL. Cysts of the lung and mediastinum. In: Grosfeld JL, O'Neill JA, Fonkalsrud EW, *et al.*, editors. *Pediatric Surgery. Vol. 1.* 6th ed. Philadelphia, PA: Mosby; 2006. pp. 955–70.

Azizkhan RG, Crombleholme TM. Congenital cystic lung disease: contemporary antenatal and postnatal management. *Pediatr Surg Int.* 2008; 24(6): 643–57.

Cromblehome TM, Coleman B, Hedrick H, *et al.* Cystic adenomatoid malformation volume ratio predicts outcome in prenatally diagnosed cystic adenomatoid malformation of the lung. *J Pediatric Surg.* 2002; 37(3): 331–8.

Stanton M, Njere I, Ade-Ajayi N, *et al.* Systematic review and meta-analysis of the postnatal management of congenital cystic lung lesions. *J Pediatr Surg.* 2009; 44(5): 1027–33.

# CHAPTER 22

# Acquired lung disease

## MATIAS BRUZONI, CRAIG T ALBANESE

**From the choices below each question, select the single best answer.**

Q1   An otherwise healthy 3-year-old male presented to the hospital 7 days ago with a diagnosis of right lower lobe pneumonia. He has been treated with intravenous antibiotics and continues to have a fever. The patient is on room air. An ultrasound is performed which shows a pleural effusion that layers in the decubitus position. What is the *most* appropriate management at this point?

   A   chest physiotherapy and extending the coverage of the antibiotics
   B   thoracoscopic debridement and pleurodesis
   C   continue to observe and complete 14 days of intravenous antibiotics
   D   thoracostomy tube placement
   E   thoracotomy and debridement of empyema

A1   **D**   Primary therapy for empyema is the administration of high-dose intravenous antibiotics. However, failure to respond to the initial treatment such as the presence of persistent fevers requires effective drainage of the pleural space. Fluid that layers in the decubitus position may be treated with chest tube drainage alone. Loculated fluid collections may not be sufficiently drained in such a way, and the optimal management of these patients is still debated. This patient probably has an empyema in its exudative phase given the fact that there are no loculations on ultrasound. Thoracoscopy or thoracotomy is not indicated at this time, and postural drainage alone has not shown to be effective in treating empyema. If fevers persist despite 7 days of antibiotic treatment, it is unlikely that the empyema will resolve by extending coverage or treatment time.

**Q2** The most common pathogen affecting the lungs in children under 1 year of age with cystic fibrosis is:

A *Staphylococcus aureus*

B *Streptococcus pneumoniae*

C *Haemophilus influenzae*

D pseudomonas

E anaerobes.

**A2** **D** Cystic fibrosis is the most common autosomal recessive disease affecting Caucasians and occurs in approximately 1 in 3500 live births. In the first decade of life, the most common organism isolated from cystic fibrosis patients is *S. aureus*, followed by *H. influenzae*. However, pseudomonas is usually the first pathogen isolated in children younger than 1 year of age, and over 80% are infected with this organism by 18 years of age. Sodium is also thought to facilitate increased bacterial binding to the airway mucosa, particularly pseudomonas. Clinically, pseudomonas is the most important pathogen in cystic fibrosis, since it also produces exotoxins that contribute to its virulence, increasing the viscosity of secretions and further impairing ciliary transport.

**Q3** Which of the following statements is true regarding bronchiectasis in children?

A Localised damage to the elastic fibres of the bronchi in association with oedema and inflammation, result in the saccular phase of bronchiectasis.

B The digital clubbing associated with this disease is usually irreversible.

C Surgical resection is indicated once the diagnosis is made.

D Patients with tuberculosis usually present with bilateral lung involvement.

E Saccular bronchiectasis is considered an irreversible condition.

**A3** **E** Bronchiectasis is the irreversible dilatation of the airways secondary to the inflammatory destruction of bronchial and peribronchial tissue. The pathogenesis of bronchiectasis follows three progressive stages. Initially, the ciliary epithelium is replaced with cuboidal squamous epithelium. In the next stage, called cylindrical bronchiectasis, there is localised damage to the elastic tissue of the airway in addition to oedema and inflammation. The last, irreversible stage is called saccular bronchiectasis, and the damage involves the muscle and cartilage layers of the airways, with neovascularisation between pulmonary and bronchial arteries in the areas of saccular dilatation. Up to 50% may have digital clubbing, which is reversible after appropriate treatment. The mainstay of treatment is medical. However, there are surgical indications such as localised disease with severe and debilitating symptoms, massive haemoptysis from localised disease, resectable disease in the context of failure to thrive, and resectable disease in an area of recurrent lower respiratory tract infections. Lastly, patients with pulmonary tuberculosis tend to have unilateral involvement.

**Q4** A 4-year-old male patient with cystic fibrosis presents to the emergency department with massive haemoptysis. After sedation and intubation the patient is resuscitated with intravenous fluids and his vital signs remain stable. There is still active bloody discharge through the endotracheal tube. What is the most appropriate next step in management?

A angiography and embolisation of the bleeding bronchial vessel

B thoracotomy in the operating room with lobectomy

C clinical observation in the intensive care unit

D intravenous vasopressin drip

E emergency room thoracotomy and damage control surgery

**A4** **A** Massive haemoptysis is defined in children as the expectoration of at least 240 mL of blood in 24 hours or recurrent episodes involving substantial amounts of blood (>100 mL/day) over days to weeks. It occurs in approximately 1% of patients with cystic fibrosis and is more frequent in those patients with severe lung disease. The pathogenesis is related to the enlargement and tortuosity of the bronchial arteries and the multiple anastomoses that form between these vessels and the pulmonary arteries. Several treatments have been proposed such as vasopressin drips, endobronchial balloon tamponade and topical alpha agonists without encouraging success. However, bronchial artery embolisation has emerged as a highly successful non-surgical intervention for the short-term control of haemoptysis. Several series have demonstrated that this technique is safe and effective for the control of massive haemoptysis. Clinical observation would not be appropriate in this patient given the evidence of ongoing massive haemoptysis. Surgery with lobectomy may be life-saving for patients who fail embolisation, or those who present with haemodynamic instability due to fulminant haemoptysis.

**Q5** A 3-year-old female patient developed a right upper lobe pneumatocele secondary to *S. aureus* pneumonia. There is no associated pneumothorax or pleural effusion. What is the next most appropriate step in management?

  **A** thoracoscopic marsupialisation of the cyst

  **B** right upper lobectomy

  **C** clinical observation

  **D** percutaneous drainage of the cyst

  **E** bronchoscopy and transbronchial drainage of the cyst

**A5** **C** Pneumatoceles are small, thin-walled structures consisting of single or multiple cysts within an air-lined cavity secondary to alveolar and bronchiolar necrosis. These abnormalities are seen frequently as a consequence of infection by *S. aureus* and group A Streptococcus. Complications of pneumatoceles such as pneumothorax or empyema usually require surgical intervention. However, non-complicated pneumatoceles often resolve spontaneously. Follow-up chest radiographs are required until the resolution of the pneumatocele, and computed tomography may be useful in difficult situations. In uncomplicated cases, there is usually no residual pulmonary disease.

**Q6** Which one of the following statements is *true* regarding empyema in children?

  **A** Anaerobes are the most common isolated organisms in empyema.

  **B** Thoracostomy and fibrinolytics have shown to be equally as effective as thoracoscopic debridement in the treatment of empyema.

  **C** The diagnosis is confirmed by an elevated glucose and a pH < 7 in the pleural fluid.

  **D** The fibrinopurulent phase results in a thick pleural 'peel' which is usually refractory to antibiotic treatment.

  **E** Fibrinolytic therapy is usually reserved for the organising phase of empyema.

**A6** **B** An empyema is the accumulation of purulent fluid in the pleural cavity secondary to different disease processes such as pneumonia, trauma, neoplasms, intrathoracic oesophageal perforation, or surgeries on the chest. Close to 30% of children with pneumonia will develop an empyema. Currently, the most common organisms in childhood empyema are *S. pneumoniae*, *S. aureus* and *H. influenzae*. The diagnosis is confirmed by analysis of the pleural fluid, which shows a pH of less than 7 and a glucose level less than 40 mg/dL. Empyema exhibits three characteristic stages: (1) an exudative stage when the fluid is thin and of low cellular content; (2) a fibrinopurulent stage during which large numbers of polymorphonuclear cells and fibrin are deposited in the pleural space, progressively impairing lung expansion and leading to the formation of fluid loculations; and (3) a fibrotic and organising empyema during which a thick peel forms around the pleural surface, entrapping the lung. Patients who present with loculations during the second stage usually cannot be managed with chest tube alone. A randomised prospective trial showed no difference in outcomes or hospital stay when these patients are treated with thoracoscopic debridement or thoracostomy tube and fibrinolysis. Currently, the recommendation is to place a chest tube and treat with tissue plasminogen activator for 3 days and reserve the thoracoscopy or thoracotomy for refractory cases.

 **Q7** Spontaneous pneumothorax occurs frequently in patients with cystic fibrosis. The recurrence rate after a first episode treated with thoracostomy tube is:

  **A** 5%–10%

  **B** 20%–30%

  **C** <5%

  **D** 40%–60%

  **E** 75%.

 **A7** **D** Primary spontaneous pneumothorax is defined as a pneumothorax occurring secondary to apical blebs without evidence of other lung pathology. On the other hand, secondary spontaneous pneumothoraces occur in the context of underlying lung disease, such as cystic fibrosis. A pneumothorax less than 15% can usually be treated with observation alone; however, larger pneumothoraces need drainage initially. Adolescents with spontaneous pneumothorax have been reported to have a recurrence rate of 40%–60%. The indications for surgical management include recurrence, persistent air leak, bilateral disease, and possibly the presence of large blebs. The recurrence rate after thoracoscopy with bleb resection and pleurodesis ranges from 2% to 10%.

**Q8** What is the appropriate initial management of lung abscesses in children?

  **A** percutaneous drainage and antibiotics

  **B** thoracoscopic drainage and antibiotics

  **C** antibiotics only

  **D** antibiotics and postural or bronchoscopic drainage

  **E** wedge resection of the affected area

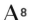 **A8** **D** Appropriate intravenous antibiotic therapy combined with postural or bronchoscopic drainage is the initial approach to lung abscesses in children. Percutaneous drainage would be the next step in case of treatment failure. Bacterial organisms recovered from most cases have been susceptible to penicillin. Most isolates

include both aerobic and anaerobic flora. *S. aureus* is the most common organism found. Improved results can usually be achieved with a combination of ampicillin and metronidazole or clindamycin. Patients who fail therapy may be immunocompromised or have fungal isolates and often require pulmonary resection.

**Q9** Which of the following statements regarding the thoracic duct is *true*?
   **A** It enters the chest through the oesophageal hiatus.
   **B** It crosses the midline from left to right at the level of the fifth thoracic vertebra.
   **C** It ascends posterior to the aortic arch towards the neck.
   **D** Anatomical variations are rare.
   **E** At the level of the diaphragm, it is located in the left chest.

**A9** **C** The thoracic duct originates in the abdomen at the cisterna chyli located over the second lumbar vertebra. The duct travels into the chest through the aortic hiatus and then passes upward into the posterior mediastinum via the right chest. It then crosses the midline towards the left at the level of the fifth thoracic vertebra. It ascends posterior to the aortic arch and into the posterior neck where it drains at the junction of the subclavian and internal jugular veins. Many variations are present in the entire ductal system, and the typical course of the thoracic duct is present in approximately 50% of individuals.

**Q10** Which is the *correct* progression of treatment steps for a chylothorax?
   **A** chest drainage, octreotide, dietary modification and surgical ligation of the thoracic duct
   **B** dietary modification, postural drainage, octreotide and thoracoscopic pleurodesis
   **C** surgical intervention and chest-tube drainage, octreotide, nil by mouth and TPN until resolution
   **D** chest drainage, dietary modification, TPN, octreotide, and surgical ligation of the thoracic duct
   **E** octreotide, pleura-peritoneal shunt, dietary modification, and surgical ligation of the thoracic duct

**A10** **D** The initial approach to a chylothorax is thoracentesis. It is used for diagnosis and may also be sufficient to relieve spontaneous chylothorax. In addition, tube drainage allows quantification of the daily output and promotes pulmonary re-expansion, which may enhance healing. The next step in management is dietary modification. Between 80% and 90% of all fat absorbed from the gut is transported by the thoracic duct as chylomicrons. Short- and medium-chain fatty acids are transported directly into the portal circulation. Thus, feeding restricted to medium- or short-chain triglycerides theoretically results in reduced lymph flow in the thoracic duct and may enhance spontaneous healing of a thoracic duct leak. Recently, octreotide has been found useful in several reports. Octreotide can be given subcutaneously every 8 hours, starting at a dose of 10–20 mg/kg/day. If non-operative management is effective, external intake should be reinstituted first with medium-chain triglycerides, followed by an age-appropriate diet after 2 weeks.

If drainage persists after 2–3 weeks, despite the above treatment steps, ligation of the thoracic duct on the side of the effusion may be necessary.

Q11 Which of the following is *not* an indication for surgical intervention in children with tuberculosis?

A cavitary disease with massive haemoptysis

B cavitary disease with continued positive sputum cultures after 6 months of therapy

C compression of the airway refractory to antibiotics and steroids

D solitary and peripheral lobar caseous nodule

E entrapped lobe with associated empyema

A11 D First-line therapy for patients with pulmonary tuberculosis consists of multi-drug antibiotic therapy for at least 6 months. In otherwise healthy children who are compliant with the antibiotic therapy, a cure rate close to 100% is be expected. Surgery for tuberculosis in children is indicated to treat complications and reduce bacillary load. Examples include refractory bronchial obstruction, cavitary lesions with either massive haemoptysis or persistent positive cultures after 6 months of treatment, and associated empyema. Actual pulmonary resection should be avoided whenever possible given its morbidity in these patients. Surgical intervention can be very challenging because of the degree of intrathoracic scarring from chronic infection.

Q12 Which of the following statements is *true* regarding chylothorax?

A Spontaneous chylothorax in the neonatal period is more likely to resolve than postoperative chylothorax.

B This condition rarely causes malnutrition given that the protein content of chyle is low.

C Chemical pleurodesis is usually effective as first-line therapy.

D Prematurity is a risk factor for the development of chylothorax.

E The diagnosis is made by a pleural triglyceride level of greater than 40 mg/dL.

A12 A One of the most common causes of pleural effusion in the newborn period is spontaneous chylothorax. It can sometimes be related to traumatic vaginal deliveries; however, most of the time its aetiology is unclear. Compared with postoperative or neoplastic chylothorax, spontaneous chylothorax in the neonate is more likely to heal with conservative treatment. The chyle contained in the thoracic duct carries three-quarters of the ingested fat from the intestine to the systemic circulation. The fat content of chyle varies from 0.4 to 4.0 g/dL. The total protein content of thoracic duct lymph is also high and persistent leaks can cause severe malnutrition. In addition, the thoracic duct carries white blood cells such as lymphocytes and eosinophils. Loss of lymphocytes through a thoracic duct fistula may lead to immunosuppression. Initial treatment with pleurodesis is not effective given the high fluid circulation, preventing the formation of adhesions. Finally, a triglyceride level of greater than 110 mg/dL is considered diagnostic of chylothorax.

Q13 The three most common organisms that cause empyema in children are:

A  *S. aureus*, *H. influenzae* and anaerobes

B  *S. pneumoniae*, *S. aureus* and atypical mycobacteria

C  *H. influenzae*, *S. pneumoniae* and pseudomonas

D  *S. aureus*, *S. pneumoniae* and *H. influenzae*

E  *S. pneumoniae*, atypical mycobacteria and *H. influenzae*.

A13  D  Currently, the most common organisms in childhood empyema are *S. pneumoniae*, *S. aureus* and *H. influenzae*. Although pneumococcal species were considered the most common organisms associated with thoracic empyemas, the introduction of penicillin and the pneumococcal vaccine has resulted in *S. aureus* now being the predominant pathogen. Pseudomonas can be a cause of thoracic empyema, mainly in cystic fibrosis patients. Other causative organisms include *Bacteroides* spp. and mycobacteria. Tuberculous empyema is associated with a high bacterial load within the pleural space.

Q14 Which is not a surgical indication in patients with cystic fibrosis?

A  massive haemoptysis

B  persistent productive cough with cultures positive for pseudomonas

C  end-stage lung disease

D  recurrent pneumothorax

E  refractory localised bronchiectasis

A14  B  Pulmonary complications of cystic fibrosis, such as localised bronchiectasis, massive haemoptysis, and pneumothorax require surgical intervention. Lung transplantation remains the ultimate resort for patients with end-stage pulmonary disease. Bilateral, sequential lung transplantation is the preferred approach for children with cystic fibrosis. Although long-term survival is still a problem for most patients, 1- and 2-year survival rates between 65% and 85% have been reported.

**Q15** Which of the following statements is *true* regarding chronic interstitial lung disease?

　　**A** It is characterised by an obstructive pattern on spirometry.

　　**B** It is usually caused by an infectious process.

　　**C** Refractory disease commonly mandates surgical resection.

　　**D** If tissue diagnosis is needed, a percutaneous core biopsy is indicated.

　　**E** Corticosteroids are indicated once infectious causes are ruled out.

**A15** **E** Chronic interstitial lung disease may result from both infectious and non-infectious causes. The precise pathophysiology is poorly understood, but current evidence suggests that its aetiology is related to an intense inflammatory reaction at the level of the interstitial and perialveolar tissues. It is characterised by a restrictive lung physiology and abnormal gas exchange. Usually paediatric surgeons are asked to confirm the diagnosis by lung biopsy. The current recommendation for tissue specimen is at least a 1 cm³ sample from anywhere in the lung except for the lingula and the right middle lobe, unless there is obvious radiographic disease in specific locations. The right middle lobe and the lingula often show disproportionate histological changes and might confuse the clinical picture. A core biopsy is not recommended. Surgical resection (e.g. lobectomy) can result in further deterioration and is not indicated. Steroids are the most commonly used agent once infectious causes have been excluded, followed by hydroxychloroquine, cyclosporine and methotrexate. In severe cases, extracorporeal membrane oxygenation might be necessary.

## Further reading

Adzick NS, Farmer DL. Cysts of the lung and mediastinum. In: Grosfeld JL, O'Neill JA, Fonkalsrud EW, *et al.*, editors. *Pediatric Surgery. Vol. 1.* 6th ed. Philadelphia, PA: Mosby; 2006. pp. 955–70.

Rodgers BM, Michalsky MP. Acquired lesions of the lung and pleura. In: Holcomb GW, Murphy JP. *Pediatric Surgery.* 5th ed. Philadelphia, PA: Saunders-Elsevier; 2010. pp. 290–303.

St Peter SD, Tsao K, Spilde TL, *et al.* Thoracoscopic decortication vs tube thoracostomy with fibrinolysis for empyema in children: a prospective, randomized trial. *J Pediatr Surg.* 2009; **44**(1): 106–11.

# CHAPTER 23

# Diseases of mediastinum and mediastinal masses

## DAVID SIGALET, MARY BRINDLE

From the choices below each question, select the single best answer.

**Q1** The three mediastinal compartments are shown diagrammatically in Figure 23.1. Which of the subsequent options describes the correct association between zone and pathology?

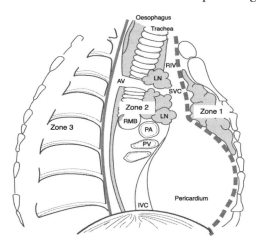

**FIGURE 23.1 The mediastinal compartments**

**A** Zone 1: ganglioneuromas
**B** Zone 1: foregut cysts and duplications
**C** Zone 2: teratomas
**D** Zone 3: thymic cysts
**E** Zone 3: neuroblastomas

**A1** **E** The anterior mediastinum (Zone 1) is bounded by the posterior surface of the sternum, the thoracic inlet, and the anterior surface of the great vessels, heart and pericardium. The middle mediastinum (Zone 2) extends to the anterior border of the vertebrae. The posterior mediastinum (Zone 3) is the area posterior to the anterior border of the vertebrae. A thorough understanding of the anatomy and embryology of the mediastinum is important for the surgeon when evaluating, planning, diagnosing and operating on patients. Conditions that can present within Zone 1 include teratoma, thymic hyperplasia, thymic cysts, non-Hodgkin's lymphoma, Hodgkin's lymphoma and lymphangioma. In Zone 2, non-Hodgkin's lymphoma, Hodgkin's lymphoma, lymphangioma and foregut cysts and duplications can be seen. Similarly the conditions that can develop within Zone 3 include ganglioneuroma and neuroblastoma.

Q2 Which of the following symptoms of airway obstruction is considered to be of greatest concern?

  **A** dyspnoea when lying flat

  **B** noisy breathing

  **C** dyspnoea on exertion

  **D** dyspnoea

  **E** haematemesis

A2   **A** The most worrisome symptoms are dyspnoea on laying flat, and dyspnoea when sleeping.

Q3 In a patient being evaluated for a mediastinal tumour, which of the following signs on physical exam would be of most concern?

  **A** plethora of the facies

  **B** venous distension in the upper neck

  **C** fullness and swelling with masses in the supraclavicular and cervical areas

  **D** inspiratory wheeze

  **E** splenic enlargement

A3   **B** Venous distension in the upper neck, which may also be associated with enlarged veins across the upper chest, indicates obstruction of the venous return from the head and neck. The potential consequences of superior vena caval obstruction are so severe that they should be reviewed with every patient who is evaluated for a mediastinal mass.

4 Symptomatic patients with a mediastinal mass may require a biopsy for definitive diagnosis (*see* Figure 23.2) In order of *increasing* risk what would be the best option for obtaining tissue?

A biopsy of an involved node at a distant site, e.g. cervical or axillary node

B needle (or core) mediastinal biopsy (under local anaesthetic)

C Chamberlain's procedure (under local anaesthetic)

D empiric treatment with irradiation and steroids, and biopsy out of the field of irradiation

E thoracoscopic or open biopsy of mass

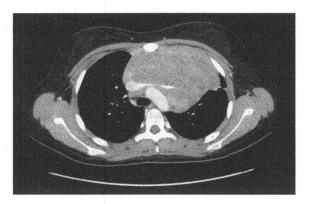

FIGURE 23.2 CT scan of the chest, showing a mediastinal mass

4 A The rapidly growing malignancies of the mediastinum include non-Hodgkin's lymphoma, which can have a doubling time of 30 minutes. Thus those patients who present with symptoms of vena caval obstruction *do* require biopsy, despite the anaesthetic risk. However, these patients will almost always have lymph nodes at other sites which are palpable, are involved in the disease process, and will provide a tissue diagnosis. These, then, provide the diagnosis and facilitate planning of therapy, without requiring the direct sampling of the mediastinal compartment, or the induction of general anaesthetic. In the rare instances where biopsy of a more peripheral node is not possible, the options of biopsy of the mass following the scheme B, C, D and finally E are appropriate. The appropriate selection of biopsy techniques is critical to the safe management of the patient. The use of thoracoscopic techniques is not any safer than open techniques.

**5** What is the most common cause of the mass seen in Figure 23.3?

 A neuraoenteric cyst

 B lymphatic malformation

 C neuroblastoma/ganglioneuroma

 D oesophageal duplication cyst

 E bronchogenic cyst

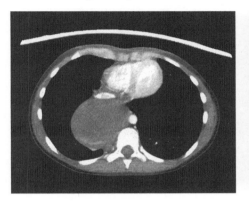

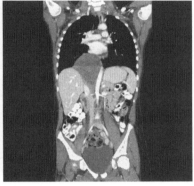

FIGURE 23.3A CT scan of the chest (horizontal view)

FIGURE 23.3B CT scan of the chest (coronal view)

**A5** C The most common masses in the posterior mediastinum are ganglioneuromas and neuroblastomas. (Approximately 20% of ganglioneuromas and neuroblastomas present in the chest.) Because of their benign behaviour, the outlook is significantly better than neuroblastomas presenting in the abdomen. Anterior thoracic meningoceles are rare lesions associated with severe vertebral abnormalities; they are progressive in size and symptoms. They typically present with weakness that progresses to paraplegia and require operative correction. The other rare lesion in this region is the neuroenteric cyst; these connect the central nervous system and the gastrointestinal tract. They occur embryologically as a result of failure of separation of the primitive neural tube and foregut. The lesions typically have well-differentiated muscular layers with intestinal mucosal lining, typically gastric. They are optimally imaged using MRI.

Q6 What is the most common cause of the lesion seen in Figure 23.4?
  A neuroenteric cyst
  B lymphatic malformation
  C neuroblastoma/ganglioneuroma
  D foregut duplication cyst
  E sarcoma

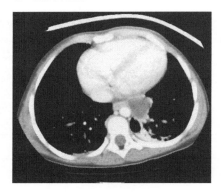

FIGURE 23.4 CT scan of the chest

A6 **D** Foregut duplication cysts: oesophageal duplication cysts and broncho-genic cysts. Oesophageal duplication cysts are usually found arising within the oesophageal wall near the carina. There is a great deal of variation in the location of these cysts. They share the muscular layer with the oesophagus and often have a respiratory epithelial lining, sometimes with rudiments of cartilage. Bronchogenic cysts are lined by respiratory epithelium. These lesions are most commonly discovered in asymptomatic patients who have a chest X-ray done for other reasons. The CT scan is best for delineating the extent and location of these lesions. Treatment consists of excision, if possible. More-peripheral lesions can be resected completely; central lesions often share a common wall with the underlying structure and require careful planning prior to surgery.

Q7 Regarding the biology and behaviour of thoracic neuroblastomas:
  A despite an increased histological grade, the lesions are less likely to behave aggressively with improved survival
  B histological grade and staging tend to be less advanced, and the lesions are less likely to behave aggressively with improved survival
  C histological grade does not correlate with survival
  D in keeping with an increased histological grade, the lesions are more likely to behave aggressively with reduced survival
  E despite a less aggressive histological grade and less advanced staging, the lesions are more likely to behave aggressively with reduced survival.

A**7**   **B**  Neuroblastomas (and ganglioneuromas) arise from the sympathetic chains along each side of the spine, and exhibit varying degrees of differentiation; from malignant neuroblastoma to mature ganglioneuroma. It is not clear why, but thoracic neuroblastoma tends to be less malignant than those originating in the abdomen; the histology, the staging, and biologic markers of aggressiveness such as *nMYC* and ploidy are all better than typically seen in the abdomen. However, the principles of surgical resection for cure remain the same. There may be local pressure effects on the spine, neural foramina and ribs. In extreme cases with intraspinal extension, the patient may develop neurologic symptoms including paraplegia; this should mandate laminectomy (although some groups do not advocate laminectomy). Ideally, the primary tumour should be resected, with use of adjuvant chemotherapy as required to deal with residual disease. Regardless of the presenting symptoms and histology, the long-term results are significantly better than seen with equivalent abdominal primaries. Unfortunately, spinal cord damage, if it occurs, tends to be permanent.

Q**8**   A 13-year-old girl is referred with a mass as shown in Figure 23.5. What is the most likely diagnosis?

   **A**  lymphoma
   **B**  thymic cyst
   **C**  teratoma (germ cell tumour)
   **D**  duplication cyst
   **E**  neuroblastoma

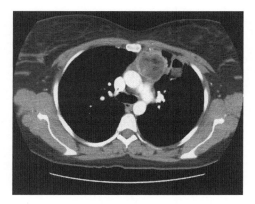

**FIGURE 23.5** CT scan of the chest, showing a mass in the mediastinum

A**8**   **C**  Primitive germ cell tumours may occur in the mediastinum: these include the general categories of tumours arising from pure extraembryonic tissues (seminoma, embryonal carcinoma, yolk sac tumour or choriocarcinoma), which are very rare, or of embryonic tumours (teratomas) containing tissues for all three embryonic cell lines (ectoderm, endoderm and mesoderm), which are uncommon but comprise roughly 16% of all tumours in this region. However, teratomas are the only tumour with a solid or circumscribed morphology. They arise from thymus or pericardial tissues. Depending on their location, they may be asymptomatic (detected on a chest X-ray done for other reasons (most common), vascular effects, airway compression, or specific hormonal effects.

**Q9** In the evaluation and treatment of the lesion in Figure 23.5, which of the following treatment plans is most likely to be effective?

  **A** needle biopsy, followed by chemotherapy

  **B** radiation, followed by biopsy and likely chemotherapy

  **C** thoracoscopic resection

  **D** median sternotomy (or lateral thoracotomy) and resection

  **E** resection, followed by chemotherapy

**A9**   **D** Most teratomas are benign; surgical excision is the treatment of choice. Usually the best approach is via a median sternotomy, but depending on the growth pattern, a lateral thoracotomy may be preferable. In the unusual situation of a locally advanced and aggressive malignancy (which is more likely with the totipotential cell lines, e.g. yolk sac, seminoma, choriocarcinoma), then biopsy, chemotherapy and a secondary resection is likely the most effective therapy.

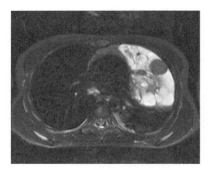

**FIGURE 23.6** CT scan of the chest

**Q10** The lesion in Figure 23.6 has developed in a 5-year-old female, 2 years after resection of a cervical cystic hygroma. She has intermittent short-ness of breath, with exertion, but is otherwise well. What would your treatment strategy be?

  **A** embolisation

  **B** cautious resection

  **C** sclerotherapy: OK-432 or bleomycin injection

  **D** interferon-2α therapy

  **E** steroid therapy followed by vincristine if necessary

**A10  B** Cystic hygromas are progressive in some cases. The mixed nature of this lesion may suggest it might respond to sclerotherapy, but with this there is the risk of increased swelling in the injected cysts, which in this case, may worsen the respiratory compromise. Cautious resection is indicated, with meticulous attention to preserving any vital neuronal or vascular structures.

## Further reading

Akwari OE, Payne WS, Onofrio BM, *et al*. Dumbbell neurogenic tumours of the mediastinum: diagnosis and management. *Mayo Clin Proc.* 1978; **53**(6): 353–8.

Alqahtani A, Nguyen LT, Flageole H, *et al*. 25 years' experience with lymphangiomas in children. *J Pediatr Surg.* 1999; **34**(7): 1164–8.

Billmire D, Vinocur C, Rescorla F, *et al*. Malignant mediastinal germ cell tumours: an intergroup study. *J Pediatr Surg.* 2001; **36**(1): 18–24.

Burt M, Ihde JK, Hajdu SI, *et al*. Primary sarcomas of the mediastinum: results of therapy. *J Thorac Cardiovasc Surg.* 1998; **115**(3): 671–80.

Castellote A, Vazquez E, Vera J, *et al*. Cervicothoracic lesions in infants and children. *Radiographics.* 1999; **19**(3): 583–600.

Dehner LP. Germ cell tumors of the mediastinum. *Semin Diagn Pathol.* 1990; **7**(4): 266–84.

Ricketts RR. Clinical management of anterior mediastinal tumors in children. *Semin Pediatr Surg.* 2001; **10**(3): 161–8.

## CHAPTER 24

# Tracheobronchial and oesophageal foreign bodies

### ROBERT BAIRD, PRAMOD S PULIGANDLA

**From the choices below each question, select the single best answer.**

**Q1** Emergency retrieval is indicated for a:
  **A** battery in the oesophagus
  **B** battery in the stomach
  **C** battery in the intestine
  **D** a single magnet in the stomach
  **E** a single magnet in the intestines.

**A1** **A** Objects found within the oesophagus should generally be considered impacted. Because impacted oesophageal foreign bodies may lead to significant morbidity (and even mortality), removal of impacted oesophageal foreign bodies is mandatory. Batteries located in the oesophagus should be removed urgently because of the risk of oesophageal burns and resultant complications. The procedure of choice is flexible fibreoptic endoscopy. Most swallowed foreign bodies pass harmlessly through the GI tract once they have reached the stomach. Button (disc) batteries in the stomach or intestines do not need to be removed immediately, as they generally pass through the lower GI tract without difficulty. Button batteries retained in the stomach or at a fixed spot in the intestines should be removed. The ingestion of multiple magnets may lead to the development of pressure necrosis and subsequent perforation as the opposite poles of the magnets will become attracted to one another. This may be particularly true when the magnets are ingested at intervals. However, a single magnet poses no such risk and should spontaneously pass.

Q2 Which of the following is true regarding impaction of oesophageal foreign bodies?

A There is an equal distribution of sites of impaction along the entire length of the oesophagus.

B The most common site of impaction is at the lower oesophageal sphincter (LOS) at the gastro-oesophageal junction.

C The most common site of impaction is at the mid-oesophagus, in the region where the aortic arch and carina compress the oesophagus.

D The most common site of impaction is at the anatomical change from oesophageal skeletal muscle to smooth muscle.

E Most oesophageal foreign body impaction occurs in children with a pre-existing oesophageal abnormality.

A2 **D** Most complications of paediatric foreign body ingestion are due to oesophageal impaction, and this usually occurs at one of three typical locations. The most common site of oesophageal impaction is at the thoracic inlet. This is defined as the area between the clavicles on chest radiograph, and the site of anatomical change from the skeletal muscle to the smooth muscle of the oesophagus. The cricopharyngeus sling at C6 is also at this level and may 'catch' a foreign body. About 70% of blunt foreign bodies that lodge in the oesophagus do so at this location. Another 15% become lodged at the mid-oesophagus, in the region where the aortic arch and carina overlap the oesophagus on chest radiograph. The remaining 15% become lodged at the LES at the gastro-oesophageal junction. Children with pre-existing oesophageal abnormalities (e.g. repair of a tracheo-oesophageal fistula) are likely to have foreign body impaction at the site of the abnormality. If a child with no known oesophageal pathology has a blunt foreign body lodged at a location other than the three typical locations described above, the possibility of a previously unknown oesophageal abnormality should be considered. This latter population makes up a small minority of oesophageal ingestions overall.

Q3 Two hours ago, during dinner, a healthy 3-year-old child swallowed a coin that is confirmed on X-ray to be located in the mid-oesophagus. He is in no distress and is asymptomatic. Which of the following is *not* a reasonable treatment plan?

A use of a Foley catheter under fluoroscopy to extract the coin

B use of an oesophageal bougie to advance the coin into the stomach

C emergency flexible endoscopy

D flexible endoscopy in 6 hours

E allow clear fluids and reassess in 12 hours with a repeat X-ray

**A³** **C** Endoscopy (oesophagoscopy) is by far the most commonly used means of oesophageal foreign body removal and is usually the procedure of choice. Most children with oesophageal foreign bodies are stable from a cardiovascular and respiratory standpoint. Endoscopy usually can be delayed until the child's stomach is emptied and a surgical team is assembled. However, pointed objects and batteries should be removed as rapidly as possible to avoid further injury to the oesophageal mucosa and subsequent mediastinitis. Because endoscopy is relatively invasive and expensive, other methods of oesophageal foreign body removal have been investigated and are probably more cost-effective when used appropriately. These have been performed most commonly on children with oesophageal coins, and should be performed only in previously healthy children whose ingestion of a blunt object was witnessed less than 24 hours prior to the procedure.

**Foley catheter method:** blunt foreign bodies may be removed by use of a Foley catheter. Typically, the patient is restrained in a head-down position on a fluoroscopy table, and an uninflated catheter is inserted distal to the object. The catheter balloon is then inflated and gently withdrawn, drawing the foreign body with it. On some occasions, the object is dislodged and passed into the stomach. Progress is typically monitored fluoroscopically. This procedure is performed without radiographic monitoring at some centres with extensive experience and does not require general anaesthesia.

**Bougienage method:** blunt oesophageal foreign bodies may be advanced into the stomach with a bougie. While the child is sitting upright, the lubricated instrument is gently passed down the oesophagus, dislodging the object. The object is then expected to pass through the rest of the GI tract; thus, this procedure should not be performed on children with known lower GI tract abnormalities. A brief observation period and a repeat radiograph should follow any removal procedure to rule out retained foreign bodies and other complications (e.g. pneumomediastinum). In recent studies, the bougienage method has been shown to be far more cost-effective than endoscopy, for properly selected patients.

**Spontaneous passage:** blunt foreign bodies located at the LES often pass spontaneously within several hours of ingestion. This has been best studied in coin ingestions. Previously healthy children may be given food and drink and have repeat radiographs 24 hours following ingestion. Often, the coin passes through the LES, and a removal procedure can be avoided. Although blunt foreign bodies located in other areas of the oesophagus are less likely to spontaneously pass, this strategy may be an appropriate alternative for stable children with normal oesophageal anatomy and a foreign body in the thoracic inlet or the mid-oesophagus. This may be most successful in asymptomatic children. Follow-up imaging should be arranged to ensure transit, and once the oesophagus is clear, nearly all foreign bodies are evacuated – 97% in one large series.

**Q4** A 3-year-old presents with acute wheezing after being held down and fed peanuts by her older brother. A normal chest X-ray is obtained in the emergency department. What should the next step be?

**A** spiral CT of the chest

**B** bronchodilators

**C** Heimlich's manoeuvre

**D** bronchoscopy

**E** oesophagoscopy

 **A4** **D** Bronchoscopy should be performed in *any* patient with a definitive or suspected diagnosis of a tracheobronchial foreign body in order to confirm the diagnosis and to remove the foreign body. Most practitioners recommend rigid bronchoscopy, which should be done as soon as the patient is deemed stable. Spiral CT of the chest would not contribute to the care of this child and would subject her to unnecessary radiation. Bronchodilators are of benefit in a child with reactive airway disease, but this history indicates a probable ingested foreign body as a cause of the wheezing. The Heimlich manoeuvre is widely recommended as a first-aid measure but is of dubious efficacy in the stable patient and can sometimes displace an inhaled object into a relatively riskier location. It should be reserved for complete airway obstruction without other available resources. Oesophagoscopy is of no value in this context, as the child's symptomatology indicates the foreign body is affecting the tracheobronchial tree.

 **Q5** The most common radiographic finding on chest X-ray after aspiration of a foreign body is:

**A** a normal study

**B** unilateral hyperlucency

**C** atelectasis

**D** identification of the foreign body

**E** post-obstructive pneumonia.

 **A5** **B** A wide variety of radiological findings are possible after aspiration of a foreign body. As recently reported by Bittencourt *et al.* (2006) the most common finding is unilateral hyperlucency distal to the obstructing material (*see* Table 24.1). Identification of the foreign body is relatively rare (<25%), and the development of pneumonia is a late finding.

| Radiological findings | % |
|---|---|
| Unilateral hyperlucency | 30.1 |
| Atelectasis | 21.7 |
| Radio-opaque foreign body | 24.3 |
| Reduction of the bronchovascular markings | 14.0 |
| Shift of the mediastinum | 12.5 |
| Normal chest or neck radiograph | 15.7 |
| Infiltrate | 14.3 |
| Other findings | 2.5 |

**TABLE 24.1  Radiological findings of foreign body aspiration**

*From* Bittencourt *et al.*, 2006

Q⁶  The most common site of an aspirated foreign body is:

A  the trachea

B  the left mainstem bronchus

C  the right mainstem bronchus

D  at the vocal cords

E  all sites equally common.

A⁶  C  The most common location of aspirated foreign bodies is the right main bronchus as indicated by several investigators on the subject. The proposed mechanism for this asymmetrical distribution is the more direct course that the right bronchus follows after the tracheal bifurcation when compared with the left bronchus.

A recent review (Saki *et al.*, 2009) found the distribution of aspirated foreign bodies to be as follows:

- right mainstem bronchus in 560 (55.1%)
- left mainstem bronchus in 191 (18.8%)
- trachea in 173 (17.1%)
- vocal cords in 75 (7.4%)
- both bronchi in 16 (1.6%).

Q⁷  The most common presenting complaint after aspiration of a foreign body is:

A  asymptomatic

B  coughing

C  wheezing

D  dyspnoea

E  stridor.

$A^7$ **B** Saki *et al.* (2009) review the presenting symptoms in their series, as well as in the available data reported in literature. In their review, coughing was the most common symptom (73%), and this was seen consistently in the publications on the subject. It is important to note, however, that a significant minority of patients will present late with no appreciable history. These patients may manifest persistent pneumonia or lung abscesses, in which case a high index of suspicion of a foreign body aspiration needs to be maintained.

$Q^8$ Which of the following complications can occur following ingestion of multiple magnets?

**A** intestinal perforation

**B** malabsorption

**C** intestinal obstruction

**D** acute volvulus

**E** all of the above

$A^8$ **E** Numerous reports have recently been published illustrating the many complications associated with the ingestion of multiple magnets. If more than one magnet is ingested, the magnets may be attracted to one another leading to pressure necrosis between two loops of intestine. Ultimately, this may result in a perforation or an enteric fistula. Should an enteroenteric fistula occur, malabsorption and diarrhoea may ensue. Intestinal obstruction has also been reported, both secondary to the magnets themselves, and as a consequence of an acute intestinal volvulus.

$Q^9$ A 2-year-old boy presents to the emergency department with stridor and drooling; the parents cannot provide any additional history. An upright chest radiograph confirms that a coin has become impacted in the subglottic area. Which of the following is *not* appropriate management?

**A** topical anaesthesia to the respiratory mucosa

**B** emergency rigid bronchoscopy

**C** possible tracheotomy

**D** racemic adrenalin

**E** corticosteroids

$A^9$ **D** Long-standing foreign bodies are at risk of embedding themselves within the surrounding tissues, making them particularly challenging to remove by endoscopic means. Rigid bronchoscopy under general anaesthesia is the treatment of choice as it provides optimal conditions for foreign body removal. Sufficient anaesthesia is required for the procedure in order to prevent laryngospasm, for which topical anaesthesia with tetracaine or lidocaine is an important adjunct.

The presence of localised oedema is an indication for systemic corticosteroid therapy, either before or after the procedure. Tracheostomy is occasionally indicated in foreign body extraction, especially when the foreign object is impacted in the subglottic region, or if the foreign body is large and obstructs the glottis during removal. Racemic adrenalin is useful in the treatment of laryngotracheitis as it leads to mucosal vasoconstriction and the reduction of oedema via alpha-adrenergic receptors located in the airway. However, it has not been shown to be of benefit in the context of an airway foreign body.

**Q10** A button battery is noted on abdominal X-ray (AXR) to be in the stomach of an otherwise asymptomatic 2-year-old boy. Treatment options include all *except*:

   **A** endoscopic removal

   **B** repeat AXR in 6 hours

   **C** administration of ipecac (emetic agent)

   **D** discharge with a repeat AXR in 48 hours

   **E** discharge and have parents strain the stool.

**A10** **C** Button batteries within the stomach or intestine do not need to be removed immediately, as the vast majority will pass through the lower GI tract without difficulty. Button batteries retained in the stomach or at a fixed point in the intestine should be removed. Generally, these patients may be managed on an outpatient basis. Serial daily radiographs are not required, and as long as the patient remains asymptomatic, weekly radiographs may be obtained if it cannot be recovered after straining the stool. Intervention is required when symptoms arise (e.g. peritonitis, bowel obstruction), or if the foreign body has been retained more than 2 weeks in the same location. It is important to realise that it is often difficult to clearly define its location based on plain radiographs. If the battery is suspected to be in the stomach, it should be removed by endoscopy. The administration of ipecac or other emetic agent is not indicated and may result in aspiration.

**Q11** Which patient is at highest risk for a foreign body aspiration?

   **A** an unwitnessed 18-month-old girl

   **B** a witnessed 6-month-old girl

   **C** an unwitnessed 6-year-old boy

   **D** a witnessed 18-month-old boy

   **E** a witnessed 6-year-old girl

**A11** **D** In the year 2000, in the United States, foreign body aspiration accounted for more than 17 000 emergency department visits and 160 deaths in children aged 14 years or younger. Airway foreign bodies are the fifth most common cause of death in children younger than 1 year. The peak ages during which aspiration of foreign bodies occur are the toddler through preschool ages, although foreign bodies have been found in the airways of patients of all ages and sizes. Foreign body aspiration occurs with a slight male predominance and is typically (although not always) witnessed by a friend or family member.

**Q12** Regarding the pathophysiology of oesophageal injury in a button battery ingestion, which of the following is *not* true?

  **A** Liquefaction necrosis typically occurs because sodium hydroxide is generated by the current produced at the anode.

  **B** Injury occurs as a consequence of multiple mechanisms including thermal, caustic and toxic phenomena.

  **C** Maximal effects typically occur in less than 6 hours.

  **D** The alkali of a button battery is effectively neutralised by stomach contents.

  **E** Because lithium batteries contain no alkali, they do not pose the same risk as other button batteries.

**A12** **E** Disc batteries do not usually cause problems unless they become lodged in the GI tract. The most common location that disc batteries become lodged, resulting in clinical consequences, is the oesophagus. Batteries that successfully traverse the oesophagus are unlikely to lodge at any other location, and are effectively neutralised by GI secretions. They can be managed expectantly. Oesophageal damage can occur in a relatively short period of time when a disc battery is lodged in the oesophagus. Liquefaction necrosis may occur as a result of the production of sodium hydroxide when current is produced by the battery (usually at the anode). However, the necrosis is multifactorial as electrochemical analysis *ex vivo* suggests that thermal, caustic and toxic phenomena are all contributing factors. Perforation has occurred as rapidly as 6 hours after ingestion, with maximal effects occurring in as little as 2 hours. Lithium batteries make up only 1% of all battery ingestions overall, but although they contain no alkaline material they tend to be larger and have a greater voltage, and have been shown to cause similar mucosal damage as alkaline batteries.

**Q13** Therapeutic manoeuvres that may aid in tracheobronchial foreign body retrieval include all *except*:

  **A** laryngoscopic examination of the oropharynx under conscious sedation with possible extraction with Magill forceps

  **B** extraction with a Fogarty balloon catheter via a rigid bronchoscope

  **C** extraction using telescopic forceps with a rigid bronchoscope

  **D** a repeat bronchoscopy to retrieve and to reassess for foreign body fragments

  **E** segementectomy of the affected lung lobe.

**A13** **A** General anaesthesia provides optimal conditions for the removal of most airway foreign bodies. In patients with laryngeal foreign bodies (not tracheo-bronchial), removal without anaesthesia can be attempted. Rigid bronchoscopy is the primary tool for evaluating and treating aspirated foreign bodies. Forceps remain the most commonly employed instrument for retrieval, but the Fogarty catheter has been described to aid in extracting material inaccessible to grasping instruments. In cases that result in fragmentation of the foreign body, a second endoscopy may be required. Should foreign material completely obstruct the airway of a pulmonary segment on repeat bronchoscopy, the surgeon should be prepared to perform a segmentectomy as required.

**Q14** Which of the following factors makes an underlying oesophageal pathology more likely?
  **A** impaction at the level of the cricopharyngeus
  **B** the child is older than 5 years
  **C** the child is female
  **D** the foreign body is a tack
  **E** the ingestion was unwitnessed

**A14** **B** Typical foreign body impaction occurs in the area of the cricopharyngeus muscle, at the level of the aortic arch, or at the LOS. Impaction at another site may indicate an underlying anatomical abnormality, but is non-specific. In one series of patients, an impacted food bolus was associated with an abnormality in 70% of cases; tacks or other solid objects are more commonly seen in children without underlying pathology. Impaction at an older age (>5 years) has been noted to be associated with an increased likelihood of detecting an underlying anatomical abnormality. A follow-up oesophagram may be indicated if the diagnosis remains a possibility. The male-to-female ratio for aspirated foreign bodies in young children is 1 : 1, although in adolescents, males are more commonly affected than females. There is no correlation with an underlying anatomical abnormality based on gender or if the aspiration is witnessed.

**Q15** You are consulted to evaluate a 33-week premature neonate with slowly worsening abdominal distension, non-bilious emesis and a palpable mass in the epigastrium. He has stable vital signs and had previously been taking breast milk. Abdominal plain film reveals considerable gastric air and an intraluminal soft tissue mass within the stomach air bubble. After an abdominal ultrasound, management should include:

**A** nil by mouth, parenteral fluids and repeat imaging after several days

**B** laparotomy, gastrotomy and resection of the mass

**C** laparotomy, antrectomy and Bilroth I reconstruction

**D** CT scan of the abdomen

**E** upper endoscopy.

**A15** **A** This description is classic for a lactobezoar, which is a compacted mass of undigested milk concretions. Although case series describing this entity are small, prematurity is a consistently described risk factor. It has been reported with virtually every milk product available, including breast milk and soy-based formulae. They frequently present with partial or complete gastric outlet obstruction in neonates or infants. AXR findings include a soft-tissue mass within a large stomach air bubble. Ultrasound and contrast radiographs can further support the diagnosis. CT scan of the abdomen subjects the child to needless radiation and is not indicated. Upper endoscopy is technically demanding in neonates and is not justified given the working diagnosis. The preferred treatment for a presumed lactobezoar is initiation of intravenous hydration, and the cessation of enteral feedings. Resolution of symptoms and the radiological findings provide confirmatory evidence of the diagnosis. While gastric perforation has been reported in the context of a lactobezoar, laparotomy should only be reserved for rare cases of complication.

## Further reading

Bittencourt PF, Camargos PA, Scheinmann P, *et al.* Foreign body aspiration: clinical, radiological findings and factors associated with its late removal. *Int J Pediatr Otorhinolaryngol.* 2006; **70**(5): 879–84.

Centers for Disease Control and Prevention. Nonfatal choking-related episodes among children: United States, 2001. *MMWR Morb Mortal Wkly Rep.* 2002; **51**(42): 945–8.

Litovitz T, Whitaker N, Clark L. Emerging battery-ingestion hazard: clinical implications. *Pediatrics.* 2010; **125**(6): 1168–77.

Little D, Shah S, St Peter S, *et al.* Esophageal foreign bodies in the pediatric population: our first 500 cases. *J Pediatr Surg.* 2006; **41**(5): 914–18.

Saki N, Nikakhlagh S, Rahim F, *et al.* Foreign body aspirations in infancy: a 20-year experience. *Int J Med Sci.* 2009; **6**(6): 322–8.

# CHAPTER 25

# Congenital anomalies of the oesophagus

## ASHWIN PIMPALWAR

**From the choices below each question, select the single best answer.**

**Q1** The commonest type of oesophageal atresia is:
- **A** oesophageal atresia (OA) with distal tracheo-oesophageal fistula (TOF)
- **B** OA without TOF
- **C** TOF without OA
- **D** OA with fistula to both pouches
- **E** OA with a proximal TOF.

**A1** **A** OA is of five types. The commonest type is OA with distal TOF, with an incidence of 85.8%. This is also known as type 'C' OA. The next common type is the pure OA with no fistula. The incidence of this anomaly is 7%–8%.

**Q2** VACTORL association includes the following *except*:
- **A** vertebral anomalies
- **B** anorectal malformation
- **C** cardiac anomalies
- **D** tracheo-oesophageal anomalies
- **E** liver anomalies.

**A2** **E** VACTORL association is a spectrum of clinical conditions in the human neonate that includes vertebral (V), anorectal (A), cardiac (C), tracheo-oesophageal (TO), renal (R) and limb (L) defects. This spectrum of anomalies has not been recognised as a specific syndrome in humans but rather represents a non-random association of congenital defects of poorly known aetiology and pathogenesis and its components have been variable.

**Q3** Which of the following is *not* true about prenatal diagnosis of oesophageal atresia?
   **A** It is associated with maternal polyhydramnios.
   **B** Ultrasound shows an anechoic area in the middle of the fetal neck.
   **C** Small or absent stomach bubble on ultrasound.
   **D** Predictive value of prenatal ultrasonography is around 40%–50%.
   **E** Rarely diagnosed antenatally.

**A3** **D** The predictive value of prenatal ultrasonography in the diagnosis of OA is only 20%–40%. Presence of anechoic shadow in the fetal neck with a small or absent stomach bubble on ultrasound associated with the maternal polyhydramnios is suggestive of OA antenatally. Fetal MRI may be an important adjunct for the prenatal diagnosis of oesophageal anomalies. OA is rarely diagnosed antenatally.

**Q4** Which one of these statements about oesophageal atresia is true?
   **A** Most cases are diagnosed very late in life.
   **B** It is usually associated with excessive salivation.
   **C** Feeding is followed by regurgitation, choking and coughing.
   **D** A and B are correct.
   **E** B and C are correct.

**A4** **E** Most neonates with OA are diagnosed early in life. The earliest clinical sign is excessive salivation. Feeding is followed by regurgitation, choking and coughing. There may be associated cyanosis, respiratory distress, inability to swallow and inability to introduce a nasogastric tube into the stomach. Some babies with distal fistula may distend their stomach, leading to elevation of the diaphragm and subsequent pulmonary compromise.

Q5 Which of the following investigations is essential before taking a neo-nate with OA to the operating room (OR)?

 A renal ultrasound (US)

 B MRI of the neck

 c ECG

 D echocardiogram (ECHO)

 E spinal US

A5 D An ECHO is essential before taking the patient to the OR. ECHO is useful in diagnosing associated cardiac anomalies that could alter the prognosis in these patients. It also reveals the site of the aortic arch. Babies with right-sided aortic arch may need a left thoracotomy for TOF repair.

Q6 In neonates with OA and TOF, bronchoscopy may be useful for which of the following purposes?

 A to locate the site of distal fistula

 B to determine the number of fistulas

 c for temporary occlusion of fistula

 D to inject glue in recurrent TOF

 E all of the above

A6 E In babies with OA and TOF, bronchoscopy is useful. Bronchoscopy is performed using a rigid bronchoscope. It is usually done just before positioning the patient for the OA and TOF repair. Bronchoscopy has several advantages. It provides informa-tion about the site, size, location and number of fistulas. It allows placement of guide wire through the fistula allowing for better identification of the fistula during repair. In babies who have a distal TOF with severe gastric distension and inef-fective ventilation, bronchoscopy can be used to block the fistula site temporarily using a Fogarty catheter and save the baby. In patients with recurrent TOF repair following previous open or thoracoscopic repair of OA and TOF, bronchoscopy can be used for injection of glue at the recurrent fistula site.

Q7 Which of the following factors is not implicated in the pathogenesis of oesophageal stricture after OA repair?

 A excessive tension on the anastomosis

 B two-layered anastomosis

 c anastomotic leak

 D gastro-oesophageal reflux (GOR)

 E transpleural approach

**A7** **E** Oesophageal stricture is a common problem after OA repair. Most babies benefit from a few dilatations. The factors implicated in the pathogenesis of these stricture are tension on the anastomosis, two-layered anastomosis, anastomotic leak, use of non-absorbable silk suture, GOR and ischaemia at the site of repair. A single-layered interrupted absorbable-suture anastomosis with minimum tension is preferred and helps prevent this complication. Anastomotic leak after OA repair produces scarring in the area of anastomosis and forms a stricture that may need several dilatations or even resection. There is a high incidence of GOR in patients with OA and TOF. Antireflux treatment should be considered in all these patients after TOF repair. Some of these patients may have recurrent strictures and may need fundoplication with dilatation of the stricture or even resection of the stricture. There is no evidence that either the transpleural or extrapleural approach increases/decreases incidence of stricture formation.

**Q8** All of these statements are true about OA *except*:

A GER disease (GORD) is a common complication

B GORD may be due to shortened intra-abdominal portion of the oesophagus

C short, floppy Nissen's wrap is considered to be better than traditional Nissen's wrap

D GORD is contributing factor for recurrent strictures

E most patients with GORD and recurrent strictures can be managed with antireflux medications.

**A8** **E** There is a high incidence of GOR in patients with OA and TOF. This may be because of the shortened intra-abdominal portion of the oesophagus. Also, there is altered motility at the site of anastomosis leading to reduced clearance which makes the effects of reflux more permanent. Medical antireflux treatment should be considered in all these patients after TOF repair. Some of these patients may have recurrent strictures and may need fundoplication with dilatation of the stricture or even resection of the stricture. A short, floppy Nissen's wrap has been shown to be better than the traditional Nissen's wrap. This has shown to produce less dysphagia than the original technique.

**Q9** Which of the following is true about tracheomalacia in OA?

A It is defined as a weakness in the tracheal wall.

B Symptoms may be difficult to distinguish from recurrent TOF.

C It commonly requires surgery for correction.

D A and B are correct.

E A and C are correct.

**A9**   **D**   Tracheomalacia is defined as a weakness in the wall of the trachea. It may be mild, moderate and severe in variety. Most cases are mild to moderate, and usually get better as the child grows. The severe variety is where there is a complete collapse of the anterior and posterior walls of the trachea at expiration or when the child coughs. This type may benefit from surgical treatment. Although almost 75% of patients with OA and TOF have tracheomalacia, only about 20%–25% of patients are symptomatic from it. Typical presentation is with 'barking' cough. Symptoms may be difficult to distinguish from recurrent TOF, oesophageal stricture or GOR. In severe cases the child may have acute, life-threatening apnoeic spells and may benefit from aortopexy. The weak trachea is compressed between dilated oesophagus and aorta, and this pressure can be relieved by doing an aortopexy that fixes the aorta to the sternum and prevents it from compressing trachea.

**Q10**   In OA and distal TOF associated with duodenal atresia, which of the following is true?

    **A**   Duodenal atresia should be repaired first.

    **B**   Gastrostomy should be performed first.

    **C**   Gastric perforation does not occur.

    **D**   TOF should be ligated first.

    **E**   Upper GI contrast is required for diagnosis.

**A10**   **D**   OA and distal TOF associated with duodenal atresia is a difficult problem to manage. Since there is a communication between the trachea and distal oesophagus the air tends to take the path of least resistance and it escapes from the trachea into the distal oesophagus and then into the GI tract. If the child is intubated it is difficult to ventilate the child because of the reason mentioned above. If there is an associated duodenal atresia the problem becomes worse; the stomach and duodenum continue to distend till they burst/perforate making the child very sick. Therefore OA and distal TOF associated with duodenal atresia is an emergency and needs immediate treatment – emergency thoracotomy and ligation of fistula. The other option is to do an immediate bronchoscopy and place a Fogarty balloon catheter in the fistula to block it as a temporising manoeuvre. Performing a gastrostomy would complicate the problem even more and may lead to immediate demise of the child from inability to ventilate. Diagnosis is mostly clinical and based on plain X-rays. Upper GI contrast studies are not required to make a diagnosis.

**Q11** Regarding H-type TOF, which of the following is false?

    **A** Prone cine oesophagram is diagnostic.

    **B** Bronchoscopy and placement of guide wire through the fistula may be useful to identify the fistula during surgery.

    **C** It usually presents later than the other OA anomalies.

    **D** Most cases can be closed through a neck incision.

    **E** The ansa cervicalis may be damaged.

**A11**   **E**   H-type TOF is an anomaly where there is a connection between the trachea and the oesophagus without oesophageal atresia. Babies with this type of anomaly usually present late with symptoms of choking with feeds, excessive gas in the GI tract with distension, or with recurrent pneumonia. The overall incidence of this anomaly is about 4.2% of all the OA anomalies. Diagnosis can be made by cine prone oesophagram or by rigid bronchoscopy. At the time of bronchoscopy, a guide wire is placed through the fistula to help identify the fistula at the time of surgery. Surgical repair is usually performed through a cervical approach and the fistula is divided and closed. During the surgical repair the recurrent laryngeal nerve (contralateral more than ipsilateral) is at risk of injury.

**Q12** Regarding surgical repair of oesophageal atresia, which of the following is true?

    **A** It is usually accomplished through a left thoracotomy.

    **B** The intrapleural approach prevents empyema.

    **C** Usually a double-layer anastomosis is recommended.

    **D** An upper pouch flap may be required to bridge the gap in some cases.

    **E** All the above are correct.

**A12**   **D**   Surgical repair of OA can be accomplished by either the open thoracotomy approach or the by the thoracoscopic approach. The right side is the usual site of entry. In cases where there is a right-sided aortic arch, a left-sided approach is used. The most preferred route is the extrapleural approach because leakage from the anastomosis with potential infection would be contained outside the pleura thus preventing an empyema. The first step is to identify the fistula and divide it. Next the upper pouch is mobilised and an end-to-end interrupted single-layer absorbable suture anastomosis is performed without tension. In cases where the gap between the two ends is greater, a flap from the upper pouch may help bridge the gap.

**Q13** In babies with a large distal TOF the following may be necessary to prevent gastric perforation *except*:

- **A** endotracheal intubation beyond the fistula
- **B** bronchoscopic occlusion of the fistula
- **C** emergency gastrostomy
- **D** emergency thoracotomy and ligation of fistula
- **E** emergency thoracotomy, ligation of the fistula and repair of OA.

**A13 C** In patients with type 'C' anomaly with a large TOF the air follows the path of least resistance and bypasses the lung. This distends the stomach and creates a risk of gastric perforation. Pushing the endotracheal tube beyond the fistula is an important first step to solve this problem. This may not always be successful since the fistula may be low or at the bifurcation of the trachea. The other options are to perform either an emergency bronchoscopy with balloon occlusion of the fistula or an emergency thoracotomy and ligation of the fistula. Performing a gastrostomy would complicate the problem even more and may lead to immediate demise of the child from inability to ventilate. If the child's condition permits and the anaesthetist is happy with intraoperative patient stability, both a ligation of fistula and oesophageal anastomosis may be accomplished.

**Q14** Which of the following is *not* true about congenital stenosis of the oesophagus?

- **A** It can be of three types.
- **B** The tracheobronchial remnant requires surgical excision.
- **C** In most cases the stenosis is longer than 3 cm.
- **D** A and B are correct.
- **E** B and C are correct.

**A14 D** Congenital stenosis of the oesophagus is a rare condition. There are three types: (1) a membranous web or a diaphragm, (2) fibromuscular thickening and (3) narrowing secondary to tracheobronchial remnants. The length of the narrow segment is usually less than 3 cm. Types 1 and 2 are located in the mid-portion of the oesophagus while type 3 is seen in the distal third of the oesophagus. Type 1 is the rarest and type 2 is the commonest variety of oesophageal stenosis. The first two conditions may be treated with dilatation but the third type usually needs surgical excision and end-to-end oesophageal anastomosis.

Q15 All of the following is true about laryngotracheo-oesphageal cleft (LTOC) *except*:

A type IV may involve one or both main bronchi

B risk of injury to the recurrent laryngeal nerve is higher with the anterior pharyngotomy approach of repair

C may be associated with OA and TOF

D type II extends beyond the cricoid lamina to the cervical trachea

E type I anomaly may not require surgical correction.

A15 B LTOC is a rare anomaly. It involves a midline communication between the larynx, trachea and oesophagus. It is classified into four types: type I is limited to the larynx; type II extends beyond the cricoid lamina to the cervical trachea; type III involves the entire trachea down to the carina; type IV extends beyond the carina to involve one or both of the main bronchi. Several other anomalies may be associated with LTOC. OA with TOF may occur in 20%–36% of patients with LTOC. Type I anomaly may not require surgical correction, but types II, III and IV do need surgical correction. A right thoracotomy and extrapleural approach is used for repair. The approach may be lateral through the tracheo-oesophageal groove or anterior by opening the anterior wall of trachea. There is a high risk of injury to the recurrent laryngeal nerve, which is greater with the lateral approach than with the anterior approach. Treatment of this anomaly is complex and needs a multidisciplinary approach. Survival is poor and ranges from 50% to 75%. It is also associated with a lot of morbidity. Inability to wean the patient from the ventilator, pharyngo-oesophageal dysfunction and GOR are common postoperative problems.

## Further reading

El-Gohary Y, Gittes GK, Tovar JA. Congenital anomalies of the esophagus. *Semin Pediatr Surg.* 2010; **19**(3): 186–93.

Mortell AE, Azizkhan RG. Esophageal atresia repair with thoracotomy: the Cincinnati contemporary experience. *Semin Pediatr Surg.* 2009; **18**(1): 12–19.

Ron O, De Coppi P, Pierro A. The surgical approach to esophageal atresia repair and the management of long-gap atresia: results of a survey. *Semin Pediatr Surg.* 2009; **18**(1): 44–9.

# CHAPTER 26

# Caustic injuries of the oesophagus

## BRICE ANTAO, MICHAEL S IRISH

From the choices below each question, select the single best answer.

**Q1** Which of the following is true regarding caustic ingestion in children?
  **A** It is always accidental.
  **B** Most cases occur in children <3 years.
  **C** It occurs more commonly in girls.
  **D** It occurs more commonly in boys in all age groups.
  **E** It is always associated with oesophageal injuries.

**A1** **B** Caustic ingestion in children is a major health hazard with around 5000 cases per year in the United States. It most commonly occurs in children aged 1–3 years. Boys are more frequently involved than girls. In children older than 5 years, non-accidental injury is very likely. Among adolescents, females predominate and the cause is usually intentional. Approximately 20% of caustic ingestions result in some degree of oesophageal injury.

**Q2** Which of the following is true regarding caustic ingestion?
  **A** Acid and alkali ingestion can cause the same degree of injury.
  **B** Acid ingestion causes more severe injuries than alkali ingestion.
  **C** Ferrous sulphate tablets may induce caustic injury to the oesophagus.
  **D** Acid injuries are more common in children.
  **E** Acid injuries cause most damage in the duodenum and proximal small bowel.

**A2** **C** The pH and physical form of the substance ingested play an important role in the site and type of injury. A pH >12 or <1.5 is associated with severe corrosive injuries. Strong alkalies in both liquid and granular form are the principal cause of severe injuries. These include sodium hydroxide (lye), potassium hydroxide and sodium carbonate. Unlike alkalies, which do not have much taste, strong acids are bitter, burn on contact and are usually expectorated. When they are swallowed, they pass rapidly through the oesophagus and cause most substantial damage in the antrum of the stomach. This is due to pooling of swallowed acid proximal to the pylorus, which goes into spasm on contact with acid. The injury tends to be worse when the stomach is empty. The duodenum and proximal small intestine are relatively protected by pylorospasm. Ferrous sulphate in both tablet and capsule form may induce caustic injury to the oesophagus and stomach.

**Q3**  Which of the following is not true regarding acid ingestion?
  **A**  The duodenum and small bowel are relatively protected.
  **B**  A hard eschar is formed.
  **C**  It usually results in full-thickness injury.
  **D**  Injury is worse when the stomach is empty.
  **E**  Most substantial damage occurs in the antrum of the stomach.

**A3**  **C**  In cases of acid ingestion, the duodenum and proximal small bowel are relatively protected by pylorospasm. Most injuries occur in the antrum of the stomach and tend to be worse when the stomach is empty. Acid ingestion causes coagulation necrosis with a hard eschar formation. The protective coagulum layer at the site limits acid penetration through the mucosa.

**Q4**  The characteristic features of alkali ingestion include all of the following *except*:
  **A**  tissue destruction continues until alkali is neutralised
  **B**  destruction extends beyond the muscle layer
  **C**  coagulation necrosis occurs
  **D**  the common sites of injury are the entrance to oesophagus, mid-oesophagus and proximal to the oesophagogastric junction
  **E**  in the solid form, the injuries are usually limited to the oropharyngeal and supraglottic region.

**A4**  **C**  Alkalis tend to be tasteless and odourless, so large quantities can be ingested. The solid form results in more oropharyngeal and supraglottic injuries because of limited quantities of ingestion. In cases of alkali ingestion, liquefactive necrosis occurs with destruction of the epithelium and submucosa, and may extend through the muscle layer. A friable discoloured eschar forms, beneath which tissue destruction continues until all the alkali has neutralised. The principal sites of damage are the areas of hold up such as cricopharyngeal area, the mid-oesophagus where it is crossed by the aortic arch and left main stem bronchus, and immediately proximal to the gastro-oesophageal junction.

**Q5** Which of the following is not true regarding the clinical presentation of caustic ingestion?

    **A** Drooling is an indication of pharyngeal injury.

    **B** Oesophageal injury can occur without evidence of oropharyngeal injury in 20% of cases.

    **C** Clinical presentation depends on the concentration and form of the ingested substance.

    **D** Can present with surgical emphysema.

    **E** Most cases remain asymptomatic.

**A5**   **B** Most children with caustic ingestion remain asymptomatic and do not develop signs of corrosive injuries. Others present with signs of oral burns, retrosternal pain, tachycardia, dyspnoea and agitation. The extent and severity of injury depends on the concentration and form of the ingested substance. Oesophageal injury without any evidence of oropharyngeal injury can occur in up to 10% of cases. Drooling and inability to swallow indicate severe posterior pharyngeal or upper oesophageal injury. Acute respiratory distress may occur as a result of posterior pharyngeal oedema or upper airway burns. Severe injuries can also result in oesophageal perforation with mediastinitis, shock and surgical emphysema in the neck and chest.

**Q6** Which of the following is most urgent in the initial management of caustic ingestion in children?

    **A** maintaining airway and oxygenation

    **B** inducing vomiting

    **C** fibre-optic endoscopy

    **D** urgent surgery

    **E** chest radiograph

**A6**   **A** Initial management, irrespective of the type of caustic ingestion, is directed at achieving haemodynamic and respiratory stability. Attempts to remove the ingested substance by emesis or lavage are strictly contraindicated as they may reintroduce the corrosive material onto the epiglottis, vocal cords and larynx. No neutralising chemicals should be given as they produce heat when interacting with the ingested substance, which may increase the severity of the injury. After stabilisation of the patient, chest and abdominal radiographs are obtained as a baseline and to rule out free air in the mediasternum or abdomen. Likewise, contrast oesophagram is not helpful in the early stages of acute injury, unless there is a strong suspicion of perforation, or endoscopy cannot be performed for some reason. Water-soluble contrast should always be used in case perforation is present. Urgent surgery is reserved for rare cases of severely charred oesophagus when oesophagectomy is performed and cervical oesophagostomy and feeding jejunostomy or gastrostomy is established. Upper gastrointestinal endoscopy is usually performed 24–48 hours after injury (*see* answer 7).

 **Q7** All of the following are true regarding the use of endoscopy in caustic ingestions *except*:

   **A** it is best recommended between 24 and 48 hours after injury
   **B** it helps in staging and management of oesophageal injuries
   **C** it is vital to visualise the entire upper gastrointestinal tract
   **D** there is a high risk of perforation associated with this procedure
   **E** it is contraindicated in cases of severe pharyngeal burns.

 **A7**   **C**   The timing of fibre-optic endoscopy is not universally agreed, but it is thought to be safe and more accurate if done within 24–48 hours after injury. This is because it takes 12–24 hours for the injured areas of the oesophagus and stomach to demarcate. The risk of perforation is high after 4–7 days, as there is completion of necrotic tissue sloughing and early granulation.

Endoscopy helps to grade the severity of the injury, plan management and predict long-term outcomes.

| Grade | Description | Management |
|-------|-------------|------------|
| 0 | Normal | No specific treatment |
| I | Oedema and hyperaemia of mucosa | |
| IIa | Friability, haemorrhage, erosion blisters, exudates or whitish membranes, superficial ulcers | Treatment to prevent stricture formation |
| IIb | Grade IIa plus deep, discrete or circumferential ulcerations | |
| IIIa | Small scattered areas of necrosis, areas of brownish black or grey discolouration | |
| IIIb | Extensive necrosis | Immediate surgery |

**TABLE 26.1  Endoscopic grading of injury severity**

Perforation is a severe complication that may be accompanied by mediastinitis and even mortality. In the presence of pharyngeal burns with stridor, early oesophagoscopy is contraindicated because of the risk of aggravating the airway obstruction. Indirect laryngoscopy is useful in these cases. Although an attempt is made to visualise the entire upper gastrointestinal tract, it is not always necessary and can be potentially dangerous and increases the risk of perforations. This can be avoided by examining the oesophagus only to the level of first significant injury.

**8** Which of the following is true regarding the use of steroids in caustic ingestion?

A Long-term treatment with high dosage of steroids is indicated.

B Steroids definitely help in reduction of stricture formation.

C Steroids should always be used concomitantly with antibiotics in all cases.

D Stricture formation is related to degree of burns irrespective of steroid treatment.

E It reduces incidence of malignancy post caustic injuries of oesophagus.

 **8**  **D** The role of steroids in caustic injuries is still a mater of debate. Animal experiments have suggested that steroids inhibit inflammatory response and decrease the risk of stricture formation and perforation. However clinical trials and retrospective reviews showed no statistical difference in prevention of strictures. Anderson *et al.* (1990) showed that with first- and second-degree oesophageal injuries, strictures developed in 5% of the steroid-treated patients and none of the controls, with third-degree injuries strictures occurred in 90% of the steroid-treated children and 100% of the controls. Stricture formation is thus related to the degree of burn irrespective of steroid treatment. It has been suggested that antibiotics should be used concomitantly along with steroids. This is based on animal studies where the risk of steroid-induced complications was shown to be higher. There is no evidence that it decreases incidence of malignancy.

 **9** Which of the following is true regarding the use of antibiotics in caustic ingestion?

A They are routinely indicated in caustic injuries.

B They are indicated in cases of oesophageal or gastric perforation.

C They decrease the incidence of oesophageal or gastric perforation.

D They reduce the risk of stricture formation.

E They are indicated only when steroids are used.

**A9**  **B** The routine use of broad-spectrum antibiotics in caustic injuries still remains a matter of debate. They are definitely indicated where there is clinical evidence of oesophageal or gastric perforation. There is no evidence to show any decrease in rate of stricture formation or perforation following antibiotic usage. Some authors advocate use of antibiotics along with steroids to decrease steroid-induced complications. If considered, their use may more be justified in full-thickness injuries because of the risk of mediastinitis or peritonitis secondary to loss of mucosal and muscular barrier. However, the role of both steroids and antibiotics in caustic ingestion is still controversial.

**Q10** Which of the following is true regarding the feeding regimen for caustic ingestion?

    **A** A nasogastric tube is recommended in all cases.

    **B** The patients are kept *ne per oris* for 7–10 days.

    **C** Oral feeding is commenced as soon as patient can swallow saliva.

    **D** Total parenteral nutrition is used until endoscopic evidence of healing has occurred.

    **E** Nasogastric tubes are contraindicated in caustic ingestion.

**A10** **C** The routine use of a nasogastric tube is not recommended in all cases of caustic ingestion. Introduction of a nasogastric tube before endoscopy should be avoided as it may result in a perforation. It should be passed only after the degree and severity of caustic injury has been assessed at endoscopy. For patients with severe injuries, nasogastric tube may be passed for early feeding. It can also function as an intraluminal stent. There is no evidence to show that a period of nil by mouth is of any benefit. Oral feeding should be commenced as soon as the patient is able to swallow saliva.

**Q11** Complications of caustic ingestion include which of the following?

    **A** oesophageal strictures

    **B** oesophageal carcinoma

    **C** gastric outlet obstruction

    **D** Barrett's oesophagus

    **E** all of the above

**A11** **E** The severity of complications relates to the depth of injury. Superficial mucosal injuries are painful but resolve without long-term sequelae. Deep caustic injuries result in healing by fibrosis and subsequent stricture formation. Full-thickness injuries can result in perforation and posterior fistula formation with either the trachea or aorta. Gastric outlet obstruction is less common, but can occur specially after strong-acid ingestion resulting in the need for a partial gastrectomy. The risk of oesophageal cancer after caustic strictures is around 5% with a latent period of 15–40 years. Hence lifelong surveillance is important in these cases. Barrett's oesophagus has also been reported following sodium hydroxide ingestion (lye).

**Q12** The management of oesophageal strictures includes all of the following *except*:
  **A** oesophageal dilatation
  **B** resection and anastomosis
  **C** colonic patch procedures
  **D** pyloroplasty
  **E** gastric tube oesophagoplasty.

**A12** **D** Oesophageal dilatations are the mainstay treatment of oesophageal strictures. These are usually commenced 3–4 weeks after injury. These should be done at least once a week, commencing with catheters that are at least one or two French sizes smaller than the estimated diameter of the stricture. If dilatations fail and a dense stricture develops, it requires further management. Localised strictures may be resected with end-to-end anastomosis. Local steroid injections have been combined with dilatation with some success. In those cases that have failed dilatation, various oesophageal bypass/substitution procedures such as colonic interposition, gastric tube oesophagoplasty, jejunal interposition, gastric advancement and colonic patch procedures have been used. Pyloroplasty is often combined with some of these procedures, but in itself is not a method for treatment of oesophageal strictures.

**Q13** Poor prognostic factors for oesophageal dilatation in caustic strictures include all of the following *except*:
  **A** older children
  **B** delay in presentation
  **C** stricture greater than 5 cm
  **D** ongoing oesophageal ulceration
  **E** extensive grade III injury on initial endoscopic assessment.

**A13** **A** Generally oesophageal dilatation is quite effective in moderate oesophageal injuries. Poor prognostic factors include delay in presentation, extensive grade III injury, ongoing oesophageal ulceration, a dense fibrotic stricture that cracks on dilatation, a stricture longer than 5 cm, and inadequate lumen patency despite repeated dilatations over a 9–12 month period. There is no difference in outcome or severity based on age at presentation.

Q14 Which of the following is true regarding long-term management of caustic injuries?

A  Long-term surveillance with endoscopy is recommended.

B  Surgical management of associated gastro-oesophaeal reflux is not recommended.

C  Oesophageal stents are indicated in all cases of caustic strictures unresponsive to dilatations.

D  Prolonged use of antireflux medications.

E  Oesophageal strictures can be avoided if dilatations are commenced immediately after the injury.

A14  A  Oesophageal dilatation should not be performed immediately following ingestion, as it has an increased risk of perforation. It is usually best to wait for 3–4 weeks until the acute lesion has healed and fibrosis has developed. Once commenced, to be effective, routine weekly dilatations are recommended. A water-soluble contrast study is usually done 7–10 days following injury to assess the presence of a stricture. The incidence and severity of gastro-oesophageal reflux must be investigated and excluded as a contributing cause of persisting stricture. Gastro-oesophageal reflux must be managed surgically before definitive procedures are attempted. There is no need for prolonged antireflux medications once gastro-oesophageal reflux is surgically corrected. Because of an increased risk of oesophageal cancer following caustic strictures (5%) and a long latent period of 15–40 years, lifelong surveillance is necessary. Oesophageal stents can be used to maintain the patency of the lumen and prevent adhesions of the de-epithelialised area of the oesophagus. If used, stents should be left in place for at least 6 weeks. Not all cases of failed dilatation respond to stents and in many cases these are not tolerated well.

## Further reading

Anderson KD, Rouse TM, Randolph JG. A controlled trial of corticosteroids in children with corrosive injury of the esophagus. *N Engl J Med.* 1990; **323**(10): 637–40.

Hawkins DB, Demeter MJ, Barnett TE. Caustic ingestion: controversies in management: a review of 214 cases. *Laryngoscope.* 1980; **90**(1): 98–109.

Spitz L, Lakhoo K. Caustic ingestion. *Arch Dis Child.* 1993; **68**(2): 157–8.

# CHAPTER 27

# Gastro-oesophageal reflux disease

**VICTORIA LANE, MARK POWIS**

**From the choices below each question, select the single best answer.**

**1** Regarding gastro-oesophageal reflux, which of the following is true?
  **A** It features uncontrolled vomiting caused by noxious stimuli.
  **B** All newborns have a degree of gastro-oesophageal reflux.
  **C** Gastro-oesophageal reflux always requires investigation.
  **D** It is always pathological.
  **E** There is an increased incidence in neurologically impaired children.

**A1** **E** Gastro-oesophageal reflux is the passage of gastric contents into the oesophagus, not caused by noxious stimuli, and is an extremely common, usually self-limiting condition, which is not pathological. The peak incidence is around 4 months of age and resolves by 1–2 years of age in most patients. Gastro-oesophageal reflux should be of concern only when associated with complications when it is termed gastro-oesophageal reflux disease. Early detection and treatment of gastro-oesophageal reflux in children may prevent associated problems.

In infants gastro-oesophageal reflux most commonly manifests as regurgitation, vomiting and 'spitting up'. These symptoms occur in up to 67% of otherwise healthy infants aged 4–5 months, declining to 21% by 6–7 months of age and to less than 5% by 12 months of age. In older children the incidence has been reported to be 1.8%–22% in those aged 3–18 years.

Neurologically impaired children are affected more commonly than normal children; studies show gastro-oesophageal reflux in up to 75% of neurologically impaired children. The severity of the reflux has also been shown to be related to the severity of the neurological dysfunction.

**Q2** With regard to the natural barriers to gastro-oesophageal reflux , which of the following is false?

**A** The lower oesophageal sphincter is a high-pressure zone near the gastro-oesophageal junction.

**B** Oesophageal peristalsis plays a role in the prevention of gastro-oesophageal reflux .

**C** The presence of an intra-abdominal segment of oesophagus is not required in antireflux surgery.

**D** The angle of His is the junction between the oesophagus and stomach.

**E** There is a mucosal rosette at the gastro-oesophageal junction which acts as a weak valve.

**A2** **C** Pathophysiology

Four components of gastric juice can damage the oesophageal epithelium. These are:

- hydrochloric acid
- pepsin
- bile salts
- pancreatic enzymes.

In typical circumstances, however, hydrochloric acid and pepsin are the main factors, as the bile salts and pancreatic enzymes are inactivated at acidic pH.

A small amount of acid/pepsin reflux is normal; however, in gastro-oesophageal reflux disease a combination of defects in the antireflux barrier and luminal clearance mechanisms allows the refluxate to be in direct contact with the oesophageal epithelium for a prolonged period and to damage the epithelium.

There are three lines of defence against damage from acid reflux, the first being the antireflux barrier consisting of a lower oesophageal sphincter, the diaphragmatic pinchcock and the angle of His. This barrier serves to limit the frequency and volume of refluxed gastric contents. When this line of defence fails the second becomes more important, namely, gastric clearance together with salivary and oesophageal secretions to neutralise the acid. The third mechanism is tissue or oesophageal mucosal resistance.

### The antireflux barrier
#### *The lower oesophageal sphincter*

The lower oesophageal sphincter is a high-pressure zone near the gastro-oesophageal junction, although there is no anatomical structure.

Oesophageal peristalsis normally begins at the pharynx and progresses down the oesophagus and produces, at an appropriate time, relaxation of the lower oesophageal sphincter to allow the food bolus to pass into the stomach. It is thought that this is controlled by afferent and efferent vagal pathways. It is vital that an adequate length of intra-abdominal oesophagus is present, as this is compressed when the intra-abdominal pressure increases and therefore acts as a valve preventing reflux from the stomach into the lower oesophagus. The greater the length of the intra-abdominal oesophagus the more effective the lower oesophageal sphincter becomes.

The key to antireflux procedures is ensuring an adequate length of intra-abdominal oesophagus (>2 cm).

### The pinchcock action

The oesophagus passes through the diaphragm at the hiatus, a sling-shaped orifice in the right crus of the diaphragm. The crural diaphragm constitutes the external mechanism of the lower oesophageal sphincter. As the oesophagus passes through the hiatus it is surrounded by the phreno-oesophageal membrane. The insertion of this membrane marks the junction of the intrathoracic and intra-abdominal oesophagus.

### Angle of His

The angle of His is the angle formed by the juncture of the oesophagus and the stomach. In children with a normal length of abdominal oesophagus, the angle is acute. This acute angle creates a double antireflux mechanism, so that when a patient attempts to vomit, the vomitus is forced into the fundus, increasing the already acute angle further, thereby reducing the amount able to escape in the oesophagus. If the angle is obtuse however, the oesophagus is turned into a funnel and the vomit is channelled into the oesophagus.

### Mucosal rosette

In the presence of a normal angle of His, a convoluted fold of mucosa with a rosette-like configuration is seen at the gastro-oesophageal junction. When there is an increase in the intra-abdominal pressure the folds are squeezed together and it acts as a weak antireflux valve.

 The incidence of gastro-oesophageal reflux disease is increased in which of the following conditions?

  A  gastroschisis

  B  cerebral palsy

  C  congenital diaphragmatic hernia

  D  oesophageal atresia

  E  all of the above

   E  Patients with abdominal wall defects (gastroschisis, omphalocele, prune belly syndrome) are at increased risk of developing gastro-oesophageal reflux, as are those with congenital diaphragmatic hernia.

Sandifer's syndrome is associated with gastro-oesophageal reflux and oesophagitis. This syndrome includes voluntary dystonic contortions of the head, neck and trunk. These movements have been shown to increase the peristalsis in the lower oesophagus.

As mentioned, neurologically impaired children have an increased risk of developing gastro-oesophageal reflux and are more likely to suffer complications.

## Asthma and gastro-oesophageal reflux

Asthma is a well-recognised disease and one of the most common illnesses in childhood, with an estimated 5 million children or more having asthma in the United States. Gastro-oesophageal reflux disease is also a common disease and the two diagnoses often present together, but with a frequency greater than one would expect by chance alone.

Asthma is a disorder caused by chronic inflammation of the airways in which, in addition to increased airway mucus secretion and smooth muscle hyperactivity, a number of inflammatory cells including eosinophils, mast cells, macrophages and T-lymphocytes play a critical role. These different cell types secrete a wide variety of mediators. The natural history of asthma, irrespective of the age of onset is one in which chronic inflammation can result in airway remodelling, irreversible airflow obstruction and an accelerated decline in lung function. In short, the longer the history of asthma the greater the risk of irreversible lung damage.

Asthma is known to promote gastro-oesophageal reflux by a number of mechanisms including cough-induced increase in intra-abdominal pressure, hyperinflation of the lungs leading to alteration in the angle of His, airway obstruction leading to negative intrathoracic pressure, and specific asthma medications that reduce the pressure of the lower oesophageal sphincter.

Several theories have been proposed to explain the association between asthma and gastro-oesophageal reflux. These include the theory that acid reflux causes direct stimulation of the airways and promotes inflammation on the basis that the common embryological origin of the respiratory and gastrointestinal systems results in a shared innervation via the vagus nerve and thereby shared autonomic reflexes. Therefore, stimulation of receptors in the distal oesophagus can lead to a vagal reflex and bronchial constriction.

There are numerous clinical clues suggestive of pulmonary symptoms being due to reflux, including asthma occurring after 3 years of age, symptoms of reflux preceding asthma, failure to exhibit an improvement in pulmonary function despite good compliance with standard asthma medications, and a family history negative for pulmonary disease and positive for gastro-oesophageal reflux–related disorders.

Respiratory symptoms suggestive of asthma can arise from a number of different disorders including gastro-oesophageal reflux, which often results in symptoms that are consistent with asthma or pneumonia. Asthma management focuses on the regulation and control of chronic airway hyperactivity and inflammation. Those children who do not respond to standard asthma medication should be investigated for other causes of their pulmonary symptoms including gastro-oesophageal reflux.

Up to 75% of adults with asthma report symptoms of gastro-oesophageal reflux. In addition among those individuals with asthma, abnormal oesophageal pH studies were observed in 55%–83% of adults, and 50%–63% of children. Mathew *et al.* (2004) noted that the severity of the asthma was directly related to the degree of reflux. Twenty-four-hour pH studies in 68 children demonstrated a reflux prevalence of:

- 0% in those with mild intermittent asthma
- 11% in those with mild persistent disease
- 23% in children with moderate persistent asthma
- 57% in those with severe persistent asthma.

The reverse also seems to be true in that the relative risk of pulmonary disease is increased in individuals with gastro-oesophageal reflux. Other studies have confirmed that children with gastro-oesophageal reflux are at increased risk of developing sinusitis, laryngitis, pneumonia and bronchiectasis.

## Oesophageal atresia and gastro-oesophageal reflux

Gastro-oesophageal reflux after repair of oesophageal atresia is common, occurring in at least 50%. A previous report of nine children reported 100% gastro-oesophageal reflux in those with oesophageal atresia not associated with a tracheo-oesophageal fistula. The mechanism for this may be due to the mobilisation of the lower oesophagus leading to shortening of the intra-abdominal portion of the oesophagus and widening of the angle of His. It may also be related to a congenital defect in the motor function of the lower oesophagus. A study looking at the prevalence of gastro-oesophageal reflux in 40 adults who had undergone correction for oesophageal atresia more than 28 years previously, identified 34% having difficulty swallowing solid food, 18% reported heartburn and 21% retrosternal pain. Sixty-one per cent of the patients agreed to undergo an oesophagogastroduodenoscopy and biopsy, which identified Barrett's oesophagus in one and oesophageal squamous cell carcinoma in another patient. They were unable to confirm that patients with oesophageal atresia should undergo routine screening.

In 1993, a study looked at 80 patients with oesophageal atresia and tracheo-oesophageal fistula treated from January 1974 to December 1988. Thirty-four (55%) were identified as having gastro-oesophageal reflux. After an unsuccessful trial of medical therapy, 21 underwent a Nissen fundoplication. Only eight patients had an uncomplicated postoperative course. Wrap disruption occurred in 33%, and 8 of 21 developed severe dysphagia, requiring prolonged feeding with gastrostomy, probably due to the inability of the dyskinetic oesophagus to overcome the increased resistance caused by the wrap. Three out of 21 (14%) died from complications related to antireflux surgery. Seventy-one per cent of the children who underwent a Nissen fundoplication eventually had excellent long-term results, but the authors did question whether a Nissen was appropriate in those with a previous history of oesophageal atresia considering the significant morbidity and mortality.

 **Q4** Which of the following is a presenting feature for gastro-oesophageal reflux?

**A** recurrent pneumonia

**B** asthma

**C** choking

**D** chest pain

**E** all of the above

**A4** **E** **Symptoms of gastro-oesophageal reflux**

Children with gastro-oesophageal reflux classically complain of abdominal pain. A key component in differentiating acid-related disorders in children with chronic or recurrent abdominal pain is the location, quality and timing of the pain. When taking a history from the patient, it is useful to have the child standing as they will often point to the site of pain. Pointing to the epigastrium or mesogastrium is suggestive of gastro-oesophageal reflux. Children may find it difficult to articulate the feeling of heartburn, which may be a reason for epigastric pain being a more common presenting feature.

One study of 76 children found the presenting symptoms to be recurrent abdominal pain in 64%, heartburn in 34%, respiratory symptoms in 29%, regurgitation in 22%, retrosternal pain in 18% and vomiting in 16%.

Review of a child's medical history may be helpful in reinforcing the diagnosis of gastro-oesophageal reflux because recurrent ear infections, sore throats and dental problems are consistent with known extraoesophageal manifestations of gastro-oesophageal reflux .

Symptoms of gastro-oesophageal reflux:

- vomiting
- rumination
- failure to thrive
- oesophageal manifestations
  — anaemia, haematemesis
  — chest pain, heartburn
  — dysphagia
  — stricture
- respiratory manifestations
  — aspiration pneumonia
  — laryngospasm, hoarseness
  — reactive airway disease
  — chronic cough

- choking
- apnoea
- neurological problems
  - infantile irritability
  - seizure-like events
  - Sandifer's syndrome
- other symptoms
  - glue ear
  - increased dental carries
  - halitosis.

## Q5 Which of the following investigations is able to detect anatomical abnormalities of the upper gastrointestinal tract?

A  upper gastrointestinal barium study

B  chest radiograph

C  24-hour oesophageal pH monitoring

D  upper gastrointestinal endoscopy and biopsy

E  scintigraphy

## A5  A  Investigations

Diagnostic procedures other than clinical evaluation should be used when the results will strongly influence treatment or will identify complications. For the infant with frequent regurgitation who is otherwise thriving, no investigations are necessary.

Despite a number of diagnostic methods ranging from upper gastrointestinal series with barium or technetium scans to 24-hour oesophageal pH monitoring or endoscopy, there is no gold standard for the investigation of acid-related disease in children.

### Upper gastrointestinal barium study

Upper GI studies may detect anatomical abnormalities but are insensitive and non-specific for the diagnosis of gastro-oesophageal reflux and *Helicobacter pylori*-associated mucosal injury. Associated conditions such as hiatus hernia, pyloric obstruction and malrotation may be identified. An experienced radiologist may be able to evaluate the oesophagus for structural and mucosal irregularities, and may also be able to comment on oesophageal peristalsis.

### Scintigraphy

Episodes of gastro-oesophageal reflux are demonstrated on scintigraphy through the presence of the isotope in the oesophagus, using serial images 30–60 minutes after the instillation of the isotope into the stomach. The sensitivity is higher than conventional barium studies and exposes the patient to lower doses of radiation.

It has three clinical applications.

1 Diagnosis of gastro-oesophageal reflux.
2 Detection of pulmonary aspiration.
3 Assessment of the rate of gastric emptying.

### 24-hour oesophageal monitoring

This technique was developed in the 1970s for use in adults but it was quickly adapted for use in children. A pH probe of appropriate size is positioned transnasally at the junction of the middle and lower thirds of the oesophagus. The pH is continuously measured and recorded. A pH of less than 4 denotes reflux of gastric contents. The frequency and duration of reflux episodes are recorded. A diary is also kept to document what the patient is doing at certain times (e.g. sleeping, feeding, coughing, and so forth). The test has been found to have a sensitivity and specificity of at least 94%. However, pH studies are unable to identify non-acid-related or alkaline-reflux-related disease.

The test is indicated in the following circumstances.

1 Infants who have respiratory symptoms.
2 Infants who are irritable, crying and poor feeders.
3 Children with reactive airway disease.
4 Children who are unresponsive to medical therapy and in whom the role of gastro-oesophageal reflux is uncertain.
5 Children who become symptomatic after fundoplication.

### Upper gastrointestinal endoscopy and biopsy

Clinical suspicion of oesophagitis and dysphagia are indications for this procedure. An upper gastrointestinal endoscopy alone has a low sensitivity for oesophagitis, therefore biopsies are taken. Biopsy and microscopic diagnosis are both highly specific and sensitive in the diagnosis of oesophagitis (95%).

Oesophagoscopy can also identify Barrett's, strictures and ulcers.

Routine gastric biopsies are taken in children undergoing endoscopy to identify those with *H. pylori*. When testing for *H. pylori*, serological testing should be avoided as antibody responses in children differ from those of an adult. Antibody levels in children may remain elevated for years after the infection has been eradicated.

### Manometry

Oesophageal manometry studies the contractile activity of the oesophagus and the upper and lower sphincters. This investigation is important in research of gastro-oesophageal disease, but is of little value as a diagnostic tool.

**Q6** Gastro-oesophageal reflux and neurological impairment. Which of the following is false?

   A It is present in 70% of children with neurological impairment.

   B The severity of reflux is directly related to the severity of neurological impairment.

   C Reflux is improved with a gastrostomy.

   D Reflux is worse due to abdominal spasticity.

   E Neurologically impaired children are more likely to have complications following antireflux surgery.

 **A6** C Difficulty in feeding and feed refusal is a common problem in neurologically impaired children and in those with gastro-oesophageal reflux. The most difficult clinical problem is managing the severely neurologically impaired child with persistent vomiting. Vomiting is common in this group with 15% of severely impaired institutionalised children having recurrent vomiting. Seventy-five per cent of these children have been shown to have gastro-oesophageal reflux, and the severity of the neurological dysfunction is directly related to the degree of gastro-oesophageal reflux.

Many of these children are unable to communicate verbally, making diagnosis difficult and these children are often non-ambulatory, confounding the problem of gastro-oesophageal reflux because of the lack of gravitational forces to aid stomach emptying. Increased abdominal pressure also probably plays a role, with an increased incidence of scoliosis, spastic quadriplegia and seizures all contributing to an increase in the intra-abdominal pressure leading to the normal antireflux barrier being overcome. Neurologically impaired children also have more associated complications of gastro-oesophageal reflux with oesophageal strictures and oesophagitis being more common as well as pneumonia. These children are also more likely to encounter postoperative complications following antireflux surgery.

 **Q7** Gastrostomy and gastro-oesophageal reflux. Which of the following is true?

   A Gastrostomy decreases the risk of gastro-oesophageal reflux because it opens the angle of His.

   B Development of postgastrostomy gastro-oesophageal reflux in neurologically impaired children is reported as 66%.

   C Greater-curvature tubes are associated with less gastro-oesophageal reflux than lesser-curvature tubes.

   D It is possible to place a gastrostomy in the lesser curve percutaneously.

   E None of the above.

**A7** **B** The placement of a gastrostomy increases the risk of gastro-oesophageal reflux due to opening of the angle of His, lowering of the lower oesophageal sphincter and a reduction in the lower oesophageal length. The development of post-gastrostomy gastro-oesophageal reflux has been shown to be as high as 66% in neurologically impaired children with normal preoperative studies.

Lesser curvature gastrostomy tubes are associated with less gastro-oesophageal reflux than greater curve tubes, because there is no change in the angle of His. It is not possible to place a percutaneous gastrostomy tube in the lesser curve of the stomach.

**Q8** Which of the following is not a treatment for gastro-oesophageal reflux?

**A** ranitidine

**B** cisapride

**C** omeprazole

**D** metoclopramide

**E** domperidone

**A8** **B** **Medical therapy**

The major treatment options for those with gastro-oesophageal reflux disease are medical, and antireflux surgery.

### Drugs that inhibit or neutralise gastric acid

The principal clinical indications for reducing acid secretion are peptic ulceration and reflux oesophagitis.

Therapy for peptic ulcers and reflux oesophagitis aims to decrease the release of gastric acid with $H_2$-receptor antagonists or proton pump inhibitors, and/or neutralise the acid with antacids.

#### Proton pump inhibitors

The first proton pump inhibitor was the substituted benzimidazole, omeprazole, which irreversibly inhibits $H^+/K^+$-ATPase (the proton pump), the terminal step in the acid secretory pathway. Both basal and stimulated gastric acid secretion is reduced. Omeprazole is currently the only proton pump inhibitor licensed in the UK for the treatment of gastro-oesophageal reflux disease in children over 2 years of age.

#### Histamine $H_2$-receptor antagonists

The histamine $H_2$-receptor antagonists competitively inhibit histamine actions at all $H_2$-receptors, but their main clinical use is the inhibitors of gastric acid secretion. They can inhibit histamine, gastrin and acetylcholine-stimulated acid secretion; pepsin secretion also falls with the reduction in volume of gastric juice.

Drugs include ranitidine, nizatidine, famotidine and cimetidine.

### Drugs that increase gastrointestinal motility

#### Domperidone

Primarily used as an antiemetic but it also increases gastrointestinal motility (mechanism unknown). Clinically it also increases the pressure at the lower oesophageal sphincter, thus inhibiting gastro-oesophageal reflux. It also increases gastric emptying and enhances duodenal peristalsis. It is therefore useful in disorders of gastric emptying and gastro-oesophageal reflux disease. A recent review, however, concluded that there was no robust evidence of efficacy of domperidone for the treatment of gastro-oesophageal reflux in young children.

#### Metoclopramide

Metoclopramide is a $D_2$-receptor antagonist closely related to the phenothiazine group. It acts centrally on the chemoreceptor trigger zone and also has a peripheral action on the gastrointestinal tract itself, stimulating gastric motility and causing a marked acceleration in gastric emptying. It is useful in gastro-oesophageal reflux disease and in disorders of gastric emptying.

It is a similar drug to domperidone but has more tendency to cross the blood brain barrier and cause the unwanted central side effects due to its blockade of dopamine receptors, including disorders of movement, fatigue, motor restlessness, spasmodic torticollis and oculogyric crises.

#### Cisapride

Cisapride was used until 2000. Guidelines (1993) in ESPGAN (the European Society of Paediatric Gastroenterology Hepatology and Nutrition) cited cisapride as a first-line treatment for gastro-oesophageal reflux/gastro-oesophageal reflux disease. However, a more recent systematic Cochrane Review in 2000, and a large multicentre Canadian trial in 1999, have shown that there is little evidence of efficacy in its use. It has now been withdrawn after being found to have had no advantage over placebo for relief of symptoms of gastro-oesophageal reflux and also because of side effects including fatal cardiac arrhythmias. Cisapride stimulates acetylcholine release in the myenteric plexus in the upper gastrointestinal tract through $5-HT_4$-receptor-mediated effect. This raises oesophageal sphincter pressure and increases gut motility.

#### Histamine $H_1$-receptor antagonists

Alimemazine/trimeprazine is a phenothiazine $H_1$-receptor antagonist commonly used for its antipruritic effect and in high dose for its sedative effect. It is also known to have antiemetic properties and antispasmodic effect on smooth muscle. It has been shown to decrease the frequency of retching after a Nissen fundoplication in neurologically impaired children.

**Q9** During a Nissen fundoplication which of the following steps is not performed?

    **A** Fundus of the stomach is passed posteriorly around oesophagus to form a 360-degree wrap.

    **B** A window is created anterior to the gastro-oesophageal junction.

    **C** Gastrophrenic ligaments are divided.

    **D** Short gastric vessels are divided.

    **E** The gastrohepatic ligament is divided.

**A9**   **B** In the **Nissen fundoplication** the following steps are performed.

1 The gastrohepatic ligament is divided with the peritoneal covering of the oesophagus.

2 The oesophagus is mobilised ensuring an adequate length.

3 The gastrophrenic ligaments are divided to mobilise the posterior aspect of the fundus of the stomach.

4 Division of the short gastric vessels is often required.

5 A window is then created posterior to the oesophagus.

6 The right and left leaves of the right crus of the diaphragm are approximated.

7 The fundus is passed from left to right posterior to the oesophagus.

8 A 360-degree wrap is created.

9 The left and right margins of the wrap are sutured anteriorly including the anterior wall of the oesophagus in the sutures.

10 The superior margin of the wrap is sutured to the hiatus.

**Q10** Which of the following is true following a Nissen fundoplication?

    **A** More than 90% of children have long-term resolution of symptoms with a Nissen fundoplication.

    **B** Emesis is improved.

    **C** Gas bloat occurs in 10%.

    **D** Asthma is improved.

    **E** All of the above.

**A10**   **E** More than 90% of children have long-term resolution of their symptoms with Nissen's fundoplication, with the cure rate for emesis approaching 100%. Pulmonary symptoms are improved in 96% of children and weight gain is improved in the majority, especially if a gastrostomy is positioned at the same time. Asthma is improved in 92% of patients.

    Neurologically impaired children have an increased risk of developing complications following antireflux surgery and neurological status is a major predictive factor in the success of antireflux surgery. Dedinsky *et al.* (1987)reported the results of 429 Nissen operations in children, 297 of whom were neurologically impaired. This group accounted for all four deaths, 24/28 wrap herniations. Spitz and Kirkane had a 20% morbidity and 12% mortality rate among children with neurological impairment undergoing Nissen fundoplication.

**Q11** Which of the following antireflux procedures involves a 270-degree wrap, positioned posterior to the oesophagus?

   **A**  Toupet's repair

   **B**  Boix–Ochoa's repair

   **C**  Thal's repair

   **D**  Boerema's repair

   **E**  Hill's repair

**A11**  **A**  **Other antireflux procedures**

### Thal and Boix–Ochoa

In the Thal and Boix–Ochoa techniques, the lower oesophagus is mobilised in a similar fashion to the Nissen procedure and the crus is approximated posterior to the oesophagus to re-establish a hiatus of a normal size. The stitch is also used to attach the hiatus to the posterior wall of the oesophagus. A partial 180-degree anterior fundal wrap is then constructed, plicating the upper fundus to the anterior oesophageal wall. This procedure does not require division of the short gastric vessels, is technically easier, and has a shorter operating time. The Boix–Ochoa procedure differs from the Thal in that the remaining fundus is fixed by interrupted sutures to the underside of the left hemidiaphragm to maintain the angle of His. In both the Thal and the Boix–Ochoa techniques there is a reduced incidence of gas bloat.

### Toupet's technique

Another partial-wrap technique is the Toupet procedure also developed to mini-mise gas bloat. In this operation a partial 270-degree wrap is positioned posterior to the oesophagus. After the crura have been approximated to restore the size of the hiatus, the gastric fundus is passed posterior to the oesophagus. Division of the short gastric vessels is often necessary. The posterior aspect of the wrap is sutured to the right crus. The margins of the wrap are then sutured to the left and right margins of the oesophagus, leaving the anterior wall of the oesophagus free.

    The **Boerema** is an anterior gastropexy, and the **Hill** is a posterior gastropexy.

Q12 Which of the following is a recognised complication of surgical therapy for gastro-oesophageal reflux disease?

A  dysphagia

B  wrap breakdown

C  intestinal obstruction

D  splenic injury

E  all of the above

A12  E  Reported complications following antireflux surgery include wrap breakdown, dysphagia secondary to a slipped wrap, a wrap that is too tight, torsion of the wrap and gas bloat. Early intestinal obstruction occurs in 2%–6%. Splenic injury and perforation of the oesophagus are rare. As mentioned, complications following Nissen fundoplication in neurologically impaired children are higher than in neurologically normal children.

Q13 Which of the following is a minimally invasive approach to the control of gastro-oesophageal reflux in children?

A  laparoscopic Nissen fundoplication

B  Stretta's procedure

C  TIF with EsophyX

D  EndoCinch procedure

E  all of the above

A13  E  All of the above procedures are minimally invasive and are being used/evaluated at centres around the world.

- **Laparoscopic Nissen fundoplication** is perhaps the most commonly performed minimally invasive therapy for gastro-oesophageal reflux. It has become the 'gold standard' against which other procedures are compared.
- **The Stretta procedure** (Curran Medical Inc) uses endoluminal radiofrequency energy to cause collagen contraction at the level of the lower oesophageal sphincter. This modulates the physiology of the sphincter and so reduces gastro-oesophageal reflux.
- **TIF with EsophyX** (EndoGastric Solutions) is transoral incisionless fundoplication. Under endoscopic guidance a former is used to reduce any hiatus hernia and fold the fundus of the stomach. The fundus is then secured with endoscopically applied fasteners to form a partial wrap.
- **EndoCinch** (Bard) is another endoscopically guided device that allows pleats to be stitched into the lower oesophagus below the sphincter. These pleats reduce symptoms and medication usage in mild gastro-oesophageal reflux.

- Other endoluminal therapies involve the injection of bulking materials submucosally into the lower oesophagus at the level of the sphincter to reduce gastro-oesophageal reflux.

## Further reading

Dedinsky GK, Vane DW, Black T, *et al.* Complications and reoperation after Nissen fundoplication in childhood. *Am J Surg.* 1987; **153**(2): 177–83.

Hassall E. Decisions in diagnosing and managing chronic gastroesophageal reflux disease in children. *J Pediatr.* 2005; **146**(3 Suppl.): S3–12.

Kimber C, Kiely E, Spitz L. The failure rate of surgery for gastro-oesophageal reflux. *J Pediatr Surg.* 1998; **33**(1): 64–6.

Mathew JL, Singh M, Mittal SK. Gastro-oesophageal reflux and bronchial asthma: current status and future directions. *Postgrad Med J.* 2004; **80**(950): 701–5.

Nelson SP, Chen EH, Syniar GM, *et al.* Prevalence of symptoms of gastroesophageal reflux during infancy: a pediatric practice-based survey; Pediatric Research Practice Group. *Arch Pediatr Adolesc Med.* 1997; **151**(6): 569–72.

Rothenberg SS. Experience with 220 consecutive laparoscopic Nissen fundoplications in infants and children. *J Pediatr Surg.* 1998; **33**: 274–8.

Wheatley MJ, Coran AG, Wesley JR. Efficacy of the Nissen fundoplication in the management of gastroesophageal reflux following esophageal atresia repair. *J Pediatr Surg.* 1993; **28**(1): 53–5.

# SECTION VI

# Cardiovascular

# CHAPTER 28

# Congenital cardiac anomalies

## BASSEM N MORA

**From the choices below each question, select the single best answer.**

**Q1** The most common primary cardiac tumour in children is:
 **A** fibroma
 **B** angiosarcoma
 **C** rhabdomyoma
 **D** teratoma
 **E** myxoma.

**A1** **C** Cardiac tumours are classified as primary (arising from the heart, more than 90% of which are benign) or secondary (representing metastases, which are uniformly malignant). Most cardiac tumours in children and adults represent metastatic disease. In children, these are secondary to non-Hodgkin's lymphoma, leukaemia and neuroblastoma. The most common primary cardiac tumour in children is rhabdomyoma, accounting for 50%–80% of all paediatric primary cardiac tumours. Other benign primary cardiac tumours vary according to age: in neonates and infants, fibroma and intrapericardial teratoma may occur, while in older children and adolescents, myxoma and fibroma are seen. Rhabdomyomas are multiple, well-circumscribed, white, intracavitary or intramural masses that may occur anywhere in the heart. Most are diagnosed in the newborn period and may present with respiratory distress or heart failure, especially if large. Tuberous sclerosis, an autosomal dominant mutation with variable expressivity, is a common association, with approximately 50% of patients with tuberous sclerosis having rhabdomyomas. Approximately 30% of rhabdomyomas will regress spontaneously. Rhabdomyosarcoma is the most common primary malignant cardiac tumour in children whereas angiosarcoma is the most common primary malignant cardiac tumour in adults; both portend a poor prognosis. Myxomas, arising from the interatrial septum, are the most common primary benign cardiac tumours in adults, usually diagnosed in the third to sixth decade of life. Treatment is by surgical excision with reconstruction of the interatrial septum. Fibromas represent the second most common primary benign cardiac tumour in children, and present usually as solitary large white non-encapsulated tumours in the left ventricular septum or free wall. Presentations include left ventricular outflow tract obstruction and ventricular tachyarrhythmias. Treatment is by surgical enucleation on cardiopulmonary bypass. Intrapericardial teratomas are solitary, encapsulated tumours that are attached to the base of the heart. As with other teratomas, all three embryonic germ cell layers may be present. Treatment is by surgical excision.

**Q2** All of the following may be found in scimitar syndrome *except*:
- **A** dextrocardia
- **B** haemoptysis
- **C** aortopulmonary collateral artery
- **D** bronchopulmonary sequestration
- **E** ventricular septal defect.

**A2** **E** Scimitar syndrome is a form of partial anomalous pulmonary venous return where the right pulmonary veins drain into the inferior vena cava, with subsequent drainage into the right atrium. The left pulmonary veins drain normally into the left atrium. There is often an associated atrial septal defect (ASD) that is low in the interatrial septum, close to the orifice of the inferior vena cava. The chest radiograph in the anteroposterior projection shows the scimitar sign, which is a crescent-like shadow in the right lower lung field, parallel to and distinct from the right heart border. This extra shadow is similar to a scimitar, which is a curved Turkish sword. Right pulmonary artery hypoplasia may be present, as well as right lung hypoplasia. As a result, the heart may be shifted to the right; cases of mesocardia (midline heart) or dextrocardia (cardiac apex pointing to the right) have also been described. Pulmonary parenchymal abnormalities include sequestration, with an anomalous systemic arterial blood supply, usually from the descending thoracic aorta to the sequestered lung. A ventricular septal defect is not associated with this defect, whereas an ASD is often found. If no ASD is present, those patients typically present later in life, often in adulthood, with right atrial enlargement and right ventricular volume overload. An ASD results in an earlier presentation because of the increased right atrial and right ventricular volume overload from left-to-right shunting across the interatrial septum, in addition to the anomalous drainage of the right pulmonary veins into the right atrium. This results in exercise intolerance and palpitations from atrial tachyarrhythmias, although a number of patients may be asymptomatic. Treatment is by rerouting the anomalous right pulmonary veins into the left atrium, either through a baffle across the ASD, or by direct anastomosis of the pulmonary veins to the left atrium.

**Q3** A child was a restrained passenger in a high-speed head-on motor vehicle collision. Of the following injuries after blunt cardiac trauma, which is the least likely to occur?

A  ASD

B  cardiac free-wall rupture

C  coronary artery thrombosis

D  ventricular septal defect

E  myocardial contusion

**A3** **A** Cardiac trauma is classified as blunt or penetrating, with most penetrating cardiac trauma resulting in death at the scene. Blunt cardiac trauma is most often due to high-speed motor vehicle collisions, usually from impact of the chest and sternum against the steering wheel or the dashboard. Other causes include direct blows to the chest from an object, a fall or a kick. Although most patients are asymptomatic and free of injury, blunt cardiac trauma may be life-threatening. Clinical presentations include free-wall rupture of the atria or ventricles, coronary artery trauma with thrombosis, tachyarrhythmias, rupture of the chordae tendinae or papillary muscles, pericardial rupture with cardiac herniation, pericardial effusions and aortic transection, typically at the ligamentum arteriosum in the proximal descending thoracic aorta from a sudden deceleration injury. Of those with blunt cardiac injuries who survive the injury to present in the emergency room, myocardial contusion is the most common presentation. This may result in cardiac enzyme elevations, premature ventricular contractions and arrhythmias on electrocardiography, and regional wall-motion abnormalities on echocardiography. Pericardial effusions may be present, and delayed myocardial rupture may occur. Of the choices presented, all involve the ventricular myocardium except ASDs, which are not recognised as common sequelae of blunt cardiac trauma.

**Q4** The vascular structure that has the highest oxygen saturation in the fetal circulation is:

A  aorta

B  umbilical vein

C  ductus arteriosus

D  umbilical artery

E  ductus venosus.

**A4** **B** The fetal circulation is characterised by several shunts: the ductus venosus in the liver that shunts blood from the umbilical vein into the inferior vena cava, the foramen ovale that shunts blood from the right atrium to the left atrium, and the ductus arteriosus that shunts blood from the right ventricle into the descending thoracic aorta. Fetal haemoglobin binds oxygen more avidly than mature haemoglobin, and holds onto oxygen more strongly as well. As a result, the arterial oxygen saturation in the fetal aorta is only 60%–65%. Blood travels from the fetal descending thoracic aorta through the right and left fetal common iliac arteries, into the right and left fetal internal iliac arteries, then into the right and left umbilical arteries into the placenta, which has low vascular resistance. After oxygenation, the blood travels from the placenta into the fetal umbilical vein, a solitary structure that drains into the ductus venosus in the liver. Blood from the ductus venosus drains into the inferior vena cava then the right atrium. Streaming within the right atrium directs the inferior vena cava blood towards the foramen ovale and into the left atrium, thence into the left ventricle and the ascending aorta. This ensures that the fetal brain and heart receive blood with the highest possible oxygen saturation. The blood from the superior vena cava will enter the right atrium and preferentially stream into the right ventricle, then into the main pulmonary artery. Fetal pulmonary vascular resistance is high because of the collapse of the fetal lungs and the muscularisation of the pulmonary arterioles. As a result, most of the blood in the main pulmonary artery will drain into the descending thoracic aorta via the ductus arteriosus. The blood in the transverse aortic arch will mix with the blood from the ductus arteriosus and return to the placenta for oxygenation. Immediately following birth, the paired umbilical arteries close first, allowing a brief period of autotransfusion from the placenta into the umbilical vein. Within a week of birth, the umbilical vein will become a fibrous cord, knows as the round ligament of the liver. This passes from the umbilicus to the transverse hepatic fissure, where it joins the ligamentum venosum (remnant of the ductus venosus) to separate the liver into right and left hepatic lobes.

**Q5**  The most common congenital cardiac anomaly is:
  A  ASD
  B  bicuspid aortic valve
  C  ventricular septal defect
  D  D-transposition of the great arteries
  E  tetralogy of Fallot.

**A5**  **B**  The most common cyanotic congenital heart disease lesion in the neonatal period is D-transposition of the great arteries, where the aorta and main pulmonary artery are transposed, with the aorta connecting to the right ventricle, and the main pulmonary artery connecting to the left ventricle. The most common cyanotic congenital heart disease lesion beyond the neonatal period is tetralogy of Fallot, manifested by hypoplasia of the outflow of the right ventricle with the presence of a ventricular septal defect below the aortic valve. Ventricular septal defects are common in congenital heart disease, and are divided into four types: muscular, perimembranous, inlet and conal septal types. ASDs are also common, and are also of four types: secundum defects, primum defects, coronary sinus septal defects and sinus venosus defects. A bicuspid aortic valve is by far the most common congenital cardiac anomaly, occurring in 1%–2% of the population, more commonly in males. While fusion of any of the three commissures of the aortic valve is possible, the most common fusion site is between the right and left sinuses of Valsalva. At birth, most patients with bicuspid aortic valves are asymptomatic, although some will present with critical neonatal aortic stenosis requiring intervention. A bicuspid aortic valve is associated with aortic coarctation, which is a narrowing of the aorta at the insertion of the ductus arteriosus in the proximal descending thoracic aorta. In adulthood, bicuspid aortic valves predispose to the development of aortic stenosis, with some patients requiring aortic valve replacement. In addition, there is an association between bicuspid aortic valves and the development of ascending aortic aneurysms and aortic dissections.

Q6 Which statement regarding the aorta and aortic arch is correct?

**A** In a left aortic arch, the aortic isthmus lies proximal to the left subclavian artery.

**B** The most common aortic arch anomaly is a right aortic arch with an aberrant left subclavian artery.

**C** The ascending aorta normally arises posterior and to the right of the main pulmonary artery.

**D** Patients with a double aortic arch become symptomatic late in infancy or young adulthood.

**E** Truncus arteriosus is commonly associated with an interrupted aortic arch.

A6 **C** The aortic arch is divided into three segments. In a left aortic arch, the proximal arch is the segment between the right innominate (brachiocephalic) artery and the left common carotid artery; the distal arch is the segment between the left common carotid artery and the left subclavian artery; the aortic isthmus is the segment between the left subclavian artery and the patent ductus arteriosus (PDA) (or ligamentum arteriosum). The most common aortic arch anomaly is a right aortic arch with mirror-image branching, where the aortic arch vessels are a mirror image of the left aortic arch. The first branch off a right aortic arch with mirror-image branching is the left innominate (brachiocephalic) artery, the second branch is the right common carotid artery, and the third branch is the right subclavian artery. The descending thoracic aorta in this setting descends in the right chest, reflecting a mirror image of what takes place in a normal left aortic arch, where the descending thoracic aorta descends in the left chest. The vast majority of those patients (approximately 90%) have associated congenital heart disease. Patients with vascular rings most commonly have a double aortic arch, where there are two aortic arches. Typically, the left aortic arch in a double aortic arch is the smaller of the two arches, and may even be atretic, represented by a fibrous cord. Since the constriction of the trachea and oesophagus is complete

(360 degrees), patients with a double aortic arch present early in infancy, often within the neonatal period. Another common vascular ring is the right aortic arch with an aberrant left subclavian artery and a left ligamentum arteriosum, the latter two structures arise from a diverticulum of Kommerell. In patients with truncus arteriosus, there is a common arterial trunk arising from the ventricular mass. The pulmonary arteries arise off this common trunk, which continues as the ascending aorta. There is no pulmonary valve. In truncus arteriosus, the aortic arch is left-sided in 65%, and right-sided in 35%. The aortic arch is interrupted in only 10%–15% of patients with truncus arteriosus. In normal cardiac development, the ascending aorta arises posterior and to the right of the pulmonary artery, with the ascending aorta arising from the left ventricle, and the main pulmonary artery arising from the right ventricle. In D-transposition of the great arteries, there is ventriculoarterial discordance, meaning that the ascending aorta arises from the right ventricle, and the main pulmonary artery arises from the left ventricle. In most cases of D-transposition of the great arteries, the aorta arises anterior and to the right of the main pulmonary artery.

**Q7** PDA in premature infants is characterised by each of the following *except*:

  **A** cardiopulmonary deterioration in one-third of patients

  **B** increased cardiac size on chest X-ray

  **C** pharmacological responsiveness to indomethacin

  **D** an absence of clinical findings on cardiovascular examination

  **E** non-invasive evidence of shunting before physical exam findings are apparent.

**A7**   **D** In premature infants, the ductus arteriosus is patent at birth. In some, it closes spontaneously, but in the majority the PDA persists for a prolonged period of time. Approximately one-third of patients will develop heart failure symptoms and require increased ventilator support. Pharmacological treatment with non-steroidal anti-inflammatory drugs, such as indomethacin, results in closure of the PDA in most premature infants. In approximately 10%, surgical ligation is needed for ductal closure. The left-to-right shunt across the PDA results in increased left-heart return, correlating with cardiomegaly and increased pulmonary interstitial vascular markings on chest radiography. The premature lungs exacerbate this. The physical examination is notable for a machinery-type murmur, heard throughout systole and in early-to-mid diastole, also known as Gibson's murmur. Other findings include bounding peripheral pulses from run-off of blood into the pulmonary arteries during diastole, resulting in a widened pulse pressure. A hyperactive precordium and hepatomegaly may be present. Echocardiography is diagnostic and reveals left-to-right shunting across the PDA, as well as dilatation of the left atrium and the left ventricle at end diastole. Echocardiography may reveal a PDA before the development of symptoms, especially in the first few days after birth, or if the PDA is small.

**Q8** Concerning aortic coarctation, which of the following statements is correct?

   **A** The most common location of an aortic coarctation is preductal.

   **B** Aortic coarctation is associated with Turner's syndrome.

   **C** The aortic valve is bicuspid in 10% of patients.

   **D** Inferior rib notching affects the first to eighth ribs.

   **E** Repair is typically via median sternotomy.

**A8**   **B** Aortic coarctation is a narrowing of the aorta at the insertion of the ductus arteriosus into the proximal descending thoracic aorta. The most common location of coarctation is juxtaductal, and not proximal to the ductus arteriosus. A bicuspid aortic valve is present in approximately 50% of patients. Collateral arteries develop primarily from intercostal vessels, and provide blood flow to areas distal to the coarctation. Over time, the enlarged intercostal vessels result in notching of the inferior aspect of the ribs, where the neurovascular bundle runs. These intercostal vessels arise from the subclavian arteries and their branches, including the internal mammary arteries. Notching is not seen in the first or second ribs, since the upper intercostal arteries in those ribs are not supplied by the subclavian artery. Aortic coarctation is present in approximately 20% of patients with Turner's syndrome, and is the major congenital cardiac anomaly in Turner's syndrome. In patients with a left aortic arch, which represents the majority of patients, repair is through a left thoracotomy, and not a median sternotomy. If there is associated proximal aortic arch hypoplasia, then repair is via median sternotomy on cardiopulmonary bypass with enlargement of the aortic arch with a patch.

**Q9** Which one of the following is the most reliable indicator of right atrial morphology?

   **A** Drainage of the superior vena cava into the atrium.

   **B** Drainage of the inferior vena cava into the atrium.

   **C** Presence of an atrial appendage that is triangular with a broad base.

   **D** Outflow into the tricuspid valve.

   **E** Presence on the right side of the heart.

**A9**   **B** In normal hearts, all of the choices listed are correct. However, in complex congenital heart disease, only choice B definitively identifies the right atrium. Patients may have bilateral superior vena cavae, with the right superior vena cava draining into the right atrium and the left superior vena cava draining into the left atrium. In some patients, there is only one left-sided superior vena cava draining into the left atrium, which could be a morphological right atrium. The inferior vena cava, when present, will always drain into the right atrium. In patients with heterotaxy syndrome, the inferior vena cava may be interrupted below the liver, with continuation into the azygos vein that drains into the superior vena cava. The hepatic veins in those cases would drain directly into the atrium. In those cases, it may be difficult to determine which atrium is the morphological right atrium, a condition known as situs ambiguus. The right atrial appendage is triangular with a broad base, in contradistinction to the left atrial appendage, which is finger-like and long with a narrow base. In patients with heterotaxy of the asplenia variety (also known as right atrial isomerism), both atrial appendages are triangular with broad bases, requiring the presence of other anatomical landmarks to determine which atrium is the morphological right atrium. While the coronary sinus usually drains into the right atrium, it may be absent, or may be unroofed and drain into the left atrium. The atrium that is located on the right side of the heart may often be the morphological right atrium, although that is not a uniform finding. In patients with situs inversus totalis, the morphological right atrium is left-sided and the morphological left atrium is right-sided. In corrected transposition of the great arteries, the morphological right atrial outflow is through the mitral valve into the left ventricle then through the pulmonary valve into the pulmonary arteries. The morphological left atrial outflow is through the tricuspid valve into the right ventricle then through the aortic valve and aorta.

## Q10 A secundum ASD is a hole in which of the following structures?

**A** atrioventricular septum

**B** superior vena cava junction with the right atrium

**C** septum secundum

**D** septum primum

**E** endocardial cushions

## A10 **D** ASDs are defects in the interatrial septum that result in left-to-right shunting of blood. This results in dilatation of the right atrium and right ventricle, with cardiomegaly on chest X-ray and right ventricular volume overload on echocardiography. Secundum ASDs are the most common type of ASDs, and represent defects in septum primum. In the embryonic heart, septum secundum forms to the right of septum primum; after birth it fuses with septum primum to close the foramen ovale and form the interatrial septum. Defects in the interatrial septum at the junction of the superior vena cava with the right atrium represent sinus venosus defects. Ostium primum ASDs, also known as primum ASDs, represent defects within the endocardial cushions at the posterior and inferior aspects of the interatrial septum, at the junction of the tricuspid valve with the interatrial septum. The atrioventricular septum is the small part of the membranous septum

of the heart just above the septal cusp of the tricuspid valve, separating the right atrium from the left ventricle.

**Q11** Partial anomalous pulmonary venous drainage is most commonly associated with which congenital cardiac abnormality?

   A   atrioventricular canal defect

   B   sinus venosus ASD

   C   ventricular septal defect

   D   secundum ASD

   E   tetralogy of Fallot

**A11**   **B**   Anomalous pulmonary venous return represents abnormal drainage of the pulmonary veins into the heart. Patients with total anomalous pulmonary venous return (TAPVR) have all four pulmonary veins draining abnormally. Those are divided into supracardiac types (the most common subtype), intracardiac types and infracardiac types; the latter are invariably obstructed. Patients with partial anomalous pulmonary venous return have some pulmonary veins draining normally into the left atrium (often the left-sided veins), while one or more pulmonary veins drain abnormally, usually ending in the right atrium or inferior vena cava (the latter are associated with scimitar syndrome). While all of the choices listed may have anomalous pulmonary venous return, the most common congenital cardiac anomaly with partial anomalous pulmonary venous return is sinus venosus ASD. In that lesion, there is a defect in the interatrial septum at the junction of the superior vena cava with the right atrium. The right upper pulmonary vein is located in the normal anatomical position, but, because of the absence of the interatrial septum at the site where this vein normally drains into the atrium, the resultant drainage of blood is into the right atrium. Secundum ASDs are located in the central portion of the interatrial septum and are not typically associated with partial anomalous pulmonary venous return. Patients with endocardial cushion defects, also known as atrioventricular canal defects or atrioventricular septal defects, often, but not always, have normal pulmonary venous drainage. Tetralogy of Fallot is an anomaly of the right ventricular outflow tract with pulmonary stenosis and a ventricular septal defect; it is not usually associated with partial anomalous pulmonary venous return.

**Q12** Which of the following ventricular septal defects is least likely to close spontaneously?

   A   perimembranous ventricular septal defect

   B   muscular ventricular septal defect

   C   inlet ventricular septal defect

   D   apical ventricular septal defect

   E   restrictive ventricular septal defect

A12 **C** Ventricular septal defects are holes in the interventricular septum, which separates the right ventricle from the left ventricle. There are four types of ventricular septal defects: perimembranous defects (located in the membranous interventricular septum at the junction of the septal and anterior leaflets of the tricuspid valves), muscular defects (located anywhere in the muscular interventricular septum), inlet defects (located below the septal leaflet of the tricuspid valve), and conal septal defects (located in the conal septum that separates the aortic valve from the pulmonary valve). Perimembranous defects are the most common defects that are closed surgically. The bundle of His penetrates at the posterior inferior aspect of the ventricular septal defect and care should be taken at the time of surgical closure not to damage the conduction tissue, which may result in complete heart block. Muscular ventricular septal defects are further subdivided into anterior muscular (located inferior to the pulmonary valve), mid-muscular (located close to the moderator band), posterior muscular (located at the posterior septal tricuspid valve leaflet) and apical muscular (located in the apex of the ventricular septum). Restrictive defects are those that have a pressure gradient across the defect, which would be consistent with partial spontaneous closure of the defect. Spontaneous closure may be a result of hypertrophy of muscle bundles within the right ventricle, aortic valve prolapse, presence of tricuspid valve chordae and accessory tricuspid valve tissue, or the presence of a subaortic membrane on the left ventricular aspect of the ventricular septal defect. All of the defects listed may close spontaneously except for inlet ventricular septal defects, which never close. Conal septal defects, also known as outlet defects or supracristal defects, also do not close spontaneously, and require surgical closure.

Q13 A patient has a chest X-ray that shows increased pulmonary arterial markings, mild to moderate cardiomegaly, prominent pulmonary arteries, and lack of left atrial dilatation. Of the following congenital cardiac lesions, which is the most likely?

**A** ventricular septal defect

**B** tetralogy of Fallot

**C** aortic coarctation

**D** PDA

**E** ASD

A13 **E** The chest radiograph may be used to discriminate between various aetiologies of congenital heart disease. The presence of increased pulmonary arterial markings is consistent with increased pulmonary blood flow, as is seen with ventricular septal defects and PDA. These result in cardiomegaly, although cardiomegaly may also result from systemic hypertension, cardiomyopathy and obstruction to systemic blood flow. Prominent pulmonary arteries, and prominent pulmonary artery convexity, are often due to a left-to-right shunt, resulting in increased pulmonary blood flow and dilatation of the pulmonary arteries. Dilated and aneurysmal pulmonary arteries are also seen in tetralogy of Fallot with absent pulmonary valve syndrome. The left atrium is dilated in patients with ventricular septal defects and PDA due to increased left atrial return from pulmonary overcirculation. The left atrium is not dilated in ASDs due to the presence of the ASD and the decreased relative compliance of the left atrium compared with the right atrium. As a result, the blood shunts from the left atrium to the right atrium, resulting in right atrial dilatation and right ventricular volume overload. Patients with tetralogy of Fallot have a characteristic boot-shaped heart ('coeur en sabot') where the cardiac apex is displaced upwards. Tetralogy patients also have decreased pulmonary vascular markings due to decreased pulmonary blood flow from right ventricular outflow tract obstruction. The pulmonary arteries are not prominent and the left atrium is not dilated.

**Q14** Which of the following is *not* a true statement regarding tetralogy of Fallot?

**A** A right aortic arch is present in 25% of patients with tetralogy of Fallot.

**B** Tetralogy of Fallot is the most common cause of cyanosis in infants and children.

**C** The ventricular septal defect is usually non-restrictive, large and anteriorly malaligned.

**D** The degree of right-to-left shunting depends on the severity of obstruction to pulmonary blood flow.

**E** The ventricular septal defect is located in the anterior muscular septum below the pulmonary valve.

**A14 E** Tetralogy of Fallot is characterised by the presence of four features: (1) obstruction to pulmonary blood flow that may be valvar (at the level of the pulmonary valve), subvalvar (below the pulmonary valve, within the right ventricular infundibulum or outflow tract) and supravalvar (above the pulmonary valve, in the main pulmonary artery or its branches) – often, all three sites of obstruction to pulmonary blood flow are present concomitantly; (2) presence of an anteriorly malaligned ventricular septal defect that shunts blood from the right ventricle into the left ventricle due to the presence of right ventricular outflow tract obstruction, resulting in cyanosis – occasionally the obstruction to pulmonary blood flow is minimal, and the shunting will be left-to-right across the ventricular septal defect; (3) override of the aortic valve so that part of the aortic valve will lie over the right ventricle, while most (>50%) of the aortic valve will lie over the left ventricle; (4) development of right ventricular hypertrophy due to obstruction to pulmonary blood flow.

Tetralogy of Fallot is further subdivided into three types, depending on the aetiology of obstruction to pulmonary blood flow: (1) tetralogy of Fallot with pulmonary stenosis, the most common type; (2) tetralogy of Fallot with pulmonary atresia, also known as pulmonary atresia with ventricular septal defect, where the main pulmonary artery and branch pulmonary arteries may be very small; and (3) tetralogy of Fallot with absent pulmonary valve, associated with congenital absence of the ductus arteriosus and to-and-fro passage of blood *in utero* across the absent pulmonary valve, resulting in aneurysmal dilatation of the pulmonary arteries and air trapping from bronchial obstruction due to the dilated pulmonary arteries. A right aortic arch is present in one-quarter of all patients, especially those with tetralogy of Fallot with pulmonary atresia, where collateral arteries develop from the aorta and provide additional sources of pulmonary blood flow. Tetralogy of Fallot is the most common cause of cyanosis beyond the neonatal period, and is present in approximately 10% of congenital heart disease patients. The ventricular septal defect is large and non-restrictive. There is anterior deviation (i.e. malalignment) of the distal conal septum compared with the proximal interventricular septum, such that the two ends of the interventricular septum (where the ventricular septal defect is located) are not in the same anatomical two-dimensional plane. The degree of right-to-left shunting across the ventricular septal defect depends on the severity of obstruction to pulmonary blood flow. The ventricular septal defect is located in the subaortic region, and is described as a perimembranous defect with anterior malalignment, also known as a conoventricular defect. It is not an anterior muscular ventricular septal defect (which would be located in the muscular interventricular septum below the pulmonary valve).

Q15 Concerning the Blalock–Taussig shunt, which one of the following statements is correct?

   A  It connects the subclavian artery to the pulmonary artery.

   B  It is a conduit between the right atrium and the pulmonary artery.

   C  It is an intra-atrial tunnel that connects the inferior vena cava to the pulmonary artery.

   D  It connects the superior vena cava to the pulmonary artery.

   E  It is a connection between the systemic right ventricle and the pulmonary artery.

A15  A  The Blalock–Taussig shunt was originally described by Drs Blalock and Taussig to provide increased pulmonary blood flow in patients with tetralogy of Fallot. The classic Blalock–Taussig shunt involved division of the subclavian artery with anastomosis end to side to the ipsilateral pulmonary artery. This allowed blood to bypass the obstruction in the right ventricular outflow tract, so that it may be oxygenated and subsequently pumped into the systemic circulation. The original Blalock–Taussig shunt continued to grow with the child, resulting in torrential pulmonary blood flow with time. This is now modified by placement of a polytetrafluoroethylene (PTFE) tube between the subclavian artery and the pulmonary artery, obviating the need for division of the subclavian artery. It is used for palliation of cyanotic congenital heart disease, including patients with tetralogy of Fallot and those with single ventricle physiology with decreased pulmonary blood flow. It is not a conduit between the right atrium and the pulmonary artery, as was done in earlier versions of the Fontan procedure. A lateral tunnel Fontan would consist of the placement of an intra-atrial tunnel that connects the inferior vena cava to the undersurface of the right pulmonary artery. This serves as the third and final palliation of single ventricle patients. The second-stage palliation of single ventricle patients is the Glenn shunt, which is an anastomosis between the superior vena cava and the right pulmonary artery. The Sano shunt is a conduit between the systemic right ventricle and the pulmonary artery bifurcation in patients with hypoplastic left heart syndrome.

**Q16** All of the following statements are true regarding long-term complications following the Fontan procedure *except*:

   **A** atrial arrhythmias are common

   **B** progressive clinical deterioration is uncommon

   **C** protein-losing enteropathy may occur and carries a high mortality

   **D** plastic bronchitis is a recognised complication

   **E** heart failure is a common cause of death.

**A16** **B** Single ventricle patients have either a dominant systemic right ventricle or left ventricle. Surgical palliation consists of a series of operations that eventually result in passive flow of blood into the pulmonary circulation, with active pulsatile flow from the ventricular mass into the systemic circulation. Typical palliation consists of three stages: the first stage involves augmenting or limiting pulmonary blood flow, depending on whether there is a decrease or increase in pulmonary blood flow, respectively. Operations performed during this stage consist of the Norwood procedure for hypoplastic left heart syndrome, pulmonary artery banding for patients with increased pulmonary blood flow, or placement of a modified Blalock–Taussig shunt for patients with decreased pulmonary blood flow who are dependent on the PDA for pulmonary blood flow. Second-stage palliation consists of the Glenn shunt, also known as a superior cavopulmonary anastomosis, whereby the right superior vena cava is transected at the atrium and sutured directly to the right pulmonary artery. A bilateral Glenn procedure is indicated if there are bilateral superior vena cavae. A hemi-Fontan procedure is an alternative to the Glenn procedure and consists of a side-by-side anastomosis of the superior vena cava to the right pulmonary artery, with patch closure of the orifice of the superior vena cava within the atrium. Third-stage palliation consists of the Fontan procedure, which baffles blood from the inferior vena cava to the pulmonary arteries. Two types of Fontan operations are done: the lateral tunnel Fontan procedure, which involves placement of a piece of PTFE within the right atrium to baffle the inferior vena cava to the cardiac end of the superior vena cava, along with re-establishment of a connection between the right atrium and the undersurface of the right pulmonary artery. An alternative is the extracardiac Fontan procedure which consists of a tube of PTFE that is anastomosed end to end to the transected inferior vena cava, then anastomosed end to side to the right pulmonary artery. Complications following the Fontan procedure are common, and often result in progressive clinical deterioration, influenced by the systolic and diastolic function of the single ventricle, the degree of pulmonary vascular resistance, and the anatomical type of systemic ventricle. Atrial arrhythmias are common, and a number of patients will develop a slow junctional rhythm, requiring the implantation of an epicardial pacemaker. One dreaded long-term complication is protein-losing enteropathy, where protein is lost in the stool, as documented by a stool trypsin test. Treatment options are limited and may involve construction of a fenestration between the pulmonary and systemic venous chambers to result in a decrease in the elevated pressures in the systemic venous chamber. Cardiac transplantation is usually curative. Plastic bronchitis is another dreaded complication where bronchial casts develop that may be removed during bronchoscopy. Recurrence is the rule and survival is poor without cardiac transplantation. Heart failure is a common cause of death, due to dysfunction of the single systemic ventricle.

**Q17** Polysplenia is characterised by which one of the following features?

A Bilateral atrial appendages with triangular morphology and wide ostia.

B More severe and complex cardiac anomalies than asplenia.

C An association with azygos continuation of the inferior vena cava.

D Bilateral eparterial bronchi.

E Three lobes in each of the right and left lungs.

**A17** C Polysplenia and asplenia represent the two forms of heterotaxy syndrome, which involves abnormalities of sidedness. Normally, the liver is on the right and the spleen is on the left, with the right atrium receiving inferior vena caval blood. The right lung has three lobes while the left lung has two lobes. Polysplenia is also known as bilateral left-sidedness, or left atrial isomerism. There are multiple spleens present on the left side of the abdomen. The right lung has two lobes, and so does the left lung. The atrial appendages are both left atrial appendages, with long finger-like morphology and narrow ostia. The inferior vena cava may be normal or may be interrupted with azygos vein continuation into the superior vena cava. Associated cardiac malformations are usually less severe than in asplenia, which is characterised by the absence of a spleen. In both asplenia and polysplenia, splenic function is depressed; as a result, patients are susceptible to infections with encapsulated organisms, and lifelong amoxicillin prophylaxis has been advocated. In asplenia, also known as bilateral right-sidedness or right atrial isomerism, the atrial appendages are both right atrial appendages, characterised by triangular morphology with a broad base and wide ostia. There are three lobes in each of the right and left lungs. The right superior lobar bronchus is the only bronchus that is superior to the right pulmonary artery, and is termed an eparterial bronchus. In asplenia, there are bilateral eparterial bronchi because of the presence of bilateral right-sided lungs. In polysplenia, the bronchi are hyparterial, i.e. below (inferior) to the ipsilateral pulmonary arteries.

**Q18** The most common type of obstructed TAPVR is:

    **A** infracardiac type

    **B** supracardiac type

    **C** intracardiac type

    **D** mesocardiac type

    **E** mixed type.

**A18** **A** TAPVR is characterised by drainage of all four pulmonary veins into a pulmonary venous confluence, which subsequently drains into the right atrium via a supracardiac connection, an intracardiac connection or an infracardiac connection. Supracardiac TAPVR is the most common type, representing approximately 45% of patients. There is an ascending vertical vein that drains the pulmonary venous confluence into the left innominate vein, the azygos vein or the superior vena cava. When drainage is into the azygos vein, there is uniformly obstruction of pulmonary venous return. When drainage is into the superior vena cava, obstruction develops in approximately 65% of patients, while obstruction develops in 40% of patients when drainage is into the left innominate vein. Only approximately 20% of TAPVR is of the intracardiac type, typically draining into the coronary sinus, or less often directly into the right atrium. Obstruction develops in approximately 20% of those patients. Infracardiac TAPVR is characterised by a descending vertical vein that penetrates the diaphragm and connects with the portal vein or its branches. Obstruction is invariably present, resulting in elevated pulmonary venous pressures, white-out on the chest radiograph, poor oxygenation and metabolic acidosis. Surgery is the only option as these patients do not respond to nitric oxide or to prostaglandins. Mixed TAPVR is a combination of any of the three types of drainage; obstruction is present in approximately 40% of mixed TAPVR. There is no entity known as mesocardiac TAPVR.

**Q19** When present, a left superior vena cava most often drains directly into which of the following structures?

    **A** left atrium

    **B** coronary sinus

    **C** pulmonary vein

    **D** inferior vena cava

    **E** innominate vein

**A19** **B** There are two drainage patterns to a left superior vena cava. Typically, the left superior vena cava travels in the left atrioventricular groove posterior to the heart and joins the coronary sinus to drain into the right atrium. This normal variant has no physiologic consequence, although it does limit visibility within the heart when the right atrium is opened during open-heart surgery. There may be an innominate vein of normal size, although often the innominate vein is small or absent. The other drainage pattern of the left superior vena cava is directly into the roof (superior aspect) of the left atrium, close to the orifice of the left upper pulmonary vein and the base of the left atrial appendage. In those cases, known as the Raghib association, the left superior vena cava needs to be baffled to the right atrium, usually by construction of a pathway on the superior aspect of the left atrium to drain it into the right atrium at the interatrial septum. The other sites mentioned are not drainage sites of the left superior vena cava.

**Q20** All of the following are complications of closure of PDA *except*:

    **A** pulmonary artery injury

    **B** chylothorax

    **C** diaphragmatic paralysis

    **D** hoarseness

    **E** Horner's syndrome.

**A20** **E** Surgical closure of a PDA, typically performed via a left thoracotomy, may result in a number of surgical complications. If the PDA is not identified accurately, the wrong vessel may be ligated. Accidental closure of the aortic isthmus, transverse aortic arch and left pulmonary artery have been described, and usually involves misidentification of the anatomical landmarks. The left subclavian artery invariably enters the distal aortic arch; this should identify the aortic arch, and distinguish it from the ductus arteriosus, which should be inferior (caudad) to the arch. When the PDA is large, the ductal arch may be confused with the aortic arch, resulting in ligation of the aortic arch. The left recurrent laryngeal nerve, a branch of the left vagus nerve, lies in close proximity to the undersurface of the PDA. It encircles the PDA before ascending into the neck to innervate the left vocal cord. If the left recurrent laryngeal nerve, or the vagus nerve superior to the takeoff of the left recurrent laryngeal nerve, is injured (by electrocautery, traction, ligation or division), hoarseness will result, as well as feeding intolerance, as manifested by aspiration in the neonate. The left phrenic nerve may be injured by overzealous retraction of the lung and pleura for surgical exposure. There are a number of small lymphatic vessels that may be injured during surgery, resulting in chylothorax. Invariably, this is a self-limited condition that resolves with time. Injury to the stellate ganglion of the sympathetic nervous system results in Horner's syndrome, manifested by ptosis (drooping of the upper eyelid from loss of sympathetic innervation to the superior tarsal muscle), miosis (pupillary constriction) and anhidrosis (decreased sweating on the affected side of the face). This typically arises following extensive dissection of the left subclavian artery, which is not done during surgical PDA ligation.

## Further reading

Allen HD, Driscoll DJ, Shaddy DE, *et al. Moss and Adams' Heart Disease in Infants, Children, and Adolescents: including the fetus and young adult.* 7th ed. Philadelphia, PA: Lippincott Williams & Wilkins; 2008.

Castaneda AR, Jonas RA, Mayer JE, *et al. Cardiac Surgery of the Neonate and Infant.* New York, NY: WB Saunders; 1994.

Jonas RA, Dodson R, DiNardo J, *et al. Comprehensive Surgical Management of Congenital Heart Disease.* London: Arnold; 2004.

Keane JF, Fyler DC, Lock JE. *Nadas' Pediatric Cardiology.* 2nd ed. New York, NY: WB Saunders; 2006.

Kouchoukos NT, Blackstone EH, Doty DB, *et al. Kirklin and Barratt-Boyes' Cardiac Surgery.* 3rd ed. New York, NY: Churchill Livingstone; 2003.

Nichols DG, Ungerleider RM, Spevak PJ, *et al. Critical Heart Disease in Infants and Children.* 2nd ed. Philadelphia, PA: Mosby; 2006.

# CHAPTER 29

# Vascular disorders

## ALAN P SAWCHUK, GARY LEMMON, RAGHU MOTAGANAHALLI

**From the choices below each question, select the single best answer.**

**Q1** A 16-year-old female with a 3-year history of hypertension is referred with a diastolic blood pressure of 118 mmHg. It has been refractory to treatment with diuretic and beta-blocker therapy. A CT arteriogram reveals bilateral, focal, main renal artery stenoses near their ostia. What treatment should be recommended for this patient?

  **A** addition of an ACE inhibitor to her medical management

  **B** surgical bypass of the renal artery stenoses

  **C** angioplasty of the renal artery stenoses

  **D** bilateral renal artery uncovered stent placement

  **E** bilateral renal artery covered stent placement

**A1**   **B** This patient has bilateral renal artery stenosis from renal artery fibrodysplasia. The diagnosis can be suspected by the appearance of significant hypertension in a paediatric patient as well as by the development of diastolic hypertension with a diastolic pressure greater than 115 mmHg. Many paediatric patients do not present with the classic chain-of-lakes appearance seen in adult cases of renal fibrodysplasia.

Although many cases of mild to moderate hypertension caused by renal artery fibrodysplasia may be amenable to treatment with medication, this patient's hypertension is severe, occurred at an early age, and has not responded to treatment with two medications. With bilateral, significant renal artery stenosis, renal function may deteriorate with the addition of an ACE inhibitor. Unfortunately, percutaneous therapies in paediatric patients with ostial lesions are frequently unsuccessful and there is a high incidence of nephrectomy in these patients with unsuccessful treatment. This patient would be less likely to have a successful result in view of the ostial nature of the lesions. The optimal treatment in this paediatric patient with severe diastolic hypertension unresponsive to medical management and with lesions near the renal artery ostia, is surgical renal artery bypass.

**Q2** A 14-year-old male is referred with a right thigh mass. It has recently progressively enlarged. It is warm to the touch, with a thrill and bruit present. There are prominent veins present throughout the thigh and lower right pelvis. The mass has been painful and has intermittently bled. An MRI disclosed a diffuse vascular mass extending into several muscle planes. What treatment would you recommend for this patient?

  **A** compression stocking therapy

  **B** surgical excision

  **C** leg amputation

  **D** embolisation therapy of the main feeding vessels

  **E** embolisation of distal vessels leaving the feeding vessels intact

**A2** **E** This patient has a classic presentation for an arteriovenous malformation. The MRI indicates that this is not a discrete lesion that would be easily amenable to a standard surgical resection. Compression therapy is often helpful, but this patient is quite symptomatic with pain and bleeding. An amputation is definitely not indicated without a trial of more conservative therapy. Embolisation or sclerotherapy of the distal vessels leaving the feeding vessels intact is the preferred treatment in this patient. The average patient requires two or three treatments for reasonable symptom control. Ligation or embolisation of the feeding vessels will not prevent growth of the lesion and will prevent successful distal embolisation techniques to be used in the future, although there may still be options for percutaneous sclerotherapy

**Q3** A 16-year-old male was referred after a family practitioner was asked to do a history and physical examination prior to the student joining his high school basketball team. The student's father died in his mid-forties. The child is tall, thin and has mild pectus excavatum. The referring physician obtained a chest CT scan, which demonstrated that the lad's aortic root measured 3.9 cm in diameter (normal up to 3.6 cm in diameter). What follow-up and treatment would you recommend for this patient?

  **A** No follow-up or treatment is needed for this mild abnormality.

  **B** Surgical replacement of the aortic root and ascending aorta should be done.

  **C** Follow-up CT scans should be done on a routine basis with no other intervention.

  **D** Follow-up CT scans should be done and the patient should be placed on beta-blocker therapy.

  **E** Follow-up CT scans should be done and the patient should be placed on antihypertensive medication if he is found to have high blood pressure.

**A³**  **D**  This patient has Marfan's syndrome. It is inherited as an autosomal dominant with limited penetrance. It is caused by a mutation in the gene for fibrillin 1. The student has the classic body habitus, an enlarged aortic root diameter and a family history of a parent dying at an early age.

   The student has an aortic root diameter less than 4.0 cm. Most authors recommend repair of an adult aorta when it reaches 5.0–5.5 cm in diameter. The risk of rupture or dissection increases more than eightfold in a patient with an aortic root diameter of 6–7 cm. Surgical repair would not be indicated at this time. Follow-up studies to assess the aortic root diameter should certainly be done. A prospective randomised study has shown that putting these patients on lifelong beta blockers decreases the risk of aortic dissection by half and slows enlargement of the aortic root. The long-term benefit of beta-blocker therapy is highest in young patients with mild aortic root enlargement.

**Q⁴**  A 14-year-old female presents with progressively enlarging right leg varicose veins. Her right leg is swollen and slightly longer than her left. Her left leg appears to be normal. The leg is painful and the symptoms have not been adequately treated with compression therapy. What would you recommend for this patient?

   **A**  There are no alternatives to treatment other than continued compression therapy.

   **B**  Proceed with ablation of the right greater saphenous vein and stab phlebectomies of the secondary venous varicosities.

   **C**  Obtain a duplex venous ultrasound, coil embolise abnormal connections between the deep and superficial system with greater saphenous ablation and stab phlebectomies.

   **D**  Obtain a duplex venous ultrasound and proceed with stab phlebectomies of the superficial vein branches if the deep system is intact.

   **E**  Obtain a duplex venous ultrasound and treat incompetent superficial vein branches with sclerotherapy if the deep system is intact.

**A⁴**  **C**  This patient has Klippel–Trénaunay's syndrome, which is a capillary–lymphatic–venous malformation. Its appearance is sporadic in the population. It may present with enlarged veins, limb hypertrophy, lymphatic hypoplasia and anomalous, enlarged superficial veins. The deep venous system may not be intact.

   There are treatment options other than compression therapy. Prior to ablating any major superficial veins, it is important to ascertain that the deep system is intact. This can be done with a duplex venous ultrasound. If the deep system is not intact, any venous ablation should be done in a highly selective fashion in order to preserve venous limb drainage. If the deep system is intact, ablating the symptomatic segments of the superficial system is often not adequate because of abnormal connections between the deep and superficial systems.

These connections can be treated by the placement of microcoils in the aberrant connecting vessels. Following this treatment, the symptomatic superficial veins can be ablated. Sclerotherapy of the superficial system alone will not treat these abnormal connections between the deep and superficial systems.

**Q5** A 5-year-old child sustains a deep laceration to his right leg from a boat propeller. The limb is neurologically intact. The foot is cool to the touch and painful. During wound exploration, there are long segments of injured superficial femoral artery and vein. What would be your plan of treatment?

   **A** wound closure, anticoagulation and observation

   **B** repair of the superficial femoral artery with a prosthetic graft

   **C** repair of both the superficial femoral artery and vein using saphenous vein

   **D** repair of the superficial femoral artery using a saphenous vein graft/vein ligation

   **E** leg amputation if vessels too small to repair

**A5** **D** In general, paediatric vascular trauma is managed similarly to adult vascular trauma and the expected long-term results are equivalent to repairs in adults. At 5 years of age, the femoral vessels are large enough to surgically repair with the anticipation of having a good outcome if there are no significant associated orthopaedic or neurologic injuries. The saphenous vein is generally a large enough conduit in this patient age group and a prosthetic graft is not needed or beneficial. Repair of the superficial femoral artery alone will result in a viable limb. The vein should only be repaired if it is a reasonable undertaking and the patient is stable.

## Further reading

Rutherford RB. *Rutherford Vascular Surgery*. 6th ed. Philadelphia, PA: Elsevier Saunders; 2005.

# CHAPTER 30

# Vascular tumours and malformations

## CAMERON C TRENOR III, STEVEN J FISHMAN, ARIN K GREENE

**From the choices below each question, select the single best answer.**

Q1  A 5-year-old healthy male has an asymptomatic, enlarged upper lip at birth. The skin is normal. The lip has continued to steadily increase in size over the course of his lifetime. Which of the following is the most likely diagnosis?

   **A** infantile haemangioma

   **B** congenital haemangioma

   **C** pyogenic granuloma

   **D** lymphatic malformation

   **E** kaposiform haemangioendothelioma (KHE).

A1  **D** Lymphatic malformation is present at birth and slowly enlarges over time. Infantile haemangioma is usually noted 2 weeks after birth and grows rapidly over the first few months of life; by 1 year of age the tumour begins to regress. Congenital haemangioma is fully grown at birth and does not enlarge postnatally. Pyogenic granuloma does not appear at birth. It usually appears in early childhood as a rapidly growing, red lesion that frequently bleeds. KHE often presents at birth or in infancy and nearly 90% have cutaneous, reddish-purple lesions. KHE is frequently associated with Kasabach–Merritt's phenomenon (severe thrombocytopenia due to intralesional trapping).

**Q2** A 3-month-old girl has a rapidly enlarging, 10 cm facial haemangioma causing ulceration and a nasal deformity. Which of the following is the most appropriate treatment?

**A** interferon

**B** corticosteroid

**C** resection

**D** pulsed dye laser

**E** sclerotherapy

 **A2** **B** First-line treatment for a large, problematic infantile haemangioma is pred-nisolone, a corticosteroid. Almost all infantile haemangiomas will respond as long as the correct dose is given (3 mg/kg/day). Response is considered either stabilisation (the tumour no longer enlarges) or accelerated regression (the lesion becomes smaller). Corticosteroid is very safe. Unlike patients who receive chronic, high-dose corticosteroid for transplants or autoimmune disorders, infants with infantile haemangioma are treated for only a few months and the dose is rapidly weaned as they gain weight and the physician lowers the dose. Interferon is no longer used for patients with infantile haemangioma because it causes spastic diplegia. Resection of this large, proliferating tumour is contraindicated; during infancy the tumour is highly vascular and the patient is at risk for major blood loss and facial nerve injury. Pulsed dye laser treatment for a cutaneous, proliferating infantile haemangioma is contraindicated; the laser cannot penetrate into the deep dermis or subcutaneous tissue and thus has minimal efficacy. In addition, the laser delivers a thermal injury to the already compromised skin and has been shown to increase the risk of ulceration, pain and scarring. Sclerotherapy is effective treatment for lymphatic or venous malformations, not for infantile haemangioma.

 **Q3** What is first-line management of a painful, diffuse venous malformation involving the left cheek, orbit and lip?

**A** resection

**B** embolisation

**C** corticosteroid

**D** interferon

**E** sclerotherapy

**A3** **E** Sclerotherapy, the injection of the malformation with a sclerosant (e.g. sodium tetradecyl sulphate, ethanol), causes endothelial damage, scarring and shrinkage of the lesion. It is first-line treatment for a large, symptomatic venous malforma-tion. Resection of a diffuse venous malformation of the face would leave a worse deformity than the lesion, and the patient would be at risk for major blood loss and facial nerve injury. Resection is reserved for small venous malformations that may be removed for cure, or when sclerotherapy is no longer possible because all vascular spaces have been obliterated. Corticosteroid and interferon are indicated for some vascular tumours. Embolisation is used to treat high-flow arteriovenous malformations.

**Q4** Each of the following is a possible treatment for KHE *except*:
A resection
B sclerotherapy
C vincristine
D corticosteroid
E interferon.

**A4** **B** Sclerotherapy is used to treat venous and lymphatic malformations, not vascular tumours. Resection is rarely indicated for KHE, but is possible for small or localised lesions. Vincristine and corticosteroids are first-line options for KHE, though steroids are much less efficacious than vincristine. Interferon may be used to treat KHE, but as a second-line agent because of side effects such as spastic diplegia in infants.

**Q5** A mutation in each of the following genes is associated with inherited vascular anomalies except:
A *RASA1*
B *PTEN*
C *BRCA1*
D *VEGFR3*
E *TIE2.*

**A5** **C** Mutations in *BRCA1* have not been found to cause vascular anomalies. *RASA1* mutation causes capillary malformation-arteriovenous malformation. *PTEN* mutations can cause arteriovenous malformations. *VEGFR3* mutations can cause primary lymphoedema. Mutations in *TIE2* may result in venous malformations.

**Q6** First-line operative management for a symptomatic child with a moderately enlarged lower extremity from primary lymphoedema is:
A liposuction
B excision and skin grafting
C lymphaticovenous anastomosis
D staged skin/subcutaneous excision
E omental flap transfer.

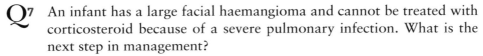

A**6**   **A**  Liposuction effectively removes, with low morbidity, the subcutaneous adipose tissue that develops from lymphoedema. Excision and skin grafting is a radical approach and is only considered in extreme disease because the procedure is associated with significant morbidity. Lymphaticovenous anastomosis may improve lymphatic flow in patients with secondary lymphoedema, but has minimal effects on limb size because the subcutaneous adipose tissue is not removed. Staged skin/subcutaneous excision is indicated for patients with severely enlarged legs when significant skin excess would be expected following liposuction. Omental flap transfer has not been shown to improve lower extremity lymphoedema and is associated with significant complications.

Q**7**   An infant has a large facial haemangioma and cannot be treated with corticosteroid because of a severe pulmonary infection. What is the next step in management?
  **A**  vincristine
  **B**  cyclophosphamide
  **C**  propranolol
  **D**  thalidomide
  **E**  interferon

A**7**   **C**  Propranolol, a beta blocker, recently has been shown to have activity in infantile haemangioma. However, its efficacy and safety compared with corticosteroid has not been studied. Complications such as hypotension and hypoglycaemia have been reported, and infants require close monitoring after the initiation of therapy. Vincristine and cyclophosphamide have been reported to slow haemangioma growth, but they require intravenous administration and have greater toxicity and less efficacy than propranolol. Thalidomide has antiangiogenic activity but has not been used to treat infantile haemangioma. Although interferon is effective, it is avoided in infants because it can cause spastic diplegia.

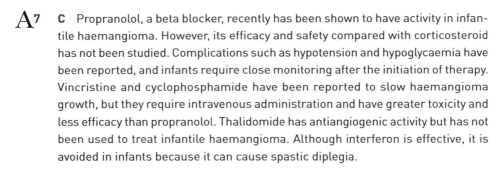

Q**8**   A 5-year-old male has a large upper lip microcystic lymphatic malformation causing a deformity. What is the most appropriate management?
  **A**  corticosteroid
  **B**  pulsed dye laser
  **C**  sclerotherapy
  **D**  resection
  **E**  embolisation

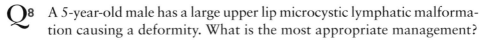

A**8**   **D**  Resection is the only current treatment for microcystic lymphatic malformation; the cysts are too small to be accessed for sclerotherapy. Sclerotherapy is first-line treatment for macrocystic lymphatic malformation. Corticosteroid is used to treat problematic infantile haemangioma. Pulsed dye laser can effectively lighten capillary malformations. Embolisation is indicated for arteriovenous malformations.

**Q9** A 3-month-old healthy female has a 1 cm superficial infantile haemangioma on the buttock. What is the most appropriate management?

**A** corticosteroid

**B** resection

**C** observation

**D** embolisation

**E** sclerotherapy

**A9** **C** More than 90% of infantile haemangiomas are non-problematic and are observed; lesions will regress after 12 months of age. Corticosteroid is reserved for problematic lesions threatening vital structures or at risk for causing a significant deformity. Resection is rarely indicated for proliferating lesions during infancy, but may be performed in early childhood to correct residual deformities caused by the tumour. Embolisation is rarely used for large haemangiomas causing congestive heart failure. Sclerotherapy is indicated for lymphatic or venous malformations.

**Q10** A 7-year-old female has a 4 cm, pedunculated infantile haemangioma of the right cheek. What is the most appropriate management?

**A** corticosteroid

**B** pulsed dye laser

**C** sclerotherapy

**D** resection

**E** embolisation

**A10** **D** After involution, infantile haemangiomas often leave behind fibrofatty residuum, redundant skin or damaged structures that require resection and/or reconstruction. Corticosteroid is effective for problematic infantile haemangiomas during the proliferative phase in infancy. Pulsed dye laser is used to treat residual cutaneous telangiectases following involution. Sclerotherapy is indicated for lymphatic or venous malformations. Embolisation is rarely indicated for large haemangiomas in infancy causing congestive heart failure.

Q11 You are planning to biopsy a large, firm, purple cutaneous mass on the chest of a 6-month-old and notice a platelet count of $8 \times 10^9$/L. Immediately after platelet transfusion, the mass painfully enlarges and becomes dark purple. What is the diagnosis of the mass?

A infantile haemangioma

B KHE

C arteriovenous malformation

D venous malformation

E epithelioid haemangioendothelioma

A11 B KHE is a vascular tumour typically presenting in infancy. KHE may behave aggressively, crossing adjacent tissue planes. The majority of lesions manifest severe thrombocytopenia known as Kasabach–Merritt's phenomenon, due to intralesional platelet trapping. Platelet transfusions are rapidly consumed by trapping in the lesion, as described in this case. Venous malformations may have localised intralesional coagulation leading to low fibrinogen, high D-dimer, prolonged prothrombin time (PT) and activated partial thromboplastin time (aPTT), but the platelet count is usually normal. Infantile haemangioma, arteriovenous malformations and epithelioid haemangioendothelioma are not associated with thrombocytopenia.

Q12 Possible complications from infantile haemangiomas include all of the following *except*:

A ulceration

B visual impairment

C airway compromise

D hypothyroidism

E hypokalaemia.

A12 E Infantile haemangiomas are benign, self-resolving tumours identified in 4%–8% of Caucasian infants. Despite their self-resolving natural history, certain locations are at risk of complications during the rapid proliferative phase. Infantile haemangioma in locations susceptible to incidental trauma, such as lips, nasal tip, perineum and hand are prone to ulceration. Periorbital lesions can occlude vision during a critical developmental period, leading to strabismus, amblyopia and even monocular blindness. Subglottic lesions may present with stridor and can progress to airway obstruction if untreated. Very large haemangiomas, often including diffuse hepatic haemangiomas, overproduce type III iodothyronine deiodinase leading to severe consumptive hypothyroidism requiring aggressive repletion. Electrolyte abnormalities are not associated with infantile haemangiomas.

Q13 Soon after menarche, a 12-year-old girl develops an enlarging painful mass over her right deltoid. Imaging confirms a high-flow lesion and you suspect an arteriovenous malformation. Which of the following is recommended prior to excision?

A $CO_2$-laser therapy

B embolisation

C sclerotherapy

D pulsed dye laser therapy

E bevacizumab (antiangiogenic medical therapy)

A13 **B** Arteriovenous malformations are often present at birth and present with periods of rapid growth, onset of pubertal hormones or pregnancy or after trauma. These high-flow, densely vascular lesions are surgically challenging to remove and require wide, complete excision to prevent recurrence. Preoperative embolisation of feeding arteries may shrink the malformation, reduce intraoperative bleeding and increase the chance of curative surgery.

Q14 Which of the following best describes the natural history of an infantile haemangioma?

A present at birth, proliferation for 5 months, slow involution over several years

B prenatal diagnosis, proliferation for 5 months, rapid involution by 1 year

C presenting 2 weeks after birth, proliferation for 5 months, slow involution over several years to residuum of fibrous and adipose tissue

D presenting weeks after birth, proliferation for 5 months, rapid involution by 1 year

E presenting any time through childhood, variable progression and involution

A14 **C** Infantile haemangioma may have a faint precursor lesion visible at birth, though prenatal or fully formed tumours at birth exclude this diagnosis. The median age of presentation for infantile haemangioma is 2 weeks after birth. Infantile haemangiomas exhibit rapid proliferation for 3–5 months and then slowly involute from 12–15 months through 5–7 years of age, leaving behind skin with reduced elasticity, increased fibrofatty tissue, scarring and hypopigmentation. Lesions varying from this natural history require further evaluation.

**Q15** Complications of extensive, diffuse hepatic haemangioma in a 3-month-old include all of the following *except*:

  **A** poor growth

  **B** severe consumptive hypothyroidism

  **C** restrictive lung disease due to poor diaphragm excursion

  **D** severe thrombocytopenia

  **E** massive hepatomegaly and abdominal compartment syndrome.

**A15** **D** Hepatic haemangiomas may be focal, multifocal or diffuse. Focal hepatic haemangiomas are Glut-1 negative, may be present prenatally and undergo rapid spontaneous involution. Multifocal hepatic haemangiomas are Glut-1 positive and may include arteriovenous shunting leading to high-output cardiac failure. Diffuse hepatic haemangiomas are Glut-1 positive and may efface the entire liver. Hepatomegaly can lead to inferior vena cava compression, respiratory compromise, abdominal compartment syndrome, multiorgan system failure and rarely lead to hepatic transplantation. Diffuse hepatic haemangiomas overproduce an enzyme that consumes thyroid hormone. The resulting severe hypothyroidism requires aggressive replacement to prevent mental retardation associated with congenital hypothyroidism. Thrombocytopenia is not associated with infantile haemangioma.

**Q16** Which of the following statements regarding vascular malformations is *not* true?

  **A** Vascular malformations form during embryologic vasculogenesis.

  **B** Vascular malformations may present at any age.

  **C** Vascular malformations are more amenable to interventional or surgical therapies than to medical therapies.

  **D** Vascular malformations may include combinations of venous, arterial, capillary and/or lymphatic structures.

  **E** Haemangiomas are one type of vascular malformation.

**A16** **E** Vascular anomalies are currently classified into tumours and malformations. Tumours are proliferative and present at different ages, though often in infancy. Malformations represent dysfunctional embryologic vasculogenesis. While malformations may enlarge, it is currently unclear if this occurs through enlargement of existing channels, angiogenesis or vasculogenesis. Because they are less proliferative than tumours, they are less amenable to antiangiogenic and antiproliferative therapies and are generally managed by sclerotherapy, embolisation and/or resection.

Q17 You are evaluating a dark-red cutaneous chest lesion in a healthy 4-month-old infant. Which of the following features supports the diagnosis of infantile haemangioma?

   **A** initial presentation at 1 month of age

   **B** no significant change in appearance throughout infancy

   **C** needle biopsy evaluation reveals negative Glut-1 staining

   **D** platelet count $12 \times 10^9/L$

   **E** slow vascular flow on Doppler evaluation

A17 **A** Infantile haemangioma typically presents in the first few weeks of life, though presentation in early infancy is not diagnostic. Not following the natural history of infantile haemangioma (proliferation, slow involution and fibrofatty residuum), the absence of Glut-1 positive immunostaining, and severe thrombocytopenia, each rule out infantile haemangioma. Infantile haemangiomas are often warm and are invariably high-flow lesions during the proliferative phase of growth.

Q18 You are evaluating a 12-year-old boy with a large lipovascular hamartoma in his thigh with associated arteriovenous malformations. You notice frontal bossing and penile freckling on exam and recommend testing for what genetic syndrome and why?

   **A** Li–Fraumeni's syndrome (*p53*) – high risk of adenocarcinomas early in life

   **B** Fanconi's anaemia – risk of aplastic anaemia and haematological malignancies

   **C** *PTEN* mutation – risk of thyroid, breast and other malignancies through life

   **D** trisomy 21 (Down's syndrome) – risk of congenital heart disease, cognitive impairment and leukaemias

   **E** Beckwith–Wiedemann's syndrome – risk of hemihypertrophy, Wilms's tumour, hypoglycaemia and hepatoblastoma

A18 **C** Among these cancer predisposition choices, benign vascular hamartomas with significant lipomatous composition, associated arteriovenous malformations, frontal bossing and penile freckling are distinctive phenotypically for patients with *PTEN* mutations. Multiple syndromes in the literature are now known to be allelic, including *PTEN* hamartoma tumour syndrome, Cowden's syndrome, Bannayan–Riley–Ruvalcaba's syndrome, Proteus and Proteus-like syndrome and adult-onset Lhermitte–Duclos's disease. Increased risk of breast and thyroid cancer require regular screening. Macrocephaly, intestinal hamartomatous polyps and mucocutaneous lesions are very common.

Q19 The following patterns of infantile haemangioma warrant additional consideration of associated underlying or associated anomalies *except*:
   A  nasal tip haemangioma
   B  extensive facial haemangioma
   C  submandibular 'beard' distribution haemangioma
   D  midline haemangioma overlying the lumbosacral spine
   E  more than 20 multifocal cutaneous haemangiomas.

A19  A  Nasal tip haemangiomas are associated with ulceration, but not with any underlying or associated anomalies. Extensive facial haemangiomas should be evaluated for PHACE syndrome (Posterior cranial fossa abnormalities, Haemangioma, Arterial anomalies, Cardiovascular defects and Eye abnormalities). 'Beard' distribution haemangiomas are associated with subglottic haemangiomas and risk of airway compromise. Lumbosacral midline haemangiomas are associated with underlying spinal cord dysraphisms. Multifocal cutaneous infantile haemangiomas (>5) are associated with visceral haemangiomas, particularly hepatic.

Q20 The best initial therapy for a newborn with a large, prenatally identified, submandibular macrocystic lymphatic malformation (previously called 'cystic hygroma') is:
   A  elective tracheostomy
   B  aspiration of fluid followed by sclerotherapy
   C  close observation without intervention until older than 5 years
   D  treatment with either corticosteroid or propranolol
   E  simple aspiration of fluid.

A20  B  Some prenatal macrocystic lymphatic malformations cause concern around methods of delivery and protection of the neonatal airway. Tracheostomy is rarely indicated since needle aspiration will decompress these macrocysts effectively. These malformations tend to be compressible and wrap around structures without compressing them. Aspirated fluid will simply re-accumulate if a sclerosant is not administered. Deferral of sclerotherapy allows intralesional haemorrhage to convert these to solid, scarred masses no longer treatable with sclerotherapy and instead, require more difficult surgical resection/debulking. Corticosteroid or propranolol therapy is used for some patients with infantile haemangioma, but these therapies have no role in macrocystic lymphatic malformations.

**Q21** A 1-month-old with a severely swollen and purple right leg, severe thrombocytopenia (8000 × 10⁹/L), is referred to you with the diagnosis of 'haemangioma'. What is the cause of the thrombocytopenia?

    **A** autoimmune idiopathic thrombocytopenia with purpura

    **B** sepsis with disseminated intravascular coagulation

    **C** intralesional platelet trapping

    **D** alloimmune (maternal antibody against fetal platelet) thrombocytopenia

    **E** congenital amegakaryocytic thrombocytopenia

**A21** **C** The case describes Kasabach–Merritt's phenomenon associated with KHE. This consumptive thrombocytopenia is due to intralesional platelet trapping and may be seen in some biopsy samples. Platelet transfusion leads to rapid painful expansion of the vascular tumour due to engorgement behind occlusive platelet thrombi. Sepsis should always be considered in a young infant with thrombocytopenia, though prolonged PT and aPTT are the main laboratory findings in sepsis and disseminated intravascular coagulation, thrombocytopenia is rarely this severe. Other choices are rare causes of neonatal/infant thrombocytopenia with no association to vascular anomalies.

**Q22** A 3-month-old presents with a purple 6 cm cutaneous chest lesion with a surrounding halo present at birth and now much smaller and paler. What is the diagnosis?

    **A** infantile haemangioma

    **B** non-involuting congenital haemangioma (NICH)

    **C** congenital lymphoedema

    **D** KHE

    **E** rapidly involuting congenital haemangioma (RICH)

**A22** **E** The natural history of this lesion is critical to making the diagnosis of RICH. The pale halo signifies involution. NICH does not change over time. Infantile haemangiomas proliferate over the first 3 months of life and do not have a halo present at birth. KHE lesions may involute spontaneously over a few years and would not have a halo present at birth. Congenital lymphoedema presents with swollen legs and genitalia and some cases are caused by autosomal dominant inheritance of *VEGFR3* mutations.

**Q23** Which of the following is the most likely cause of progressive osteolysis involving bone cortex, sparing joints between involved bones and often affecting the skull and cervical spine?

**A** Gorham–Stout's syndrome
**B** metastatic neuroblastoma
**C** microcystic lymphatic malformation
**D** multiple myeloma
**E** Langerhans's cell histiocytosis

**A23** **A** This is a classic definition of Gorham–Stout's disease, also called 'disappearing bone disease' because of the loss of bony cortex and, therefore, even entire bones. Metastatic malignancies, such as neuroblastoma or multiple myeloma, may manifest 'punched-out' lytic bone lesions, but the cortex is preserved. Langerhans's cell histiocytosis has painful lytic bone lesions with a sclerotic or inflammatory rim. Microcystic lymphatic malformations are typically confined to soft tissue, although generalised lymphatic anomalies or lymphangiomatosis may involve bone, though again with preserved bone cortex.

**Q24** An adolescent with massive right leg and overlying port-wine discoloured stain, leg-length discrepancy, limited range of knee movement and elevated D-dimer is most consistent with which diagnosis?

**A** microcystic lymphatic malformation
**B** CLOVES syndrome
**C** diffuse capillary malformation with overgrowth (DCMO)
**D** mixed capillary-lymphatic-venous malformation (Klippel-Trénaunay)
**E** *PTEN* syndrome

**A24** **D** Microcystic lymphatic malformations may present with enlarged extremities, but do not have overlying capillary stains. CLOVES is a recently described syndrome with Congenital Lipomatous Overgrowth, Vascular anomalies, Epidermal naevi and Spinal arteriovenous malformations and Scoliosis. DCMO comprises limb overgrowth secondary to diffuse capillary malformation. Enlarged veins may be associated with DCMO, but elevated D-dimers and joint problems are not. Klippel–Trénaunay's describes a mixed capillary–lymphatic–venous malformation. Extremity overgrowth can be massive and severely debilitating. Involvement of the knee with venous or lymphatic malformations may cause pain and haemarthrosis. Intralesional thrombosis is common, leading to elevated D-dimers, low fibrinogen, prolonged PT and aPTT and these patients may have significant thromboembolic risk because of large-calibre draining veins. *PTEN* syndrome is associated with lipovascular hamartomas with unusual arteriovenous malformations, breast and thyroid cancer risk, penile freckling and frontal bossing.

# Further reading

Christison-Lagay ER, Burrows PE, Alomari A, *et al*. Hepatic hemangiomas: subtype classification and development of a clinical practice algorithm and registry. *J Pediatr Surg.* 2007; **42**(1): 62–8.

Enjolras O, Mulliken JB. Vascular tumours and vascular malformations (new issues). *Adv Dermatol.* 1997; **13**: 375–423.

Finn MC, Glowacki J, Mulliken JB. Congenital vascular lesions: clinical application of a new classification. *J Pediatr Surg.* 1983; **18**(6): 894–900.

Frieden IJ, Rogers M, Garzon MC. Conditions masquerading as infantile hemangioma: part 1. *Australas J Dermatol.* 2009; **50**(2): 77–97, quiz 98.

Mulliken JB, Glowacki J. Hemangiomas and vascular malformations in infants and children: a classification based on endothelial characteristics. *Plast Reconstr Surg.* 1982; **69**(3): 412–22.

# SECTION VII

# Abdomen

# CHAPTER 31

# Congenital abdominal wall defects

## BRICE ANTAO, MICHAEL S IRISH

From the choices below each question, select the single best answer.

**Q1** Which of the following is not true regarding the embryogenesis of abdominal wall defects?

    **A** Exomphalos represents a failure of migration of the body folds.

    **B** Gastroschisis is due to failure of the umbilical coelom to develop.

    **C** Umbilical cord hernia is a failure of the midgut to return to the peritoneal cavity.

    **D** Most exomphali are medial fold defects.

    **E** Insult in exomphalos occurs early in embryogenesis.

**A1**  **D** The abdominal wall forms during the fourth week of gestation from differential growth of the embryo causing infolding in the craniocaudal and mediolateral directions. The lateral abdominal folds of the embryo meet in the anterior midline and surround the yolk sac, eventually constricting the yolk sac into a yolk stalk that becomes the site of the umbilical cord. During the sixth week of gestation, rapid growth of the intestine causes herniation of the midgut into the umbilical cord. By week 10, the midgut returns to the abdomen and undergoes rotation and fixation.

Exomphalos or omphalocele represents a failure of the body folds to complete their journey. Most exomphali are lateral-fold defects and are always at the umbilicus. The rectus muscles often insert far apart on the costal margins. The insult occurs early in embryogenesis, hence they are frequently associated with other anomalies. The exact aetiology of gastroschisis is not clear. It is thought to be caused by a failure of the umbilical coelom to develop. The elongating intestine then has no space in which to expand and ruptures out of the body wall just to the right of the umbilicus, which is unsupported as a result of resorption of the right umbilical vein. Umbilical cord hernia is a simple failure of the midgut to return to the peritoneal cavity at 10–12 weeks.

**Q2** Which of the following is true regarding gastroschisis?
  **A** The defect is usually to the left of the midline.
  **B** It is usually associated with chromosomal anomalies.
  **C** The most common association is intestinal atresia.
  **D** Cardiac anomalies are seen in 10% of cases.
  **E** All of the above.

**A2** **C** Gastroschisis occurs in four in 10 000 live births, and is often diagnosed by antenatal ultrasonography by 20 weeks' gestation. There is an increased incidence in younger mothers, and pre-term delivery is more frequent in infants with gastroschisis. Most cases of gastroschisis are isolated defects and associated anomalies are uncommon (10%), the most common being intestinal atresia, which is seen in around 10% of cases of gastroschisis. This is in contrast to exomphalos where associated anomalies are more common (50%), most commonly being cardiac and chromosomal abnormalities. The defect in gastroschisis is usually around 4 cm and to the right of the umbilical cord, without any sac.

**Q3** Which of the following is true regarding associations of exomphalos?
  **A** OEIS syndrome
  **B** Gershoni-Baruch's syndrome
  **C** Beckwith–Wiedemann's syndrome
  **D** Donnai–Barrow's syndrome
  **E** all of the above

**A3** **E** The incidence of exomphalos is lower than gastroschisis, around one in 5000 live births, and the defect is covered with a sac. More than half the cases of exomphalos have associated anomalies such as cardiac and chromosomal anomalies. Most common chromosomal anomalies are trisomies 13 and 18, and it is also associated with Down's syndrome. The risk of chromosomal abnormalities is higher with central defect, and those containing only bowel, compared with neonates with epigastric exomphalos or those containing liver and bowel. Pulmonary hypoplasia is also common and may result in early respiratory distress. An unusual form of exomphalos is cephalic fold defect or pentalogy of Cantrell (exomphalos, anterior diaphragmatic hernia, sternal cleft, ectopia cordis and intracardiac defect such as a ventricular septal defect or a diverticulum of the left ventricle).

Q4   Which of the following is *false* regarding umbilical cord hernia?
  A The contents include midgut and liver.
  B The abdominal wall above the defect is normal.
  C It is associated with malrotation.
  D It occurs due to failure of the midgut to return to the peritoneal cavity.
  E The defect is covered with a sac.

A4   **A** Umbilical cord hernia is an uncommon defect that is small and occurs at the umbilicus; it is covered with a sac and is often confused with an exomphalos. The differences are that it contains only midgut, never liver, and the abdominal wall above the defect is normal, with the rectus muscles meeting in the midline at the xiphoid. These patients have malrotation, as the midgut fails to return to the abdominal cavity to complete rotation and fixation.

Q5   The management of gastroschisis includes all of the following *except*:
  A early delivery of the fetus is advocated
  B all cases delivered by caesarean section
  C central venous catheter for parenteral nutrition
  D silo placement in the neonatal unit
  E primary closure in the operating theatre.

A5   **B** Most cases of gastroschisis are born by spontaneous vaginal delivery. Induction of labour at term is usually preferred to reduce the risk of late third-trimester fetal loss. After birth, patients are initially managed with nasogastric tube, and fluid resuscitation to compensate for serous fluid loss from the exposed bowel and defect. Exposed bowel is wrapped with cling film, before definitive treatment is planned. Various treatment options include silo placement in the neonatal unit or operating theatre, serial reductions and delayed abdominal wall closure, primary reduction with operative closure, and primary or delayed reduction with umbilical cord closure. Intestinal hypomotility is usually seen in cases of gastroschisis, hence central venous access should be established early for parenteral nutrition (usually takes 30 days before full enteral feeding is established).

  If an atresia is encountered at the time of abdominal wall closure, if the bowel is not too matted, resection and primary anastomosis can be done. If condition of the bowel makes primary anastomosis inadvisable, the bowel can be reduced with the atresia intact and repair can be undertaken 4–6 weeks after initial abdominal wall closure. Some surgeons have elected to create a stoma, particularly in cases of distal atresia.

**Q6** The management of exomphalos includes all of the following *except*:
 **A** staged silo repair
 **B** elective primary closure
 **C** delayed primary closure
 **D** pentalogy of Cantrell abnormalities (sternal cleft and pericardial defect) need to be treated before closure of exomphalos
 **E** tissue expanders.

**A6** **D** Cases of exomphalos can be born by either normal vaginal delivery or caesarean section, and neither mode of delivery has been found to be superior. However, with a large exomphalos, many prefer delivery by caesarean section because of fear of liver injury. After delivery a thorough search for associated anomalies should be undertaken. Treatment options in infants with omphalocele depend on the size of the defect, gestational age and presence of associated anomalies. In infants with small defects, the loss of abdominal domain may not be excessive and primary closure may be appropriate. In many cases, the defect is large and the loss of domain in the peritoneal cavity prevents primary closure without an undue increase in intra-abdominal pressure. In such cases, various methods such as muscle flaps, prosthetic patch repair and tissue expanders can be used to obtain primary fascial closure of the abdominal wall. In those cases, where primary closure is not possible, a staged silo repair can be done. Escharotic therapy with silver sulfadiazine or other non-toxic antibacterial dressing, which results in gradual epithelialisation of the exomphalos sac, is another form of delayed closure that can be used in neonates who cannot tolerate an operation because of prematurity, pulmonary hypoplasia, congenital heart disease or other anomalies.

In the cephalic fold defect (pentalogy of Cantrell), the sternal cleft and pericardial defect need no special treatment. The exomphalos defect can be managed with primary skin closure, and the intracardiac defect can be treated later. A non-tension repair of the central tendon of the diaphragm can be done using a Gore-Tex patch and the fascia of the abdominal wall can be closed once cardiorespiratory stability has been achieved.

**Q7** Which of the following is *false* regarding the outcome of gastroschisis?
 **A** Intestinal atresia is seen in 10% of cases.
 **B** Intestinal atresia is a prognostic determinant for a poor outcome.
 **C** There is a higher frequency of necrotising enterocolitis in full-term infants.
 **D** The incidence of cryptorchidism is 15%–30%.
 **E** When testes are in the defect they are less likely to descend.

**E** The long-term outcome for patients with gastroschisis is excellent, with an overall survival of more than 90%. The presence of intestinal atresia, which is found in 10% of cases, is the most important prognostic determinant for a poor outcome. Mortality is mainly related to intestinal failure, associated liver disease, and factors associated with small-bowel and/or liver transplantation. Necrotising enterocolitis has been encountered in full-term infants with gastroschisis in higher-than-expected frequencies (up to 18.5%). Cryptorchidism is associated with gastroschisis with an incidence of 15%–30%, and gastro-oesophageal reflux in 16% of cases. Most cases of cryptorchidism, even after replacement of herniated testes into the abdominal cavity, will result in normal testicular descent. Most long-term survivors of gastroschisis will lead normal lives.

**Q8** Which of the following is true regarding the outcome of exomphalos?
  **A** There is a higher incidence of gastro-oesophageal reflux than gastroschisis.
  **B** Most cases of gastro-oesophageal reflux will improve with age.
  **C** Respiratory insufficiency is secondary to pulmonary hypoplasia.
  **D** Mortality is mainly related to associated anomalies.
  **E** All of the above.

 **E** Survival rates for exomphalos range from 70% to 95%, with most of the mortality being related to the associated cardiac and chromosomal anomalies. Most infants with smaller defects recover well without any long-term issues. A number of long-term medical problems occur in patients with larger defects, such as gastro-oesophageal reflux, pulmonary insufficiency, recurrent lung infections or asthma and feeding difficulty with failure to thrive. A high incidence of gastro-oesophageal reflux of around 43% can be seen in cases of exomphalos, most of which improves with age. The respiratory insufficiency associated with larger defects may be secondary to abnormal thoracic development with a narrow thorax and small lung area leading to pulmonary hypoplasia.

## Further reading

Christison-Lagay ER, Kelleher CM, Langer JC. Neonatal abdominal wall defects. *Semin Fetal Neonatal Med.* 2011; **16**(3): 164–72.

Grosfeld JL, O'Neill JA, Fonkalsrud EW, *et al.*, editors. *Pediatric Surgery. Vol. 1.* 6th ed. Philadelphia, PA: Mosby; 2006.

Holcomb GW, Murphy JP. *Ashcraft's Pediatric Surgery.* 5th ed. Philadelphia, PA: Saunders; 2010.

# CHAPTER 32

# Hernia and hydrocele

## BRICE ANTAO, MICHAEL S IRISH

**From the choices below each question, select the single best answer.**

**1** Which of the following is true regarding the anatomy of the inguinal canal?

 **A** The canal of Nuck leads to the labia minora.

 **B** A direct hernia bulges medial to the inferior epigastric artery.

 **C** The superficial inguinal ring is a defect in transversalis fascia.

 **D** The deep inguinal ring corresponds to the mid-inguinal point.

 **E** A patent processus vaginalis (PPV) is posterolateral to the spermatic cord structures.

**1** **B** The inguinal canal is an oblique passage in the lower abdominal wall that passes from deep to superficial inguinal rings. It transmits the spermatic cord and ilioinguinal nerve in the male and the round ligament of the uterus and ilioinguinal nerve in the female.

Its relations are:

- anteriorly – skin, Camper's fascia, Scarpa's fascia, external oblique aponeurosis, internal oblique in lateral third of canal
- posteriorly – conjoint tendon (medially), transversalis fascia (laterally)
- above – lower arching fibres of internal oblique and transversus
- below – lower recurved edge of external oblique (inguinal ligament).

The deep inguinal ring is a defect in the transversalis fascia 1 cm above the mid-point of the inguinal ligament, lateral to inferior epigastric vessels. The superficial inguinal ring is a defect in the inguinal ligament, which lies above and medial to the pubic tubercle. An indirect hernia passes through the deep inguinal ring along the inguinal canal into the scrotum, while a direct hernia bulges through the posterior wall of the canal medial to the inferior epigastric artery through the Hasselbach's triangle. The boundaries of the Hasselbach's triangle are: inferior epigastric artery (laterally), inguinal ligament (inferiorly) and lateral border of rectus abdominis (medially). An indirect hernia in a child is due to a PPV, which is a peritoneal diverticulum extending through the internal inguinal ring into the canal. The female anlage of the PPV is the canal of Nuck, a structure that leads to the labia majora. The mid-inguinal point is halfway between the anterior superior iliac spine and the pubic symphysis and is the location of the femoral artery.

**Q2** Regarding the incidence and association of inguinal hernia, which of the following is true?

**A** The overall incidence in premature infants is 3%–5%.

**B** There is an increased incidence in Hunter's syndrome.

**C** There is an increased incidence in cases of retractile testes.

**D** Patients with a right-sided inguinal hernia have a higher risk than those with a left-sided hernia of developing a metachronous contralateral inguinal hernia.

**E** There is a higher incidence in female twins than in male twins.

**A2** **B** The overall incidence of inguinal hernia in a term newborn is 3%–5%, whereas in a premature infant this increases to 10%–30%. Other conditions associated with an increased incidence of inguinal hernia include cryptorchidism, abdominal wall defects, connective tissue disorders (Ehlers–Danlos's syndrome), mucopolysaccharidoses such as Hunter's or Hurler's syndrome, cystic fibrosis, ascites, peritoneal dialysis, ventriculoperitoneal shunts, congenital hip dislocation and myelomeningocele.

Approximately 60% of hernias are right sided, and 10% are bilateral. Approximately 11.5% have a family history of hernia, and there is an increased incidence in twins (10.6% in male twins vs. 4.1% in female twins). The overall incidence of metachronous contralateral inguinal hernia (MCIH) is 7.2%, 6.9% in boys and 7.3% in girls. Children with a left-sided inguinal hernia had a significantly higher risk of developing an MCIH than those with a right-sided hernia (10.2% vs. 6.3%).

**Q3** Which of the following is not true regarding the clinical manifestation of inguinal hernias?

**A** The risk of incarceration is higher in girls than boys.

**B** Prematurity is a risk factor for incarceration.

**C** The younger the age, the greater the risk of incarceration.

**D** Littre's hernia refers to a Meckel's diverticulum in a hernia sac.

**E** Amyand's hernia refers to an appendix in a hernia sac.

**A3** **A** Most hernias are asymptomatic, except for an inguinal bulge while straining. Incarcerated hernias result from entrapment of bowel or other viscera within the hernia sac. The risk of incarceration ranges from 12% to 17%, and is similar in boys and girls. Younger age and prematurity are risk factors for incarceration. On clinical examination, a bulge can be provoked using Valsalva's manoeuvre, and at times a thickened spermatic cord can be palpated (silk glove sign).

Occasionally other structures can be found within a hernia sac, such as the appendix (Amyand's hernia) or a Meckel's diverticulum (Littre's hernia).

**Q4** Regarding management of inguinal hernia, which of the following is true?

  **A** All hernias in children can be done as a day-case procedure.

  **B** Premature infants with inguinal hernias are best operated on once they are full term.

  **C** Bilateral exploration should routinely be performed in females.

  **D** Infants less than 60 weeks' post-conceptual age require overnight monitoring after surgery.

  **E** None of the above.

**A4**   **D** Most surgeons recommend repair of the hernia soon after diagnosis. In premature infants, there is an increased risk of incarceration and the recurrence rate is higher in smaller infants. Hence many institutions recommend repair prior to discharge from the neonatal unit, after the child has attained a weight of 2 kg in asymptomatic and otherwise relatively healthy newborns. Overnight stay is not necessary after inguinal hernia repair for healthy children or term infants. However, the risk of postoperative apnoea and bradycardia is increased in premature infants and hence overnight monitoring is essential. This risk decreases to less than 1% in premature infants more than 56 weeks' post-conceptual age (gestational age + chronological age). Hence many institutions will recommend overnight stay for patients under 60 weeks' post-conceptual age. The overall incidence of MCIH is 7.2%, 6.9% in boys and 7.3% in girls. Although contralateral exploration for unilateral inguinal hernia has been controversial, there is no evidence from the literature that routine contralateral exploration is justified.

**Q5** Regarding female inguinal hernias, which of the following is false?

  **A** Sliding hernias are more common in girls.

  **B** Between 1% and 2% of female infants with inguinal hernias have congenital androgen insensitivity syndrome (CAIS).

  **C** 75% of CAIS patients present with an inguinal hernia.

  **D** Bilateral hernias are associated with a higher risk of CAIS than unilateral hernias.

  **E** All of the above.

**5** **D** The male-to-female ratio of inguinal hernia is between 3 : 1 and 10 : 1. Sliding hernias are more common in girls, where a fallopian tube or mesosalpinx is frequently found in the wall of the hernia sac in girls and is at risk for injury. The finding of a testis during repair of a female hernia should raise the suspicion of congenital androgen insensitivity syndrome (CAIS) or true hermaphroditism. The reported incidence is 1.6% of female infants with inguinal hernias will have CAIS, while as many as 75% of CAIS patients present with a hernia. Bilateral hernias in girls are not associated with a higher risk of CAIS than is a unilateral hernia. If a testis is discovered at operation, most surgeons advocate repairing the hernia and leaving the gonads for the time being. Karyotyping and pelvic ultrasonography is then performed. The gonads would eventually need to be removed, although the timing is controversial.

**Q6** Which of the following is false regarding complications of inguinal hernia?

**A** The incidence of testicular atrophy is higher in cases of emergency hernia surgery than in elective cases.

**B** The incidence of testicular atrophy following surgery is higher in premature infants.

**C** Persistent scrotal hydrocele following high ligation of patent processus vaginalis indicates a recurrence.

**D** Patients with Hunter–Hurler's syndrome have a higher recurrence rate following high ligation.

**E** Patients with Ehlers-Danlos's syndrome have a higher recurrence rate following high ligation.

 **6** **C** Testicular vessels are vulnerable to operative injury, especially in small infants. However, testicular atrophy after routine hernia repair is rare (1%). With incarcerated hernia, the blood supply to the testis may be compromised leading to testicular atrophy (2%–3%). These cases are often operated on as an emergency procedure. The risk of recurrence in an elective inguinal hernia repair is less than 1%. It is higher in premature infants, children with incarcerated hernias and children with associated diseases (mucopolysaccharidoses such as Hurler's and Hunter's diseases and connective tissue disorders such as Ehlers–Danlos's and Marfan's syndromes). Hence in these disorders some surgeons recommend a high ligation and a formal herniorrhaphy to prevent recurrences.

Postoperative infection rates range from 1% to 3%. After hernia repair, scrotal swelling may develop as a result of fluid accumulating in the distal sac, forming a hydrocele. This does not always indicate a recurrence and most of these resolve spontaneously.

**Q7**   Which of the following is false regarding hydrocele in children?

   **A**   It is more common on the right side.

   **B**   It can occur following diarrhoeal illness.

   **C**   It can be associated with a torted hydatid of Morgagni.

   **D**   It can occur following an upper respiratory tract infection.

   **E**   Most communicating hydroceles close by 2 years of age.

**A7**   **E**   A hydrocele is a collection of fluid in the space surrounding the testicle between the layers of the tunica vaginalis. Hydroceles may be communicating (patent processus vaginalis with free flow of fluid) or non-communicating (usually scrotal in males). Hydroceles are usually bilateral, with a higher rate of occurrence on the right side. If a hydrocele was not present at birth, or dramatically changes in size or shows daily fluctuation in size (communicating hydrocele), this is suggestive of a PPV. A hydrocele may be secondary to torsion of the testis or its appendages. Alternatively, an acute hydrocele may be seen concurrently with or following an acute upper respiratory tract infection or diarrhoeal disease. Most cases of congenital hydrocele resolve by 2 years of age. Hence most surgeons would observe these children in the first 1–2 years of life, and operate on those that persist. If a hydrocele is communicating (which indicates a PPV), or a hernia cannot be ruled out, early operation is indicated.

**Q8**   Which of the following is true regarding femoral hernia?

   **A**   It usually lies below and medial to the pubic tubercle.

   **B**   It usually lies inferior and posterior to the inguinal ligament.

   **C**   The lateral boundary of the femoral canal is the femoral artery.

   **D**   The lacunar ligament forms the posterior boundary of the femoral ring.

   **E**   Management is best performed using Bassini's repair.

**A8**   **B**   A femoral hernia occurs through the femoral canal, which is the medial compartment of the femoral sheath, and is entered via the femoral ring. It contains fat and lymph nodes (Cloquet's node). The relations of the femoral ring are: inguinal ligament (anteriorly), lacunar ligament (medially), pectineal ligament (posteriorly) and femoral vein (laterally). Femoral hernias lie below and lateral to the pubic tubercle (unlike inguinal hernias, which lie above and medial), and are inferior and posterior to the inguinal ligament. Because the femoral ring is narrow and the lacunar ligament forms a sharp medial border, irreducibility and strangulation are more common in a femoral hernia.

   Femoral hernias can be repaired via either the open or the minimally invasive route.

   Three approaches have been described for open surgery.

   •   Lockwood's infrainguinal approach

- Lotheissen's transinguinal approach
- McEvedy's high approach.

The infrainguinal approach is the preferred method for elective repair. The transinguinal approach involves dissecting through the inguinal canal and carries the risk of weakening the inguinal canal. McEvedy's approach is preferred in the emergency setting when strangulation is suspected. This allows better access to, and visualisation of, bowel for possible resection. Repair is either performed by suturing the inguinal ligament to the pectineal ligament (Cooper's ligament repair) using strong non-absorbable sutures or by placing a mesh plug in the femoral ring. With either technique care should be taken to avoid any pressure on the femoral vein. Bassini's repair (conjoint tendon is approximated to the inguinal ligament) is a type of tension herniorrhaphy for the management of direct inguinal hernia.

**Q9** Which of the following is false regarding umbilical hernia?
  **A** There is an increased incidence with Beckwith–Wiedemann's syndrome.
  **B** There is an increased incidence with Hurler's syndrome.
  **C** There is an increased incidence with congenital hypothyroidism.
  **D** It has a similar aetiology as hernia of the umbilical cord.
  **E** All of the above.

**A9** **D** Umbilical hernias in childhood occur with an equal frequency in boys and girls. Premature and low-birthweight infants have a higher incidence than full-term infants. Similarly, infants with other conditions such as Beckwith–Wiedemann's syndrome; Hurler's syndrome; various chromosomal disorders such as trisomy 13, 18 and 21; congenital hypothyroidism and children requiring peritoneal dialysis. The umbilical hernia of childhood is distinguished from a 'hernia of the umbilical cord', in which there is a defect in the peritoneum, as well as an open fascial defect at the umbilicus – intestines herniate into the substance of the umbilical cord itself and are covered only by amnion. A hernia of the umbilical cord is in effect a small omphalocele. The majority of umbilical hernias will close spontaneously by 3–4 years of age. Those persisting beyond that period can be repaired through an infraumbilical approach.

**Q10** Which of the following is true regarding abdominal wall hernias?
  **A** Most epigastric hernias will resolve by 3 years of age.
  **B** Content of an epigastric hernia is usually incarcerated omentum.
  **C** Spigelian hernia is more common in girls.
  **D** Lumbar hernias usually resolve spontaneously.
  **E** All of the above.

A10 C  Epigastric hernias are hernias through the midline linea alba. They present as a small mass, usually with incarcerated properitoneal fat, between the umbilicus and xiphoid process. They have no communication with the peritoneal cavity and do not resolve and hence should be repaired. A spigelian hernia occurs through a defect at the intersection of the linea semicircularis and the lateral border of the rectus abdominis muscle. These hernias are more frequent in girls and more commonly occur on the right side below the umbilicus. Pain in that area and fullness or an actual mass are most common symptoms. These are difficult to detect and diagnose, and an ultrasonography or computed tomography may be needed. Repair is usually done with a tension-free closure through a transverse incision over the defect. Lumbar hernias are usually visible shortly after birth as a bulge (properitoneal fat) in the area bordered by the 12th rib, sacrospinalis muscle, and internal oblique muscle. These hernias tend to develop at the site of penetration of the intercostal nerves and vessels or of the ilioinguinal, iliohypogastric and lumbar nerves. Although they are asymptomatic, repair is advisable because the defect never resolves spontaneously and incarceration is possible. Repair may sometimes require a prosthetic mesh.

## Further reading

Grosfeld JL, O'Neill JA, Fonkalsrud EW, *et al.*, editors. *Pediatric Surgery. Vol. 1.* 6th ed. Philadelphia, PA: Mosby; 2006.

Holcomb GW, Murphy JP. *Ashcraft's Pediatric Surgery.* 5th ed. Philadelphia, PA: Saunders; 2010.

Ron O, Eaton S, Pierro A. Systematic review of the risk of developing a metachronous contralateral inguinal hernia in children. *Br J Surg.* 2007; **94**(7): 804–11.

# SECTION VIII

# Gastroenterology

# CHAPTER 33

# Lesions of the stomach

## VICTORIA LANE, BRICE ANTAO, MICHAEL S IRISH

From the choices below each question, select the single best answer.

Q1 Embryology of the stomach. Which of the following is false?
  A The blood supply to the midgut is from the superior mesenteric artery.
  B During the fifth week of gestation the greater curvature of the stomach becomes apparent.
  C The stomach rotates 90 degrees during the seventh and eighth weeks so that the greater curvature lies to the left.
  D The pylorus lies in the transpyloric plane at the level of L2.
  E The greater curvature derives its blood supply from the right and left gastroepiploic vessels.

A1  D  The stomach develops from the foregut and is recognisable by the fifth week of gestation. During the fifth week of gestation the dorsal wall of the stomach grows rapidly compared with the ventral wall, giving rise to the greater curvature of the stomach. During the seventh and eighth weeks of gestation the stomach rotates 90 degrees (craniocaudal) and the greater curvature lies to the left. The blood supply of the gastrointestinal tract (foregut, midgut, hindgut) is based on the coeliac trunk, the superior mesenteric and the inferior mesenteric artery, respectively. The stomach is supplied by the right and left gastric arteries along the lesser curvature, the right and left gastroepiploic arteries along the greater curvature, and the short gastric vessels from the spleen. There is also a contribution from posterior gastric artery (branch of splenic artery), as well as the phrenic arteries. The transpyloric plane lies at the level of L1 vertebra and the gastro-oesophageal junction typically lies at T10.

**Q2**  Pyloric atresia. Which of the following statements is true?

    **A**  A common presentation is bilious vomiting in first few days of life.

    **B**  Radiological features are similar to duodenal atresia.

    **C**  It is associated with epidermolysis bullosa.

    **D**  Pyloromyotomy is the treatment of choice.

    **E**  It is more common in males.

**A2**  **C**  Pyloric atresia is rare and accounts for 1% of all intestinal atresias. Its incidence is about one per 100 000 live births. There is an equal male-to-female ratio. There are three recognised forms of pyloric atresia, types A, B and C. In type A (57%) there is a pyloric membrane or web occluding the lumen; in type B (34%) the pyloric channel is a solid cord, and in type C (9%) there is a complete gap between the stomach and duodenum.

    Pyloric atresia is seen in association with other congenital defects in 30%–50% of cases (malrotation, cardiac defects, vaginal agenesis and tracheo-oesophageal anomalies). Eighteen per cent of cases of pyloric atresia are associated with epidermolysis bullosa, which is a cutaneous genetic disease of variable severity. There is usually a maternal history of polyhydramnios, and affected infants present in the first few days of life with non-bilious vomiting and complete gastric outlet obstruction. Unlike duodenal atresia, which has a classic double-bubble appearance on plain radiograph, pyloric atresia is diagnosed with a single gastric bubble with no distal gas beyond pylorus. If distal gas is seen, the diagnosis may be confirmed with a contrast study to rule out an incomplete pyloric membrane.

    In type A, excision of a complete or partial diaphragm with Heineke-Mikulicz's or Finney's pyloroplasty is the most straightforward corrective procedure. In types B and C, with atretic ends separated by a cord or discontinuous segment, a repair is usually with a Billroth type I (gastroduodenostomy) anastomosis.

**Q3**  Regarding gastric duplications, which of the following is true?

    **A**  Gastric duplication cysts account for 20% of all duplications of the gastrointestinal tract.

    **B**  Gastric duplication tends to occur along the greater curvature.

    **C**  Gastric duplications usually communicate with the gastric lumen.

    **D**  Gastric duplications are more common in males.

    **E**  Gastric duplications do not contain all layers of the gastric wall.

**A3**  **B**  Gastric duplications are rare and represent 3%–4% of all intestinal duplications and are classically seen along the greater curvature. They are slightly more common in females. They tend to contain all layers of the gastric wall but do not usually communicate with the gastric lumen. Common clinical features include failure to thrive, gastro-oesophageal reflux, abdominal distension, vomiting and a palpable mass. The cysts may rupture causing peritonitis, peptic ulceration and haemorrhage. If the lesion is near the pylorus, the presentation is similar to hypertrophic pyloric stenosis. The treatment of choice is extramucosal excision of the cyst. Occasionally a cyst-gastrostomy may be necessary.

**Q4** All of the following are associated with congenital microgastria *except*:
   **A** VACTORL association
   **B** malrotation
   **C** asplenia
   **D** situs inversus
   **E** oligohydramnios.

**A4** **E** Congenital microgastria is a rare congenital anomaly of the caudal part of the embryologic foregut, characterised by a small, tubular stomach, megaoesophagus and incomplete gastric rotation. It is usually associated with other congenital anomalies and occasionally can occur as an isolated microgastria. Associated anomalies include VACTORL association, tracheo-oesophageal cleft, malrotation, asplenia, situs inversus and megaoesophagus. It can also be associated with skeletal anomalies such as micrognathia, radial and ulnar hypoplasia, vertebral anomalies, oligodactyly and hypoplastic nails. Antenatal polyhydramnios and a small stomach may be noted.

**Q5** Regarding congenital microgastria, which of the following is true?
   **A** Diarrhoea is a common finding.
   **B** Endoscopy is the most reliable diagnostic test.
   **C** Most cases require augmentation using the Hunt–Lawrence gastric augmentation.
   **D** Most cases with associated gastro-oesophageal reflux disease, require a fundoplication.
   **E** Schilling's test is positive.

**A5** **A** Postnatally, the most frequent presenting signs are vomiting, aspiration pneumonia, diarrhoea and failure to thrive. As a result of an ill-defined gastro-oesophageal junction, they are prone to gastro-oesophageal reflux. Also, malnutrition and developmental delay can occur. Bacterial overgrowth and a blind-loop-like syndrome has been postulated to be the cause for diarrhoea and malnutrition, but the results of Schilling's test for vitamin $B_{12}$ malabsorption is normal. Upper GI contrast is usually diagnostic, and endoscopy is usually difficult and yields confusing results. Medical treatment with continuous or night-time orogastric feeds is the first line of management. This allows the patient to grow and stomach to enlarge, until they can tolerate normal feeds. If the infant's stomach fails to enlarge, the stomach capacity can be augmented using Hunt–Lawrence's gastric augmentation. Gastro-oesophageal reflux is managed with prokinetic drugs and antireflux medications, nasojejunal feeding tubes or jejunostomy tubes. Because of the megaoesophagus and small stomach, a fundoplication is not a viable option.

 **Q6** With regard to gastric volvulus which of the following is false?

**A** Organoaxial gastric volvulus is rotation about the gastric short axis.

**B** In mesenteroaxial volvulus the pylorus is seen to lie higher than the gastro-oesophageal junction.

**C** In organoaxial volvulus the greater curvature lies higher than the lesser curvature.

**D** It is associated with Ivemark's syndrome.

**E** Borchardt's triad is diagnostic of acute volvulus.

 **A6** **A** Gastric volvulus is a rare but important differential in those presenting with features of gastric outlet obstruction. It can occur from primary or secondary causes. Primary gastric volvulus is due to laxity of the gastric ligaments, while secondary volvulus is due to paraoesophageal hernia or other diaphragmatic hernia. Gastric volvulus is described as organoaxial or mesenteroaxial, depending which axis it has rotated around.

Organoaxial is rotation on the longitudinal axis through the pylorus and gastro-oesophageal junction, mesenteroaxial is rotation on an imaginary line through the lesser and greater curvatures.

Gastric volvulus tends to present with the following triad (Borchardt's) in around 70% of cases.

1 Inability to vomit.

2 Severe epigastric distension.

3 Inability to pass a nasogastric tube.

Other presenting features include chest pain, dysphagia, dyspnoea and borborygmi.

A distended stomach in an abnormal position should raise suspicion of gastric volvulus. A single radiograph may be diagnostic. Acute mesenteroaxial volvulus is seen on a plain radiograph by identifying the pylorus/antrum being higher than the gastro-oesophageal junction. In organoaxial volvulus the greater curvature is seen to lie higher than the lesser curvature

The asplenia (Ivemark's) syndrome is the association of congenital absence of the spleen with a variety of visceral abnormalities, predominantly of the cardio-vascular system. It is present in 3% of neonates with structural heart disease. Varying degrees of malrotation and malfixation of the bowel are also common in this condition.

Treatment consists of patient resuscitation, nasogastric decompression and surgical correction. The surgical options after reduction of volvulus include anterior gastropexy or a tube/button gastrostomy.

 **7** Which of the following is true regarding gastric perforation in the newborn?

**A** Most cases are secondary to stress-related peptic ulcer disease.

**B** Perforation due to duodenal ulcer occurs on the posterior wall of duodenum.

**C** Perforation due to gastric ulcer occurs along the greater curvature.

**D** Spontaneous gastric perforations usually occur along the greater curvature.

**E** Spontaneous gastric perforation can be managed by peritoneal drainage.

 **7** **D** Gastric perforation in the newborn is either spontaneous or a result of peptic ulcer disease or iatrogenic trauma. There are two main theories for gastric perforation in newborns. The first is an ischaemic insult associated with peri-natal stress resulting in a hypoxic mucosal injury progressing to perforation. The second theory is related to gastric overinflation as a result of overaggressive mask resuscitation, accidental oesophageal intubation and vigorous insufflation, trauma from passage of an orogastric tube, and perforation due to a distal outlet obstruction from pyloric atresia. Occasionally gastric ischaemia and perforation may be observed in premature infants with extensive necrotising enterocolitis. Most spontaneous gastric perforations occur along the greater curvature of the stomach distal to the oesophagus. Perforation due to a duodenal ulcer in infancy occurs on the anterior wall of the duodenum or near the pyloroduodenal junc-tion, whereas gastric ulcers may perforate along the lesser curvature near the antralfundic junction. There is a subset of premature neonates in whom bowel perforation develops spontaneously; it is not associated with necrotising entero-colitis, but is isolated, focal, idiopathic and usually indomethacin related. These cases respond well to peritoneal drainage. Spontaneous gastric perforations need prompt operative repair and peritoneal drainage is not appropriate in such cases. These patients usually present with abdominal distension and signs of sepsis or shock. The condition of an infant with gastric perforation can deteriorate rapidly, and therefore early recognition, active resuscitation and prompt surgical treat-ment is necessary. The perforation can usually be closed primarily with or without an omental patch.

Q8    Which of the following is true regarding hypertrophic pyloric stenosis?
A    The male-to-female ratio is identical.
B    Premature infants are diagnosed later than term/post-term infants.
C    It is more common in first-born female infants.
D    The risk is greater with older maternal age.
E    Offspring risk is higher if father had hypertrophic pyloric stenosis.

A8    **B**    Hypertrophic pyloric stenosis occurs at a rate of 1–4 per 1000 live births with a male-to-female ratio of 4 : 1. Risk factors include family history, younger maternal age, first-born infant (more common in males), maternal feeding pattern (breast feeding protective), erythromycin exposure and transpyloric feeding of premature infants. Premature infants are diagnosed with hypertrophic pyloric stenosis later than post-term infants. The risk of hypertrophic pyloric stenosis in offspring of mothers who had pyloric stenosis as a baby is greater than if the father has pyloric stenosis.

Q9    Which of the following is true regarding the metabolic derangement seen in hypertrophic pyloric stenosis?
A    hypochloraemia
B    hyperkalaemia
C    hypernatraemia
D    metabolic acidosis
E    respiratory alkalosis

A9    **A**    The cardinal features of pyloric stenosis is non-bilious projectile vomiting, visible peristaltic waves in the left upper quadrant, and metabolic derangement of hypokalaemic, hypochloraemic metabolic alkalosis in a full-term neonate between 2 and 8 weeks of age. There are large losses of hydrogen and chloride ions due to vomiting of gastric secretions.

The chloride loss results in hypochloraemia, which impairs the kidney's ability to excrete bicarbonate. This is the significant factor that prevents correction of the alkalosis. Secondary hyperaldosteronism develops because of the hypovolaemia. The high aldosterone levels cause the kidneys to:
- avidly retain Na+ (to correct the intravascular volume depletion)
- excrete increased amounts of K+ into the urine (resulting in hypokalaemia).

As potassium depletion worsens, sodium is reabsorbed across the renal tubules in exchange for hydrogen ions. Hence, despite having a metabolic alkalosis, the child will develop a 'paradoxical aciduria'. The compensatory response to metabolic alkalosis is hypoventilation resulting in elevated arterial $PCO_2$ (respiratory acidosis).

The only means of breaking this cycle is to rehydrate the child, and surgery should be deferred until the metabolic derangement has been reversed.

Q10 Which of the following is true regarding management of hypertrophic pyloric stenosis?

A Diagnostic feature on ultrasonography is length of pylorus >14 mm.

B Diagnostic feature on ultrasonography is the pylorus muscle thickness >3 mm.

C Urgent pyloromyotomy is the treatment of choice.

D Postoperative emesis is a common occurrence.

E Postoperative contrast study is useful in the evaluation of completeness of myotomy.

A10 D A definitive diagnosis can be made on clinical examination in 75% of cases, by palpating a pyloric mass. However, if the diagnosis is unclear after a thorough physical examination, radiological evaluation is warranted. Ultrasonography is the gold standard investigation for confirming the diagnosis of pyloric stenosis. The diagnostic criteria are a combination of a muscle thickness greater than or equal to 4 mm and a length of greater than or equal to 16 mm. In neonates younger than 30 days, a thickness of more than 3 mm is considered positive. Pyloric stenosis is not a surgical emergency, and the mainstay of therapy is initial resuscitation and correction of metabolic and electrolyte abnormality. Once the metabolic derangement is corrected the operative procedure of choice is a Ramstedt pyloromyotomy. This can be performed via an open approach or laparoscopically. Complications after pyloromyotomy are minimal and include mucosal perforation (1%–2%), wound infection (1%–2%) and incisional hernia (1%). Postoperative emesis is common and can occur in up to 80% of cases. However, prolonged emesis is less common (2%–26%) and is usually secondary to gastro-oesophageal reflux (24%–31%), but can be secondary to incomplete myotomy (0%–6%). Frequent vomiting persisting beyond 3–4 days may suggest an incomplete myotomy or an unsuspected perforation. A postoperative contrast study may demonstrate a leak but is not helpful in evaluating the completeness of the myotomy. It can take several weeks for the radiographic appearance of the pylorus to improve. Persistent and frequent vomiting 1 week beyond the pyloromyotomy may require re-exploration.

## Further reading

Cribbs RK, Gow KW, Wulkan ML. Gastric volvulus in infants and children. *Pediatrics*. 2008; **122**(3): e752–62. Epub 2008 Aug 4.

Grosfeld JL, O'Neill JA, Fonkalsrud EW, *et al.*, editors. *Pediatric Surgery. Vol. 1*. 6th ed. Philadelphia, PA: Mosby; 2006.

Hayashi AH, Galliani CA, Gillis DA. Congenital pyloric atresia and junctional epidermolysis bullosa: a report of long-term survival and review of the literature. *J Pediatr Surg*. 1991; **26**(11): 1341–5.

Holcomb GW, Murphy JP. *Ashcraft's Pediatric Surgery*. 5th ed. Philadelphia, PA: Saunders; 2010.

St Peter SD, Holcomb GW, Calkins CM, *et al*. Open versus laparoscopic pyloromyotomy for pyloric stenosis: a prospective, randomized trial. *Ann Surg*. 2006; **244**(3): 363–70.

# CHAPTER 34

# Intestinal atresia

## JASON S FRISCHER, RICHARD G AZIZKHAN

From the choices below each question, select the single best answer.

**Q1** Which of the following is true regarding the prevalence of jejunoileal atresia?

   **A** The worldwide prevalence is approximately one case per 1000 live births.

   **B** The prevalence is greatest in Spain.

   **C** A higher prevalence is noted in twins, regardless of race.

   **D** The prevalence is higher in Caucasians than East Asians.

   **E** Male infants are more commonly affected than female infants.

**A1** **C** The prevalence of jejunoileal atresia varies widely across the globe, ranging from 1.3 cases per 10 000 live births in Spain to as high as 2.9 cases per 10 000 live births in the United States. A higher prevalence is noted in twins, regardless of race, and consistent with this finding, a population-based study conducted in the Netherlands found a higher incidence of small-bowel atresia in fraternal twins. Population-based studies from Hawaii demonstrated a higher incidence of jejunoileal atresia in East Asians than white people. Multiple studies have noted that boys and girls are equally affected by intestinal atresia.

**Q2** Jejunoileal atresia has been associated with maternal use of all of the following *except*:

   **A** non-steroidal anti-inflammatory drugs (NSAIDs)

   **B** pseudoephedrine

   **C** pseudoephedrine in combination with acetaminophen

   **D** caffeine

   **E** ergotamine tartrate.

**A2** **A** Studies have demonstrated that the use of pseudoephedrine, either alone or in combination, increases the risk of developing small intestinal atresia. The mechanism is likely due to an interruption of blood supply to that segment of bowel. The treatment of migraine headaches during pregnancy with ergotamine tartrate and caffeine has also been implicated in the development of intestinal atresia. No studies to date have linked the use of NSAIDs to jejunoileal atresia.

**Q3** Which of the following is true of clinical presentation of jejunoileal atresia?

**A** Duodenal atresia occurs more frequently than jejunoileal atresia.

**B** Girls develop small-bowel atresia twice as frequently as boys.

**C** Trisomy 21 is often associated with jejunoileal atresia.

**D** Extraintestinal anomalies occur in 25%–35% of patients with jejunoileal atresia.

**E** Extraintestinal anomalies are more often associated with ileal atresia than jejunal atresia.

**A3** **D** Studies indicate that jejunoileal atresia occurs in 50%–66% of cases of bowel atresia, while duodenal atresia occurs in 33%–44% of cases and colonic atresia (6%) is uncommon. Boys and girls are equally affected by intestinal atresia. Trisomy 21, although frequently associated with duodenal atresia, is rarely seen in patients with jejunoileal atresia. The incidence of extraintestinal anomalies in patients with intestinal atresia ranges from 25% to 35%, with a higher incidence of anomalies associated with jejunal atresia than with ileal atresia.

**Q4** There is an increased incidence of the following associations with jejunoileal atresia *except*:

**A** biliary atresia

**B** duodenal atresia

**C** imperforate anus

**D** Hirschsprung's disease

**E** colonic atresia.

**A4** **C** Most cases of jejunoileal atresia are sporadic, but there is an association with other conditions such as:

- biliary atresia – 14 reported cases in the last 20 years
- duodenal atresia – fewer than five reported cases. Always test patency downstream after repair of duodenal atresia
- colonic atresia – test colonic patency either with a preoperative contrast enema or intraoperative confirmation
- gastric atresia
- Hirschsprung's disease – 19 reported cases
- arthrogryposis
- identical twins – seven pairs of twins have been reported.

Gastrointestinal anomalies in association with jejunoileal atresia are extremely rare.

**5** Which of the following is *not* true regarding the mechanism of intestinal atresia?

    **A** Epithelial plugging and failure of recanalisation is the likely aetiology of duodenal atresia.

    **B** Bile pigments, squames and lanugo hairs are often found distal to atretic jejunoileal segments.

    **C** Ligation of fetal dog mesenteric vessels produced a pattern of intestinal atresia similar to that seen in human neonates.

    **D** Intrauterine midgut volvulus can be the cause of jejunoileal atresia

    **E** A rat model using tetracycline is associated with multiple intestinal atresias.

**A5**   **E** Epithelial plugging and failure of recanalisation is the aetiology likely to apply to duodenal atresia, but not jejunoileal atresia. A common observation in jejunoileal atresia is that the proximal and distal bowel segments are often separated by either a cordlike structure or a gap between the segments of bowel with an obvious mesenteric defect. It has been documented by a number of authors that bile pigments, squames and lanugo hairs are often found distal to atretic segments. This implicates that events other than epithelial plugging may cause intestinal atresia and that these events occur later *in utero*. Moreover, fetal bile secretion and the swallowing of amniotic fluid begin in weeks 11 and 12 of intrauterine life, well after the luminal revacuolisation process. In 1955, Louw and Barnard subjected dog fetuses to ligation of mesenteric vessels and strangulation obstruction late in the course of gestation. Examination of affected fetal intestine 10–14 days later showed a variety of atretic conditions similar to those seen in human neonates. These findings strongly suggest that most jejunoileal atresias are the result of late intrauterine mesenteric vascular occlusions. Intrauterine midgut volvulus can cause an interruption of the mesenteric blood supply thereby leading to intestinal atresia. A rat model using doxorubicin reported a teratogenic mechanism of the developing midgut leading to multiple intestinal atresias.

**6** Intestinal atresias secondary to late intrauterine insults are often seen in all of the following clinical scenarios *except*:

    **A** appendicitis

    **B** midgut volvulus

    **C** intussusception

    **D** internal hernia

    **E** gastroschisis

**A6**  **A**  Intrauterine appendicitis has not been implicated in the cause of jejunoileal atresia. Intestinal atresias secondary to late intrauterine mesenteric vascular insults are often seen in patients with volvulus, intussusception, internal hernia, and tight anterior abdominal wall defects. Studies have found that volvulus was detected in 33%–35% of patients, malrotation in 16%, intussusception in 3%, internal hernia in 1%–5% and gastroschisis in 2%–14%.

**Q7**  Which of the following has been associated with a postnatal cause for small-bowel atresia?

    **A**  umbilical arterial catheter placement

    **B**  umbilical venous catheter placement

    **C**  internal hernia

    **D**  iatrogenic umbilical clamping of an occult omphalocele

    **E**  umbilical hernia

**A7**  **D**  The placement of umbilical artery or venous catheters has not been associated with the postnatal development of jejunoileal atresia. These lines are linked to high rates of thrombosis, and umbilical venous catheters can lead to portal vein thrombosis and therefore threatening injury to the intestine. Internal hernias have been linked to intrauterine intestinal atresia in 1%–5% of cases. In the rare instance of an internal hernia occurring during the neonatal period, bowel ischaemia would be the clinical presentation not atresia. Unfortunately, iatrogenic postpartum ileal atresia as a result of umbilical clamping of an occult omphalocele has been reported. Many neonates are born with an umbilical hernia but this has not been connected to intestinal atresia.

**Q8**  Complex jejunoileal atresia (multiple atresias, apple-peel deformity) has been linked to all of the following *except*:

    **A**  placental vascular anomalies

    **B**  intrauterine intussusception

    **C**  congenital immunodeficiency

    **D**  acquired immunodeficiency

    **E**  genetic contribution.

**A8**  **B**  The association of placental vascular anomalies and complex jejunoileal atresia (multiple atresias, apple-peel deformity) has been demonstrated. All of these patients had low birthweight, consistent with the impact of placental vascular compromise on fetal growth. Multiple atresias have also been noted in patients with congenital and acquired immunodeficiency. It has been noted that patients with a genetic link to jejunoileal atresia can present with multiple atresias or an apple-peel deformity and that these patients are often immunocompromised.

**Q****9** All of the following are true regarding the genetic aspects of intestinal atresia *except*:

   **A** autosomal recessive and autosomal dominant transmission

   **B** combined duodenal and jejunal atresia have a familial link

   **C** multiple atresias or the apple-peel deformity are the most common variants of genetically associated jejunoileal atresia

   **D** a familial pattern of multiple atresias has been reported in French Canadians near the St John River in Quebec

   **E** a distinct gene has been linked to intestinal atresia.

**A9**   **E** A number of studies have focused on the genetic aspects of multiple atresias. In 1973, Guttman and colleagues reported a familial pattern of multiple atresias affecting the stomach, duodenum, small intestine and colon occurring in French Canadians near the St John River in Quebec. Because of the high degree of consanguinity observed in this group, a number of authors proposed that extensive multiple atresias is most likely an expression of a rare autosomal recessive gene. A report describing the natural history of these patients found that all had an Immunoglobulin M deficiency and had died, but the aetiology remains unclear; a specific gene mutation has not yet been elucidated. The genetic contribution to jejunoileal atresia is unclear. Reports have been published regarding the familial instances of combined duodenal and jejunal atresia. Numerous authors have also reported hereditary multiple intestinal atresias and both autosomal recessive and autosomal dominant transmission has been documented. Five distinct types of familial atresia have been documented to date (i.e. pyloric atresia, duodenal atresia, hereditary multiple atresia syndrome, apple-peel atresia and colonic atresia).

**Q10** Prenatal and postnatal clinical signs of jejunoileal atresia include all of the following *except*:

   **A** passage of meconium on the first day of life

   **B** maternal polyhydramnios

   **C** bilious emesis

   **D** abdominal distension

   **E** jaundice.

**A10**   **A** Polyhydramnios is observed in 24% of intestinal atresia cases and is more common in patients with proximal jejunal atresia (38%). Bilious emesis is slightly more common in patients with jejunal atresia (84%), whereas abdominal distension is more common in patients with ileal atresia (98%). Jaundice, which is characteristically associated with elevated indirect bilirubin, occurs in 32% of infants with jejunal atresia and 20% of those with ileal atresia. Although most infants with jejunoileal atresia fail to pass meconium in the first 24 hours of life, either meconium or necrotic tissue is occasionally passed. Upper abdominal distension is often associated with more-proximal atresia; more-generalised distension usually indicates a more-distal obstruction (e.g. distal small bowel or colon) in which many loops of bowel are filled with air proximal to the level of obstruction.

**Q11** Which of the following is true regarding the prenatal imaging of jejunoileal atresia?

   **A** MRI should be the initial imaging modality in suspected cases of bowel obstruction.

   **B** Ultrasound is more reliable in detecting distal vs. proximal small-bowel atresia.

   **C** Over 75% of patients with jejunoileal atresia are diagnosed prenatally by ultrasound.

   **D** Ultrasound findings do not affect neonatal outcomes in patients with intestinal atresia.

   **E** Mothers with oligohydramnios should be suspected of having a small bowel obstruction, possibly due to intestinal atresia.

**A11** **D** Prenatal ultrasonography (US) in mothers with polyhydramnios has identified small-bowel obstruction associated with atresia, volvulus, and meconium peritonitis. The presence of small-bowel atresia is suspected when US reveals multiple distended loops of proximal bowel with vigorous peristalsis. In these patients, the distal bowel is decompressed. Ultrasound is more reliable in detecting proximal vs. distal intestinal atresia. Overall, only 31% of patients with small-bowel atresia were diagnosed during antenatal US and it has been noted that the later in gestation the US is performed, the more likely it is to detect the malformation. When recognised, the atresia was more often in a proximal location and the infants required prolonged postnatal treatment. Studies suggest that antenatal US findings have a relatively poor predictive value for bowel abnormalities and are unreliable in detecting or excluding fetal gastrointestinal malformations. Moreover, these findings do not affect neonatal outcomes in patients with intestinal atresia. The utility of fetal MRI indicates that this modality can identify gastrointestinal abnormalities and suggest that it may be more accurate than US in the prenatal diagnosis of bowel atresia.

**Q12** The pathological findings associated with jejunoileal atresia include all of the following *except*:
  **A** the distribution between the jejunum and ileum is similar
  **B** most atresias occur in the proximal ileum
  **C** approximately 90% of intestinal atresias are a single event
  **D** multiple atresias most often involve the proximal jejunum
  **E** malrotation is observed in 10%–18% of patients.

**A12** **B** Malrotation has been observed in approximately 10%–17% of patients with jejunoileal atresia. Jejunoileal atresias are nearly equally distributed between the jejunum (51%) and the ileum (49%). Most atresias (36%) occur in the distal ileum; 13% occur in the proximal ileum; 31% occur in the proximal jejunum, and 20% occur in the distal jejunum. Intestinal atresias are generally a single event (>90%); however, multiple atresias can occur (6% to 20%) and most often involve the proximal jejunum.

**Q13** In jejunoileal atresia the apple-peel deformity is associated with all of the following *except*:
  **A** it is also known as the Christmas tree deformity or classified as a type IIIb atresia
  **B** it presents with a proximal atresia near the ligament of Treitz
  **C** the blood supply is provided in antegrade fashion
  **D** it has been associated with a familial pattern of inheritance
  **E** it is often associated with prematurity.

**A13** **C** The apple-peel or Christmas tree deformity occurs in 11%–32% of all jejunoileal atresia cases. These patients present with a very proximal atresia near the ligament of Treitz, a large mesenteric defect, and foreshortened bowel. The blood supply that contributes to the distal bowel is quite precarious as it is supplied in a retrograde fashion by arcades from the ileocolic, right colic or inferior mesenteric arteries. This variant of atresia is associated with a familial pattern of inheritance. Patients with this form of atresia typically are premature (70%), of low birthweight (70%), have a high rate of malrotation (54%) and an increased number of congenital anomalies.

**Q14** All of the following are true regarding the classification system for jejunoileal atresia *except*:
  **A** type I and II atresias have a V-shaped gap within the mesentery
  **B** type II has two atretic blind ends connected by a fibrous cord
  **C** type III occurs most commonly
  **D** type III atresias have a shortened bowel length
  **E** type IV lesions occur in 6%–20% of all atresia cases.

**A14** **A** The contemporary classification of jejunoileal atresia has been modified to include four different types. Type I refers to a mucosal (septal) atresia with an intact bowel wall and its mesentery. Type II refers to two atretic blind ends connected by a fibrous cord with an intact mesentery, and type III comprises two separated segments of bowel with a V-shaped gap within the mesentery. Type III atresias have been subdivided into type IIIa, which describes the previously designated type III lesion, and type IIIb, which refers to the apple-peel or Christmas tree anomaly. Multiple atresias are referred to as type IV lesions. In a study evaluating 559 cases of jejunoileal atresia, de Lorimier and colleagues reported that 19% were type I, 31% were type II, and 46% were type III. The authors noted that type I and type II atresia typically have a normal length of intestine as compared with the type III lesions, which are associated with a shorter bowel length caused by resorption of the fetal gut after a vascular accident.

**Q15** The proximal segment of atretic bowel is known to have ineffective peristalsis due to all of the following *except*:

**A** increased bacterial colonisation of the dilated segment
**B** significant smooth muscle hypertrophy
**C** hyperplasia of the intestinal smooth muscle
**D** hypoplasia of the enteric intramural nerves
**E** decreased number of interstitial cells of Cajal.

**A15** **A** Studying the pathophysiology of the proximal segment of atretic bowel has provided convincing evidence that this segment has ineffective peristalsis and fails to function properly. At the microscopic level, it has been noted that the proximal atretic segment of bowel demonstrated significant smooth muscle hypertrophy and enlargement of the bowel diameter. Other authors have suggested that hyperplasia was the primary change occurring to the intestinal smooth muscle proximal to an obstruction. This hyperplasia may become so extreme proximal to a complete obstruction (as seen in an atresia) that the bowel may decompensate to the point that even a very strong contraction cannot approximate the intestinal walls sufficiently to generate a luminal pressure that permits efficient propulsion. Several studies have also demonstrated an effect on the enteric nervous system in association with jejunoileal atresia. In neonatal human specimens of the excised proximal atretic bowel, the presence of hypoplasia of the enteric intramural nerves has been demonstrated. Also, a remarkable decrease of interstitial cells of Cajal (pacemaker cells of the gastrointestinal tract) was noted in the wall of the small bowel of patients with intestinal atresia.

**Q**16 Which of the following is true regarding the treatment of jejunoileal atresia?

    **A** It is not necessary to test for distal atresias once the dilated proximal segment is identified.

    **B** Resection of the proximal dilated segment in ileal atresia is contraindicated.

    **C** In the case of a proximal jejunal atresia, the dilated segment should be resected back to the ligament of Treitz.

    **D** Preservation of bowel in type IV atresia is not necessary.

    **E** If bowel preservation is required, tapering of the dilated proximal segment should be performed on the mesenteric side of the bowel.

**A**16 **C** When dealing with a jejunoileal atresia, resection of the proximal dilated atretic segment of bowel up to the ligament of Treitz is necessary, but only far enough to allow an anastomosis to be fashioned without difficulty. This is typically followed by an end-to-oblique anastomosis. This scenario is typically successful and often avoids the complications of functional anastomotic obstruction. If inadequate bowel length is noted that could potentially lead to dependence on parenteral nutrition (short bowel syndrome), tapering of the dilated bowel on the antimesenteric border should be performed. This is accomplished by using either a hand-sewn or stapling enteroplasty. The most bulbous portion of the proximal atretic segment is resected and the remaining bowel is tapered over a 24–26 French catheter guide, which is placed within the lumen on the mesenteric side of the intestine. Assessment of the distal segment of bowel is essential to rule out distal atresias and this is performed by placing a purse-string suture in the distal atretic segment of bowel; this segment is opened to allow for the placement of an 8 French red rubber catheter within the lumen of the distal bowel. The bowel is then injected with saline to rule out another atretic segment or distal mucosal membrane or web. In the case of multiple atresias (type IV) especially when intestinal length is in question, a concerted effort is made to preserve as much bowel as possible. To accomplish this goal, multiple anastomoses may be necessary. Typically, the distal atretic segments are decompressed, and if the lumina are patent, end-to-end anastomoses can be fashioned.

**Q17** Which of the following is false with regard to the morbidity and mortality of jejunoileal atresia after repair?

   **A** Anastomotic leak and functional intestinal obstruction are the two most significant postoperative complications.

   **B** Overall survival rates are greater than 80%.

   **C** Over the past 3 decades, morbidity is increasing and mortality is decreasing.

   **D** A recent study noted that 25% of patients required a second operation.

   **E** Malabsorption of fat, bile salts, vitamin $B_{12}$ and calcium are associated with proximal jejunal atresia.

**A17** **E** Functional intestinal obstruction at the site of the anastomosis and anastomotic leak are the two most significant postoperative complications and are associated with a reported mortality rate of 15%. A number of reports published from 1985 to 2001 describe overall survival rates in patients with jejunoileal atresia that range from 80% to 90% or greater. A recent study found that infants with intestinal atresia, a birthweight less than 2 kg, and associated anomalies are at an increased risk for prolonged hospital stay and mortality. The same study commented that 25% required a second operation, including lysis of adhesions (33%), a tapering enteroplasty (33%), and resection of a stenotic segment of bowel with tapering (33%). Despite these complications, overall mortality was only 3.3%. Infants with more-distal ileal resections are more prone to malabsorption (fat, bile salts, vitamin $B_{12}$, calcium and magnesium), diarrhoea (steatorrhoea), and increased bacterial proliferation and overgrowth. Although many infants with short bowel syndrome survive, they require ongoing monitoring for renal stones, gallstones, and malabsorption. Late anastomotic ulcers presenting as either melaena or iron-deficiency anaemia have also been reported.

## Further reading

DeLorimier AA, Fonkalsrud EW, Hays DM. Congenital atresia and stenosis of the jejunum and ileum. *Surgery.* 1969; 65(5): 819–27.

Grosfeld JL. Jejunoileal atresia and stenosis. In: Grosfeld JL, O'Neill JA, Fonkalsrud EW, *et al.*, editors. *Pediatric Surgery. Vol. 1.* 6th ed. Philadelphia, PA: Mosby; 2006. pp. 1269–87.

Guttman FM, Braun P, Garance PH, *et al.* Multiple atresias and a new syndrome of hereditary multiple atresias involving the gastrointestinal tract from stomach to rectum. *J Pediatric Surg.* 1973; 8(5): 633–40.

Louw JH, Barnard CN. Congenital intestinal atresia: observations on its origin. *Lancet.* 1955; 269(6899): 1065–7.

Nixon HH, Tawes R. Etiology and treatment of small intestinal atresia: analysis of a series of 127 jejunoileal atresias and comparison with 62 duodenal atresias. *Surgery.* 1971; 69(1): 41–51.

# CHAPTER 35

# Malrotation and midgut volvulus

## SHIRLEY CHOU, MARCOS BETTOLLI

From the choices below each question, select the single best answer.

**Q1** Which statement describes *normal* rotation of the duodenojejunal loop?
  A The fourth portion of the duodenum is to the right of the superior mesenteric vessels.
  B The ileum and caecum are in the right lower quadrant of the abdominal cavity.
  C The ileal caecal loop passes clockwise upon re-entry into the abdominal cavity.
  D The small bowel is ventral to the colon in the final position.
  E The duodenum is ventral to the superior mesenteric vessels in the final position.

**A1** B In normal rotation, the second portion of the duodenum is to the right of the superior mesenteric vessels, the third portion is beneath the vessels, and the fourth is to the left of the vessels. The ileocaecal junction is in the right lower quadrant, giving the root of the mesentery its maximal length. Malposition, on the other hand, cannot be excluded without demonstrating both ends of the mesenteric attachment.

**Q2** The base of the mesentery is defined by which of the following structures?
  A The second portion of the duodenum and mid-transverse colon.
  B The ileocaecal junction and the rectosigmoid junction.
  C The fourth portion of the duodenum and the hepatic flexure of the right colon.
  D The duodenojejunal junction and the ileocaecal junction.
  E The ligament of Treitz and the falciform ligament.

**A2**   **D**  The base (or root) of the mesentery is defined by the duodenojejunal junction (ligament of Treitz) and the ileocaecal junction. The former is in the left upper quadrant and the latter in the right lower quadrant. This is the maximal length available in the abdominal cavity.

**Q3**   Which of the following does not describe an acute midgut volvulus?
   **A**  sudden onset of bilious vomiting
   **B**  blood per rectum
   **C**  antenatal diagnosis of 'double bubble'
   **D**  metabolic alkalosis
   **E**  shock

**A3**   **D**  In an acute midgut volvulus, there may be metabolic acidosis due to intestinal ischaemia, hypovolaemia and shock.

**Q4**   Which of the following best describes a chronic midgut volvulus?
   **A**  jaundice
   **B**  intermittent sepsis
   **C**  protein–calorie malnutrition
   **D**  massive ascites
   **E**  hyperkalaemia

**A4**   **C**  In chronic midgut volvulus, there is venous and lymphatic obstruction, which may lead to protein–calorie malnutrition.

**Q5**   Ladd's bands are:
   **A**  congenital bands from a high caecum to the lateral peritoneal wall, causing obstruction of the duodenum
   **B**  congenital bands along the lateral border of the duodenum that retroperitonealises the duodenum
   **C**  bands across the transverse colon in the case of reverse rotation
   **D**  bands along the caecum and ascending colon predisposing to caecal volvulus
   **E**  bands between the caecum and the superior mesenteric vessels causing a right mesocolic hernia.

**A5**   **A**  When the caecum returns to the abdominal cavity at 11 weeks' gestational age, it may form bands to the lateral abdominal wall, which bowstrings the duodenum, causing obstruction.

**Q6** Which of the following intraoperative findings occur in chronic volvulus?

   **A** dilated mesenteric lymphatic vessels and veins

   **B** multiple chylous cysts in the mesentery

   **C** enlarged mesenteric lymph nodes

   **D** thickened mesentery

   **E** mesenteric oedema

**A6**   **B** Although there is chronic venous and lymphatic stasis in chronic midgut volvulus, chylous cysts are not found in this entity. Chylous cysts are thought to be due to congenital malformations of lymphatic channels in the small bowel.

**Q7** Which radiological finding is the most accurate in diagnosis of malrotation?

   **A** caecum in the right upper quadrant

   **B** duodenojejunal junction is below the pylorus, and to the right of the left vertebral pedicle

   **C** partial duodenal obstruction

   **D** inverted superior mesenteric artery (SMA) and vein (SMV)

   **E** proximal jejunal loops on the left of the abdomen

**A7**   **B** The most helpful feature in the radiological diagnosis of malrotation is a duodenojejunal junction below the pylorus, and to the right of the left vertebral pedicle. Care must be taken to decompress a distended stomach. Seventy per cent with this finding had malrotation confirmed at operation. Misleading anatomical variations in the position of the mesenteric vessels exist in patients with no abnormality. Although inversion of the vessels suggest malrotation, a normal relationship between the SMA and the SMV does not exclude malrotation.

**Q8** Possible radiological findings seen with volvulus in a 6-week-old infant include all of these *except*:

   **A** normal radiographic image

   **B** distension of the stomach and proximal duodenum with a paucity of gas in the distal intestine

   **C** distension of the stomach and proximal duodenum with no gas distally

   **D** incomplete obstruction of the descending duodenum with the appearance of extrinsic compression and torsion

   **E** none of the above.

A8   C   Complete absence of distant gas is typical of duodenal atresia, while dimin-ished but discernible distal small-bowel gas is characteristic of malrotation. Duodenal stenosis with incomplete obstruction, particularly if located in the more distal location may be indistinguishable from malrotation radiographically, even using intraluminal contrast. Uncertainty requires immediate operative exploration.

Q9   Which of the following investigations is most specific to determine the breadth of the SMA vascular pedicle?
   A   upper GI series
   B   CT with IV contrast
   C   abdominal US
   D   MRI with contrast
   E   none of the above

A9   E   Although in most circumstances, an upper gastrointestinal series is the definitive imaging study for rotational abnormalities, there is no reliable imaging technique to determine whether the breadth of the SMA vascular pedicle places a particular patient at risk for volvulus. Because the potential consequences of malrotation with volvulus include death and short bowel syndrome, and because the corrective surgery is relatively straightforward, timely repair is generally indicated.

Q10   In the management of malrotation associated with congenital heart disease in the heterotaxy syndromes, which of the following is true?
   A   The propensity for volvulus is greatest in newborns and infants, therefore Ladd's procedure is indicated regardless.
   B   Correct cardiac defects first and follow with Ladd's procedure.
   C   Repair both defects simultaneously.
   D   Repair cardiac abnormalities and regular review of the malrotation in outpatient clinic.
   E   None of the above.

A10   B   In the presence of midgut rotational abnormalities associated with congenital heart disease in the heterotaxia syndromes, careful observation of the asympto-matic patient and the deferral of the Ladd's procedure until the cardiac physiology is surgically stabilised, appear to be appropriate.

Q11 Which of the following is true regarding the development of the primitive gut?

A The primitive gut is initially a flat structure.

B The embryonic midgut is defined as the portion of the primitive gut opening ventrally in the yolk sac.

C The omphalomesenteric duct develops in the fourth gestational week.

D Elongation of the midgut begins in the sixth gestational week.

E The embryonic postarterial midgut segment gives rise to the proximal jejunum.

A11 **A** The primitive gut is initially a tubular structure composed of endodermal tissue and centred within the embryo. In the human, the embryonic midgut is defined as that portion of the primitive gut opening ventrally into the yolk sac. By the fifth week of gestation, the ventral opening into the yolk sac has narrowed and is referred to as the omphalomesenteric duct. The elongation of the midgut begins in the fifth gestational week, resulting in three distinct processes that relate to rotational abnormalities of the gut.

Q12 The three stages of gut development are:

A growth and elongation of the midgut; 270 degrees counterclockwise rotation; retraction of the intestine

B herniation of the foregut; 180 degrees clockwise rotation of the midgut; 270 degrees rotation of the hindgut

C elongation and herniation of the midgut; 270 degrees counterclockwise rotation of the midgut; fixation of the root of the mesentery

D herniation of the primary midgut loop; retraction of the extracoelomic intestine; fixation of the intestine to the posterior body wall

E none of the above.

A12 **D** First, herniation of the primary midgut loop occurs into the base of the umbilical cord. The second stage of midgut development is the retraction of the extracoelomic intestine; this occurs between gestational weeks 10 and 12. The third final step in the normal midgut positioning process is fixation of the intestine to the posterior body wall. This occurs after 12 weeks of gestation, upon completion of caecal descent.

**Q13** Ladd's procedure includes:

**A** clockwise detorsion; division of Ladd's band; positioning the caecum on the left

**B** counterclockwise detorsion; division of Ladd's bands; bowel fixation and appendicectomy

**C** clockwise detorsion; division of Ladd's bands; positioning and fixation of the caecum on the left

**D** counterclockwise detorsion; division of Ladd's bands; broadening the SMA mesentery; appendicectomy

**E** counterclockwise detorsion; division of Ladd's bands; broadening the SMA mesentery; positioning of the caecum on the left; appendicectomy.

**A13** **D** The operative technique for malrotation is the procedure described by William E Ladd. A transverse supraumbilical incision is widely used, providing a generous exposure of the right upper quadrant. Following abdominal entry and rapid exploration, complete exteriorisation of the intestine and the mesentery is essential in order to visualise and assess the anatomical abnormality. The midgut volvulus is relieved by rotating the intestine in a counterclockwise direction. Ladd's peritoneal bands must be divided to relieve any extrinsic obstruction of the duodenum, this is achieved by performing an extensive Kocher's manoeuvre. Recurrence of the volvulus is prevented by broadening the base of the mesenteric vascular pedicle, and by dividing the peritoneal bands that tether the caecum, small-bowel mesentery, mesocolon, and duodenum around the base of the SMA. Appendicectomy is considered standard because of the malposition of the caecum. At the end of the procedure, the intestine is replaced into the abdomen, generally with the small intestine on the right and the caecum and the colon on the left.

**Q14** Which of the following anomalies is found in patients with malrotation?

**A** duodenal atresia

**B** diaphragmatic hernia

**C** gastroschisis

**D** omphalocele

**E** all of the above

**A14** **E** Malrotation is an integral part of congenital diaphragmatic hernia (CDH) and abdominal wall defects. Infants with CDH or omphaloceles have varying degrees of normal rotation and fixation, depending on the extent of intestinal displacement. In gastroschisis the midgut is non-rotated and may be suspended and stretched outside the fetal abdominal cavity, leading to ischaemic injury without volvulus. Duodenal atresia has been found in conjunction with malrotation and perinatal volvulus. Cardiac abnormalities are also associated with intestinal malrotation.

**Q15** Which of the following best describes non-rotation?

    **A** The caecum is behind the superior mesenteric vessels and the duodenum is anterior.

    **B** The duodenum is normally rotated, but the caecum is in the subhepatic region.

    **C** The duodenum descends vertically downwards, so that the small bowel is on the right side of the abdomen, and the colon is to the left of the midline.

    **D** The duodenum dangles vertically on the right but the caecum is in the right lower quadrant.

    **E** The duodenum is normally rotated but the caecum is to the left of the midline.

**A15** **C** The duodenum dangles vertically, and the caecum is to the left of the midline in non-rotation, thus creating a narrow base of the mesentery. Option A is termed reverse rotation and option B is termed malrotation.

**Q16** Which of the following is *not* a complication of operative treatment of malrotation with midgut volvulus?

    **A** recurrence

    **B** postoperative intussusception

    **C** caecal volvulus

    **D** small bowel obstruction secondary to adhesions

    **E** short gut syndrome

**A16** **C** Recurrent volvulus rate is around 5%. Small-bowel obstruction from adhesions can be as high as 15%. Postoperative intussusception has been reported in 3%. If massive bowel resection was required, short gut syndrome may develop. However, caecal volvulus is not associated with surgical correction of malrotation and volvulus.

## Further reading

Dilley AV, Pereira J, Shi ECP, *et al*. The radiologist says malrotation: does the surgeon operate? *Pediatr Surg Int*. 2000; **16**(1–2): 45–9.

Lampl B, Levin TL, Berdon WE, *et al*. Malrotation and midgut volvulus: a historical review and current controversies in diagnosis and management. *Pediatr Radiol*. 2009; **39**(4): 359–66.

Millar AJ, Rode H, Cywes S. Malrotation and volvulus in infancy and childhood. *Semin Pediatr Surg*. 2003; **12**(4): 229–36.

# CHAPTER 36

# Meconium ileus

## STEPHANIE A JONES, MORITZ M ZIEGLER

**From the choices below each question, select the single best answer.**

Q1 A plain abdominal radiograph may be pathognomonic for meconium
ileus when disparate-sized bowel loops are associated with:
  A small-bowel air–fluid levels with absence of gas in the rectum
  B portal venous gas in the liver and free intra-abdominal air
  C soap-bubbly appearance in the right lower quadrant and absence
    of small-bowel air–fluid levels
  D left upper quadrant speckled calcifications and distension of the
    stomach and duodenum
  E a dilated colon and intrascrotal calcifications.

A1 C After delivery, uncomplicated meconium ileus is characterised by a typical
plain obstruction series on radiographic assessment of the abdomen. In addition
to the supine and erect films appearing remarkably similar, the characteristic
findings include the following: (1) great disparity in the size of the intestinal loops
because of the configuration of the different segments of the bowel; (2) no or few
air–fluid levels on the erect film because swallowed air cannot layer above the
thickened inspissated meconium; and (3) a granular, 'soap-bubble', or 'ground-
glass' appearance seen frequently in the right half of the abdomen, a finding
that requires swallowed air bubbles to intermix within the sticky meconium. This
'soap-bubble' appearance was described by Neuhauser in 1946, and is also known
as 'Neuhauser's sign'. Each of these features alone is not exclusively diagnostic
of meconium ileus and may be seen with other causes of intestinal obstruction.
Collectively, however, they strongly suggest meconium ileus. Plain radiography
done for differential diagnosis will include any cause of a distal small bowel
obstruction, including ileal atresia, Hirschsprung's disease, or the meconium
plug/small left colon syndrome.

**Q2** Histopathological findings that might confirm the diagnosis of cystic fibrosis (CF)–associated meconium ileus in the neonateinclude:

   **A** absent sweat glands on skin biopsy

   **B** islet cell inflammation on pancreatic biopsy

   **C** an anatomically normal Meckel's diverticulum.

   **D** an appendix characterised by submucosal gland mucus accumulation

   **E** mid-small-bowel segmental hypoganglionosis.

 **A2**   **D** The diagnosis of CF is aided by the finding of pathognomonic changes in appendiceal and intestinal specimens, including goblet cell hyperplasia and accumulation of secretions within the crypts or within the lumen. If operation is done for putative meconium ileus and an appendicostomy is used as a bowel intraluminal irrigation site, appendicectomy may be warranted to obtain such a diagnostic pathological specimen.

 **Q3** Pathognomonic signs seen at the time of radiographic contrast enema for the diagnosis of meconium ileus, include:

   **A** an unused or microcolon

   **B** an elongated and redundant colon

   **C** a colon free of intraluminal material

   **D** the failure of the contrast to reflux into the distal small bowel

   **E** a rectal-to-descending colon diameter ratio of 1 : 2.

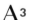 **A3**   **A** A confirming study that may support the plain radiographic diagnosis of meconium ileus is the contrast enema. A contrast enema (whether with barium, Gastrografin, or any water-soluble contrast agent like Cysto-Conray II will out-line a normally positioned colon of appropriate length but of small calibre. It will be empty or will contain pellets of inspissated meconium. The colon will be the typical 'unused' colon or 'microcolon'. If reflux of contrast agent into the terminal ileum occurs, it will outline pellets of inspissated meconium. If the contrast agent refluxes more proximally into the ileum, the transition into dilated loops of small bowel will be encountered. Failure to reflux contrast medium into the proximal dilated small bowel will neither prove the diagnosis of meconium ileus nor determine the exact level of the intestinal obstruction; and with this failure of the contrast medium to reflux into the dilated segment, operative intervention for diagnosis and treatment becomes necessary. The differential diagnosis at this point would include meconium ileus and distal small-bowel (ileal) atresia.

**Q4** Gastrografin (meglumine diatrizoate) is characterised by:

    **A** hypotonicity (osmolality <350 mOsm/L)

    **B** containing a mucosal-protecting factor

    **C** the inclusion of a solubilising agent 'Tween 80'

    **D** inducing secondary hypervolaemia

    **E** an adverse systemic effect on the vas deferens

**A4**    **C**  A Gastrografin enema has been the standard non-operative treatment. Gastrografin (meglumine diatrizoate + sodium diatrizoate) is a hyperosmolar, water-soluble, radio-opaque solution containing 0.1% polysorbate 80 (Tween 80), a solubilising or wetting agent, and 37% organically bound iodine. The meglumine is a 76% aqueous solution of sodium-methyl-glucamine salt of N,N1-diacetyl-3,5-diamino-2,4,6-triiodobenzoic acid, and this hypertonic solution has an osmolality of 1900 mOsm/L, a property that draws fluid into the intestinal lumen and aids in the release of the inspissated meconium. Because of the risk of dehydration it is recommended that the enema solution be diluted before use. After administration, both a transient osmotic diarrhoea and a putative osmotic diuresis occur, factors that emphasise the importance of aggressive fluid resuscitation. In addition, the product is radio-opaque, which enables a safe fluoroscopically monitored administration. Polysorbate 80 (Tween 80) is a non-ionic surface-active emulsifier that not only may better define the bowel mucosal pattern radiographically but may also facilitate passage of the hypertonic Gastrografin between the mucosa and the adherent meconium at the site of the obstruction. Polysorbate 80 as a 10% solution has been administered intraoperatively by way of an enterostomy to liquefy meconium. Other hypertonic water-soluble agents (e.g. 40% sodium diatrizoate (40% Hypaque), with or without polysorbate 80, or Cysto-Conray) are also effective in relieving the obstruction and preclude the potential adverse mucosal effects of Gastrografin on the colon.

 **Q5** Which of the following laboratory test results indicates that a patient will likely have CF as the aetiology of their meconium ileus?

    **A** an increased acetylcholinesterase concentration on rectal biopsy

    **B** a sweat chloride value of >5 mEq/L

    **C** a stool trypsin level of >500 mg per gram of stool

    **D** a stool albumin value of <5 mg per gram of stool

    **E** a genetic profile on *CFTR* gene mutation analysis for carrier status on paternal testing

 **A5**    **E**  The definitive study to confirm the diagnosis of CF is the sweat test. With the use of pilocarpine iontophoresis method, sweat is collected from the infant's forearm, leg or back; the amount is quantified, and the concentration of sodium and chloride in the sample is measured. The minimum amount of sweat to be collected is 100 mg, and a measured concentration of sweat chloride in excess of 60 mEq/L is diagnostic of CF. The adequacy of the size of the sweat sample is the factor that usually precludes the application of this test to the newborn, despite reports to the contrary.

Genetic testing for CF can be done by analysing cellular DNA for *CFTR*, thus establishing the carrier status of parents of a child with putative CF presenting with features of meconium ileus. However, because of the minimum number of mutations tested by these commercial analyses, negative results become less meaningful. If a family has known *CFTR* mutations, then amniocentesis with fetal DNA restriction fragment length polymorphism analysis may predict a fetal CF diagnosis.

The pathophysiologic alteration of an increased albumin concentration of meconium may prove useful as a diagnostic screening tool for meconium ileus. This test, which uses a tetrabromophenolethylester blue indicator, detects meconium albumin concentration in excess of 20 mg/g of stool; however, a persisting incidence of false-positive results was seen from such factors as prematurity, melaena, gastroschisis and intrauterine infection. Meconium from normal neonates has an albumin concentration of less than 5.0 mg/g of stool, whereas meconium from neonates with CF has values at times in excess of 80 mg/g.

Stool trypsin and chymotrypsin analysis has historically been a popular screening test for meconium ileus. A trypsin level less than 80 mg/g of stool, coupled with operative findings, supports the diagnosis of meconium ileus.

 **6** In the absence of CF, meconium ileus can occur as a result of which of the following?

**A** pancreatic ductal stenosis

**B** meconium plug syndrome

**C** a heterozygote father

**D** the sweat chloride sample was insufficient at 120 mg

**E** ileal ischaemia with an acquired secondary ileal atresia

**6** **A** Meconium ileus may occur in the absence of CF in term or pre-term infants with pancreatic or intestinal insufficiency from a variety of causes. These intraluminal obstructions result from accumulation of inspissated sticky meconium in the terminal ileum or right colon, but the meconium is neither tar-like nor resistant to conventional enema irrigation that usually proves to be therapeutic. Whether intestinal secretion insufficiency or a pancreatic achylia is aetiologic is variable, but rarely has pancreatic insufficiency been documented. Definitive exclusion of CF clinically requires a sweat chloride analysis, DNA analysis, or both. A series of 44 infants in Amsterdam identified only 53.5% of these patients as having CF. Although the clinical manifestations of meconium ileus are the same, some differences exist in the patients with and without CF. Patients with

CF presenting with meconium ileus are more likely to be born at term, whereas those with meconium ileus and prematurity or low birthweight do not have CF. Additionally, those patients with complex meconium ileus or meconium peritonitis were likely not to have CF, a small comfort to the parents of these children. Other series have described higher than expected incidence of meconium ileus in patients without CF, anywhere from 21.6% to 53.5%. These findings highlight the diversity of genetic mutations and influence of modifiers on this disease.

**Q7** The *CFTR* gene is characterised by:

**A** localisation to the long arm of chromosome 9

**B** physiologic action as a potassium ion channel blocker

**C** testability to determine carrier status

**D** autosomal dominant behaviour with variable penetrance

**E** inducing a 10-fold greater pathological influence on the pancreas than on intestinal glands.

**A7** **C** In 1989, the genetic mutation that codes for the cell membrane protein termed the CF transmembrane regulator (CFTR) was identified by Francis Collins as the locus associated with the diagnosis of CF. This locus was identified on the long arm of chromosome 7, band q31. The protein was identified as a cyclic adenosine monophosphate-induced chloride channel that regulates ion flow across the apical surface of epithelial cells. There are more than 1300 identified mutations of the *CFTR* gene that ultimately produces abnormal electrolyte content along the external apical environment of epithelial membranes. Tubular structures lined by such affected epithelia will be characterised by desiccation and reduced clearance of their secretions, and include epithelial cells of respiratory, gastrointestinal, biliary, pancreatic and reproductive systems. The clinical correlate of this pathophysiology has included pancreatic insufficiency (90%), meconium ileus (10%–20%), diabetes mellitus (20%), obstructive biliary disease (15%–20%) and azoospermia (nearly 100%). There are varying mechanisms for the epithelial glandular abnormality to be expressed, and the elaboration of a hyperviscous mucin is the result of such mutations. The tenacious meconium protein and water content and its increased viscosity have been described long before the genetic factors were identified.

The delta F508 mutation is the most common of the many *CFTR* gene mutations, occurring as a homozygous pair in almost 50% of CF patients, whereas another 25%–30% of patients will carry one copy of this mutation. Thus, up to more than 70% of patients with CF have this mutation resulting in the in-frame deletion of a phenylalanine residue at position 508 of the polypeptide chain. Homozygous individuals nearly always phenotypically express pancreatic exocrine insufficiency, and they also present with a higher incidence of meconium ileus.

A similar higher frequency of meconium ileus is also seen in delta F508 patients who also carry the G542X mutation.

 **Q8** A pathognomonic physical finding in patients with CF-induced meconium ileus is:

   **A** a bitter/sweet 'taste' of the baby's sweat

   **B** the 'putty sign' when compressing a distended bowel loop on abdominal exam

   **C** a large rectal stool ball on digital exam

   **D** an enlarged testes on scrotal exam

   **E** aniridia.

 **A8** **B** Neonates with meconium ileus often are born with abdominal distension. In fact, meconium ileus is the only variety of neonatal intestinal obstruction that produces abdominal distension at birth before the neonate swallows air. Visible peristaltic waves and palpable, doughy bowel loops are often present. Finger pressure over a firm loop of bowel may hold the indentation, the so-called 'putty sign'. In simple or uncomplicated meconium ileus, no findings of peritoneal irritation are present. The findings on rectal examination are unremarkable, and characteristically on withdrawal of the examining finger a spontaneous expulsion of meconium does not follow. In the presence of an *in utero* perforation with meconium peritonitis and 'cyst' formation, a palpable abdominal mass, discolouration of the abdominal wall, and signs of peritoneal irritation are often observed. Physical evidence of hypovolaemia may rapidly develop in infants with peritonitis. On passage of a nasogastric tube the quantity of bile-stained gastric fluid usually exceeds 20 mL.

 **Q9** Which of the following represents optimal contemporary therapy for the intestinal obstruction of simple (uncomplicated) meconium ileus?

   **A** T-tube ileocolic lavage with mucomyst

   **B** Bishop–Koop's enterostomy with subsequent bedside ligation of the stomal 'chimney'

   **C** transanal ileocolic solubilisation of inspissated meconium with Gastrografin

   **D** nasogastric tube lavage with mucomyst

   **E** gross enterostomy with extracorporeal resection of the obstructed ileocolic loop

**A9** **C** Non-operative management of meconium ileus depends on the dissolution of the inspissated intraluminal meconium in an otherwise patent and uncompromised ileocolon. Although various solubilising agents historically have been administered by mouth, intraoperatively or by rectum, the mainstay of meconium ileus treatment remained an operative procedure. In 1969 several additional reports suggested that solvents were effective and the value of non-operative application of such solvents was suggested both clinically and experimentally. Noblett reported the successful use of a hypertonic contrast enema in four neonates with uncomplicated meconium ileus. Since that report, a Gastrografin enema has been the standard of non-operative treatment (*see* explanation for question 4).

The success of non-operative treatment is variable. The initial report of Noblett suggested that as many as two-thirds of patients were successfully treated by this technique. Advantages of the non-operative therapy include a reduction in pulmonary morbidity and a reduced length of hospital stay. Disadvantages of therapy include a delay in operative intervention for those unsuccessfully treated by the enema, the risk of immediate and delayed intestinal injury or perforation, and the induction of hypovolaemia. Bowel injury leading to a potential perforation may be a product of repeated enemas, injudicious inflation of an enema catheter balloon, or a direct mucosal injury induced by the enema agent. The mechanism of such an injury may be related to bowel distension or to the polysorbate 80 content. The latter injury may be prevented by using a solubilising enema agent containing 1%–2% polysorbate 80 with isotonic Gastrografin diluted with water to a final osmolality of 320–340 mOsm/L or by using an alternative isotonic contrast agent. Reports have been published of diminishing success of the contrast enema in simple meconium ileus. One retrospective analysis compared a contemporary group of neonates receiving enemas with a historical control. The success rate for relieving the obstruction in the historical group was 39%, whereas the success in the contemporary group was only 5.5%. This discrepancy in success rates was because of fewer attempts at contrast enema compared with the historical control. Also there was a wider use of other contrast agents like Cysto-Conray (400 mOsm/kg water) and non-Tween 80–containing agents, compared with the highly osmotically active Gastrografin (1940 mOsm/kg water). The conclusion was that in stable patients, repeated enemas should be attempted prior to surgical exploration.

Q10 The diagnosis of 'complicated' meconium ileus is likely in the face of:
 A abdominal distension at birth
 B failure of transanal contrast to reflux into dilated distal ileum
 C reddish-bluish abdominal wall discolouration with radiographically proven intraperitoneal calcifications
 D high-grade proximal small bowel obstruction
 E an empty microcolon on contrast enema with 'boxcar' inspissated meconium confined to the distal ileum.

A10  C  In the presence of an *in utero* perforation with meconium peritonitis and 'cyst' formation, a palpable abdominal mass, discolouration of the abdominal wall, and signs of peritoneal irritation are often observed. Physical evidence of hypovolaemia may rapidly develop in infants with peritonitis. On passage of a nasogastric tube the quantity of bile-stained gastric fluid usually exceeds 20 mL.

Meconium peritonitis may be seen as one of several varieties. A meconium pseudocyst is a result of meconium accumulating in the peritoneal cavity for weeks to months. A calcified 'pseudocyst' fibrous wall forms around an accumulation of meconium, and spared bowel loops are peripheral to this cyst. Adhesive meconium peritonitis follows meconium contamination of the peritoneal cavity for days to weeks before delivery. Dense and vascular adhesions make operative relief of the adhesive intestinal obstruction difficult. Scattered calcifications may be present. When intestinal perforation occurs only a few days before delivery, an abdomen filled with meconium ascites results and calcification is absent. The fourth variant of meconium peritonitis is bacterially infected ascites, which occurs when colonised intestinal organisms penetrate from the perforated intestine into the peritoneal cavity.

Q11  The optimal intraoperative irrigant to solubilise tenacious intraluminal meconium is:

A  undiluted Gastrografin

B  warmed physiologic saline

C  4% acetylcysteine

D  1% Viokase

E  isotonic sodium bicarbonate.

A11  C  Irrigating solutions may include warmed saline, a 50% diatrizoate solution, a 1% solution of pancreatic enzymes (Viokase; AH Robbins Co, Richmond, VA), hydrogen peroxide, and, most commonly, either a 2% or a 4% solution of N-acetylcysteine (Mucomyst; Apothecon, Princeton, NJ). More concentrated solutions of N-acetylcysteine or Gastrografin, or the use of hydrogen peroxide with its attendant risk of air embolism, may produce greater risk than benefit. After solubilisation by the irrigant, injected through the enterotomy catheter, the meconium is gently milked distally into the colon or evacuated through the enterotomy. The enterotomy and the abdomen may then either be closed and an enterostomy created; or the site can be controlled by insertion of a T-tube. This last treatment has been designed to be located at the junction of proximal distended ileum with distal (more collapsed) ileum where intraluminal balls of inspissated meconium are found. Leaving this tube in place and attaching the enterotomy site to the anterior abdominal wall ensures a controlled fistula as well as a route of gastrointestinal access for the instillation of pancreatic enzyme solutions beginning on the first postoperative day. By postoperative days 7–14, the irrigant should pass freely into the colon, the obstruction should be relieved, and therefore the catheter can be removed. This avoids the need for reoperation and enterostomy closure. A 40-year experience with T-tube ileostomy use has been reviewed. Once the patient was on adequate oral intake and had spontaneous stooling, the T-tube could be removed at bedside without significant problems. Eighty-seven per cent of the patients with a T-tube had relief of the obstruction with T-tube solubilising irrigations. An alternative technique is appendicectomy with appendicostomy, with meconium evacuation or irrigation through this route. A temporary indwelling tube caecostomy may alternatively be left in place. For such an irrigant technique to be successful, the bowel must be handled gently, not overdistended, and not excessively massaged or 'milked' in an effort to evacuate the inspissated meconium. Additionally, there have been case reports of N-acetylcysteine-associated liver injury after oral or rectal administration.

**Q12** The operative procedure that would most likely limit the patient to a single operation (and anaesthetic) for obstructive simple meconium ileus is:

   **A**  segmental resection with a proximal diverting stoma

   **B**  a Santulli Roux-Y enterostomy

   **C**  a Gross double-barrelled Mikulicz's enterostomy

   **D**  T-tube ileostomy

   **E**  Bishop–Koop's Roux-Y enterostomy.

**A12**  **D**  The enterostomy site can be controlled by insertion of a T-tube, which is used for instillation of pancreatic enzyme solutions (*see* explanation for question 11).

An alternative operation to enterotomy irrigation is placement of a temporary obstruction-relieving stoma with or without an associated partial resection. Gross initially advocated placement of the Mikulicz's double-barreled enterostomy, which could be performed quickly and which did not require intraoperative meconium evacuation The exteriorised bowel loop can be opened and/or resected after the abdominal incision has been closed, thereby minimising intraperitoneal contamination. After the obstruction is relieved and the infant has recovered, a spur-crushing Mikulicz's clamp can be applied externally at the stoma to complete a side-to-side enteral anastomosis. It may be necessary to return to the operating room to close the stoma: after the clamp-induced anastomosis the residual enterocutaneous fistula may not spontaneously close. An alternative to such an 'extraabdominal resection' and delayed stoma closure is primary resection and anastomosis. After meconium had been evacuated, a primary intraperitoneal anastomosis could be performed, or the infant could be allowed to recover more fully, after which the stoma could be closed in a delayed fashion by an end-to-end anastomosis.

An alternative operation is resection coupled with a distal chimney enterostomy, the so-called Bishop–Koop's procedure. Intraoperatively, a No 8 French rubber catheter is passed through the ostomy chimney into the distal ileum. Within 12–24 hours after the operation, catheter irrigations are commenced with a pancreatic enzyme solution (1 teaspoon Viokase per 30 mL water) repeated every 4–6 hours until the distal intraluminal obstruction is relieved, at which time the catheter is removed. After an initial large volume of enterostomy output, the ostomy drainage will diminish as the more distal obstruction is relieved. The transcolonic passage of stool will follow. Thereafter, the output from the stoma may cease altogether. Eventually the chimney may be treated by one of two techniques. At the bedside the 'stoma' may be ligated. If the result of this non-invasive technique is a persistent enterocutaneous fistula, then a formal intraperitoneal or extraperitoneal stomal closure can be performed with the patient under a general anaesthetic. The latter procedure is necessary in approximately 75% of patients treated by this technique.

Santulli described a proximal chimney enterostomy, an operation that in essence is the reverse of the resection coupled with a distal chimney enterostomy. The distal ileal end is anastomosed end-to-side to the proximal ileum at a level corresponding to an immediate subfascial plane, and the proximal ileum is exited as an end enterostomy. With this stoma arrangement, irrigation and decompression of the proximal ileum is enhanced. As with Bishop–Koop's procedure, an intraoperative catheter passed through the stoma is positioned into the distal ileum for the postoperative instillation of solubilising agent. Because a high-output functional end enterostomy has been created, it is necessary to close such a stoma early to avoid the complications induced by excessive fluid and electrolyte losses.

**Q13** The non-operative treatment of meconium ileus was first described by:
- **A** Wilson
- **B** Noblett
- **C** Neuheiser
- **D** Bishop
- **E** Gross.

**A13** **B** Non-operative management of meconium ileus depends on the dissolution of the inspissated intraluminal meconium in an otherwise patent and uncompromised ileocolon. Although various solubilising agents historically have been administered by mouth, intraoperatively, or by rectum, the mainstay of meconium ileus treatment remained an operative procedure. In 1969, several additional reports suggested that solvents were effective and the values of non-operative application of such solvents was suggested both clinically and experimentally. Noblett reported the successful use of a hypertonic contrast enema in four neonates with uncomplicated meconium ileus. She described the need to fulfil the following criteria before applying such therapy: (1) an initial diagnostic contrast enema should exclude other causes of distal intestinal obstruction; (2) the complications of volvulus, atresia, perforation or peritonitis must be excluded; (3) the enema must be performed with careful fluoroscopic control; (4) intravenous antibiotics should be administered; (5) the patient should be attended by a paediatric surgeon during the procedure; (6) the patient should have a full fluid resuscitation with fluids given aggressively (one to three times maintenance) during the procedure; and (7) the patient should be prepared for imminent operation should complications develop. Since that report, a Gastrografin enema has been the standard of non-operative treatment. After administration, both a transient osmotic diarrhoea and a putative osmotic diuresis occur, factors that emphasise the importance of aggressive fluid resuscitation. In addition, the product is radio-opaque, which enables a safe fluoroscopically monitored administration. Polysorbate 80 is a non-ionic surface-active emulsifier that not only may better define radiographically the bowel mucosal pattern but also may facilitate the passage of the hypertonic Gastrografin between the mucosa and the adherent meconium at the site of the obstruction. Polysorbate 80 as a 10% solution has been administered intraoperatively by way of an enterostomy to liquefy meconium. Complications can arise from enema use and include hypovolaemic shock from the osmotic fluid shifts, inflammation, perforation and ischaemic enterocolitis.

The technique of solubilising enema treatment of meconium ileus continues to use the aforementioned guidelines of Noblett. After fluid resuscitation and nasogastric decompression have been performed, and after physical examination and plain abdominal radiographs have excluded the diagnosis of peritonitis or perforation, the diagnostic contrast enema with barium or water-soluble agent is administered. When the preliminary diagnostic study has been completed, an enema-tip, non-balloon catheter is inserted into the anorectum and the buttocks are taped together around the catheter. With fluoroscopic guidance and an initial solution of 50% Gastrografin in water, the contrast agent is slowly injected via the catheter-tipped syringe. When contrast medium traverses the colon and reaches the dilated meconium-impacted ileum, the study is terminated and the infant is returned to a bed for monitoring, fluid administration (two times maintenance) and normalisation of body temperature. Spontaneous passage of the inspissated meconium per rectum should follow. An abdominal radiograph should be repeated in 8–12 hours to determine whether the obstruction has been relieved. If instead the evacuation is incomplete and obstruction persists, the enema may be repeated with the same concentration of Gastrografin. If either no evacuation occurs after a successfully refluxing enema or if contrast medium cannot be refluxed into dilated bowel, then this technique should be abandoned and operative intervention planned. Similarly, signs of worsening obstruction, clinical distension, greater distension of loops on radiograph, or signs of peritonitis resulting from a possible perforation are also indication for operative intervention.

Noblett suggests that after a successful enema, 5 mL of a 10% N-acetylcysteine solution should be administered every 6 hours through a nasogastric tube to liquefy upper gastrointestinal secretions. Furthermore, when formula feedings are begun, supplemental pancreatic enzymes must be administered with each feeding.

**Q14** A combination that is difficult to treat is CF associated meconium ileus combined with:

  **A** acquired short bowel syndrome (intestinal failure)

  **B** pancreatic insufficiency

  **C** recurrent urinary tract infections

  **D** right upper lobe atelectasis

  **E** delta-F508 mutation on DNA analysis.

**A14** **A** The outcome of the treatment of patients with meconium ileus, whether the condition is complicated or simple, has steadily improved over the last 3 decades; the most recently reported survival rates approaching 100%. In a series of patients treated both non-operatively and operatively, survival rate at 5 and 10 years for the two categories improved steadily from the 1960s (30% and 70%, respectively) through the 1970s (80% and 70%, respectively) and 1980s (100% at 5-year follow-up). In the past, non-operative treatment contributed to an improved survival rate, but in the past decade the survival rate for both operative and non-operative treatment was 100%. The significant improvement in operative survival has come since the 1960s when the 6-month survival rate was only 33%. The operative survival rate had improved to 60% before 1979 and to 100% after 1979 and 1989. No significant overall differences in outcomes were observed with regard to the patient gender, whether complication of meconium ileus was present, or with regard to the type of operation performed (ileostomy, resection with primary anastomosis, resection and Mikulicz's ileostomy, and Bishop–Koop's enterostomy). Additionally, the long-term survival rates (measured at 6 years) of patients treated with Bishop–Koop's procedure (62% survival) did not differ from those of patients with other operations. Furthermore, all deaths in patients older than 6 months of age were cardiopulmonary or pneumonitic deaths related to underlying CF and not to complications of operation. Interestingly, both simple and complicated cases of meconium ileus had 72% 10-year survival rates.

Death occurs from multiple causes, which include intraperitoneal sepsis from unrecognised leakage, pulmonary sepsis and bronchopneumonia, or short bowel syndrome with complicating liver failure.

Q15 The diagnosis of CF in a neonate presenting with meconium ileus presents the significant concern that:

   A there will be a greater pulmonary morbidity and mortality

   B there will be long-term protein-calorie malnutrition

   C pancreatic insufficiency will result in diabetes mellitus as an additional co-morbidity

   D intestinal insufficiency will dominate pancreatic insufficiency

   E adolescent rectal prolapse will be a common morbidity.

A15 A Two simultaneous pathogenetic events in meconium ileus appear to begin *in utero* and result in intraluminal accumulation of a highly viscid and tenacious meconium: (1) the development of pancreatic exocrine enzyme deficiency and (2) the secretion of hyperviscous mucus by pathologically abnormal intestinal glands. The thickened meconium accumulates and begins *in utero* to obstruct the intestine intraluminally. This accounts for the complications of meconium ileus (i.e. a twist of a heavy loop with perforation, peritonitis and cyst or atresia) seen in the neonate. The proximal ileum dilates, and its wall thickens as it becomes filled with the tenacious and tarry meconium. Concomitantly, the narrowed distal small bowel, and at times the colon, contains beaded or 'boxcar' concretions of grey-white, putty-like inspissated meconium. The more distal colon is small or unused, a microcolon.

The past 2 decades have seen continued progress. The genetic lesion of a mutation in the CF transmembrane regulator (*CFTR*) gene was defined as the causal lesion of CF, and it is now recognised that patients with meconium ileus likely represent a distinct phenotype with earlier presentation and worse pulmonary function. Yet, the outcome of the treatment of patients with meconium ileus, whether the condition is complicated or simple, has steadily improved over the last three decades (*see* explanation for question 14).

## Further reading

Blackman SM, Deering-Brose R, McWilliams R, *et al*. Relative contribution of genetic and non-genetic modifiers to intestinal obstruction in cystic fibrosis. *Gastroenterology.* 2006; **131**(4): 1030–9.

Del Pin CA, Czyrko C, Ziegler MM, *et al*. Management and survival of meconium ileus: a 30-year review. *Ann Surg.* 1992; **215**(2): 179–85.

Dirkes K, Crombleholme TM, Craigo SD, *et al*. The natural history of meconium peritonitis diagnosed *in utero. J Pediatr Surg.* 1995; **30**(7): 979–82.

Escobar MA, Grosfeld JL, Burdick JJ, *et al*. Surgical considerations in cystic fibrosis: a 32-year evaluation of outcomes. *Surgery.* 2005; **138**(4): 560–71.

Warner BW, Ziegler MM. Management of the short bowel syndrome in the pediatric population. *Pediatr Clin North Am.* 1993; **40**(6): 1335–50.

# CHAPTER 37

# Meckel's diverticulum

## BRICE ANTAO, MICHAEL S IRISH

From the choices below each question, select the single best answer.

 **1** Which of the following is true regarding the development of Meckel's diverticulum?

   **A** Extracoelomic yolk sac forms the gut.

   **B** The fetal foregut is attached to the yolk sac via the omphalomesenteric duct.

   **C** The right vitelline artery remnant supplies the diverticulum.

   **D** It is located on the mesenteric border of the small bowel.

   **E** It is not a true diverticulum.

**A1** **C** The intracoelomic yolk sac forms the gut. The fetal midgut is attached to the yolk sac via the omphalomesenteric duct (also known as vitelline duct or yolk stalk). This regresses at 5–7 weeks' gestation. Meckel's diverticulum results from failure of proximal duct to obliterate. The right and left vitelline arteries originate from the aorta within the yolk stalk. The left involutes and the right persists as the superior mesenteric artery and terminally supplies the diverticulum. Meckel's diverticulum is a true diverticulum (containing all normal layers of the intestinal wall) located on the antimesenteric border of the small bowel.

**Q2** Omphalomesenteric duct anomalies include all of the following *except*:

   **A** omphaloileal fistula

   **B** umbilical polyp

   **C** patent vitelline sinus

   **D** vitelline duct cyst

   **E** patent urachus.

**A2** **E** Meckel's diverticulum is the most common vitelline duct (omphalomesenteric duct) abnormality. Abnormal regression of the vitelline duct can also give rise to other abnormalities.

- Persistent vitelline duct: appearing as a draining fistula at the umbilicus.
- Patent vitelline sinus: can be a source of infection with purulent discharge. It can be connected to the Meckel's diverticulum, by a fibrous band around which volvulus can occur.
- Fibrous band connecting the ileum to undersurface of the umbilicus: can cause obstruction or volvulus.
- Vitelline duct cyst: mucosal and muscular lined cyst, which persists after the proximal and distal duct obliterates.
- Umbilical polyp: most are independent anomalies, although some can connect with deeper structures. Sometimes they can be mistaken for umbilical granulomas.
- Omphaloileal fistula: persistent patency of the vitelline duct with the fetal intestine.

A urachus is a fibrous cord that originates from the allantois and extends from the bladder to the umbilicus. Abnormal obliteration and regression of the urachus gives rise to various abnormalities, unrelated to vitelline duct abnormalities.

 **Q3** Which of the following is true regarding the incidence of Meckel's diverticulum?

**A** It is twice as common in females as in males.

**B** It commonly occurs 2 feet away from the ligament of Treitz.

**C** It is 2 cm long.

**D** It contains two main types of heterotopic mucosa – namely, gastric and pancreatic.

**E** All of the above.

 **A3** **D** The 'rule of 2s' is often used as a mnemonic for Meckel's diverticulum:

- occurs in 2% of the population
- twice as common in males as in females
- usually located 2 feet from ileocaecal valve
- 2 inches long
- 2 cm in diameter
- symptomatic by 2 years of age
- contains two types of heterotopic tissue – gastric and pancreatic.

Male-to-female ratio is almost equal in asymptomatic group, but in symptomatic group males > females. Most cases become symptomatic within first 2 years. Approximately 60%–85% of heterotopic mucosa is gastric and 5%–16% is pancreatic. Other mucosa like colonic, endometrial and pancreatic islet are quite rare.

**4** There is an increased incidence of the following associations with Meckel's diverticulum *except*:

  **A** oesophageal atresia

  **B** Hirschsprung's disease

  **C** cardiovascular malformations

  **D** Down's syndrome

  **E** urachal anomalies.

 **4** **E** Most cases of Meckel's diverticulum are sporadic. There is an increased incidence with other anomalies such as:

  - oesophageal atresia
  - duodenal atresia
  - imperforate anus
  - omphalocele
  - malrotation
  - Hirschsprung's disease
  - Down's syndrome
  - congenital diaphragmatic hernia
  - congenital neurologic conditions
  - cardiovascular malformations.

Concomitant urachal and omphalomesenteric duct anomalies are rare. The presence of Meckel's diverticulum does not justify a search for other anomalies as <5% have associated anomalies. There has been a high incidence of incidental finding of Meckel's diverticulum with Crohn's disease (6%), but the presence of heterotopic mucosa in thess cases is extremely rare.

**Q5** Which of the following is true of clinical presentation of Meckel's diverticulum?

  **A** The type of presentation correlates with age.

  **B** Painful rectal bleeding is the most common presentation.

  **C** Occult bleeding with anaemia is a common feature.

  **D** Haematemesis is a common presentation.

  **E** *Helicobacter pylori* is a common causative agent for ulceration and bleeding.

 **5** **A** Most patients with Meckel's diverticulum are asymptomatic. Approximately 4%–16% of patients have related symptoms. The most common signs and symptoms of Meckel's diverticulum are bleeding, obstruction and inflammation. The type of presentation correlates with age. Intestinal obstruction due to volvulus or intussusception is the most typical presentation in newborns. In older infants and younger children, painless lower gastrointestinal bleeding is common. Older children usually present with inflammation mimicking appendicitis. Children are more likely to be symptomatic than adults. In adults inflammation and obstructive symptoms are common. Bleeding is generally painless, episodic and sometimes massive. Occult bleeding with anaemia is rare. *H. pylori* is rarely identified in the heterotopic gastric mucosa of a bleeding Meckel's diverticulum. This could be because of the bile salt toxicity, which affects the *H. pylori* microorganism.

**Q6** Possible mechanisms for intestinal obstruction seen with Meckel's diverticulum include all *except*:

 **A** intussusception

 **B** volvulus

 **C** prolapse through patent vitelline duct

 **D** Littre's hernia

 **E** ectopic gastric mucosa.

**A6** **E** The most common cause of intestinal obstruction secondary to Meckel's diverticulum is intussusception. Meckel's diverticulum acts as a pathological lead point and should be suspected in all cases of intussusception occurring in older children (>5 years). Pneumatic reduction in these cases is usually unsuccessful and the Meckel's diverticulum is identified at the time of bowel resection. Other mechanisms of intestinal obstruction include volvulus, inflammation, Meckel's diverticulum incarcerated in an inguinal hernia (Littre's hernia) and, rarely, prolapse through a patent vitelline duct. Volvulus can occur because of persistent vascular or vitelline remnants from the bowel or diverticulum attached to the abdominal wall allowing twisting, kinking or herniation. A giant Meckel's diverticulum can also cause volvulus in newborns. Ectopic gastric mucosa seen with Meckel's diverticulum usually causes bleeding and ulceration.

**Q7** Which of the following pathologies can occur with Meckel's diverticulum?

 **A** foreign body

 **B** stones

 **C** carcinoid tumour

 **D** carcinoid syndrome

 **E** all of the above

**A7** **E** Approximately 5% of patients with symptomatic Meckel's diverticulum present with umbilical abnormalities. They could manifest as an umbilical polyp, a persistent umbilical sinus connecting to the Meckel's diverticulum or an omphaloileal fistula. Rarely foreign bodies, stones and parasitic infections such as ascariasis or schistosomiasis have been reported within a Meckel's diverticulum. These can cause inflammation or can perforate through the diverticulum. Carcinoid tumours are more often seen in adults and are relatively aggressive. Tumours larger than

5mm have a significant risk for metastasis. Carcinoid syndrome can also occur with Meckel's diverticulum.

 **Q8** Which of the following factors is *not* associated with an increased risk of developing complications from Meckel's diverticulum?

   **A** age <40 years

   **B** male sex

   **C** presence of heterotopic mucosa

   **D** diverticular length >2 cm

   **E** association with Crohn's disease

**A8**   **E**  The lifetime risk of complications developing from an incidentally diagnosed Meckel's diverticulum ranges from 4.2% to 6.4%. The incidence of complications decreases with advancing age. Factors associated with increased likelihood of complications include age younger than 40 years, male sex, presence of heterotopic mucosa and diverticular length >2 cm. Most cases of Meckel's diverticulum associated with Crohn's disease are incidental findings at the time of hemicolectomy for Crohn's disease. The incidence of heterotopic mucosa seen with patients with Crohn's disease is very rare.

 **Q9** Regarding investigations for Meckel's diverticulum, which of the following is true?

   **A** Technetium-99m ($^{99m}$Tc) scan is indicated in all cases of Meckel's diverticulum.

   **B** Intestinal duplications can give rise to a positive $^{99m}$Tc scan.

   **C** Fasting decreases the yield of $^{99m}$Tc scan.

   **D** Selective angiography can detect a Meckel's diverticulum only in the presence of active bleeding.

   **E** When used, barium enema should always be performed before a $^{99m}$Tc scan.

 **A9**   **B**  $^{99m}$Tc pertechnetate scintiscan is useful when Meckel's diverticulum is complicated with episodes of bleeding. Because this scan is specific for gastric mucosa (in the stomach or ectopic) and not specifically diagnostic of Meckel's diverticulum, positive results can occur in other conditions where ectopic gastric mucosa is present. Duodenal ulcers, small intestinal obstruction, intestinal duplications, ureteric obstruction, aneurysms and angiomas of the small intestine yield false-positive results. False-negative results can occur when gastric mucosa is very slight or absent in the diverticulum, if necrosis of the diverticulum has occurred or if Meckel's diverticulum is superimposed on the bladder. The sensitivity is 80%–90%, specificity is 95% and accuracy is 90% for Meckel's diverticulum. Pentagastrin, histamine blockers and glucagons may enhance the accuracy of scanning. Likewise fasting, nasogastric suction and bladder catheterisation may increase the yield of scanning.

Barium study has a low diagnostic yield and is not routinely used. If performed, it should never precede $^{99m}$Tc scintiscan, because barium may obscure the hot spot. Selective arteriography may be helpful in patients in whom the results from scintiscan and barium studies are negative. They can detect a Meckel's diverticulum even in the absence of bleeding.

**Q10** Which of the following is true regarding treatment of Meckel's diverticulum?

**A** In cases of bleeding, a Meckel's diverticulectomy is the procedure of choice.

**B** All cases of Meckel's diverticulum require surgical resection.

**C** Elective removal of Meckel's diverticulum can result in adhesive bowel obstruction in 5%–10% of cases.

**D** Only symptomatic cases of Meckel's diverticulum need surgical resection.

**E** Meckel's diverticulum associated with intussusception do not need surgical removal.

**A10** **C** The treatment for Meckel's diverticulum is either a simple diverticulectomy or small-bowel resection with end-to-end anastomosis. Incidental appendicectomy is usually performed. The definitive treatment of complicated Meckel's diverticulum such as bleeding is by excision of the diverticulum along with adjacent ileal segment either using a stapling device of by hand-sewn anastomosis, which can also be accomplished laparoscopically. The ectopic gastric mucosa may extend along the adjacent ileum as well, on the mesenteric side opposite the ileum. Hence, in cases of bleeding, resection of a segment of adjacent ileum with end-to-end anastomosis is a safer option. A persistent right vitelline artery supplying the diverticulum is sometimes found during operation and must be identified and ligated.

The role of elective removal of asymptomatic Meckel's diverticulum is still controversial. The most common complication following elective removal of Meckel's diverticulum is adhesive bowel obstruction in 5%–10% of cases. In cases of intussusception secondary to Meckel's diverticulum, complete reduction with pneumatic or contrast enema is attempted followed by elective excision of Meckel's diverticulum. However, complete reduction is usually unsuccessful, and the diverticulum is often detected at the time of bowel resection.

**Q11** Indications for elective resection of incidentally discovered Meckel's diverticulum are:

  **A** palpable thickening suggestive of heterotopic mucosa

  **B** history of unexplained abdominal pain

  **C** in patients with abdominal wall attachments

  **D** in children less than 8 years old

  **E** all of the above.

**A11** **E** Management of asymptomatic Meckel's diverticulum is controversial. In the past, if Meckel's diverticulum was encountered in patients undergoing abdominal surgery, many surgeons recommended its removal. This has now been questioned given the overall likelihood of developing complications around 4.2%–6.4% and a decreasing risk with increasing age. A large number of Meckel's diverticulums would have to be excised to prevent one death.

On the other hand, some authors argue that the resection of Meckel's diverticulum is a simple operation, and the management of its complications is associated with high morbidity and mortality. Elective resection is recommended in cases with a palpable thickening suggestive of heterotopic mucosa, in those with unexplained abdominal pain, and in cases with abdominal wall attachment. In general, removal of incidental Meckel's diverticulum is indicated in children less than 8 years old, because infants and young children are at a greater risk for complications.

**Q12** Contraindications for elective removal of incidental Meckel's diverticulum are:

  **A** immunocompromised patients

  **B** patients undergoing insertion of prosthetic material

  **C** babies with gastroschisis

  **D** generalised peritonitis

  **E** all of the above.

**A12** **E** Elective excision of incidental Meckel's diverticulum is not recommended in cases highly susceptible to sepsis. It is generally contraindicated in immuno-compromised patients, those undergoing insertion of a prosthetic material and babies with gastroschisis, owing to the presence of a thickened serosal peel or prosthetic patch.

# Further reading

Moore TC. Omphalomesenteric duct malformations. *Semin Pediatr Surg.* 1996; 5(2): 116–23.

Park JJ, Wolff BG, Tollefson MK, *et al.* Meckel diverticulum: the Mayo Clinic experience with 1476 patients (1950–2002). *Ann Surg.* 2005; **241**(3): 529–33.

Yahchouchy EK, Marano AF, Etienne JC, *et al.* Meckel's diverticulum. *J Am Coll Surg.* 2001; **192**(5): 658–62.

Zani A, Eaton S, Rees CM, *et al.* Incidentally detected Meckel diverticulum: to resect or not to resect? *Ann Surg.* 2008; **247**(2): 276–81.

# CHAPTER 38

# Alimentary tract duplications

### BRICE ANTAO, SHAWQUI NOUR

**From the choices below each question, select the single best answer.**

**Q1** Which of the following is true regarding alimentary tract duplications (ATDs)?
A incidence of 1 in 4500 births
B well-developed coat of smooth muscle
C intimate anatomical association with some portion of the gastrointestinal tract
D epithelial lining representing intestinal tract mucosa
E all of the above

**A1** E Incidence of ATDs has been reported to be 1 in 4500 births with a male preponderance. Three common findings as above are seen regardless of its location.

**Q2** The aetiopathogenesis of ATD includes
A partial or abortive twinning
B split notochord theory
C persistent embryonic diverticulum
D aberrant recanalisation of alimentary tract lumen
E all of above.

**A2** E Multiple theories have been postulated, but no single theory can account for all known variants. A persistent embryonic diverticulum from the developing alimentary tract was the first postulated theory. It was later postulated that duplications resulted from aberrant recanalisation of the alimentary tract lumen. The coincidence of colonic and genitourinary tract duplications and similar findings in conjoined twins led to the partial twinning theory. The association of enteric duplication and spinal anomalies led to the 'split notochord theory'. Several other environmental factors such as trauma and hypoxia have also been implicated. This is supported by the presence of other anomalies like intestinal atresia, which may be induced by intrauterine vascular accidents.

**Q3** The most common location for ATD is:

    **A** colonic

    **B** rectal

    **C** jejunoileal

    **D** mediastinal

    **E** thoracoabdominal.

**A3**   **C** ATDs can occur anywhere from oropharynx to anus. Twenty per cent occur in the chest and the remainder in the abdomen, with just 2% thoracoabdominal. The various locations in decreasing order of frequency include jejunal and ileal (53%), mediastinal (18%), colonic (13%), gastric (7%), duodenal (6%), rectal (4%) and cervical (1%). Between 10% and 20% of cases are multiple and presence of one such lesion, should warrant a search for others.

**Q4** Which of the following is the most common association with ATDs?

    **A** VACTORL association

    **B** CHARGE association

    **C** spinal anomalies

    **D** Mayer–Rokitansky–Küster–Hauser's syndrome

    **E** malrotation

**A4**   **C** Vertebral, spinal and genitourinary anomalies make up the majority of associated anomalies with ATD seen in 30%–50% of cases. In oesophageal duplication, 20% of cases will have spinal communication, and 25% will also have an intestinal duplication. In thoracoabdominal duplication, there is 88% incidence of vertebral anomalies. Although vertebral, spinal and genitourinary anomalies make up the majority of associated anomalies, ATD in itself is not part of the spectrum of VACTORL and CHARGE association. They have also been associated with malrotation and intestinal atresias. Colonic duplication, which accounts for 15% of all duplications, and other duplicated structures such as bladder, vagina and external genitalia are described. Although vaginal aplasia is seen with Mayer–Rokitansky Küster–Hauser's syndrome, this is a disorder of müllerian duct anomaly and ATD is not spectrum of this syndrome.

**Q5** Which of the following is true regarding clinical manifestation of ATDs?

 A  Chest pain is most common presentation of ATD in the chest.

 B  Gastrointestinal bleeding is the most common presentation of ATD in the abdomen.

 C  Antenatal diagnosis in all cases.

 D  Malignancy is more common in antenatal diagnosed cases.

 E  The majority of cases are diagnosed in the first 2 years of life.

**A5**   **E**  ATDs do not have a classic presentation, but can manifest a variety of symptoms, which are related to the location, size, shape and type of mucosa. The majority of patients (80%) present prior to 2 years, with over half (60%) seen before 6 months of age. With increasing experience and availability of prenatal ultrasonography, antenatal diagnosis of ATD is becoming more common. A mass in the chest may present as wheezing, pneumonia, respiratory distress, vomiting, failure to thrive or dysphagia. Chest pain is a rare symptom unless the mass acutely enlarges from haemorrhage or infection. Abdominal pain, vomiting and an abdominal mass are the most common clinical presentation of ATD located in the abdomen. In cases with ectopic gastric mucosa, which is seen in 25%–30% cases, ulceration, bleeding and perforation can result. Duplications of the midgut or hindgut are more likely to cause abdominal pain, distension, melaena or perforation. Colon and hindgut duplications may simply present as a second opening on the perineum. In children duplications are considered benign lesions, but malignancy has been detected in adults.

**Q6** Which of the following complications are seen with ATD?

 A  hydrops fetalis

 B  volvulus

 C  intussusception

 D  recurrent pancreatitis

 E  all of the above

**A6**   **E**  A large duplication can cause localised volvulus of the adjacent intestine. Small-bowel duplications may also present as intussusception by acting as a lead point. Chest lesions may occasionally cause hydrops fetalis as a result of mediastinal shift and can be managed with *in utero* thoracoamniotic shunting. Duodenal duplications are mainly cystic and they may obstruct the biliopancreatic ducts causing jaundice or pancreatitis. The pancreatic duplications are the rarest form of duplication, and >50% are present in the pancreatic head and are sometimes difficult to distinguish from pseudocysts.

**Q7** Which of the following is *false* regarding the types of ATD?

    **A** The majority of small-bowel duplications are cystic.

    **B** Ectopic gastric mucosa is seen more frequently in the cystic type of duplication.

    **C** Thoracoabdominal duplications are invariably tubular.

    **D** Gastric duplications are mostly cystic.

    **E** Oesophageal duplications are mostly cystic and do not communicate with the oesophageal lumen.

**A7** **B** Enteric duplications are generally cystic or tubular masses. Most oesophageal duplications are cystic and do not share a muscular wall or communicate with the oesophageal lumen. Gastric duplications are most often cystic and located along the greater curvature. Thoracoabdominal duplications are all tubular, and a high percentage have ectopic gastric mucosa. The majority of small-bowel duplications are cystic. Ectopic gastric mucosa is seen in 80% of tubular and 20% of cystic duplications.

**Q8** Which of the following is *false* regarding diagnostic modalities for assessing ATD?

    **A** Characteristic features are noted on CT scan.

    **B** Characteristic features are noted on ultrasonography.

    **C** It can be diagnosed *in utero*.

    **D** It can be diagnosed with a technetium-99m ($^{99m}$Tc) pertechnetate scan.

    **E** Hindgut duplications have characteristic features on ultrasonography.

**A8** **E** Various imaging methods can help make the diagnosis. Plain radiographs may demonstrate a posterior mediastinal mass, suggesting an oesophageal duplication. Contrast studies may reveal a mass effect from the adjacent duplication or communication with the alimentary tract. In cases of oesophageal duplication, communication with the spinal column has been described in 20%, and 25% cases have associated abdominal duplications. Hence, further imaging with CT scan or MRI is warranted, with ultrasonography of abdomen as well. On CT scan an enhancing rim of tissue surrounding a fluid-filled cyst is diagnostic of ATD. Likewise, the typical sonographic appearance of duplications is an inner hyperechoic rim of mucosal-submucosal tissue and an outer hypoechoic muscular layer. Ectopic gastric mucosa is present in 25%–30% of cases, and in those cases presenting with bleeding or anaemia, a $^{99m}$Tc scintigraphy is useful. Most of these cases are now picked up on antenatal ultrasonography, including those in the chest and upper abdomen. Chest lesions may occasionally cause hydrops fetalis as a result of mediastinal shift. The diagnosis of hindgut duplications may be difficult. Accurate imaging and preoperative evaluation with CT scan, MRI, and sometimes barium enema, are essential to determine proper treatment.

**Q9** Which of the following is true regarding the management of small-bowel duplications?

   **A** Most cases of tubular duplication can be treated with simple enucleation of cyst.

   **B** Small-bowel resection with primary anastomosis is the usual approach.

   **C** Most cases of cystic duplication can be treated with simple enucleation of cyst.

   **D** Small cystic duplications are best treated by marsupialisation between the duplication and the adjacent intestine.

   **E** All of the above.

**A9**   **B** Surgical management of small-bowel duplications varies because of the heterogenicity of these malformations. Small-bowel resection with primary anastomosis is the usual approach. Only very small cystic duplications can be treated with enucleation without sacrificing the native blood supply. Long tubular duplications may be more difficult to manage because of the intimate blood supply to native bowel. Resection of large lengths of bowel poses risk of short gut syndrome. In these situations or in the presence of ectopic gastric mucosa, mucosal stripping or anastomosing the tubular duplication containing gastric mucosa to the stomach, allows the gastric acid to drain and preserves bowel length. Another approach to preserve bowel length in long tubular duplication is marsupialisation between the duplication and the adjacent intestine both proximally and distally.

**Q10** Which of the following is false regarding the management of ATD?

   **A** The preferred treatment for thoracoabdominal duplications is a one-stage combined thoracoabdominal approach.

   **B** Preferred approach for gastric duplication is excision without violating the lumen.

   **C** In cases with an intraspinal component, the thoracic component should be removed first.

   **D** Mucosal stripping is usually not needed in cases of colonic duplications.

   **E** External drainage rather than transrectal is the preferred approach for an abscess complicating a presacral duplication.

A10  C  It is usually recommended that the intraspinal component to a neuroenteric cyst be removed first. This is because of less morbidity from the potential for meningitis and less postoperative swelling when cyst is removed. Another approach in cases where there is a small neuroenteric cyst is application of a clip ligature to the intraspinal connection prior to excision of the thoracic/abdominal duplication. The intraspinal component can then be either left alone or dealt with at a later date. A single-staged approach is preferred for most thoracoabdominal duplications. Occasionally large thoracoabdominal cysts may be removed in a staged manner. When undertaking a staged approach, the remaining portion of the duplication must be decompressed (e.g. drainage into the intestine), avoiding postoperative sepsis due to leakage from an obstructed cyst. Most cases of gastric duplication can be removed without violating the lumen. Occasionally a partial gastrectomy may be required. Ectopic mucosa is very rare in colonic duplications, and hence mucosal striping is usually not needed. If a presacral duplication presents as an abscess, it is wise to drain it externally rather than through the rectum. Transrectal drainage leads to contamination of the lesion with faecal flora and recurrent abscess formation.

## Further reading

Chen JJ, Lee HC, Yeung CY, *et al.* Meta-analysis: the clinical features of the duodenal duplication cyst. *J Pediatr Surg.* 2010; **45**(8): 1598–606.

Conforti A, Nahom A, Capolupo I, *et al.* Prenatal diagnosis of esophageal duplication cyst: the value of prenatal MRI. *Prenat Diagn.* 2009; **29**(5): 531–2.

Keckler S, Holcomb G III. Alimentary tract duplications. In: Holcomb GW, Murphy JP. *Ashcraft's Pediatric Surgery.* 5th ed. Philadelphia, PA: Saunders; 2010. pp. 517–25.

Lund D. Alimentary tract duplications. In: Grosfeld JL, O'Neill JA, Fonkalsrud EW, *et al.*, editors. *Pediatric Surgery. Vol 1.* 6th ed. Philadelphia, PA: Mosby; 2006. pp. 1389–98.

# CHAPTER 39

# Intussusception

## VICTORIA LANE, BRICE ANTAO, MICHAEL S IRISH

From the choices below each question, select the single best answer.

**Q1** Regarding intussusception, which of the following statements is true?
  A The most common age at presentation for children with idiopathic intussusception is more than 2 years.
  B The most common age at presentation for children with secondary intussusception is 3–6 months.
  C Adenovirus is a common aetiological factor in primary intussusception.
  D The classic features of vomiting, abdominal pain, redcurrant jelly stool and an abdominal mass on presentation, are seen in 30%–40% of children with intussusception.
  E The term 'intussuscipiens' refers to the proximal invaginating intestine.

**A1**  **C** Intussusception is one of the most frequent causes of bowel obstruction in infants and toddlers. It occurs in 1 in 2000 infants and children. Male-to-female ratio ranges from 2 : 1 to 3 : 2. It was first described in 1674 by Paul Barbette and was subsequently described by Treves in 1899. The classic definition of intussusception is 'full thickness invagination of the proximal bowel (intussusceptum) into the distal contiguous intestine (intussuscipiens)'. John Hutchinson reported the first successful operation for intussusception in 1873, and Harald Hirschsprung later described hydrostatic reduction with an associated significant decrease in mortality.

Typically intussusception occurs in well-nourished healthy infants and over two-thirds of patients are male. Intussusception can be divided into primary (idiopathic) and secondary.

Primary intussusception (no pathological lead point) is the most common type of intussusception, commonly occurring soon after an upper respiratory tract infection or episode of gastroenteritis when the lead point is thought to be hypertrophied Peyer's patches in the ileal wall. Adenovirus and rotavirus have been implicated in around 50% of cases. Most cases of primary intussusception occur between the ages of 6 months and 3 years, when children are particularly susceptible to viral illnesses. There have been case reports of intussusception occurring in the premature neonate.

Secondary intussusception occurs in a slightly older age group, when an identifiable lead point is found. The incidence of definite anatomical lead point ranges from 1.5% to 12%. These anatomical lead points tend to present after 2 years of age, and commonly include Meckel's diverticulum, duplications of the bowel and polyps. Other benign lead points include the appendix, foreign bodies, hamartomas associated with Peutz–Jeghers's syndrome and lipomas. Malignant lead points do occur and are seen in lymphomas, lymphosarcomas and melanomas, and the incidence of these increases with increasing age. Small-bowel intussusception associated with indwelling feeding tubes has also been described.

The 'classic' history, as found in many textbooks, is that of an infant presenting with intermittent cramping abdominal pain, vomiting, redcurrant jelly stools and a palpable mass on abdominal examination. Less than 25% of patients will present with all features. The abdominal pain tends to be sudden in onset; there may be drawing of the knees to the chest, hyperextension and breath holding followed by vomiting. The pain may then subside quickly, with the child falling asleep. After repeated episodes the child becomes lethargic, may develop abdominal distension and bilious vomiting. The passage of blood per rectum is a late feature indicating bowel ischaemia and necrosis, placing the child at risk of overwhelming sepsis.

 **Which segment of bowel is most frequently associated with intussusception?**

A ileoileal

B colocolic

C ileocolic

D caecocolic

E jejunojejunal

 **C** The most common site for intussusception is ileocolic, with the ileum invaginating into the caecum or right ascending colon. The right lower quadrant may appear empty on examination (Dance's sign) because of the intussuscepted mass being pulled upwards. The second most common type is ileoileocolic, and has two anatomical components: first is ileoileal, which then invaginates into the caecum and colon and becomes ileoileocolic. Although this type can occasionally occur in the idiopathic group, 40% have a pathological lead point. Other rarer forms like appendicocolic, caecocolic, colocolic, jejunojejunal and ileoileal are usually associated with a pathological lead point.

**Q3** Regarding rectal prolapse and intussusception, which of the following is false?

    **A** In rectal prolapse, a lubricated tongue blade can be passed along the side of protruding mass.

    **B** Rectal prolapse can be differentiated from intussusception, based on clinical symptoms.

    **C** Prolapse of intussusceptum through the anus is a grave sign.

    **D** Prolapse of intussusception exhibit signs of systemic illness.

    **E** All of the above.

**A3**   **A** Prolapse of the intussusceptum through the anus is a grave sign, particularly when the intussusceptum is ischaemic. Such patients exhibit signs of systemic illness. On digital rectal examination it is often possible to ascertain whether this is a rectal prolapse or a prolapsed rectal intussusception. In rectal prolapse it is not possible to advance a tongue blade along the side wall of the prolapsed bowel, whereas in intussusception the blade can be advanced. Rectal prolapse, although it can present with discomfort, is not generally accompanied by vomiting or signs of sepsis. Hence, based on a good clinical history and examination, one can differentiate between the two and prompt management can be instituted. The greatest danger is the misdiagnosis of a prolapse of the intussusceptum and attempt to reduce what is thought to be a rectal prolapse.

**Q4** Which of the following is true of investigations in a case of suspected intussusception?

    **A** Abdominal radiograph is a first-line investigation to confirm the diagnosis of intussusception.

    **B** At ultrasonography, a pseudokidney sign on transverse section is diagnostic.

    **C** At ultrasonography, a doughnut sign on longitudinal section is diagnostic.

    **D** Ultrasonography can predict irreducibility of intussusception using pneumatic reduction.

    **E** All of the above are true.

**A4**   **D** The diagnosis of intussusception can be suspected on plain abdominal radiographs. Features suggestive of intussusception include an abdominal mass, abnormal distribution of gas and faecal contents, sparse large-bowel gas, and air–fluid levels in the presence of bowel obstruction. The 'meniscus' sign is a crescent-shaped lucency in the colon outlining the distal end of the intussus-ception. Although these features are suggestive of intussusception, plain films have limited value in confirming the diagnosis and cannot be used as the sole diagnostic test.

A very high accuracy rate has been reported for the use of ultrasonography in the diagnosis of intussusception. A transverse sonographic image of the bowel consisting of alternating rings of low and high echogenicity, representing the bowel wall and mesenteric fat within the intussusceptum, is diagnostic (target or doughnut sign). The 'pseudokidney' sign seen on longitudinal section appears as superimposed hypoechoic and hyperechoic layers. Other features predict the reducibility of the intussusception by enema and the presence of bowel necrosis; for example, a thick peripheral hypoechoic rim of intussusception, free intra-peritoneal fluid, fluid trapped within the intussusceptum, enlarged lymph nodes dragged with the mesentery into the intussusception, a pathological lead point and absence of blood flow in the intussusception on Doppler study. Although the presence of any of the above features may alert one to the possibility of irreducibility or necrosis, or both, it should not preclude attempting reduction by enema.

 **5** Which of the following statements is true with regard to non-operative reduction of intussusception?

**A** The maximum pressure recommended for pneumatic reduction is 180 mmHg.

**B** The risk of perforation in pneumatic reduction is 3.5%–6.3%.

**C** If the child develops a pneumoperitoneum following pneumatic reduction, the child should be taken immediately to the operating theatre.

**D** Hydrostatic reduction should always be performed under fluoroscopic control or ultrasonographic guidance.

**E** Children with significant abdominal tenderness should receive opiate analgesia prior to attempts at pneumatic and hydrostatic reduction.

 **5** **D** Prior to any attempts at non-operative/operative reduction, the infant must be adequately resuscitated with intravenous fluids and a nasogastric tube should be passed to decompress the stomach. The child should have secure intravenous access and be started on appropriate antibiotics. Persistent hypotension, peritonitis and bowel perforation are absolute contraindications to hydrostatic and pneumatic reduction.

Hydrostatic reduction involves placing a large catheter per rectum and attempts are made to form a seal by strapping the buttocks together. Under fluoroscopic/ultrasonographic control the contrast is instilled until contrast medium is seen to flow freely beyond the area of obstruction.

Pneumatic reduction uses a similar technique. Here, air is instilled to a maximum pressure of 80 mmHg for younger infants and 120 mmHg for older children, once again under fluoroscopic control. The perforation rate associated with pneumatic reduction is reported as 0.4%–2.5%. If the infant develops a tension pneumoperitoneum, a large-gauge cannula is placed immediately into the right iliac fossa to decompress the abdomen before transferring to theatre.

 **Q6** Which of the following is *not* an indication for operative management of intussusception?

**A** clinical evidence to suggest a pathological lead-point

**B** recurrence within 24 hours following non-operative management

**C** documentation of imaging confirming presence of a pathological lead point

**D** postoperative intussusception occurring 2 days post bowel resection and primary anastomosis

**E** persistence of symptoms after a successful reduction enema

 **A6** **B** Treatment of intussusception has changed over the last 50 years, with a move towards non-operative management. Non-operative reduction is performed by radiologists with pneumatic or hydrostatic pressure under fluoroscopic or sonographic visualisation and is successful in 85% of cases. Non-operative reduction of intussusception has been shown to reduce the length of hospital stay, shorten recovery, decrease hospital costs and decrease the complications associated with abdominal surgery. False-positive reductions do occur because of poor visualisation of the intussusception and reduction process.

Somme *et al.* (2006) reviewed the factors determining the need for operative reduction in children with intussusception. They reviewed 961 children aged less than 6 years, with intussusception, over an 8-year period. They had an operative rate of 25.4%. They identified that risk factors for operative management were the presence of a Meckel's diverticulum and being transferred from one institution to another over 24 hours after admission.

The French Study Group for Paediatric Laparoscopy reviewed 69 patients (48 males and 21 females) with intussusception, who were managed initially with attempted hydrostatic reduction but required operative management. In total 31.9% required an open procedure, 11 patients because of failure of laparoscopic reduction. The risk for conversion to open surgery was found to be directly linked to the length of time between the onset of symptoms and diagnosis, peritonitis at presentation (did not undergo attempts at non-operative management) and the presence of a pathological lead point. They concluded that children with a history less than 36 hours with no signs of peritonitis were the best candidates for laparoscopic reduction.

Indications for operative reduction include:
- irreducible recurrence
- clinical evidence to suggest a pathological lead point
- documentation of a pathological lead point by an imaging procedure
- persistence of symptoms after completion of the reduction enema.

Pathological lead points can be identified in about 6% of cases. Naturally, general manifestations of underlying disease indicate the specific cause of the intus-susception for example perioral pigmentation in Peutz–Jeghers's syndrome and the classic rash of Henoch–Schönlein's purpura seen over the buttocks and extensor aspects of the arms and legs. Pathological lead points are identified in the majority of children over the age of 5 years and the percentages with respect to age range are shown in Table 39.1. In a review of 3468 patients with intussus-ception, the most common lesions acting as a lead point were, in order, Meckel's diverticulum, lymphoma/lymphosarcoma, Peutz–Jeghers's, duplication cysts with an overall percentage of 6.5%.

| Age group | 0–11 months | 12–24 months | 3 years | 4 years | 5–14 years |
|---|---|---|---|---|---|
| % with pathological lead point | 5 | 10 | 15 | 23 | 58 |

TABLE 39.1 Age-related correlation of intussusception with pathological lead point

**Q7** Regarding recurrent intussusception, which of the following statements is false?

**A** Recurrence of intussusception occurs on average in 5% of patients.

**B** Recurrent intussusception (within 2 weeks of initial presentation) is less likely to reduce with non-operative methods.

**C** Thirty-three per cent of recurrences occur within 24 hours.

**D** Intussusception accounts for 3%–10% of postoperative bowel obstruction.

**E** Recurrent intussusception tends to present earlier.

**A7** **B** The recurrence rate for intussusception is quoted as occurring in 2%–20% of cases, with the average being 5%. A third of recurrences occur within the first 24 hours and the vast majority occur within the first 6 months of the initial episode. Recurrences do not usually have any defined lead point and they are less likely to occur after surgical reduction/resection. Success rates with enema reduction after one recurrence are comparable with those after the first episode, but less successful after an initial surgical reduction. This may be due to the parents presenting earlier because of early recognition of worrying symptoms.

Q8 Which of the following statements with regard to postoperative intussusception is false?

A Most postoperative intussusceptions are ileocolic.

B Postoperative intussusception is a recognised complication of Wilms's tumour resection.

C Postoperative intussusception presents at a similar time to those with adhesive obstruction.

D Postoperative intussusception occurs in 0.08% of all paediatric laparotomies.

E Most postoperative intussusceptions have a latent period of 6–8 weeks following surgery.

A8 C Postoperative intussusception is a rare but well-recognised clinical entity. The reported incidence ranges from 0.5% to 16% of all cases of intussusception and 0.08% of all paediatric laparotomies. Most cases occur after major abdominal surgery, especially in those where there has been extensive retroperitoneal dissection, such as nephrectomy for Wilms's tumour.

Postoperative intussusception accounts for 3%–10% of cases of postoperative bowel obstruction during childhood. In contrast to adhesions, which tend to occur within 2 years of laparotomy, postoperative intussusception occurs in 90% of all cases within less than 14 days (64% within the first 7 days) post laparotomy. Only 25% of patients with postoperative intussusception are infants. In postoperative intussusception the lead point tends to be proximal, involving the jejunum or proximal ileum.

The aetiology of postoperative intussusception is varied; presumed causes include a lead point from a suture line or appendiceal stump, disordered intestinal motility secondary to extensive retroperitoneal dissection, postoperative oedema, bowel handling, electrolyte disturbances, radiation and chemotherapy.

## Further reading

Blakelock RT, Beasley SW. The clinical implications of non-idiopathic intussusception. *Pediatr Surg Int*. 1998; **14**(3): 163–7.

Holcomb GW, Murphy JP. *Ashcraft's Pediatric Surgery*. 5th ed. Philadelphia, PA: Saunders; 2010.

Linke F, Eble F, Berger S. Postoperative intussusception in childhood. *Pediatr Surg Int*. 1998; **14**(3): 175–7.

Niramis R, Watanatittan S, Kruatrachue A, *et al*. Management of recurrent intussusception: nonoperative or operative reduction. *J Pediatr Surg*. 2010; **45**(11): 2175–80.

Somme S, To T, Langer JC. Factors determining the need for operative reduction in children with intussusception: a population-based study. *J Pediatr Surg*. 2006; **41**(5): 1014–19.

## CHAPTER 40

# Necrotising enterocolitis

### RODRIGO ROMAO, J TED GERSTLE

**From the choices below each question, select the single best answer.**

 **1** Regarding the occurrence of necrotising enterocolitis (NEC), which of the following is true?

    **A** There is no association between birthweight or gestational age and NEC.

    **B** Almost all patients diagnosed with NEC require surgical intervention.

    **C** The mortality rate for NEC is the same for patients managed medically or surgically and is approximately 50%.

    **D** Over 90% of patients diagnosed with NEC were previously enterally fed and breast milk can be considered protective when compared with formula.

    **E** NEC is much more common in male than female newborn babies.

 **1**   **D**   Overall frequency of NEC is estimated to be 1% of all live births but can be as high as 7% in selected populations of very low birthweight (VLBW) infants. Prematurity is present in more than 90% of the cases and incidence is inversely related to gestational age and birthweight. There is no gender predilection. The occurrence of NEC in babies who have never been fed is rare. Over 90% of babies with NEC have received enteral feeds and there is an estimated 3- to10-fold risk reduction in infants who have been fed breast milk. The overall mortality rate for NEC ranges between 15% and 30% and is significantly higher (up to 50%) in babies who undergo surgery. Surgical intervention is required in 20%–40% of patients.

**Q2** Possible pathogenic mechanisms for NEC include all *except*:

   **A** There is an association between congenital heart defects/heart surgery and NEC in full-term babies.

   **B** There is evidence to support immaturity of the intestinal barrier as the single most important factor associated with NEC.

   **C** Abnormal bacterial colonisation and immaturity of gastrointestinal tract immunity play an important role in the pathogenesis of NEC.

   **D** Currently, the aetiology of NEC can be considered largely multi-factorial with a series of events culminating in injury to the bowel mucosa in a susceptible host.

   **E** Abnormal motility patterns in premature babies can lead to a prolonged exposure of the mucosa to deleterious substances as well as inadequate clearance of bacteria with subsequent overgrowth.

**A2**   **B** The exact pathophysiology of NEC has been closely studied but is still a matter of considerable debate. At this time, it is accepted that all the following factors outlined may play a role in the development of NEC with no clear indication that one is more important than the others:

- immature intestinal motility and digestion
- abnormal intestinal barrier function
- abnormal bacterial colonisation
- immaturity of the intestinal immunological defences
- impaired circulatory regulation
- circulatory and ischaemic changes to the bowel, as can occur in pre-term and full-term infants with cyanotic congenital cardiac disease (pre- or postoperatively), may predispose these infants to NEC.

**Q3** The radiological sign known as pneumatosis intestinalis (PI) refers to which of the following?

   **A** presence of gas in the portal vein

   **B** presence of intramural gas dissecting the bowel layers

   **C** bowel perforation

   **D** presence of an ileus

   **E** none of the above

**A3**   **B** PI is the cornerstone of radiographic diagnosis of NEC. In a patient with a suggestive clinical presentation, the presence of PI confirms the diagnosis of NEC. If a patient does not have PI, NEC is still a possible diagnosis. The pathogenesis of PI involves the breakdown of mucosal integrity with air dissecting the bowel layers. Subserosal gas usually has a linear appearance whereas submucosal gas has more of a bubbly appearance and, when extensive, can be hard to differentiate from stool.

**Q4** Radiological and laboratory signs that suggest worsening NEC include all of the following *except*:

  **A** elevated CRP (C-reactive protein)

  **B** portal venous gas on abdominal X-ray

  **C** thrombocytopenia

  **D** metabolic acidosis

  **E** diffuse pneumatosis intestinalis.

**A4**  **A**  The presence of diffuse pneumatosis intestinalis and/or portal venous gas on abdominal X-rays is associated with significant NEC. Persistent thrombocytopenia and metabolic acidosis are part of Bell's modified criteria and raise the suspicion for bowel perforation. CRP is usually elevated in inflammatory states; however, it is quite non-specific for the different stages of NEC and its complications.

**Q5** A 2-week-old premature baby boy with a birthweight of 900 g, who was being fed formula, suddenly develops episodes of apnoea and bradycardia that require intubation, mild abdominal distension and tenderness, and occult blood in the stool. His abdominal X-ray shows uniformly distended loops of bowel with gas in the rectum, no pneumatosis intestinalis and no pneumoperitoneum. Based on this clinical scenario, which of the following statements is most correct?

  **A** This patient has a definite diagnosis of NEC and should be treated with bowel rest, gastric decompression and broad-spectrum antibiotics for at least 7 days.

  **B** This patient has advanced NEC and should be taken immediately to the operating room.

  **C** This patient has suspected NEC. He should be started on broad-spectrum antibiotics and abdominal X-rays should be obtained to confirm the diagnosis. Feeds should *not* be stopped unless there is clear radiological diagnosis of pneumatosis intestinalis.

  **D** This patient has a definite diagnosis of NEC and the length of treatment will depend on the progression of the disease and/or the development of complications.

  **E** This patient has suspected NEC. Initial management includes bowel rest, gastric decompression, broad-spectrum antibiotics, serial X-rays and frequent clinical re-evaluations. Septic ileus could present in a similar fashion.

**A5**  **E**  The diagnosis of NEC is based on the presence of general and gastrointestinal signs and symptoms combined with imaging findings. The staging system proposed by Bell has been slightly modified and is still largely utilised worldwide to guide diagnostic and therapeutic decisions:

| Stage | Systemic signs | Intestinal signs | Radiological signs |
|---|---|---|---|
| **Stage 1 Suspected NEC** | Temp instability, apnoea, bradycardia, lethargy | Increased pre-feed residuals, mild abdom distension, emesis, occult blood in stool | Normal or intestinal dilatation, mild ileus |
| **Stage 2A Definite NEC** | As above | Absent bowel sounds, prominent distension, grossly bloody stools | Intest dilatation, ileus, focal pneumatosis intestinalis |
| **Stage 2B Definite NEC** | Mild metabolic acidosis, thrombocytopenia | Definite abdominal tenderness, palpable loops, abdominal wall oedema | Widespread pneumatosis, ascites, portal venous gas |
| **Stage 3A Advanced NEC** | Hypotension, coagulopathy, oliguria, mixed acidosis | Abdominal wall erythema, induration and oedema | Prominent bowel loops, no free air, worsening ascites |
| **Stage 3B Advanced NEC** | Shock, deterioration | Bowel perforation | Pneumoperitoneum |

TABLE 40.1 Modified Bell's Staging Criteria for necrotising enterocolitis

Based on the criteria in Table 40.1, this case illustrates a patient who clearly has stage 1 (suspected) NEC. Close follow-up is warranted to determine if the patient will develop definite NEC (stage 2A or worse) with worsening abdominal signs and specific radiological findings such as pneumatosis intestinalis. Neonatal sepsis can cause an ileus and may be undistinguishable from a diagnosis of suspected NEC.

 **Q6** Twenty-four hours after the scenario in question 5, the baby's abdomen becomes more distended and tender, albeit without any inflammatory signs in the abdominal wall. The abdominal X-ray now shows linear pneumatosis intestinalis in the right lower quadrant and questionable portal vein gas. At this point the *best* therapeutic approach is:

**A** Repeat the abdominal X-ray in 6 hours to confirm the presence of portal vein gas. If it is confirmed, the patient should be taken to the operating room immediately.

**B** Irrespective of the presence of portal vein gas, this patient needs a laparotomy.

**C** A penrose drain should be inserted into the abdomen at the bedside.

**D** Monitor the patient's clinical status closely and repeat abdominal films at least every 8 hours looking for radiological signs of pneumoperitoneum.

**E** Repeat the abdominal X-rays every 8 hours. If the pneumatosis intestinalis does not disappear in 24 hours, a surgical procedure (placement of a drain or laparotomy) is indicated.

**A6**  **D**  The patient now has a definite diagnosis of NEC. Initial treatment for NEC is almost always medical with bowel rest, decompression (nasogastric tube) and broad-spectrum antibiotics. Surgical treatment is usually indicated when signs of perforation are evident, there is continued clinical deterioration in the setting of optimal medical management, and/or there are radiological findings of necrotic intestine. The presence of pneumatosis intestinalis alone is not an indication for surgery. Although portal venous gas has been traditionally correlated with higher mortality rates, it is not an absolute indication for surgery. This patient needs frequent re-examinations and serial X-rays looking for pneumoperitoneum.

**Q7**  All of the following are *relative* indications for surgical treatment of NEC *except*:

    **A**  fixed loops on plain abdominal film

    **B**  abdominal wall erythema

    **C**  palpable mass

    **D**  failure of medical management

    **E**  free air on abdominal X-ray.

**A7**  **E**  The only absolute indication for surgical intervention in patients with NEC is the presence of free air on abdominal X-rays. All of the alternatives are classic relative indications for surgery.

**Q8**  Which of the following statements is true regarding small (<1000 g) premature babies with intestinal perforation?

    **A**  Laparotomy with bowel resection is the treatment of choice and should eventually be undertaken in all patients.

    **B**  Primary peritoneal drainage can be used only as a temporising measure until the patient is more stable to undergo laparotomy.

    **C**  Initial bedside insertion of a Penrose drain into the abdominal cavity is acceptable and may be the only surgical treatment required.

    **D**  Primary peritoneal drainage has the same survival rate as laparotomy but the time patients spend on parenteral nutrition is significantly longer.

    **E**  Primary peritoneal drainage is a treatment of exception and should be reserved only for patients that are moribund and cannot tolerate a laparotomy.

**A8**  **C**  Primary peritoneal drainage for premature patients with NEC was described in the 1970s. The principle behind it was to avoid aggressive surgical intervention in unstable patients. Initially, it was considered a temporising measure until the patient could tolerate a full laparotomy; however, over time it has been acknowledged that in many cases drainage may be the only procedure needed. A multicentre, prospective, randomised clinical trial failed to show any difference in survival of patients below 1500 g that underwent laparotomy vs. drainage. Furthermore, no difference was documented in terms of long-term parenteral nutrition dependence. A subset of patients in the peritoneal drainage group did require laparotomy early for clinical deterioration or later for strictures or bowel obstruction. These are reasons why patients treated with a peritoneal drain should be followed closely; however, some may not require any additional surgical treatment.

**Q9** Regarding spontaneous intestinal perforation (SIP), which of the following statements is not true?

**A** It usually happens in the antimesenteric border of the terminal ileum.

**B** In general, patients are not as critically ill as patients with NEC.

**C** An association with the use of indomethacin for treatment of persistent ductus arteriosus (PDA) in premature babies has been suggested but never adequately documented.

**D** It is very easy to differentiate SIP from NEC preoperatively.

**E** Apart from the perforated site, the rest of the bowel usually looks healthy.

**A9** **D** Isolated ileal perforation (also called SIP) is often considered a separate entity from NEC. Usually, patients with SIP are not as ill as patients with NEC, although preoperative distinction between the two is very difficult; an association between SIP and the use of indomethacin for PDA closure has been suggested but never confirmed.

**Q10** When operating on a newborn with NEC, which of the following is true?

**A** It is more common to find a perforation in the small bowel.

**B** It is more common to find a perforation in the colon.

**C** The disease seldom affects multiple segments of bowel separated by normal areas.

**D** The most common finding is an isolated perforation in the terminal ileum.

**E** Although uncommon, massive necrosis of the entire bowel is possible and usually lethal.

**A10** **E** Small bowel (usually ileum) and large bowel seem to be *equally* affected by NEC. Additionally, multiple-segment disease ('patchy' bowel necrosis with normal areas in between) is as common as single-segment disease. A small subset of patients with NEC have massive, diffuse bowel necrosis for which there is not much to be offered in terms of surgical treatment and the mortality rate in these patients is very high.

**Q11** When dealing with diffuse NEC and indeterminate bowel viability, the best surgical option is:

   **A** 'clip and drop' technique

   **B** resection of all suspect areas and creation of a stoma

   **C** resection of all suspect areas and creation of multiple primary anastomoses

   **D** resection of all suspect areas and creation of multiple primary anastomoses over a silicon catheter

   **E** do nothing and close the abdomen.

**A11**  **A**  In the setting of diffuse NEC, it can be difficult to determine bowel viability. Affected areas that are not clearly necrotic may recover. The 'clip and drop' technique involves resection of only clearly necrotic bowel, stapling off areas of intermediate viability, and reoperating in 48 hours for reassessment and definitive management. Performing multiple anastomoses over a silicon catheter ('stent') is a valid option in cases of patchy small-bowel disease, where necrotic and viable segments are clearly identifiable.

**Q12** An 1100 g premature baby with free air on the X-ray is taken to the operating room and found to have a perforation in the terminal ileum with NEC involving approximately 15 cm of the distal small bowel. In addition, the left colon is mildly inflamed but not perforated. Which of the following statements is true?

   **A** Bowel resection with primary anastomosis is contraindicated.

   **B** Since surgery is being performed and the disease is not diffuse, all segments of affected bowel (ileum and colon) should be resected and the patient should get an ileostomy.

   **C** A stoma should be created proximal to the perforation to allow it to heal and prevent loss of bowel length.

   **D** Resection of the ileum including the perforation and ileostomy is probably the safest surgical approach in this case.

   **E** None of the above.

**A12**  **D**  Traditionally, patients with NEC who require a laparotomy get a stoma. During the operation, the entire bowel should be assessed and areas with obvious ischaemia, necrosis and perforation should be resected. More recently, it has been suggested that primary anastomosis is feasible even in babies <1000 g, but this hypothesis is yet to be proven in the context of a clinical trial. That is why a primary anastomosis is not formally contraindicated, but in this patient, with a perforation and more distal involvement in the colon, an ileostomy after bowel resection is probably the safest approach.

$Q$13 Long-term complications of NEC include all of the following *except*:

   **A** short bowel syndrome

   **B** bowel strictures

   **C** inflammatory bowel disease

   **D** neurodevelopmental problems

   **E** stoma-related electrolyte imbalance.

$A$13 **C** There has been no association reported between NEC and future development of inflammatory bowel disease. Short bowel syndrome is possible in cases of diffuse disease and major resection. The stricture rate after NEC is between 10% and 35% for patients managed both medically and surgically and also for patients who had peritoneal drains as their primary treatment. Neurodevelopmental problems are related to NEC as well as to the concurrent diseases associated with prematurity.

$Q$14 Possible complication of an ileostomy for NEC in a 1200 g infant include:

   **A** failure to thrive

   **B** hyponatraemia and dehydration

   **C** prolapse

   **D** skin excoriation

   **E** all of the above.

$A$14 **E** Stoma-related complications in children, especially infants, have long been recognised. They can be divided into the following:

   1 Technical (local) complications: prolapse, retraction, stricture, parastomal hernia, skin excoriation.

   2 Medical (systemic) complications: dehydration, hyponatraemia, malnutrition. These are seen frequently with ileostomies because the output is usually quite high in volume and the patient experiences significant intestinal losses of sodium and water.

## Further reading

Epelman M, Daneman A, Navarro OM, *et al*. Necrotizing enterocolitis: review of state-of-the-art imaging findings with pathologic correlation. *Radiographics*. 2007; **27**(2):285–305.

Hall NJ, Curry J, Drake DP, *et al*. Resection and primary anastomosis is a valid surgical option for infants with necrotizing enterocolitis who weigh less than 1000 g. *Arch Surg*. 2005; **140**(12): 1149–51.

Henry MC, Moss RL. Neonatal necrotizing enterocolitis. *Semin Pediatr Surg*. 2008; **17**(2): 98–109.

Lin PW, Stoll BJ. Necrotising enterocolitis. *Lancet*. 2006; **368**(9543): 1271–83.

Moss RL, Dimmitt RA, Barnhart DC, *et al*. Laparotomy versus peritoneal drainage for necrotizing enterocolitis and perforation. *N Engl J Med*. 2006; **354**(21): 2225–34.

# CHAPTER 41

# Short bowel syndrome

## DEREK WAKEMAN, JENNIFER A LEINICKE, BRAD W WARNER

From the choices below each question, select the single best answer.

**Q1** In the paediatric population, the most common cause of short bowel syndrome (SBS) is:

    **A** congenital atresia

    **B** midgut volvulus

    **C** necrotising enterocolitis (NEC)

    **D** gastroschisis

    **E** Hirschsprung's disease.

**A1**   **C**   The most common aetiology of SBS in children and infants today is NEC. Historically, the most common aetiologies of SBS were midgut volvulus and congenital intestinal atresias. However, as neonatal medicine has improved the treatment of premature lung disease, the number of premature infants with a propensity for developing NEC has increased dramatically. Most cases of SBS result after resection of infarcted bowel as is the case in children with NEC and midgut volvulus. However, functional disorders also exist wherein the bowel length is normal, but motility and the ability to provide sufficient enteral nutrition are impaired (long-segment Hirschsprung's disease and idiopathic intestinal pseudo-obstruction). Gastroschisis, another common cause of paediatric SBS, usually involves a combination of severely dyskinetic small bowel and congenitally foreshortened intestine. Inflammatory bowel diseases, such as Crohn's disease, typically affect older children. Crohn's disease may lead to SBS if its severity leads to multiple, extensive bowel resections or fistulas that bypass absorptive mucosa. Finally, mesenteric vascular occlusion is a rare cause of SBS in this patient population. In this case invasive aortic monitoring devices, neonatal aortic thrombosis, or cardiogenic emboli lead to occlusion of the mesenteric vasculature and subsequent bowel infarction.

**Q2** During intestinal adaptation after massive small-bowel resection, the following things are known to occur *except*:

   **A** increased bowel calibre

   **B** increased mucosal surface area

   **C** increased enterocyte proliferation

   **D** decreased enterocyte apoptosis

   **E** increased digestive capacity per unit length.

**A2**   **D** After massive bowel resection, there is a compensatory response known as intestinal adaptation. During adaptation the bowel increases in calibre and, to a lesser degree, length. Mucosal surface area is enhanced by increases in villus length and crypt depth. Mucosal expansion is driven by increased enterocyte turnover; both enterocyte proliferation and apoptosis increase during intestinal adaption. Functional adaptation, measured by digestive enzymatic activity per unit area, is also more robust after intestinal resection.

**Q3** Efficacy has been demonstrated in clinical trials for which of the following factors as part of multimodality or combination therapy for patients with SBS?

   **A** growth hormone (GH)

   **B** insulin-like growth factor-1 (IGF-1)

   **C** epidermal growth factor (EGF)

   **D** glucagon-like peptide-1 (GLP-1)

   **E** thyroid hormone

**A3**   **A** Many endogenous hormones have been shown to enhance intestinal adaptation after massive small-bowel resection in animal models including GH, IGF-1, EGF, GLP-2, and thyroid hormone. However, only GH and GLP-2 have been tested in clinical trials in humans. GH administration has been shown to help patients gain body mass and wean from parenteral nutrition. Some of the clinical trials on GH tested its efficacy when combined with glutamine and a modified diet (usually a high-carbohydrate, low-fat diet). In early clinical studies GLP-2 (not GLP-1) has been shown to help patients with SBS gain weight. Because of its short half-life, an analogue of GLP-2 with improved pharmacokinetics has been developed and is being tested in short bowel patients with encouraging results.

**Q4** All of the following factors are thought to be important for intestinal adaptation *except*:

**A** presence of ileocaecal valve

**B** pancreatic secretions

**C** biliary secretions

**D** presence of enteral nutrition

**E** composition of enteral nutrition.

**A4** **A** While the presence of an ileocaecal valve is correlated with decreased likelihood of developing SBS, it is not specifically known to augment intestinal adaptation. However, there is evidence in animal models that both pancreatic and biliary secretions promote adaptation. In addition, the presence of luminal nutrition is known to enhance adaptation. This is evidenced by the fact that starvation leads to mucosal atrophy, while refeeding causes mucosal expansion. The python has been used as an animal model to study adaptation; feeding causes the intestinal mucosa to grow up to 10 times thicker than in the starving state. The composition of enteral nutrition has also been found to affect adaptation with more complex nutrient sources such as long-chain and unsaturated fats providing the most trophic stimulus.

**Q5** Which of the following is the most important factor for clinical outcomes after massive small-bowel resection?

**A** presence of ileocaecal valve

**B** site of intestinal resection

**C** aetiology of small-bowel syndrome

**D** age of patient

**E** length of remnant bowel

**A5** **E** Several factors shape the clinical response that follows massive bowel resection. However, the amount of bowel removed, or conversely, the length of bowel remaining after resection is thought to be the most important predictor and has been shown to strongly correlate with achieving independence from parenteral nutrition. The age of the patient is also important, particularly in the paediatric population. Infants are born with 200–250 cm of small intestine. During fetal development, the length of small bowel increases with age. The period of greatest growth is during the third trimester, when the small-bowel length doubles. The rate of small intestinal growth remains rapid after birth until crown–heel length approaches 60 cm; growth slows between crown–heel lengths 60 and 100 cm, and little growth occurs after 100–140 cm. In this way, a neonate born prematurely with 30 cm of small bowel left after resection would be more likely to wean from parenteral nutrition than a 15-year-old with the same length of bowel. The aetiology of SBS is also felt to be important, but exactly how each disease impacts overall prognosis is still unknown. The site of bowel resection can lead to specific complications. For instance, extensive proximal resections are felt to be better tolerated than equivalent distal resections because the ileum is believed to have more adaptive capacity than the jejunum. In addition, the distal ileum has specific absorptive functions, such as bile salt and vitamin $B_{12}$ absorption. The presence of an ileocaecal valve often receives a great deal of attention from practitioners. The ileocaecal valve is thought to slow transit of intestinal contents, thereby allowing more time for nutrient absorption. The valve is also said to help prevent backwash of colonic microbes that may promote bacterial overgrowth. However, studies are mixed with regard to its true clinical significance.

 **Q6** Complications from total parenteral nutrition (TPN) include all of the following *except*:

**A** catheter sepsis

**B** cholestasis

**C** venous thrombosis

**D** immune deficiency

**E** electrolyte imbalance.

 **A6** **D** The use of TPN affords remarkable survival improvement for patients with SBS. However, TPN does lead to many complications, some of which can be life-threatening. Indeed, the most common cause of death in patients with SBS is TPN-induced hepatic dysfunction. Although new formulations of TPN being tested to reduce the extent of hepatic toxicity, this remains a serious drawback of long-term parenteral nutrition. TPN, if calculated and administered incorrectly, can lead to electrolyte imbalances and fluid shifts, particularly in smaller patients. Because TPN requires central venous access, its use can lead to venous thrombosis, subsequent extremity swelling, and catheter sepsis. Long-term TPN use can result in a lack of central venous access because of indwelling catheters causing thrombosis and stenosis of available veins. TPN would be expected to promote immune function (relative to a malnourished state) as the nutrients support immune health.

 **Q7** Resection of which portion of the alimentary tract may result in gastric hypersecretion?

**A** stomach

**B** jejunum

**C** ileum

**D** ileocaecal valve

**E** colon

**A7** **B** The site of enterectomy has important consequences on intestinal physiology. Removal of the jejunum produces minimal permanent defects in the absorption of macronutrients and electrolytes because the ileum has the greatest capacity to adapt and take over these absorptive functions. However, jejunectomy may result in gastric hypersecretion because several of the intestinal hormones responsible for gastric inhibition are produced mainly in the jejunum. Loss of the ileum, on the other hand, can result in several pathological sequelae. The ileum is the primary site for bile salt absorption, and extensive ileal resection can lead to depletion of the bile salt pool with subsequent fat malabsorption and cholelithiasis. The ileum is also the primary site for absorption of the fat-soluble vitamins (A, D, E and K). Vitamin $B_{12}$ is absorbed exclusively in the terminal ileum when bound to intrinsic factor. Resection of the ileum can lead to vitamin $B_{12}$ deficiency and megaloblastic anaemia. The colon, while not essential for any specific nutrient absorption, should be preserved, as it provides both absorptive surface area for passive nutrient absorption and a braking effect on intestinal transit. The ileocaecal valve is thought to slow transit of intestinal contents, thereby allowing more time for nutrient absorption. The valve is also said to help prevent backwash of colonic microbes that may promote bacterial overgrowth.

**Q8** The length of the small intestine in a full-term infant is:
   **A** 100–150 cm
   **B** 150–200 cm
   **C** 200–250 cm
   **D** 250–300 cm
   **E** 300–350 cm.

**A8** **C** Normal small intestine length in term infants is 200–250 cm. The growth rate of the gastrointestinal tract increases with gestational age, the most rapid growth occurring during the last trimester. In fact continual elongation of the small bowel can be expected until the crown–heel length reaches 100–140 cm. Therefore, after massive bowel resection during the neonatal period, consideration should be given to the expected rate of intestinal lengthening due to developmental growth.

**Q9** Which of the following is not true regarding effects of bacterial overgrowth?
   **A** Luminal conjugated bile acids increase.
   **B** Fat malabsorption occurs.
   **C** Short-chain fatty acids increase.
   **D** Mucosal inflammation occurs.
   **E** Patients without an ileocaecal valve are at increased risk.

A⁹    **A**  Bacterial overgrowth commonly plagues patients with SBS. It occurs in the dilated, dysfunctional segments of intestine common in these patients. This syndrome is driven by bacteria colonising the remnant bowel leading to decreased conjugated bile acids. This, in turn, results in fat malabsorption, increased short-chain fatty acids, and diarrhoea. Bacterial overgrowth also leads to mucosal inflammation which further exacerbates malabsorption. Patients without an ileocaecal valve are thought to be at an increased risk for bacterial overgrowth as bacteria in the colon are able to reflux into the intestine. This syndrome should be suspected in patients with abrupt onset diarrhoea and dilated bowel loops on radiographic imaging. Its diagnosis requires a high index of suspicion and treatment is often empiric. Antibiotics are the mainstay of treatment and are aimed at gram-positive, gram-negative and anaerobic organisms.

Q10   You are taking care of a 5-month-old child, born at 30 weeks' gestation, with a history of NEC requiring multiple small-bowel resections. His GI tract is now in continuity, but he remains TPN dependent because of SBS. When is the optimal time to perform an operative intervention for the treatment of SBS?

   **A**  When the child is less than 6 months of age.
   **B**  When the child is a year out from his original surgery and continues to progress with tolerance of enteral feedings.
   **C**  When the child is 8 months of age, has developed TPN cholestasis, and has required multiple admissions to the hospital for catheter-induced sepsis.
   **D**  When the child is a year out from his original surgeries, has had minimal complications secondary to TPN, but has had worsening tolerance of enteral feedings.
   **E**  C and D.

A10   **E**  The best surgical approach for SBS is prevention. Avoidance of SBS requires prompt surgical intervention in patients at risk for bowel ischaemia and a conservative approach to intestinal resection. After bowel resection, the ultimate goal is to provide all calories enterally and to discontinue TPN. Patients often reach a point where stool output and/or electrolyte losses limit the ability to advance enteral feeding or develop complications related to parenteral nutrition. Additionally, some patients' tolerance of enteral nutrition may actually worsen and require increasing, rather than decreasing, amounts of TPN. Operative intervention should be considered for patients who suffer complications of TPN, fail to advance on enteral nutrition, or experience decreased tolerance of enteral nutrition.

   Optimising the timing of surgical intervention is also important. Surgery performed too early may be unnecessary because normal post-resection adaptation or intestinal lengthening due to normal growth may prevent the need for long-term TPN. Surgery, if offered too late, may result in the patient suffering from complications from TPN added to the financial cost of prolonged TPN support. A reasonable minimal interval of time to allow for adaptation would be one year. However, if the patient is progressing with regard to improved tolerance of enteral feeding and complications from TPN are minimal, surgical therapy should be deferred. In the context of significant TPN complications, though, this strategy may need to be re-evaluated.

**Q11** The preferred fuel for small-bowel enterocytes is:
- **A** short-chain fatty acids
- **B** butyrate
- **C** glutamine
- **D** glucose
- **E** free fatty acids.

**A11** **C** Small-bowel enterocytes preferentially use glutamine as their major energy source. Colonocytes, however, preferentially use the short-chain fatty acid butyrate, while the brain utilises glucose.

**Q12** Which of the following patients would be a candidate for advancement of enteral feedings?
- **A** a 10 kg child with a 24-hour stool output of 100 mL yesterday and 120 mL today
- **B** a 10 kg child with a 24-hour stool output of 200 mL yesterday and 350 mL today
- **C** a 10 kg child with a 24-hour stool output of 300 mL yesterday and 200 mL today
- **D** a 10 kg child with a 24-hour stool output of 550 mL yesterday and 500 mL today
- **E** A and C.

**A12** **E** When managing SBS, the most important goal is to provide sufficient nutrition in order to support continued growth. Gastrostomy tubes allow access for continuous enteral feeding and are important for optimising nutrition in SBS patients. Continuous feeding is superior to bolus feeding, as it allows for continuous saturation of absorptive transporter proteins in the intestine. Therefore, continuous feeding results in improved nutrient absorption and more caloric intake. The ideal enteral infusion formula is isotonic and feedings should be advanced slowly (usually a few mL/hr/day). Ultimately, enteral feeding volumes can be increased gradually while decreasing the volume of parenteral feedings depending on the patient's tolerance. Stool losses increasing by more than 50% in a 24-hour period are usually a contraindication to advancing feeding volumes. Enteral feedings should not be advanced in the setting of stool losses greater than 40 mL/kg/day, especially when stools are strongly positive for reducing substances. Under these circumstances, the limit of the patient's absorptive capacity has been exceeded by the volume of feeding administered.

**Q13** Which of the following conditions is not associated with resection of the terminal ileum?

A   megaloblastic anaemia

B   decreased serum iron levels

C   choleretic diarrhoea

D   vitamin $B_{12}$ deficiency

E   none of the above

**A13**   **B**   The type of bowel removed is an important variable influencing the clinical response to intestinal resection. The ileum is a key location for the absorption of bile salts. Extensive ileal resection is associated with depletion of the bile salt pool and choleretic diarrhoea. Loss of bile salts leads to a higher incidence of cholelithiasis and fat malabsorption. The malabsorption of fat results in the deficiency of fat-soluble vitamins A, D, E, and K. Vitamin $B_{12}$ malabsorption may occur after resection of more than 60 cm of ileum. The intestine is seemingly unable to adaptively recruit new vitamin $B_{12}$ receptors into residual ileum or jejunum. The subsequent vitamin $B_{12}$ deficiency causes megaloblastic anaemia. Iron is absorbed in the proximal small bowel, mostly by the duodenum and proximal jejunum.

**Q14** Which of the following is not true about the post-small-bowel resection state?

A   Enteral nutrition is critical for small-bowel adaptation following massive small-bowel resection.

B   Resection of the ileocaecal valve results in decreased absorption by increasing intestinal transit time and promoting small-bowel bacterial overgrowth.

C   Patients who undergo proximal small-bowel resections are more likely to have deficiencies of calcium, iron and folate.

D   Gastric hypersecretion is more common after a large jejunal resection than a large ileal resection.

E   The remnant small bowel adapts by increasing villus length, rates of enterocyte proliferation and production of absorptive enzymes.

$\mathbf{A}$**14  B**  The ileocaecal valve slows intestinal transit, thereby increasing contact time between luminal nutrients and the small intestinal mucosal surface. In addition, the ileocaecal valve serves as a barrier preventing the migration of luminal colonic microorganisms into the distal small bowel.

Removal of the jejunum produces minimal permanent defects in the absorption of macronutrients and electrolytes because the ileum has the greatest capacity to adapt and take over these absorptive functions. However, jejunectomy may result in gastric hypersecretion because several of the intestinal hormones responsible for gastric inhibition are produced mainly in the jejunum. Folate is absorbed by the proximal jejunum. Iron is absorbed by the duodenum and proximal jejunum. Calcium is actively absorbed by the duodenum and passively absorbed in the jejunum and, to a lesser extent, in the ileum.

Enteral nutrients appear to stimulate intestinal adaptation via several mechanisms, including direct contact with epithelial cells, stimulation of trophic gastrointestinal hormones, and by increasing the output of pancreatic and biliary secretions. In fact, starvation induces gut mucosal atrophy that is reversed by refeeding. Not only is the presence of luminal nutrition important for adaptation, but its composition also plays a role. Adaptation is minimally affected by luminal administration of non-nutrient substrates. More complex nutrients requiring more energy for digestion and absorption appear to induce the greatest adaptation response. This concept is known as the functional workload hypothesis. Enteral fats appear to be the most trophic of the macronutrients in inducing adaptation. More specifically, longer-chain and more-unsaturated fats may provide an even greater adaptive stimulus.

Resection-induced adaptation provokes alterations that affect intestinal morphology, kinetics of cell turnover and overall function. Morphological changes include hyperplasia and hypertrophy of all intestinal layers, resulting in both lengthening of the bowel and greater bowel calibre. Villi become taller and crypts deeper, increasing mucosal surface area. In addition to the morphological changes, enterocytes have enhanced rates of turnover, as demonstrated by increased proliferation and programmed cell death (apoptosis). Functional adaptation, as gauged by digestive and absorptive enzyme activity per unit area, is augmented as well.

**Q15** Regarding the nutritional management of children with SBS, which of the following is true?

   **A** Young infants should be encouraged to practise suckling and swallowing behaviours with intermittent bottle feedings of small amounts of formula or breast milk.

   **B** The safest way to administer parenteral nutrition is via continuous intravenous infusion.

   **C** Pharmacological agents to reduce gastric acid hypersecretion should be used indefinitely in patients following massive small-bowel resection.

   **D** Pharmacological agents to slow intestinal transit time and reduce diarrhoea do not have an effect on intestinal absorption.

   **E** Older children with SBS should never be given solid foods in order to reduce stool volumes.

**A15** **A** When managing patients with SBS, particularly younger children, it is important to promote healthy feeding behaviours. Young infants should be allowed to practise sucking and swallowing and should be given intermittent bottle feedings of small amounts of formula. Older children should try eating small quantities of foods that are enjoyable and not associated with excessive stool output.

Histamine ($H_2$) receptor antagonists and proton pump inhibitors are Pharmacological agents that reduce gastric hypersecretion and are indicated in the early management of patients with SBS. Treatment later than 1 year after massive enterectomy is rarely warranted because gastric hypersecretion usually does not persist beyond 6–12 months postoperatively.

Pharmacological agents, such as opioids, can be used to slow intestinal transit in order to improve absorption. Opioid agents most commonly used to treat diarrhoea include codeine, diphenoxylate and loperamide. In several clinical trials, loperamide has been found to be more effective than diphenoxylate for controlling diarrhoea. Although its efficacy for controlling diarrhoea is desirable, codeine's side effects on the central nervous system and its potential for abuse warrant caution.

Parenteral nutrition administration should be transitioned from an around-the-clock continuous infusion to a night-time infusion cycle once the patient's condition has been stabilised. This infusion schedule is safe and results in fewer restrictions in daytime activities for both patient and caretaker.

**Q16** The best source of nutrition for neonates with SBS is:

- **A** Nutramigen
- **B** Pregestimil
- **C** Alimentum
- **D** breast milk
- **E** Neocate.

**A16** **D** Early enteral feeding is critical in patients with SBS. The ultimate goal is for the patient to eat as normal a diet as possible. Breast milk is the best source of nutrition for neonates because of its positive influences on cell proliferation and adaptive change in the remnant bowel. Breast milk's benefits likely derive from its trophic growth factors, whose effects are not yet completely understood.

Infants younger than 1 year of age have an increased risk of developing a protein allergy to commercial formulas due to the potential for increased gut permeability to food antigens. In theory, hypoallergenic formulas such as Nutramigen, Pregestimil (Mead Johnson Laboratories, Evansville, IN), and Alimentum (Ross Laboratories, Columbus, OH) have an advantage over standard formulas. Amino acid formulas, such as Neocate (SHS, Liverpool, England), can be used to further reduce the risk of allergic response. Another advantage of these formulas is that a high percentage of their calories is in the form of fat, which is better tolerated by the immature gut than carbohydrates. A major disadvantage of these formulas can be their considerable cost. Protein absorption is rarely a concern in older children, and they are usually able to tolerate more complex and less expensive feeding formulas.

**Q17** Regarding surgical procedures for the management of SBS, which of the following is true?

- **A** A recirculating loop allows for decreased transit time and increased nutrient absorption.
- **B** Before undergoing a lengthening procedure, patients should have intestinal continuity restored if possible.
- **C** In a patient with SBS and a functional obstruction due to a small segment of dilated bowel, resection of the dilated portion is the best surgical option.
- **D** The only benefit of performing a lengthening procedure, such as the Bianchi procedure or STEP, is the increase in intestinal length resulting in decreased transit time and increased nutrient absorption.
- **E** When creating a reversed intestinal segment for a child with SBS, a standard length of 10 cm should be used.

**A17** **B** The primary goal of surgical intervention is to increase intestinal absorptive and digestive capacity. If possible, patients with diverting stomas should have intestinal continuity restored. Other surgical procedures have been conceived to address the specific anatomical and physiologic anomalies of short bowel patients. These abnormalities include rapid intestinal transit, reduced mucosal surface area, dysfunctional peristalsis, and decreased intestinal length. The various surgical procedures, therefore, may be classified by the defect they were devised to address.

Recirculating intestinal loops are not advised and are addressed here only for thoroughness. Theoretically, creating a loop of intestine that allows luminal contents to recirculate several times before proceeding distally would slow intestinal transit and afford nutrients prolonged exposure to the mucosa for absorption. Unfortunately, experimental studies have failed to show benefits. Enteral contents can be radiographically shown to recirculate, but absorption is not improved. Furthermore, morbidity and mortality increase with the complexity of the loop.

Dilated intestinal segments are known to cause functional bowel obstruction. Failure of bowel-wall apposition during contraction results in ineffective peristalsis. The dilated bowel is unable to generate sufficient contraction pressure, resulting in poor forward propulsion of the enteric contents. Stasis of intestinal contents results, leading to bacterial overgrowth, toxin production, and malabsorption. Patients with only a short segment of dilated bowel and sufficient small-bowel length can simply undergo resection of the affected bowel. Unfortunately, the bowel of patients with SBS is typically dilated and short, and isolated resection of the dilated segment of bowel is rarely a tenable solution. In this case, patients should undergo either a tapering enteroplasty or a lengthening procedure.

In a tapering enteroplasty, a stapling device is used to longitudinally excise the dilated antimesenteric portion of the intestine. The remaining bowel is, therefore, smaller in calibre and demonstrates improved motility. Antimesenteric plication is an alternative surgical option to reduce bowel diameter. The bowel is folded into the lumen and plicated, which preserves absorptive surface area, while decreasing bowel calibre. Unfortunately, over time, the suture lines tend to break down and bowel dilatation recurs. Tapering has much less morbidity than a lengthening procedure and is usually the procedure of choice for patients with a reasonable length of small intestine.

The following proposed algorithm for management of patients with SBS takes into account the presence or absence of intestinal dilatation as the first decision point.

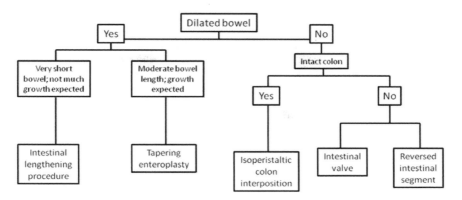

**FIGURE 41.1** Algorithm for management of patients with short bowel syndrome

A lengthening procedure not only increases intestinal transit time by increasing intestinal length but also improves peristalsis by decreasing the calibre of the bowel. The procedure of choice depends on the patient's anatomy and the surgeon's preference.

The first lengthening procedure was described by Bianchi in 1980, and takes advantage of the anatomical features of the mesenteric blood supply to the bowel. The mesenteric blood vessels bifurcate before contacting the edge of the bowel wall. Each branch supports one half of the bowel circumference. The gut's vascular configuration, therefore, allows division along its longitudinal axis into two tubes whose circumference is half that of the original bowel. Division and tubularisation of the bowel can be done using either a gastrointestinal anastomosis (GIA) stapling device or a hand-sutured technique. The two newly constructed tubes of bowel are then anastomosed in an isoperistaltic fashion. Thus, the Bianchi procedure effectively doubles the length and halves the circumference of the dilated segment. This technique not only augments bowel length for nutrient absorption, but also improves peristalsis by narrowing intestinal calibre.

The Iowa (Kimura) procedure was developed for bowel lengthening in SBS patients with limited mesentery associated with very short bowel. The procedure is performed in two stages. In the first surgery, the antimesenteric bowel wall is pexed to the undersurface of the abdominal wall to create a systemic-based blood supply for the antimesenteric side of the bowel. A seromyotomy along the bowel wall and mechanical abrasion of the abdominal wall facilitates neovascularisation. Several months later, the bowel may be longitudinally divided into two limbs. The antimesenteric limb now has a systemically derived blood supply, while the other limb continues to utilise the original mesenteric blood supply. These two limbs are then reapproximated to double the intestinal length. This procedure appears to be specifically useful in children, whose remaining bowel is limited to the duodenum. Unfortunately, the Iowa procedure is technically very difficult to perform, limiting its applicability.

The most recently developed lengthening procedure is the STEP, or serial transverse enteroplasty, described in 2003. In this procedure, the dilated small bowel is lengthened by serial transverse applications of a GIA stapler, from opposite directions, to create a zigzag channel. Proponents of the STEP cite that the procedure is technically less challenging to perform than the Bianchi procedure, can be performed multiple times in a single patient, and has comparable clinical outcomes with regard to TPN independence and avoidance of intestinal transplantation. Additionally, some studies have found the procedure efficacious for the treatment of bacterial overgrowth in dilated bowel segments of patients who do not have short gut syndrome. Further studies are needed, and a STEP registry has been created to critically evaluate this novel procedure.

A reversed intestinal segment is an operation commonly performed in patients with postvagotomy diarrhoea or dumping syndrome and has been applied to patients with SBS. A 'physiologic' valve is created by interposing a segment of bowel in which peristalsis is in the opposite direction. The antiperistaltic bowel provides a break in the peristaltic wave and slows overall gut transit. The length of bowel interposed is significant. Using too short a segment may not effectively slow peristalsis, while inserting too long a segment may result in functional bowel obstruction. In adults, 10 cm is the most common length reversed. However, in infants. beneficial effects have been derived from as little as 3 cm of gut being utilised. The segment being reversed should be anastomosed to the most distal region of gut possible to provide maximal intestinal braking and enhancement of mucosal absorption. In patients with extremely short bowel lengths, reversed segments may have limited utility because creating a reversed segment can compromise what little bowel exists.

# Further reading

Longshore SW, Wakeman D, McMellen M, *et al.* Bowel resection induced intestinal adaptation: progress from bench to bedside. *Minerva Pediatr.* 2009; **61**(3): 239–51.

McMellen ME, Wakeman D, Longshore SW, *et al.* Growth factors: possible roles for clinical management of the short bowel syndrome. *Semin Pediatr Surg.* 2010; **19**(1): 35–43.

Simeone DM. Anatomy and physiology of the small intestine. In: Mulholland MW, Lillemoe KD, Doherty GM, *et al.*, editors. *Greenfield's Surgery: scientific principles and practice.* 4th ed. Philadelphia, PA: Lippincott Williams & Wilkins; 2006.

Sudan D, Thompson J, Botha J, *et al.* Comparison of intestinal lengthening procedures for patients with short bowel syndrome. *Ann Surg.* 2007; **246**(4): 593–601.

Warner BW. Short bowel syndrome. In: Grosfeld JL, O'Neill JA, Fonkalsrud EW, *et al.*, editors. *Pediatric Surgery.* 6th ed. Philadelphia, PA: Mosby-Elsevier; 2006. pp. 1369–82.

# CHAPTER 42

# Appendicitis

## NITIN PATWARDHAN

From the choices below each question, select the single best answer.

**Q1** Which of the following is true with regard to acute appendicitis?
  **A** It is common at any age group.
  **B** It is more common in females.
  **C** It is rare in a neonatal population.
  **D** The white cell count is always raised.
  **E** It is easy to diagnose with various imaging techniques.

**A1** **C** Although appendicitis can happen at any age, it commonly affects older children above 10 years of age. Boys are at a slightly higher risk of getting appendicitis. White cell count is usually raised but it is possible to have a normal count with appendicitis. Despite various imaging modalities the diagnosis of appendicitis is best based on a combination of clinical picture, blood investigations and imaging.

**Q2** Which investigation is required to be performed for suspected appendicitis?
  **A** white cell count
  **B** ultrasound scan
  **C** CT scan
  **D** abdominal X–ray
  **E** none of the above

**A2** **E** It is possible to diagnose appendicitis in most patients simply on the basis of history and clinical examination. Investigations may be performed when the diagnosis is not clear on presentation.

**Q3** Which of the following can be considered as a definitive diagnostic test for appendicitis?

**A** CT scan

**B** ultrasound scan

**C** diagnostic laparoscopy

**D** white cell scan

**E** none of the above

**A3** **E** Ultrasound scan and CT scan are becoming increasingly popular investigations for diagnosing appendicitis. Ultrasound is commonly used in the UK while CT and ultrasonography are used in the United States. Although there are reports claiming a high sensitivity and specificity for both, their main use is for the equivocal cases where clinical diagnosis is not possible. Similarly a normal looking appendix at laparoscopy may indeed show inflammation under the microscope.

**Q4** Differential diagnosis for appendicitis does not include:

**A** pancreatitis

**B** pneumonitis

**C** urinary tract infection

**D** ectopic pregnancy

**E** gastro-oesophageal reflux disease (GORD).

**A4** **E** Abdominal pain is a common symptom in children for a variety of disorders that can mimic the clinical picture of appendicitis. GORD typically presents with heartburn, regurgitation and dysphagia.

 **Q5** While performing appendicectomy for perforated appendicitis one should always:

**A** bury the stump

**B** leave a drain

**C** look for and remove any faecoliths

**D** irrigate with saline plus antibiotic solution

**E** avoid primary skin closure.

**A5** **C** A variety of steps are employed by surgeons to prevent postoperative complications, but there is no conclusive evidence that they help. A retained faecolith is very likely to cause postoperative sepsis and it is good practice to remove it.

**Q6** Laparoscopic appendicectomy is contraindicated in:
   **A** children under the age of 5 years
   **B** perforated appendicitis
   **C** an overweight patient
   **D** an immunocompromised patient
   **E** none of the above.

**A6** E

**Q7** In the postoperative period for perforated appendicitis:
   **A** keep the patient nil oral for 48 hours
   **B** check white cell count daily
   **C** change the dressing daily
   **D** give broad-spectrum antibiotics for >24 hours
   **E** perform ultrasound of abdomen after 5 days.

**A7** **D** Antibiotic policies vary from hospital to hospital. However, most surgeons prescribe a combination of antibiotics covering a broad spectrum, for a period of 1–7 days.

**Q8** Postoperative complications following appendicectomy include:
   **A** lung consolidation
   **B** intussusception
   **C** necrotising fasciitis
   **D** intra-abdominal abscess
   **E** all of above.

**A8** E

**Q9** Appendicectomy is usually performed as part of which procedure?
   **A** gastroschisis repair
   **B** congenital diaphragmatic hernia repair
   **C** Ladd's procedure
   **D** laparotomy for meconium obstruction
   **E** pull-through procedure for Hirschsprung's disease

**A9** **C** Most surgeons advocate removal of the appendix following a Ladd's procedure for malrotation. This is because following a Ladd's procedure, the malrotated bowel is orientated such that the appendix tends to be in the left side of the abdomen. If these patients present with appendicitis at a later date, the clinical signs may be confusing and misleading. These cases are done using an inversion appendicectomy, without any contamination of the peritoneal cavity.

**Q10** A 12-year-old girl has undergone appendicectomy for perforated appendicitis with pus in the pelvis. The parents want to know about long-term problems. Which of the following statements is true?

   **A** There is an increased risk of infertility.

   **B** There is a increased risk of ovarian torsion.

   **C** There is an increased risk of adhesive intestinal obstruction.

   **D** There is an increased risk of endometriosis.

   **E** All of the above.

**A10** C

## Further reading

Adibe OO, Amin SR, Hansen EN, *et al.* An evidence-based clinical protocol for diagnosis of acute appendicitis decreased the use of computed tomography in children. *J Pediatr Surg.* 2011; **46**(1): 192–6.

Parks NA, Schroeppel TJ. Update on imaging for acute appendicitis. *Surg Clin North Am.* 2011; **91**(1): 141–54.

# CHAPTER 43

# Inflammatory bowel disease and polypoid diseases in children

## A ANISH, MIKE THOMSON

**From the choices below each question, select the single best answer.**

**Q1** Which of the following is true regarding Crohn's disease?

   **A** Between 10% and 20% of children have inflammation in the colon only.

   **B** 70% of children with the disease have inflammation of the lower part of the ileum.

   **C** In about 15%–20% of people, the disease runs in the family.

   **D** Mutations in one gene, called *CARD15*, are present in about 40% of people with Crohn's disease.

   **E** All of the above.

**A1** **E** In about 15%–20% of people, the disease runs in the family. This is especially true of people who develop the disease at a younger age. Several genes have been linked to the disease, but there is no clear pattern to how these genes interact to cause the disease. Mutations in one gene, called *CARD15*, are present in about 40% of people with Crohn's disease. However, this gene is also frequently present in healthy people who never develop this disease. As many as 70% of children with the disease have inflammation of the lower part of the ileum. More than half of these children also have inflammation in variable segments of the colon. About 10%–20% of children have inflammation in the colon only. Another 10%–15% have inflammation scattered around the small bowel, mainly in the middle section (jejunum and upper ileum). A very small number have inflammation only in the stomach and the duodenum.

**Q2** Which of the following is not a routine investigation to detect Crohn's disease?

A upper GI endoscopy

B ileo colonoscopy

C inflammatory markers

D barium enema

E all of the above

 **A2** **D** Because of advances in diagnostic modalities, barium enema is not routinely performed in Crohn's disease.

When endoscopic intubation of the intestine is not possible, radiological studies are necessary to determine disease extent and location. Small-bowel enema for small-bowel disease and double contrast barium enema for large-bowel disease are recommended. Complementary imaging procedures may be performed, including ultrasonography, CT, and/or MRI. Differentiation between inflammatory and fibrostenotic bowel stenosis would be very helpful, but current techniques do not permit an accurate distinction.

 **Q3** Which of the following investigations is least helpful in the diagnosis of Crohn's disease?

A ileo colonoscopy

B ultrasound for pelvic collection

C wireless capsule endoscopy (WCE) to diagnose strictures

D CT scan of the abdomen

E Lower GI contrast study

 **A3** **C** WCE represents an advance for small-bowel imaging, but large prospective studies are needed to confirm the diagnostic relevance in Crohn's disease. WCE may be considered in symptomatic patients with suspected small-bowel Crohn's disease in whom a stricture/stenosis has been excluded, endoscopy of terminal ileum is normal or not possible, and in whom fluoroscopic or cross-sectional imaging has not showed lesions.

 **Q4** Barium features of Crohn's disease include:

A aphthoid ulcers

B fold thickening, deformity and truncation

C long, linear mesenteric border ulcers

D deep fissuring (transmural) 'rose thorn' ulcers

E all of the above.

**A4    E**   Radiological features seen on barium enema for Crohn's disease include:
- aphthoid ulcers
- fold thickening, deformity and truncation
- long, linear mesenteric border ulcers
- deep fissuring (transmural) 'rose thorn' ulcers
- intersecting linear and transverse ulcers producing a 'cobblestone' pattern
- discontinuous disease ('skip lesions' – patchy inflammation may give false negative biopsies)
- loop separation – diseased and non-diseased loops are displaced from one another because of one or more of the following: bowel wall thickening, creeping subserosal intestinal fat, interloop fluid collections and abscesses
- rigid, straightened or kinked bowel segments
- stenoses with or without pre- and poststenotic dilatation
- pseudodiverticula or sacculations (usually antimesenteric border) caused by blowing out of spared normal patches of bowel wall in a diseased segment.

**Q5**  Regarding capsule endoscopy which of the following is not true?
- **A**  High-definition pictures are obtained.
- **B**  Strictures and dilatation can also be seen.
- **C**  Incomplete visualisation can be a problem.
- **D**  Biopsy can be freely taken.
- **E**  None of the above.

**A5    D   Advantages**

High definition pictures may be reliably obtained from areas of the small bowel previously beyond endoscopic reach. Studies involving the small numbers of patients with either known or highly likely Crohn's disease indicate that this is likely to be a sensitive way of identifying early Crohn's disease.

**Disadvantages**

Incomplete visualisation: the camera is situated at one end of the capsule. As the capsule rolls through the intestine, there is potential for lesions to be missed, as the bowel surface may not be completely examined.

Capsule retention: early trials documented failure of the capsule to re-emerge and surgical removal was necessary in a small percentage. Current publications on Crohn's disease investigation usually involve prior radiological assessment to exclude subjects with stricturing disease. A test capsule has been developed, to identify potential 'capsule retainers' – if retained it will disperse and not require surgical intervention.

Superficial information only: like other endoscopic techniques, the images are obtained of the mucosa and of the deeper layers only to the extent that these are revealed by mucosal breaks, such as ulcers and fissures. Little or no information about transmural inflammation and extraintestinal complications is obtainable.

No biopsies: capsule endoscopy is unable to provide biopsy specimens for histological analysis – the primary advantage of other endoscopic techniques.

**Q6** All of the following are ultrasound findings in Crohn's disease *except*:

   **A** ultrasonography demonstrates transmural inflammatory change and extramural complications

   **B** enlarged mesenteric lymph nodes are a common feature of active Crohn's disease

   **C** thumbprint sign can be seen

   **D** loss of normal bowel fold pattern

   **E** cobblestone appearance of bowel.

**A6**   **E** Ultrasonography demonstrates transmural inflammatory change and extramural complications that make diseased segments easier to recognise than the normal small-bowel loops. It can be recommended as the first-line test in young patients presenting with recurrent lower abdominal symptoms. Enlarged mesenteric lymph nodes are a common feature of active Crohn's disease. In the right iliac fossa, loss of normal fold pattern and small 'thumbprints' along the inferior (antimesenteric) border can be picked up by ultrasound. Cobblestone features of bowel is seen on contrast studies and not visualised on ultrasonography.

**Q7** Which of the following is *not* true of Crohn's disease?

   **A** patchy chronic inflammation

   **B** stricture formation

   **C** pancolitis

   **D** caseating granulomas

   **E** crypt distortion

**A7**   **D** The granuloma in Crohn's disease is defined as a collection of epithelioid histiocytes (monocyte/macrophage cells), the outlines of which are often vaguely defined. Multinucleated giant cells are not characteristic and necrosis is usually not apparent. Only granulomas in the lamina propria not associated with active crypt injury may be regarded as a corroborating feature of Crohn's disease. Granulomas associated with crypt injury are less reliable features. Non-caseating granulomas, small collections of epithelioid histiocytes, and giant cells or isolated giant cells can be seen in infectious colitis (granulomas suggest Mycobacterium, Chlamydia, *Yersinia pseudotuberculosis*, Treponema; microgranulomas suggest

Salmonella, Campylobacter, *Yersinia enterocolitica*; giant cells suggest Chlamydia and must not be regarded as evidence for Crohn's disease.

**Q8** Which of the following macroscopic features will not aid in the diagnosis of Crohn's disease?

**A** ileal disease

**B** strictures

**C** cobblestone appearance

**D** fistulas

**E** none of the above

**A8**   **E**   Macroscopic features for the diagnosis of Crohn's disease include:

- ileal disease*
- rectum typically spared
- confluent deep linear ulcers, aphthoid ulcers
- deep fissures
- fistulas
- fat wrapping*
- skip lesions (segmental disease)
- cobblestoning
- thickening of the intestinal wall*
- strictures.

*Typical discriminating features for a diagnosis of Crohn's disease compared with other conditions.

**Q9** Which of the following treatments is not used in the management of ulcerative colitis?

**A** steroids

**B** 5-ASA supplements

**C** azathioprine

**D** exclusive enteral nutrition

**E** all of the above

**A9**   **D**   Exclusive enteral nutrition is used in the management of Crohn's disease.

**Q10** Which of the following treatments is *not* used to maintain remission in Crohn's disease?

**A** steroids

**B** methotrexate

**C** infliximab

**D** azathioprine

**E** enteral nutrition

A10 **A**  There is no role for maintenance steroids for patients with Crohn's disease in remission. For patients who are steroid dependent, every effort must be made to find other effective treatment. Azathioprine (2–2.5 mg/kg/day) or 6-mercaptopurine (1–1.25 mg/kg/day) should be initiated as maintenance therapy in cases that relapse in less than 6 months, cases that relapse two or more times per year following initial successful therapy, and in all that are steroid dependent. There is some evidence that over half of all adults will relapse within 3 years of stopping azathioprine and hence the usual practice of stopping at 4 years may not be valid. Methotrexate 15 mg/m$^2$ once weekly by subcutaneous injection, if azathioprine or 6-mercaptopurine is ineffective or poorly tolerated, with folic acid 5 mg 24 hours after each dose to ameliorate any GI side effects. Enteral nutrition supplementary therapy may reduce the risk of relapse and may improve growth and nutritional status. If remission is induced with infliximab, maintenance with infliximab may be necessary (5 mg/kg intravenously, every 8 weeks). It may be necessary to escalate to a higher dose (10 mg/kg) for loss of responsiveness and if successful, should revert to lower dose for subsequent infusions.

Q11  Which of the following is a recognised treatment option for acute severe colitis?

**A**  intravenous (IV) steroids
**B**  cyclosporine
**C**  surgery
**D**  IV antibiotics
**E**  all of the above

A11 **E**  Early surgical opinion is essential and patient should be managed jointly between physician and surgeon. IV fluids/blood transfusion if required. IV steroids such as hydrocortisone 2 mg/kg q.i.d. (maximum dose 100 mg q.i.d.) or methylprednisolone 2 mg/kg/day (maximum dose 60 mg/day). Failure to respond by 72 hours suggests the need for escalation of therapy or colectomy. At least daily plain abdominal X-ray if toxic/unwell. IV antibiotics only if infection is suspected or sometimes prior to surgery, e.g. cefotaxime (50 mg/kg t.i.d.) and metronidazole (7.5 mg/kg t.i.d.).

Urgent surgical review is also indicated with a view to early colectomy if there is evidence of toxic megacolon (diagnosed if diameter >5.5 cm transverse colon and/or >9 cm in caecum, based on adult data) and in cases that are deteriorating. IV cyclosporine 2–4 mg/kg/day, aiming for trough levels of 100–200 ng/mL, can be considered in cases not responding to steroids as a temporary measure to delay/avoid colectomy allowing recovery and initiation of second-line immunosuppressant. Infliximab IV – there is some evidence that infliximab could be considered in non-responding acute severe ulcerative colitis.

**Q12** Which of the following is *not* true of Crohn's disease?

    **A** Surgery can be considered for isolated ileocaecal disease.

    **B** Colectomy is curative for pancolitic disease.

    **C** 30% of patients require surgery in the first 10 years of disease.

    **D** Between 70% and 80% will have surgery in their lifetime.

    **E** Stricturoplasty is a good option for isolated small-bowel strictures.

**A12**  **B**  Surgery should be considered especially for isolated ileocaecal disease, strictures or fistulas and for those in whom medical treatment has failed. It is essential that there is close collaboration between gastroenterologists and a surgeon experienced in paediatric inflammatory bowel disease. In Crohn's disease, surgery is not curative and management is directed at minimising the impact of disease. At least 30% of patients require surgery in the first 10 years of disease and approximately 70%–80% will have surgery in their lifetime.

**Q13** Which one of the following is *not* a well-recognised symptom in Crohn's disease?

    **A** constipation

    **B** growth failure

    **C** amenorrhoea

    **D** delayed puberty

    **E** none of the above

**A13**  **E**  Many children with Crohn's disease present with vague complaints such as lethargy, anorexia and abdominal discomfort or with isolated growth failure. A significant minority have markedly impaired final adult height. Neglect to record growth parameters, particularly for those not presenting to a paediatrician, has been identified. Other symptoms may include fever, nausea, vomiting, delayed puberty, psychiatric disturbance and erythema nodosum. The clinical course of Crohn's disease is characterised by exacerbations and remissions. Crohn's disease tends to cause greater disability than ulcerative colitis. Secondary amenorrhoea has been reported in few cases as a presenting symptom in Crohn's disease.

**Q14** What is the mechanism of action of infliximab in Crohn's disease?

    **A** It binds to TNF-alpha.

    **B** It blocks TNF-alpha receptors.

    **C** It reduces TNF-alpha production.

    **D** It reduces TNF-alpha secretion.

    **E** It increases hepatic metabolism of TNF-alpha.

$A$14  **A**  Infliximab is a monoclonal antibody that has a high sensitivity for and affinity to TNF-alpha. Infliximab neutralises the biologic activity of TNF-alpha by inhibiting binding to its receptors.

$Q$15  Which of the following colonic polyps are highly unlikely to be premalignant?

**A** juvenile polyps

**B** hamartomatous polyps

**C** villous adenomas

**D** tubular adenomas

**E** Peutz–Jeghers's syndrome (PJS) polyps

$A$15  **A**

$Q$16  Which of the following extraintestinal feature is associated with familial adenomatous polyposis (FAP)?

**A** epidermoid cysts

**B** osteoma

**C** adrenal gland adenomas

**D** supernumerary teeth

**E** all of the above

$A$16  **E**  Extraintestinal features of FAP include:

- congenital hypertrophy of the retinal pigmented epithelium (70%–80%)
- thyroid cancer (2%–3%)
- epidermoid cysts (50%)
- brain tumour (1%)
- osteoma (50%–90%)
- hepatoblastoma (1%)
- desmoid tumour (10%–15%)
- supernumerary teeth (11%–27%)
- adrenal gland adenomas (7%–13%).

**Q17** Regarding FAP, which of the following is not true?

    **A** Between 20% and 30% of cases are de novo mutations.

    **B** Gastric and duodenal lesions occur in approximately 45% of children with FAP.

    **C** Gastric polyps are more likely to be adenomatous than duodenal lesions.

    **D** The risk for carcinoma in the proximal GI tract is small, about 3%–5%.

    **E** Once adenomas are identified, it is generally recommended that ileal pouch anal anastomosis should be offered to patients.

**A17** **C** Once adenomas are identified, it is generally recommended that ileal pouch anal anastomosis or ileal anal anastomosis be performed.

Gastric and duodenal lesions occur in approximately 45% of children with FAP. It is generally recommended that upper endoscopic surveillance begins when colonic adenomas are identified, or at age 20–25 years. Although gastric polyps are more common than duodenal polyps, duodenal polyps are much more likely to be adenomatous.

**Q18** Which of the following statements about FAP is true?

    **A** It is inherited as an autosomal recessive condition.

    **B** It is characterised by polyp formation in late adulthood.

    **C** It is associated with osteomas and epidermoid cysts in Gardner's syndrome.

    **D** It is due to a mutation on the short arm of chromosome 12.

    **E** It cannot be screened for by rigid or flexible sigmoidoscopy.

**A18** **C**

**Q19** Regarding PJS, which of the following is true?

    **A** PJS is an autosomal dominant syndrome with high penetrance.

    **B** Hamartomatous polyps of the small intestine and colon are present.

    **C** The risk of colorectal cancer is 10%–20%.

    **D** Mutations can be identified in the gene *STK11(LKB1)*.

    **E** All of the above.

**A19** **E** PJS is an autosomal dominant syndrome with high penetrance, defined by the presence of hamartomatous polyps of the small intestine, colon and rectum, in association with mucocutaneous pigmentation. The risk of colorectal cancer is 10%–20%. In 20%–63% of cases, inactivating mutations can be identified in the gene *STK11(LKB1)*. There is evidence for genetic heterogeneity with *LKB1* involvement being formally excluded in some families.

**Q20** Which of the following is *not* true about PJS?

 A It is an autosomal recessive condition.

 B It often presents with anaemia in childhood.

 C It is characterised by circumoral mucocutaneous pigmented lesions.

 D It is associated with adenomatous polyps of the small intestine.

 E Malignant change occurs in 2%–3% of polyps.

**A20** A

**Q21** Which of the following is true about juvenile polyposis?

 A It is an autosomal dominant syndrome.

 B The incidence rate is 1 in 100 000.

 C The underlying defect is an inactivating mutation in growth inhibitory transforming growth factor beta, or bone morphogenetic protein.

 D Multiple juvenile polyps, usually 50–100, are found primarily in the colon.

 E All of the above.

**A21** E Juvenile polyposis is a rare autosomal dominant syndrome with an incidence of approximately 1 in 100 000. The underlying defect is an inactivating mutation in growth inhibitory transforming growth factor beta or bone morphogenetic protein signalling pathways, leading to multiple gastric, small-intestinal and colonic polyps.

**Q22** Which of the following is true regarding colonic polyps?

 A Metaplastic polyps are premalignant.

 B Adenomatous polyps are premalignant.

 C Villous adenomas are more common than tubular adenomas.

 D Genetic mutations can result in epithelial metaplasia.

 E Carcinomas arise only in adenomatous polyps.

**A22** B

**Q23** Which of the following is true regarding colonic polyps?

  **A** Juvenile rectal polyps are adenomatous polyps.

  **B** Metaplastic polyps are premalignant.

  **C** The risk of malignancy is higher in tubular than villous adenomas.

  **D** Villous adenomas occasionally cause hyperkalaemia.

  **E** All patients with untreated familial adenomatous polyposis will eventually develop colorectal carcinoma.

**A23** **E** Juvenile rectal polyps are hamartomatous polyps. Metaplastic polyps are not premalignant. Villous adenomas have a higher risk than tubular adenomas of being malignant. Villous adenomas occasionally present with hypokalaemia as a result of potassium loss from their mucus secretion. FAP is an autosomal dominant condition. Untreated, all patients usually develop a colonic neoplasm by the age of 40 years. All patients at risk should be screened and if polyps are identified should be offered prophylactic surgery.

**Q24** Which of the following is *not* true regarding Cowden's syndrome?

  **A** Multiple hamartomas of the skin, breast, thyroid gland, endometrium and GI tract.

  **B** The risk of colon cancer is significantly higher than the normal population.

  **C** Genetic screening by DNA sequencing for *PTEN* mutations, is widely available.

  **D** Mild mental retardation and macrocephaly are associated features.

  **E** None of the above.

**A24** **B** Cowden's syndrome is characterised by multiple hamartomas of the skin, breast, thyroid gland, endometrium and GI tract. There is an increased risk of neoplasia in breast, thyroid and other organs, although the risk of colon cancer is low and may not be more than the general population despite the presence of multiple GI polyps. Other common findings are trichilemmomas and papillomatous papules, mild mental retardation and macrocephaly. Occasional children with autism and Cowden's syndrome have been described. The GI tumours are juvenile polyps, lipomas and ganglioneuromas. Specific clinical criteria have been developed for Cowden's syndrome.

## Further reading

Barnard J. Screening and surveillance recommendations for pediatric gastrointestinal polyposis syndromes. *J Pediatr Gastroenterol Nutr.* 2009; **48**(Suppl. 2): S75–8.

Travis SP, Stange EF, Lémann M, *et al.* European evidence based consensus on the diagnosis and management of Crohn's disease: current management. *Gut.* 2006; **55**(Suppl. 1): i16–35.

Travis SP, Stange EF, Lémann M, *et al.* European evidence-based consensus on the management of ulcerative colitis: current management. *J Crohns Colitis.* 2008; **2**(1): 24–62.

# CHAPTER 44

# Gastrointestinal bleeding

## MANJULA VELAYUDHAN, MIKE THOMSON

From the choices below each question, select the single best answer.

**Q1** A previously well 3-year-old presented with an upper respiratory tract infection and had been retching and vomiting small amounts of blood. She is growing well and has a normal examination. The most likely diagnosis is:

A non-steroidal anti-inflammatory drug gastropathy

B Mallory–Weiss's tear

C haemorrhagic gastritis

D peptic ulcer

E vascular malformation

**A1** **B** A Mallory–Weiss's tear is an acute mucosal laceration of the gastric cardia or gastro-oesophageal junction. The classic presentation is haematemesis following repeated retching or vomiting. Abdominal pain is uncommon and is most likely to be musculoskeletal in origin because of the forceful retching. Vomiting episodes are usually related to a concurrent viral illness, and occur in previously well children with normal growth patterns and with no history of vomiting or loose stools.

**Q2** Most gastrointestinal (GI) stromal tumours are found in the

A mesentery

B stomach

C retroperitoneum

D omentum

E duodenum.

**A2** **B** GI stromal tumours are mesenchymal tumours arising from the GI wall, mesentery, omentum and retroperitoneum. Most GI stromal tumours are found in the stomach (60%–70%) and should be considered in a patient with neurofibromatosis.

**Q3** The investigation of choice for evaluating haematemesis is:

  **A** barium swallow

  **B** upper GI endoscopy

  **C** pH study

  **D** *Helicobacter pylori* antigen in stool

  **E** breath test for *H. pylori*.

**A3** **B** Upper GI endoscopy is the test of choice for evaluating haematemesis. The aims of endoscopy are to identify the site of bleeding and to initiate therapeutic interventions as and when necessary. Emergency endoscopy is only indicated when the bleed is ongoing and life-threatening. Most centres use general anaesthesia and control of the upper airways in children.

**Q4** The most likely diagnosis in a 18-month-old baby with an antecedent viral illness followed by sudden onset of colicky abdominal pain, tenderness and passage of 'redcurrant jelly' in stools is:

  **A** Meckel's diverticulum

  **B** intussusception

  **C** irritable bowel syndrome

  **D** portal hypertension

  **E** von Willebrand's disease.

**A4** **B** Idiopathic intussusception should be the working diagnosis for any child younger than 2 years of age who presents with abdominal pain or tenderness associated with lower GI blood loss. The sudden onset of colicky abdominal pain and vomiting with antecedent viral illness, followed by redcurrant jelly stool is intussusception until proved otherwise. Beyond 2 years, intussusception is most likely to be associated with a lead point such as Meckel's diverticulum, polyp, lymphoid nodular hyperplasia, foreign body, intramural haematoma, lymphoma or bowel wall oedema in relation to Henoch–Schönlein's purpura.

**Q5** A previously well 2-year-old has painless rectal bleeding. She has normal growth and a normal examination. She also has soft stools and opens her bowels once every day. She is haemodynamically stable. The investigation that would help make the diagnosis is:

  **A** colonoscopy

  **B** Technetium-99m ($^{99m}$Tc) scan

  **C** abdominal X-ray

  **D** cow's-milk-free trial

  **E** all of the above.

**A⁵**  **B**  In any child who presents with painless, frank bleeding per rectum, the possible diagnosis are Meckel's diverticulum, polyp, intestinal duplication, intestinal submucosal mass or angiodysplasia. Meckel's diverticulum is a vestigial remnant of the omphalomesenteric duct located on the antimesenteric border in the distal ileum that occurs in 1.5%–2% of the general population. A Meckel's diverticulum that contains gastric mucosa may present as painless acute lower GI bleed.

After exclusion of an intussusception, the next step in evaluation of haematochezia is a $^{99m}$Tc pertechnetate scan. The radionuclide binds strongly to gastric mucosa in the Meckel's diverticulum, which forms a focus in the right lower quadrant. The radionuclide may also be taken up by the gastric heterotopias in the small-bowel mucosa or enteric duplications.

**Q⁶**  Which of the following is true about Meckel's diverticulum?
  **A**  It is found in 2% of the population.
  **B**  In children who are less than 4 years old, the commonest presentation is with obstruction or bleeding.
  **C**  The commonest ectopic tissue found histologically is gastric.
  **D**  Symptomatic diverticula are more common in males.
  **E**  All of the above.

**A⁶**  **E**  Among paediatric patients, the most common presentations of symptomatic Meckel's diverticula are obstruction, intussusception, volvulus, bleeding and diverticulitis.

It is more common in males; up to 50% of those requiring surgery occur under the age of 2 years, and 80% by 10 years of age. It classically presents as massive painless frank blood loss per rectum, often requiring blood transfusion, in an otherwise healthy child. Bleeding is due to ectopic gastric mucosa, which may ulcerate, in 90% of cases. Diagnosis is made by $^{99m}$Tc pertechnetate abdominal scintigraphy to detect heterotopic gastric mucosa. The scan is positive in around 85% of cases. Treatment is prompt surgical removal.

**Q⁷**  Which of the following is *not* true about juvenile polyposis syndrome?
  **A**  It is an autosomal dominant condition.
  **B**  Diagnosis requires the presence of at least three polyps.
  **C**  Surveillance endoscopy is required every 2 years.
  **D**  Malignant change is mostly in the first and second decades.
  **E**  It usually presents in the first decade with bleeding, rectal prolapse and anaemia.

**A⁷**  **D**  Juvenile polyposis syndrome is autosomal dominant, with multiple polyps anywhere in the GI tract, especially the colon. It presents around the age of 9 years with bleeding, rectal prolapse or anaemia. Diagnosis requires the presence of between three and five polyps. Malignant change and colorectal carcinoma occur in 15% of cases under the age of 35 years. Surveillance endoscopy is required every 2 years. First-degree relatives should be screened using colonoscopy from the age of 12 years as they may be asymptomatic.

**Q8** Which of the following is *not* true of Peutz–Jeghers's syndrome?
- **A** Polyps mainly arise in the colon.
- **B** It is an autosomal dominant condition.
- **C** It is associated with melanin pigmentation of buccal mucosa, hands, feet and eyelids.
- **D** The family should be counselled regarding intussusceptions.
- **E** Screening for malignancy should start in adolescence.

**A8** **A** Peutz–Jehgers' syndrome is an autosomal dominant inherited condition, with the mutated gene on chromosome 19p13.3. It is associated with mucocutaneous melanin pigmentation of lips, buccal mucosa and, occasionally, more peripheral sites including hands, feet and eyelids. Children present with melanin pigmentation of their mucosa, and rectal bleeding. Polyps mainly arise in the small intestine, but also in the stomach and colon. Management includes removal of larger midgut polyps, and counselling the family regarding the high risk of intussusceptions. Young adults may develop malignancy in the GI tract, pancreas or ovaries/testes. Screening for malignancy should commence after adolescence.

**Q9** A 6-month-old baby has presented to the outpatient clinics with failure to thrive. He has crossed 2 centiles on his growth charts, and suffered from loose stools since birth, occasionally mixed with blood. He suffers from eczema and has episodes of vomiting. Which of the following interventions would help him most?
- **A** endoscopy to rule out varices
- **B** cow's milk exclusion diet
- **C** colonoscopy to look for causes of lower GI bleed
- **D** bloods to rule out inflammatory bowel disease and coeliac disease
- **E** all of the above

**A9** **B** This condition should be suspected in infants who present with rectal bleeding, even those who are exclusively breast fed as antigens may be passed down via the breast milk. GI manifestations may occur with skin (eczema) and respiratory manifestations (wheeze). Acute watery diarrhoea may occur with vomiting or abdominal cramps. Chronic diarrhoea and failure to thrive may follow after the ingestion of the milk because it induces a patchy villous atrophy in the small intestine. Excessive intestinal protein and blood loss may lead to hypoproteinaemia and iron deficiency anaemia. Peripheral blood eosinophilia may be present.

Stools may contain eosinophils and biopsy specimens from colon, oesophagus and small intestine contains eosinophils predominantly.

**Q10** Which of the following is true about Henoch–Schönlein's purpura?

   **A** Lower GI bleeding occurs in 25% of the cases.

   **B** Endoscopic examination may show patchy erythema, mucosal oedema and erosions.

   **C** These lesions are most prominent in the duodenal bulb and second part of duodenum.

   **D** Biopsy findings may include neutrophilic infiltration in the lamina propria around blood vessels.

   **E** All the above.

**A10** **E** Henoch–Schönlein's purpura is a multisystem disorder characterised by purpura, colicky abdominal pain, haematuria and obscure GI bleeding. Lower GI bleeding occurs in 25% of the cases. Endoscopic examination may show mucosal oedema, patchy erythema and multiple gastric erosions. The lesions are more severe in the duodenal bulb and the second part of the duodenum. Biopsies show neutrophilic infiltrates especially in the lamina propria.

**Q11** The treatment of choice for an acute variceal bleed that is not controlled by conservative measures in children is:

   **A** endoscopic sclerotherapy

   **B** endoscopic variceal ligation

   **C** portosystemic shunts

   **D** octreotide

   **E** propanolol.

**A11** **B** Where there are known varices, prompt resuscitation followed by intravenous octreotide may provide time for the child to be transferred to a paediatric liver unit where therapeutic endoscopy can be performed safely. Octreotide is a somatostatin analogue that decreases pressure within varices by decreasing splanchnic blood flow. It is safe, has few side effects and stops bleeding completely in approximately 70%–80% of patients. Endoscopically large or bleeding varices can be injected or, preferably, ligated using an endoscopic variceal ligator (EVL). EVL was first described in 1989 and is now considered to be first-line treatment for variceal haemorrhage. It is both safe and effective, even in small children, and results in less stricture formation than sclerotherapy. Regular endoscopy with banding should be performed until varices are minimal or ablated.

Q12 A 12-year-old presented with abdominal pain when passing stools, rectal bleeding and mucus in stools. He may have any of the following *except*:

**A** salmonella

**B** shigella

**C** ischaemic colitis

**D** inflammatory bowel disease

**E** Meckel's diverticulum.

A12 **E** Symptoms of colitis include acute bloody diarrhoea, tenesmus and abdominal pain. Beyond infancy, the two main causes of colitis are infectious colitis and inflammatory bowel disease. Bacterial colitis is self-limiting and usually resolves in 2 weeks; if bloody diarrhoea persists for more than 2 weeks in any patient, a paediatric gastroenterologist referral is required to rule out inflammatory bowel disease.

The presence of fever, fatigue, weight loss, arthritis or arthralgia supports the diagnosis of inflammatory bowel disease.

Ischaemic colitis should be considered in any child with collagen vascular disease, a recent history of anaesthesia, cardiac failure, uraemia, or history of taking medication for birth control or taking digitalis.

Q13 In children with obscure GI bleed, with normal endoscopic and colonoscopic findings, which of the following investigation may help in reaching a diagnosis?

**A** wireless capsule endoscopy (WCE) on its own

**B** double-balloon enteroscopy (DBE) on its own

**C** capsule endoscopy followed by DBE

**D** laparotomy with peroperative endoscopy

**E** none of the above

A13 **A** WCE is a useful tool for diagnosing small-bowel lesions in patients with obscure GI bleeding, with a yield rate of 38%–93%.

Flexible GI endoscopy is sufficient for diagnostic and therapeutic procedures in the vast majority of paediatric cases, and in adult patients with obscure GI bleeding the procedure determines the source in up to 90% of cases. However, in the small number of cases where the pathology is confined to the small bowel beyond the reach of conventional endoscopy, WCE and DBE have been recently employed. WCE has been compared favourably with intraoperative enteroscopy for the diagnosis of obscure bleeding in adults, with 95% sensitivity and 75% specificity. WCE has been found to be diagnostically superior to endoscopy and barium follow-through/CT scan in obscure GI bleeding, and has been recently evaluated in children. WCE is, however, non-therapeutic by its nature, and since the imperative in paediatric gastroenterology is the drive to diagnosis by mucosal histology, this is a shortcoming of WCE.

**Q14** Dieulafoy's lesion is best described by which one of the following?
 **A**  A submucosal artery that protrudes through a minute defect in the gastric mucosa.
 **B**  A GI stromal tumour that arises from the stomach.
 **C**  Oesophageal varices in the lower end of the oesophagus.
 **D**  Another name for hiatus hernia.
 **E**  None of the above.

**A14** **A**  Among the mucosal lesions that may be a cause for haematemesis, a Dieulafoy lesion is a submucosal artery that aberrantly protrudes through a minute defect in the mucosa. It is a very rare cause for haematemesis.

**Q15** The main disadvantage in wireless capsule endoscopy is:
 **A**  the time taken for transit through the small bowel
 **B**  the inability to get tissue for diagnosis
 **C**  that the bowel needs preparation
 **D**  that the child has to be nil by mouth for 6–8 hours
 **E**  that it can be used for treatment of lesions found during examination.

**A15** **B**  WCE has recently become the investigation of first choice for such diagnoses, while intraoperative enteroscopy, despite its invasive quality, has been the mainstay in the subsequent treatment of obscure GI bleeding in children and adults. WCE is, however, non-therapeutic by its nature, and since the imperative in paediatric gastroenterology is the drive to diagnosis by mucosal histology, this is a shortcoming of WCE.

**Q16** A 26-weeker who is 8 weeks old was feeding and growing in the transitional care area. Over a couple of days he developed diarrhoea, which was initially thought to be due to breast feeding. Over the next couple of days, he became lethargic and had one episode of blood in stools. Which of the following interventions will help him most?
 **A**  vitamin K as intramuscular injection
 **B**  septic screen, abdominal X-rays and triple antibiotics
 **C**  fresh frozen plasma
 **D**  reassure parents that it is due to breast feeding
 **E**  change the milk, as this could be cow's milk protein allergy

A16  **B**  Ex-prems are prone to develop necrotising enterocolitis. Any loose stools in an ex-prem, especially when they are establishing feeds, should be viewed with suspicion. Blood in stools is a late presentation. Any suspicion of necrotising enterocolitis warrants a septic screen and abdominal X-rays and starting triple antibiotics. Fresh frozen plasma is of help only in those with known coagulation defects. Cow's milk protein allergy presents as a chronic problem with vomiting and failure to thrive, rather than as an acute presentation.

Q17  Which of the following is not a cause of GI bleeding in a neonate?
   **A**  necrotising enterocolitis
   **B**  swallowed maternal blood
   **C**  vitamin K deficiency
   **D**  hypertrophic pyloric stenosis
   **E**  Hirschsprung's enterocolitis

A17  **D**  All of the causes present with GI bleed except hypertrophic pyloric stenosis, which presents with vomiting at 3–8 weeks of life. Swallowed maternal blood may arise from the mother's nipple or may have been swallowed during delivery, and can be proved to be maternal in origin by Apt Downey test, where, on mixing with alkali, maternal blood turns brown because of formation of haematin, whereas there is no change in colour with fetal haemoglobin, which is alkali resistant.

   All neonates who present with haematemesis should also be given vitamin K, as they may have missed the prophylaxis post delivery.

## Further reading

Arain Z, Rossi TM. Gastrointestinal bleeding in children: an overview of conditions requiring nonoperative management. *Semin Pediatr Surg.* 1999; 8(4): 172–80.

Boyle JT. Gastrointestinal bleeding in infants and children. *Pediatr Rev.* 2008; 29(2): 39–52.

Flynn DM, Booth IW. Investigation and management of gastrointestinal bleeding in children. *Curr Paediatr.* 2004; 14(7): 576–85.

Lin TN, Su MY, Hsu CM, *et al.* Combined use of capsule endoscopy and double-balloon enteroscopy in patients with obscure gastrointestinal bleeding. *Chang Gung Med J.* 2008; 31(5): 450–6.

Park JJ, Wolff BG, Tollefson MK, *et al.* Meckel diverticulum: the Mayo Clinic experience with 1476 patients (1950–2002). *Ann Surg.* 2005; 241(3): 529–33.

Thomson M, Venkatesh K, Elmalik K, *et al.* Double balloon enteroscopy in children: diagnosis, treatment, and safety. *World J Gastroenterol.* 2010; 16(1): 56–62.

# CHAPTER 45

# Disorders of colonic motility

## TAIWO A LAWAL, ALBERTO PEÑA, MARC A LEVITT

From the choices below each question, select the single best answer.

**Q1** Which of the following statements about Hirschsprung's disease is true?
  A  Hirschsprung's disease is more common in females.
  B  It occurs more commonly in black people.
  C  The incidence is 1 : 5000 live births.
  D  The first successfully treated child was reported by Harald Hirschsprung.
  E  It is the commonest cause of constipation in children.

**A1**  C  Hirschsprung's disease occurs in 1 in 5000 live births, and is more common in males with a male-to-female ratio of 4 : 1. In long-segment disease, this ratio decreases. A higher incidence has been reported in white people and in Asian children.

Harald Hirschsprung is credited with the first classic description of the disease. He was a Danish paediatrician and presented the cases of two children with the clinical and anatomical characteristics of the condition in Berlin, in 1886. The first surgical approach was reported by Swenson and Bill in 1949.

The commonest cause of constipation in children is idiopathic constipation, which affects 3% of the paediatric population.

**Q2** A 3-year-old boy underwent a Swenson's pull-through for rectosigmoid Hirschsprung's disease as an infant. His parents are thinking about having another child. Which of the following is a true statement about the familial risk?
  A  There is a 25% chance that the sibling, if male, will be affected.
  B  A female sibling has a higher risk of being affected.
  C  There is a 5% chance that the sibling, if female, will be affected.
  D  The likelihood increases with the length of aganglionosis in an older sibling.
  E  None of the above.

**A2**   **D**   There is evidence of familial involvement in Hirschsprung's disease. The incidence of familial occurrence ranges from 2% to 18%. The risk of familial involvement increases with the length of aganglionosis. The chances that a male sibling will be affected (5%) are greater than those of a female (1%) in short-segment Hirschsprung's disease. Male relatives of females with long-segment Hirschsprung's disease have the greatest risk of being affected (25% for brothers and 30% for sons).

**Q3**   With regard to the diagnosis of Hirschsprung's disease in the neonatal period, which of the following is true?

  **A**   99% of full-term neonates pass meconium within the first 24 hours of life.

  **B**   Failure to pass meconium within the first 48 hours is pathognomonic of Hirschsprung's disease.

  **C**   A bedside suction biopsy is the preferred method of diagnosis.

  **D**   A barium enema is preferred to water-soluble contrast to exclude other causes of large bowel obstruction.

  **E**   None of the above.

**A3**   **C**   Failure of passage of meconium within the first 48 hours of life is the commonest feature of patients with Hirschsprung's disease. Ninety-five per cent of full-term neonates will pass meconium within the first 24 hours of life and 10%–40% of patients with Hirschsprung's disease, in various reports, successfully pass meconium, so it is not always helpful as a clinical feature.

  A water-soluble contrast enema is preferred to barium in neonates to avoid barium peritonitis in cases of occult perforation. Water-soluble enemas are also therapeutically better at dislodging meconium plugs.

  A bedside suction biopsy is the key diagnostic study.

**Q4**   Concerning rectal biopsy for the diagnosis of Hirschsprung's disease, which of the following is true?

  **A**   A full-thickness biopsy is preferred in newborns.

  **B**   The absence of ganglion cells and the presence of hypertrophic nerves confirms the diagnosis of Hirschsprung's disease.

  **C**   The biopsy should be done at the level of the dentate line.

  **D**   A and B are both correct.

  **E**   Rectal suction biopsy has a specificity of 85%.

**A4**   **B**   To make the diagnosis of Hirschsprung's disease, a rectal biopsy for histology is vital. A suction biopsy at the bedside or in clinic offers a rapid way of obtaining the specimen without the need for anaesthesia but is difficult to do in infants after 1 year of age. The sensitivity of rectal suction biopsy is >90% and specificity is >95%. The pathological evaluation, however, is more technically difficult for a suction biopsy specimen than for a full-thickness rectal biopsy specimen.

In older children or in patients with indeterminate suction biopsy results, a full-thickness biopsy is needed. The features on hematoxylin and eosin staining that are diagnostic of Hirschsprung's disease are the absence of ganglion cells and the presence of hypertrophic nerves.

 **Q5** Which of the following is true of the transition zone?

A In this zone, there are often ganglion cells and the nerves are larger than 40 µm.

B The bowel should never be pulled through at the level of the transition zone.

C It is located between the collapsed and dilated segments of the rectosigmoid colon.

D It is more obvious, radiographically, in older children.

E All of the above.

**A5** **E** The transition zone is a segment of the colon where there is an admixture of areas with ganglion cells and areas of aganglionosis. It is easier to see on a contrast enema in older children and is a helpful guide in planning for the pull-through procedure.

It is characterised by the presence of hypertrophic nerves (nerves larger than 40 µm) against a background of reduced number of ganglion cells (hypoganglionosis). The bowel should never be pulled through until normal ganglion cells and normal-sized nerves are present and it is advisable to go a few centimetres above where the intraoperative frozen section sample was obtained and reported to be normal.

**Q6** The following statements about the extent of aganglionosis are true *except*:

A long-segment Hirschsprung's disease occurs in 10% of affected patients

B total colonic aganglionosis may involve the terminal ileum

C rectosigmoid involvement is the most common manifestation

D the extent of aganglionosis correlates well with the severity of symptoms

E the descending colon is always involved in long-segment Hirschsprung's disease.

 **A6** **D** The most common type of Hirschsprung's disease, seen in two-thirds of patients, is one in which the extent of aganglionosis includes the rectum and

sigmoid colon. Long-segment Hirschsprung's disease, which occurs in 10% of patients, signifies that aganglionosis extends proximal to the splenic flexure.

The entire colon is aganglionic in patients with total colonic aganglionosis, frequently including the terminal ileum. Total colonic aganglionosis (TCA) occurs in 10% of the patients with Hirschsprung's disease. The severity of symptoms seen in patients does not necessarily correlate with the extent of aganglionosis; in fact, TCA patients often present late and have more subtle symptomatology, such as chronic distension and failure to thrive.

 **Q7** Concerning the pathology of Hirschsprung's disease, which of the following is true?

A Ganglion cells are absent in the submucosa and muscularis of the affected segment of the bowel.

B Ganglion cells are absent in the submucosa but present in the muscularis of the affected segment of the bowel.

C There is a reduction in acetylcholinesterase in the affected segment of the bowel.

D Excessive nitric oxide synthase activity is a possible pathogenetic mechanism.

E None of the above.

 **A7** A Ganglion cells are absent in the rectum and, to a varying degree, the colon in Hirschsprung's disease. Ganglion cells are missing from Auerbach's plexus (the myenteric plexus is located between the circular and longitudinal layers of bowel wall), Henle's plexus (in the deep submucosa) and also Meissner's plexus (in the superficial submucosa).

In addition to the finding of aganglionosis, there is an increase in acetylcholinesterase in the aganglionic colon. This can be shown using acetylcholinesterase staining and can assist in the diagnosis of Hirschsprung's disease. Nitric oxide has been postulated as a neurotransmitter that is responsible for the inhibitory action that is elicited by enteric nerves, and a lack of nitric oxide synthase has been demonstrated in the myenteric plexus of the aganglionic segment of bowel.

**Q8** Which of the following is not a factor in the pathogenesis of enterocolitis?

A alteration in mucin composition

B reduction in the amount of immunoglobulin A present in the intestines

C stasis in the colon

D increased expression of *MUC2* gene in the colon

E decrease in gut-associated lymphoid tissue

**A**8 **D** The pathophysiology of enterocolitis has not been fully elucidated. However, in patients with Hirschsprung's disease, the presence of stasis resulting from aganglionosis has been associated with overgrowth of unusual anaerobic bacteria including *Clostridium difficile*, which leads to secretory diarrhoea and hypovolaemia. In contrast, stasis in the absence of aganglionosis in patients with idiopathic constipation does not produce enterocolitis.

Patients with Hirschsprung's disease have an altered mucin composition in the intestine with almost undetectable levels of MUC2, the major mucin component in the colon in humans.

Other immunologic defects include decline in the amounts and function of immunoglobulin A and T-lymphocytes.

**Q**9 With regard to enterocolitis in Hirschsprung's disease, which of the following is true?

**A** It occurs rarely after a pull-through procedure.

**B** Recurrent enterocolitis after a pull-through procedure warrants further investigation.

**C** Oral metronidazole is ineffective.

**D** Enterocolitis is better treated with enemas than irrigations.

**E** None of the above.

**A**9 **B** Enterocolitis can occur in patients with Hirschsprung's disease, both preceding and after the pull-through. It occurs in 10%–40% of patients who have undergone a definitive pull-through procedure. The mechanism of enterocolitis is still unclear.

Enterocolitis after a technically correct pull-through responds to an aggressive course of irrigations and metronidazole. If enterocolitis becomes recurrent after a pull-through procedure, further investigation for an anatomical cause (e.g. a constricting Soave's cuff) or pathological cause (retained aganglionosis or transition zone pull-through) becomes necessary. Oral metronidazole is very useful in the treatment of enterocolitis, especially when combined with irrigations.

Enemas are not effective when compared with rectal irrigations in treating enterocolitis. The administration of an enema will exacerbate the distension in a patient with enterocolitis and aggravate the condition. The fluid must be washed out of the lumen of the bowel, which can be accomplished with irrigations, to break the cycle of stasis and bacterial overgrowth.

**Q10** Concerning colostomy in the management of Hirschsprung's disease, which of the following is true?

 **A** Colostomy may be indicated as a form of decompression in severe enterocolitis unresponsive to irrigations.

 **B** Diverting colostomy is best sited in the distal sigmoid colon.

 **C** Permanent colostomy is a form of treatment for total colonic aganglionosis.

 **D** Colostomy should be performed prior to treatments with colonic irrigations.

 **E** Colostomy, if performed, should always be a loop stoma.

**A10** **A** The ideal treatment of Hirschsprung's disease nowadays is a primary pull-through, without protective colostomy. A diverting colostomy may be indicated as an emergency procedure in very ill patients or if intraoperative pathology is not available. A diverting colostomy has to be sited at an optimal location which depends on the level of aganglionosis. Without the availability of pathological correlation, in most patients the safest area is proximal to the sigmoid colon – usually in the descending or transverse colon or an ileostomy. In a centre without a paediatric pathologist, diversion with a colostomy can be life-saving, with a reconstruction planned for a future date. If frozen section is available, an option is to perform a levelling colostomy. Then the colostomy can be pulled down at the time of the definitive repair. This deprives the patient of the protection of proximal diversion, but reduces the needed operations from three to two.

 A colostomy would be ineffective in the treatment of total colonic aganglionosis. An ileostomy is the preferred form of diversion.

**Q11** Which of the following statements is correct about the definitive treatment of Hirschsprung's disease?

 **A** In Swenson's procedure, the aganglionic colon is resected and the normoganglionic bowel should be anastomosed to the anal canal precisely at the dentate line.

 **B** Soave's original procedure involves endorectal dissection, resection of the aganglionic colon, and a primary coloanal anastomosis.

 **C** The commonest complication of Duhamel's procedure is neurovascular injury.

 **D** Martin's procedure for total colonic aganglionosis incorporates the aganglionic colon in the anastomosis.

 **E** None of the above.

**A11** **D** Swenson and Bill performed the first corrective surgery for Hirschsprung's disease in 1948. The Swenson procedure involves dissection of the rectum, staying as close to the bowel wall as possible, and resection of the aganglionic as well as the dilated parts of the colon and the rectum. The coloanal anastomosis is done 1–2 cm above the dentate line. The dentate line should be protected in all forms of surgery for Hirschsprung's disease because of the risk of faecal incontinence associated with destruction of the dentate line.

In Soave's original description, there was a transabdominal dissection through the seromuscular layer, starting 2 cm above the peritoneal reflection and this was carried down to 1–2 cm above the dentate line. The aganglionic rectum and colon were then resected and the colostomy out of the anal canal pulled through a muscular cuff. The protruding colon was left dangling outside and a coloanal anastomosis performed at a later date. Boley modified this approach by performing a primary coloanal anastomosis.

The Duhamel procedure involves dissection through a presacral retrorectal space in an attempt to limit the risk of injury to pelvic nerves and urogenital structures with pull-through of ganglionic bowel, and anastomosing it to the aganglionic pouch.

Martin described the use of the aganglionic portion of the colon to treat total colonic aganglionosis by creating a long channel of anastomosed ganglionic small bowel to aganglionic colon.

Today, the most common approach is a transanal Soave-like technique, which sometimes can be completed without entering the abdomen at all.

**Q12** Regarding idiopathic constipation, which of the following is true?
  **A** It has a primary psychological component.
  **B** Symptoms are due to a hyperactive internal anal sphincter.
  **C** The contrast enema is similar to the picture seen in Hirschsprung's disease.
  **D** It is often fatal.
  **E** None of the above.

**A12** **E** Idiopathic constipation is a poorly understood entity. A secondary psychological component is a consequence of delay in the proper management of idiopathic constipation particularly when encopresis (overflow soiling) occurs. Individuals who have the incapacity to empty their colon and soil their underwear daily can have serious psychological distress. In addition, the passage of large, hard pieces of stool may provoke pain, which will make the patient afraid to have bowel movements.

The cause remains unknown; it is not thought to be due to a hyperactive internal anal sphincter, but rather related to an inherent dysmotility of the colon.

The contrast enema in idiopathic constipation typically shows a megarectosigmoid colon, the opposite of that seen in Hirschsprung's disease. Idiopathic constipation is not a fatal condition, unlike another rarer cause of constipation – intestinal pseudo-obstruction – which can have serious systemic complications.

**Q13** Which of these is true regarding Hirschsprung's disease and idiopathic constipation?

**A** Enterocolitis is common to both.

**B** Soiling is a common symptom in idiopathic constipation but is unusual in Hirschsprung's disease.

**C** A rectal biopsy taken at the dentate line will differentiate between the two.

**D** A pathological transitional zone is present in both conditions.

**E** Anal fissures commonly accompany Hirschsprung's disease but are rare in idiopathic constipation.

**A13** **B** Enterocolitis is a symptom seen in patients with Hirschsprung's disease but not those with idiopathic constipation. Even though stasis plays a role, there are other mechanisms which are poorly understood, that lead to enterocolitis in patients with Hirschsprung's disease.

Soiling is typical with idiopathic constipation (also called encopresis) and when it occurs without the patient's awareness, it is an ominous sign of bad constipation. It is unusual in patients with Hirschsprung's disease unless the anal canal or sphincters have been damaged during the pull-through. A rectal biopsy taken 1–2 cm above the dentate line for histology is the gold standard in the diagnosis of Hirschsprung's disease. If the biopsy is taken right at the dentate line, there may be a false positive result because of the natural zone of aganglionosis in the anal canal at the level of, and just above, the dentate line.

A transitional zone of hypoganglionosis and hypertrophic nerves is present in Hirschsprung's disease but is not a feature of idiopathic constipation. Fissures occur in idiopathic constipation and can lead to a vicious cycle of symptoms. As the fissures attempt to heal, constipation and passage of hard stools reopen the fissures.

**Q14** An 8-year-old boy has had constipation since infancy. He stooled normally at birth. He now soils daily despite enemas once a week. His general physical examination, except for a malleable mass in the left lower quadrant, is normal. Rectal examination reveals normal tone and stool is palpated on the examining finger. The most likely finding on radiography with water-soluble contrast material is:

A dilated colon with normal rectosigmoid

B dilated proximal colon, transition zone, contracted distal recto-sigmoid

C narrow left colon with megarectosigmoid

D normal colon and rectosigmoid

E normal colon except for megarectosigmoid.

**A14** **E** The boy has features consistent with idiopathic constipation. Hirschsprung's disease is highly unlikely because the patient stooled normally at birth, soils every day and has a normal physical examination at 8 years of age despite not having had surgery. The radiographic appearance in idiopathic constipation is a megarectosigmoid; the colon is normal proximally, which is exactly the opposite of what is found in Hirschsprung's disease, in which the distal bowel is contracted.

**Q15** Which of the following statements about chronic intestinal pseudo-obstruction is *not* true?

A Histology of the colon shows hypertrophic nerves.

B It may occur secondary to Chagas's disease.

C There is a high mortality rate.

D There is no mechanical obstruction.

E It may be drug induced.

**A15** **A** Chronic intestinal pseudo-obstruction is called different names by different authors. It is a highly fatal form of functional intestinal obstruction sometimes requiring intestinal transplantation. The histological appearance of colonic biopsy ranges from a normal appearance to specific abnormalities that are described as muscle fibrosis, vacuolar degeneration, disorganisation of myofilaments, or an arrest in the maturation of the myenteric plexus. Ganglion cells are present and nerve trunks are normal in size.

In addition to idiopathic causes, intestinal pseudo-obstruction has been associated with Down's syndrome, neurofibromatosis, multiple endocrine neoplasia 2B, Russell–Silver's syndrome, Duchenne's muscular dystrophy, viral gastroenteritis and prematurity. Secondary causes include Chagas's disease, a parasitic infection caused by *Trypanosoma cruzi* that affects the myenteric plexus. Drug-induced pseudo-obstruction can be encountered in newborns with prenatal transplacental drug exposure or with prolonged ingestion of narcotics.

**Q**16 Concerning intestinal neuronal dysplasia:
   A  it is a distinct clinical entity with clear histological distinctions from Hirschsprung's disease
   B  colonic resection and pull-through procedures are indicated once the diagnosis is made
   C  it is commonly associated with infants of diabetic mothers
   D  it is more common in patients over the age of 10 years
   E  none of the above is true.

**A**16  **E**  Intestinal neuronal dysplasia has been considered a cause of constipation in children but its histology is inconsistent and it is unclear if it is truly a distinct clinical entity. It has been described by different authors to have features such as hypertrophy of ganglion cells, normal ganglion cells, immature ganglia and hypoganglionosis, hyperplasia of the submucous and myenteric plexuses with formation of giant ganglia, hypoplasia or aplasia of sympathetic innervations of the myenteric plexus, and increased acetylcholinesterase positive nerve fibres around submucosal vessels and in the lamina propria. In postoperative Hirschsprung's patients who are experiencing obstructive symptoms, their problems may instead represent transition-zone bowel.

## Further reading

Georgeson KE. Hirschsprung's disease. In: Holcomb W, Murphy JP, editors. *Ashcraft's Pediatric Surgery*, 5th ed. Philadelphia, PA: Elsevier Saunders; 2010. pp. 456–67.

Levitt MA, Peña A. Update on pediatric faecal incontinence. *Eur J Pediatr Surg.* 2009; **19**(1): 1–9.

Levitt MA, Peña A. Pediatric fecal incontinence: a surgeon's perspective. *Pediatr Rev.* 2010; **31**(3): 91–101.

Peña A, Levitt MA. Colonic inertia disorders in pediatrics. *Curr Probl Surg.* 2002; **39**(7): 666–730.

Poenaru D, Borgstein E, Numanoglu A, *et al.* Caring for children with colorectal disease in the context of limited resources. *Semin Pediatr Surg.* 2010; **19**(2): 118–27.

Teitelbaum DH, Coran AG, Martucciello G, *et al.* Hirschsprung's disease and related neuromuscular disorders of the intestine. In: Grosfeld JL, O'Neill JA, Fonkalsrud EW, *et al.*, editors. *Pediatric Surgery. Vol 2.* 6th ed. Philadelphia, PA: Mosby Elsevier; 2006. pp. 1514–59.

# CHAPTER 46

# Anorectal continence and constipation

## KAVEER CHATOORGOON, ALBERTO PEÑA, MARC A LEVITT

**From the choices below each question, select the single best answer.**

**Q1** Under the best circumstances, the global result following the surgical treatment of anorectal malformations is:

**A** 75% chance of faecal incontinence

**B** 50% chance of faecal incontinence

**C** 25% chance of faecal incontinence

**D** 5% chance of faecal incontinence

**E** no chance of faecal incontinence.

**A1** **C** Approximately 25% of patients with anorectal malformations will have a 'high'-enough malformation that continence mechanisms (anal canal, sphincters, motility) are congenitally underdeveloped or absent. Despite optimal anatomical reconstruction, these patients will be faecally incontinent. Of the remaining 75%, most can achieve good continence, though some will have occasional soiling, especially if they have diarrhoea. Many will require laxatives to treat constipation.

**Q2** Which one of the following conditions represents a formal contraindication for a pull-through to repair an anorectal malformation?

**A** myelomeningocele

**B** absent sacrum

**C** presacral mass

**D** absent colon

**E** none of the above

**A2** **D** The only contraindication for a pull-through procedure in a patient with an anorectal malformation is the inability to produce formed stool. Such a patient with limited or no continence mechanism would have no ability to hold in the stool, and would suffer from severe intractable nappy rash. If a patient has a colostomy and is considering a pull-through procedure with only a short segment of residual colon (as in cloacal exstrophy), bowel management through the stoma, to ensure that their proximal colon can be cleaned successfully, is an ideal test. This will ensure that following the pull-through procedure, they will still remain clean with enemas.

**Q3** The best way to find out if the colon of the patient is clean after the administration of an enema is by:

**A** measuring the amount of stool that came out

**B** palpating the abdomen

**C** rectal examination

**D** taking an abdominal X-ray film

**E** none of the above.

**A3** **D** An abdominal X-ray assesses whether the patient's rectum and colon is being emptied appropriately by the enema. If the X-ray shows moderate stool burden, especially in the rectum, then the volume/potency of the enema will need to be increased. If the X-ray shows an empty colon, but the patient has been soiling, then the enema is likely too potent, and needs to be reduced.

**Q4** When a patient suffers from faecal and urinary incontinence, what is the best course of action?

**A** Treat the problem of urinary incontinence first and then manage the faecal incontinence.

**B** Take care of the faecal incontinence problem first and then evaluate the urinary tract.

**C** Take care of both problems at the same time.

**D** Offer the patient a permanent colostomy.

**E** Try a course of biofeedback prior to the bowel management.

**A4** **B** Urinary incontinence can be exacerbated by severe constipation. It is important to treat any constipation before working up a patient for urinary incontinence. In cases of severe constipation, overflow incontinence can be mistaken for true faecal incontinence. In that situation, the mistake can be to attribute the faecal and urinary incontinence to a tethered cord or other neurological problem. Treating the constipation aggressively (if it exists) will often fix both the faecal and urinary continence and avoid the need for unnecessary rectal enemas and intermittent urinary catheterisations.

**Q5** A patient who suffers from faecal incontinence comes for consultation and the decision is made to implement a bowel-management programme with enemas. The patient heard about the possibility of administering the enemas through the umbilicus or through a little orifice in the abdominal wall connected to his appendix, a procedure that is called continent appendicostomy, also known as MACE or Malone's procedure. Which of the following is the best course of action?

   **A** Perform the operation, and 1 month later start the bowel management.

   **B** Perform the operation, and 3 months later start the bowel management.

   **C** Start the bowel management, and 6 months later try the surgical procedure.

   **D** Try the bowel management with rectal enemas and only when it is demonstrated that the bowel management works, because the correct enema has been found, offer the patient the operation.

   **E** None of the above.

**A5**   **D** Faecal incontinence is managed with daily enemas. These enemas can be given retrograde (through the rectum) or antegrade (through an appendicostomy). Before performing the appendicostomy procedure, it is vital to first confirm that the patient can be managed with enemas via the retrograde approach. This will help to avoid performing surgery in the small percentage of patients who are unsuccessful with bowel management. Following the appendicostomy procedure, the same enema routine is usually employed, though occasionally adjustments will have to be made.

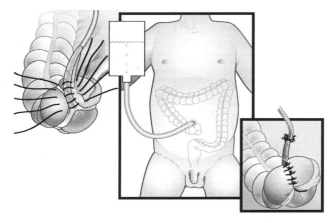

**FIGURE 46.1** Caecal plication around the native appendix: the appendix overlying the caecum, administration of the enema through the umbilicus, and the completed plication

**Q6** In which patients is the combination of enemas and laxatives indicated?
- **A** In all patients who suffer from faecal incontinence.
- **B** In the group of incontinent constipated patients.
- **C** In cases of faecal incontinence due to spina bifida.
- **D** In patients who suffer from faecal incontinence due to an operation for Hirschsprung's disease.
- **E** None of the above.

**A6** **E** Laxatives and enemas are used for two different patient populations. Laxatives are used in patients with bowel control, but who suffer from constipation. In these patients, the stimulant laxatives help propel the stool down to the rectum, where the anus then relaxes to allow the passage of a voluntary bowel movement. Enemas are used in patients without bowel control. The enemas help to mechanically empty the colon and rectum so that there is no leakage of stool for 24 hours. The next enema then cleans out any stool that has accumulated in the previous 24 hours. With this philosophy for bowel management, there is no scenario where a patient would benefit from both laxatives and enemas. In patients on daily enemas due to faecal incontinence, laxatives would promote a more rapid transit of stool, leading to soiling between enema washouts.

**Q7** What is the best way to administer an enema for the management of faecal incontinence?
- **A** with a large Foley catheter with the balloon inflated
- **B** with a large rubber tube introduced as far as possible
- **C** with a thin rubber tube introduced no more than 5 cm
- **D** with the patient in supine position
- **E** none of the above

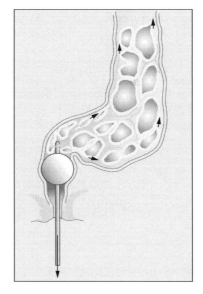

**A7** **A** Enemas should be given so that the solution can sit in the rectum for several minutes before it is allowed to evacuate. Otherwise, the full potency of the enema is lost. The best way to minimise leakage is with a large Foley catheter with the balloon inflated. Catheter insertion with the patient in prone position is very effective.

**FIGURE 46.2** Foley catheter technique with inflated balloon and traction used to avoid leakage

**Q8** What is important when beginning an enema programme?

  **A** to provide written instructions to the caregiver to administer the enema correctly at home

  **B** to demonstrate in person the correct way to give the enema as an outpatient

  **C** to sedate the patient

  **D** A and B

  **E** all of the above

**A8** **D** Families need a practical demonstration of how to administer enemas to better understand the subtleties and important tricks that can be employed. Having written literature to take home helps the family if they come across problems. Sedation is not necessary to administer enemas.

**Q9** What is the appropriate age for a continent appendicostomy or other procedure to administer antegrade enemas?

  **A** between the ages of 3 and 6 years

  **B** before 3 years of age

  **C** between the ages of 6 and 9 years

  **D** after 12 years of age

  **E** when the patient asks for it

**A9** **E** It is best to wait until the patient asks for the continent appendicostomy, so as to ensure that they are fully invested in the process. This allows them to gain their own independence. As it is only a different route for enema administration, the bowel management programme with rectal enemas must be completed first.

**Q10** A 5-year-old girl who has severe constipation and soiling and who was born with a myelomeningocele and absent sacrum, with sensory and motor dysfunction of the lower extremities, can be described as having:

  **A** aganglionosis

  **B** capability of having voluntary bowel movements

  **C** overflow faecal incontinence with constipation

  **D** true faecal incontinence with constipation

  **E** true faecal incontinence with hypermotility.

**A10** **D**

**Q11** The treatment for the previously described 5-year-old girl should include:

    **A** a daily enema

    **B** laxatives

    **C** loperamide and pectin

    **D** potty-training strategies

    **E** surgical correction.

**A11** **A** The patient has a myelomeningocele and absent sacrum, which are a poor prognostic factors for faecal continence. Additionally, she demonstrates neurological sequelae of this problem, with sensory and motor deficits. Although overflow pseudoincontinence is a possibility, her risk factors point towards faecal incontinence with elements of hypomotility. The management of faecal incontinence with hypomotility is daily enemas. None of the other options would work. It should be noted that if she had a hypermotile colon with faecal incontinence, the management would be daily enemas with loperamide and pectin to slow down the colon, so no stool passes between enemas.

**Q12** You have diagnosed severe idiopathic constipation with soiling in a 8-year-old patient. His contrast enema shows a dilated megarectosigmoid with faecal impaction. Of the following, the *most* appropriate *initial* therapy is:

    **A** aggressive use of stimulant laxatives

    **B** daily loperamide

    **C** faecal disimpaction

    **D** increased intake of bananas, apples, and pasta

    **E** stool softener twice daily.

**A12** **C** The first step in the management of idiopathic constipation is to ensure that the patient is not impacted. Starting laxatives when the colon is impacted, only leads to severe cramps and vomiting. Once the impaction has been treated with enemas, then laxatives can be started. Once the constipation is controlled, soiling will improve quickly.

**Q13** Which of the following patients is *most likely* to have faecal incontinence?

   **A** A 5-year-old male with Hirschsprung's disease, with a transition point in the splenic flexure.

   **B** A 9-year-old female patient with anorectal malformation (rectovestibular fistula), with normal sacrum and good midline groove.

   **C** A 7-year-old male patient with idiopathic constipation and occasional soiling.

   **D** A 4-year-old male patient with anorectal malformation (rectobladder neck fistula), with an abnormal sacrum (sacral ratio 0.35) and a tethered cord.

   **E** An 11-year-old female patient with cloacal malformation (common channel 1.5 cm), good sacrum (sacral ratio 0.60) and normal spine.

**A13**   **D**   Factors influencing continence in anorectal malformations include the 'height' of the malformation as well as the development of the sacrum and associated spinal cord problems. 'High' malformations include bladder neck fistula, and cloacal malformation with a common channel greater than 3 cm. 'Low' malformations include perineal fistula, vestibular fistula, bulbar urethral fistula, no fistula, and short-channel cloaca (less than 3 cm). Prostatic urethral fistula have a 50% chance of having faecal incontinence. A short, poorly developed sacrum (with a sacral ratio below 0.4), tethered cord, or other spinal anomalies all point towards poor bowel control and faecal incontinence.

**Q14** A patient comes for consultation complaining of faecal incontinence; he is 7 years old, had an abdominoperineal operation, has three sacral vertebras missing, has mislocated rectum, has a flat bottom, and passes stool constantly. The best treatment is:

   **A** biofeedback

   **B** bowel management with a daily enema

   **C** reoperation to relocate the rectum

   **D** permanent colostomy

   **E** none of the above.

**A14**  **B**

**Q15** A patient who comes for consultation complaining of faecal inconti-nence was born with imperforate anus and underwent an attempted repair in the past, his rectum is located outside the sphincter mechanism and he has a good sacrum and good-looking perineum. The best initial treatment is:

**A** bowel management with a daily enema

**B** biofeedback

**C** permanent colostomy

**D** posterior sagittal anorectoplasty redo

**E** none of the above.

**A15** **A** In patients with anorectal malformations and faecal incontinence and good potential for bowel control, a redo operation may improve continence, especially if the original operation has left them with an anus located outside of the sphincter mechanism. Patients with a good prognosis include those with a 'low' malforma-tion, good sacrum and normal spine. There is no guarantee that a redo operation will improve the faecal incontinence, and so the best initial step is to first manage the faecal incontinence with daily enemas. Once the patient is clean with bowel management, then a redo may be attempted to see if they have the capacity for voluntary bowel movements.

**Q16** Which one of the following studies is most important in the evaluation of patients suffering from faecal incontinence who underwent a previ-ous operation for the repair of imperforate anus?

**A** electromyography

**B** rectal manometry

**C** water-soluble contrast enema

**D** ultrasound of the perineum

**E** evoked potentials study

**A16** **C**

Q17 A patient suffering from faecal incontinence was born with imperforate anus, has a very poor sacrum and a normally located rectum. The water-soluble contrast enema shows absence of the rectosigmoid. The descending colon was anastomosed to the perineum. The best form of treatment is:

A biofeedback

B posterior sagittal anorectoplasty redo

C bowel management consisting of enemas, loperamide and a constipating diet

D bowel management with only colonic irrigations

E permanent colostomy.

A17 c

Q18 A patient suffering from faecal incontinence was born with imperforate anus, three sacral vertebrae missing, a flat perineum and a mislocated rectum. The Hypaque enema shows a moderate megasigmoid. The best treatment is:

A bowel management consisting of enemas, no special diet and no medication

B bowel management consisting of enemas and laxatives

C permanent colostomy

D gracilis muscle transposition

E bowel management consisting of enemas and loperamide.

A18 A When instituting bowel management with enemas, the water-soluble contrast enema can help determine if the colon is dilated (hypomotile) or non-dilated (hypermotile).

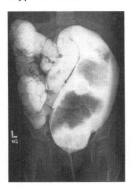

FIGURE 46.3 Contrast enema of a dilated megarectosigmoid (hypomotile)

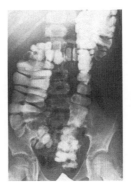

FIGURE 46.4 Contrast enema of a non-dilated colon with evidence of a previously resected rectosigmoid (hypermotile)

In patients with a dilated rectosigmoid, the bowel is hypomotile, and will retain stool until washed out by the daily enema. In patients with a previous resection of the rectosigmoid, the bowel is hypermotile, and usually requires agents to slow down bowel transit. Without these agents, the patient will soil between enemas.

Q19 A patient suffers from faecal incontinence; during the repair of his imperforate anus he lost his entire colon. He has no capacity to form solid stool, has a poor sacrum, weak sphincter muscles and has a mislocated anal opening. the best treatment is:

A permanent ileostomy

B redo posterior sagittal anorectoplasty

C biofeedback

D bowel management with loperamide and enemas

E gracilis muscle transposition.

A19 A The only contraindication for a pull-through procedure is the inability to form solid stool. In a patient who has had his entire colon removed, there is no possibility of producing solid stool. In this scenario, a permanent ileostomy would be the best option for the best quality of life.

## Further reading

Lemelle JL, Guillemin F, Aubert D, *et al*. A multicentre study of the management of disorders of defecation in patients with spina bifida. *Neurogastroentrol Motil*. 2006; **18**: 123–8.

Levitt MA, Peña A. Update on pediatric faecal incontinence. *Eur J Pediatr Surg*. 2009; **19**(1): 1–9.

Levitt MA, Peña A. Pediatric fecal incontinence: a surgeon's perspective. *Pediatr Rev*. 2010; **31**(3): 91–101.

Malone PS, Ransley PG, Kiely EM. Preliminary report: the antegrade continence enema. *Lancet*. 1990; **336**(8725): 1217–18.

# CHAPTER 47

# Anorectal disorders

## ANDREA BISCHOFF, ALBERTO PEÑA, MARC A LEVITT

**From the choices below each question, select the single best answer.**

**Q1** The most frequent anorectal defect seen in males is:
- **A** a high defect
- **B** anal membrane
- **C** rectourethral fistula
- **D** no fistula
- **E** rectal atresia.

**A1** **C** The most frequent anorectal malformation in male patients is rectourethral fistula. The correct diagnosis of the malformation is important since it predicts the prognosis for bowel control. There are two types of rectourethral fistula: rectobulbar urethral fistula (which carries the best prognosis) and rectoprostatic urethral fistula.

**Q2** The most frequent anorectal defect seen in females is:
- **A** perineal fistula
- **B** vestibular fistula
- **C** no fistula
- **D** rectovaginal fistula
- **E** persistent cloaca.

**A2** **B** The most frequent anorectal malformation in female patients is rectovestibular fistula. It is a malformation with excellent prognosis for bowel control. The most important anatomical feature during the surgical repair is the presence of a common wall between rectum and vagina that requires a very meticulous dissection.

**Q3** In the newborn with anorectal malformation, radiological studies of the location of the rectum ideally must be done:

  **A** during the first 6 hours of life

  **B** from 6 to 12 hours of life

  **C** from 12 to 18 hours of life

  **D** after 18 hours of life

  **E** after 48 hours of life.

**A3**   **D** When the patient is born, a radiological evaluation may not show the correct anatomy before 24 hours because the rectum is collapsed and it takes some time for the gas and meconium to pass through the bowel and to overcome the muscle tone of the sphincters that surround the lower part of the rectum. A radiological evaluation performed too early will show a 'high defect', which will be an incorrect diagnosis in many cases. Imaging should wait until at least 18–24 hours after birth.

**Q4** In neonates with imperforate anus, when the clinical information does not allow one to make a decision about the opening of a colostomy, the next most valuable study is:

  **A** magnetic resonance imaging (MRI)

  **B** CT scan

  **C** invertogram

  **D** cross-table lateral film with patient in prone position

  **E** ultrasound.

**A4**   **D**

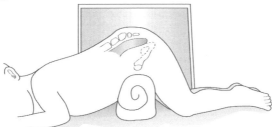

**FIGURE 47.1** Technique for a cross-table lateral radiograph: a roll has been placed beneath the hips of the infant to elevate the buttocks and allow air to migrate superiorly to the end of the rectum

A cross-table lateral film with the patient in prone position is a good tool to measure the distance between the distal rectum and the anal dimple, in order to decide whether a primary repair (air below the coccyx) or a colostomy (air above the coccyx) is appropriate. In the past, invertograms were the exam of choice, but they were very uncomfortable for the patients and there was a risk of vomiting, aspiration and cyanosis. The same information can be obtained with a cross-table lateral film.

**Q5**  The ideal colostomy in patients with anorectal malformation is:
   **A**  end colostomy with Hartmann's pouch
   **B**  divided proximal sigmoid colostomy
   **C**  double-barrelled transverse colostomy
   **D**  loop colostomy
   **E**  none of the above.

**A5**  **B**

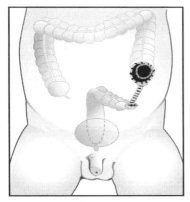

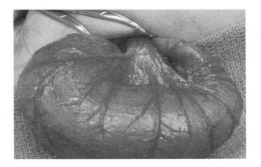

FIGURE 47.2  Diverting descending colostomy with small mucous fistula

FIGURE 47.3  A megarectosigmoid in a newborn

The ideal colostomy in patients with anorectal malformation is a divided proximal sigmoid colostomy. It is important to separate the stomas with enough distance that a bag can be adapted over the proximal stoma without including the mucous fistula in the same bag, that way faecal material coming from the proximal stoma does not enter the distal stoma. The ideal technique opens the proximal stoma in the proximal sigmoid colon, just after the descending colon is attached to the left retroperitoneum; this avoids prolapse. Placing the mucous fistula in the proximal sigmoid will provide enough distal bowel for the pull-through. It should be exteriorised as a tiny orifice to avoid prolapse of the distal segment, since this portion of the colon is not naturally fixed. Other reasons for using this type of colostomy include: performing the distal colostogram with the mucous fistula, for the correct diagnosis of the malformation, and avoiding faecal material in the urinary tract (since the majority of patients have a communication with the urinary tract).

**Q6** Which of the following studies seems to be more accurate in demonstrating the location of the fistula?

 A high-pressure distal colostogram

 B MRI with contrast

 C CT scan with contrast

 D ultrasound

 E voiding cystourethrogram

**A6** **A** The high-pressure distal colostogram is the most important exam for the surgeon. It shows the precise location of the fistula, the amount of colon available for the pull-through, and it also shows the rectum location in relation to the sacrum. When the rectum can be seen below the sacrum, it means that it can be reached posterosagittally; when it is above the sacrum it means that a laparotomy/laparoscopy will be needed.

**Q7** What is the diagnosis and what would be the best surgical approach for this patient?

 A perineal fistula, dilatation of the fistula

 B anal membrane, perforation of membrane

 C no fistula, posterior sagittal anorectoplasty

 D anal stenosis, dilatation of stenotic tract

 E anterior mislocated anus, cutback

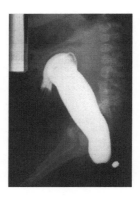

**A7** **C** This high-pressure distal colostogram shows an anorectal malformation without fistula. The distal rectum is very close (about 1–2 cm) from the anal dimple and it is also below the sacrum. This is very similar to the location of a rectourethral bulbar fistula type of anorectal malformation. With that image the surgeon can open posteriosagittally and the first structure that will be found will be the rectum. With mobilisation of the rectum an anoplasty can be performed.

FIGURE 47.4 A lateral view of a high-pressure distal colostogram

Q8   What is the diagnosis and what would be the surgical approach for this patient?

   **A**   rectoprostatic fistula, posterior sagittal approach only

   **B**   no fistula, posterior sagittal approach only

   **C**   recto-bladder neck fistula, posterior sagittal approach only

   **D**   rectoprostatic fistula, laparotomy/ laparoscopy and posterior sagittal approach

   **E**   recto-bladder neck fistula, laparotomy/ laparoscopy and posterior sagittal approach

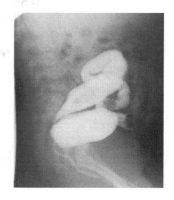

FIGURE 47.5 A lateral view of a high-pressure distal colostogram

A8   **E**   This high-pressure distal colostogram shows a recto-bladder neck fistula with plenty of distal bowel left for the pull-though. The colon is above the sacrum (as always occurs in recto-bladder neck fistulas), so a laparotomy/laparoscopy will be needed in order to reach the rectum and mobilise it. After the mobilisation, a small posterior sagittal incision and anoplasty is performed.

Q9   What is the diagnosis and how would you approach this patient:

   **A**   recto-bladder neck, posterior sagittal approach

   **B**   rectoprostatic, posterior sagittal approach

   **C**   rectobulbar, posterior sagittal approach

   **D**   rectoprostatic, laparotomy/ laparoscopy

   **E**   rectobulbar, laparotomy/ laparoscopy

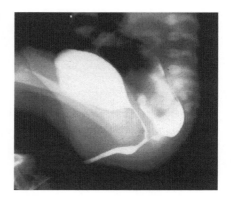

FIGURE 47.6 A lateral view of a high-pressure distal colostogram

A9   **C**   This high-pressure distal colostogram shows a rectobulbar fistula. The rectum is below the sacrum and it can be reached by a posterior sagittal approach. An important anatomical characteristic of this malformation is the fact that it is the one that shares the longest common wall with the urethra, and therefore it requires a meticulous surgical dissection.

Q10 You are asked to examine the perineum of a newborn patient, your diagnosis is:

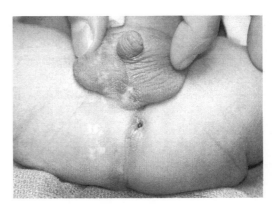

FIGURE 47.7 Perineum of a newborn patient

A imperforate anus, high malformation
B imperforate anus, unknown malformation
C rectobulbar fistula
D anorectal malformation without fistula
E perineal fistula.

A10 E Following the scrotal raphe down, one identifies a small orifice that corresponds to a perineal fistula in a male patient. A careful physical exam is the key to making this diagnosis. The surgeon can expect to find the healthy rectum within 1–2 cm of the fistulous tract. During the surgical repair, the surgeon has to be particularly careful with the dissection plane between the rectum and urethra, since these two structures are closely related.

Q11 What malformation is this?
A vestibular fistula
B rectovaginal fistula
C perineal fistula
D cloaca
E no fistula

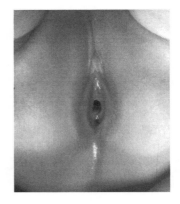

A11 A This is a vestibular fistula, the most common anorectal defect in female patients. The physical exam is key to making this diagnosis. The most important anatomical feature during the surgical repair is the common wall between rectum and vagina that requires a very meticulous dissection to achieve separation.

FIGURE 47.8 Perineum of a newborn patient

Q12 The incidence of hydrocolpos in patients with cloaca is:
A 5%
B 10%
C 30%
D 60%
E 80%.

**A12**  **C**  Hydrocolpos in patients with cloaca must be suspected, diagnosed and treated. It occurs in 30% of these patients. A pelvic ultrasound specifically looking for a cystic structure behind the bladder can make the diagnosis.

**Q13** The best treatment in a neonate patient with a persistent cloaca and a giant hydrocolpos is:

**A**  colostomy and vesicostomy

**B**  colostomy and vaginostomy

**C**  colostomy and dilatation of the single perineal orifice

**D**  colostomy and aspiration of the hydrocolpos content

**E**  colostomy and ureterostomies.

**A13**  **B**  The best treatment for a patient with cloaca and hydrocolpos is colostomy and vaginostomy performed in the newborn period. The importance of draining the hydrocolpos is to avoid perforation of the hydrocolpos with consequent peritonitis; to avoid infection (pyocolpos) that might result in vaginal tissue damage, making it unavailable for the future repair; and to relieve ureterovesical obstruction, caused by a mass effect on the trigone, resulting in megaureters and hydronephrosis, and possible kidney damage.

**Q14** During the repair of a cloaca, with two hemivaginas, where must one look for the rectal orifice?

**A**  in the right vagina

**B**  in the left vagina

**C**  on the posterior wall of the common channel

**D**  in the septum that separates the two hemivaginas

**E**  on the anterior wall of the common channel

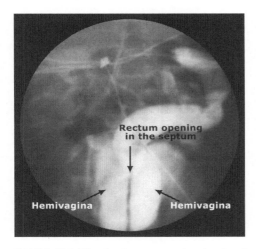

**FIGURE 47.9** Distal colostogram showing two hemivaginas in a cloaca patient

$A$14  **D**  In the presence of two hemivaginas in a patient with a cloaca, the rectum usually can be found opening in the septum between the two hemivaginas.

$Q$15  Which one of the following urologic problems is more frequently associated with an anorectal malformation?
  **A**  hypospadias
  **B**  absent kidney
  **C**  cryptorchidism
  **D**  ureteropelvic obstruction
  **E**  ureterocele

$A$15  **B**  The most frequent urologic malformation associated with anorectal malformation is absent kidney, occurring in 11%. The more complex the malformation (recto-bladder neck fistula, cloaca), the higher is the chance of having an associated urologic abnormality (90% in those complex malformations mentioned compared with 10% in perineal fistulas).

$Q$16  Which one of the following defects is more frequently associated with an anorectal malformation?
  **A**  vesicoureteral reflux
  **B**  horseshoe kidney
  **C**  ureterocele
  **D**  cryptorchidism
  **E**  hypospadias

$A$16  **A**  The most frequent urological defect in patients with anorectal malformation is vesicoureteral reflux, occurring in 21%. The first hint of this problem is the finding of hydroureter on kidney ultrasound.

$Q$17  Down's syndrome in children with imperforate anus is most frequently associated with:
  **A**  perineal fistula
  **B**  rectourethral fistula
  **C**  recto-bladder neck fistula
  **D**  cloaca
  **E**  imperforate anus with no fistula.

$A$17  **E**  Anorectal malformation without fistula occurs in about 5% of patients with anorectal malformation. When one looks specifically at patients with Down's syndrome, 95% of those born with an anorectal malformation have the no-fistula type of defect.

**Q18** Rectal atresia is a defect in which the anus and the anal canal are normal and there is an obstruction that separates the anal canal from the rectum, usually located about 1–2 cm from the skin level in the perineum. The frequency of this defect is approximately:

A  1%

B  10%

C  20%

D  30%

E  40%.

**A18  A**  Rectal atresia is an extremely unusual defect. The upper pouch is represented by a dilated rectum, whereas the lower portion is represented by a small anal canal that is in the normal location and is 1–2 cm deep. The repair involves a primary anastomosis between the upper pouch and the anal canal.

**Q19** The frequency of imperforate anus with a rectovaginal fistula is approximately:

A  1%

B  10%

C  20%

D  30%

E  40%.

**A19  A**  Rectovaginal fistulas are extremely rare, with an incidence rate of less than 1%. In the past, many rectovestibular fistulas or cloacas were erroneously named rectovaginal fistula. In a true rectovaginal fistula (extremely uncommon), the rectum opens in the posterior wall of the vagina and it can only be seen inside the vagina. The urethra and vagina must be visible as separate orifices in order to distinguish this defect from a cloaca.

**Q20** Anal dilatations post imperforate anus repair are ideally performed:

A  once a week

B  every 4 days

C  every second day

D  once a day

E  twice a day.

**A20  E**  The protocol for anal dilatation should be started 2 weeks after the repair, passing the Hegar dilator two times every day (30 seconds each time). The patient is seen in clinic and the surgeon determines with which Hegar dilator to start (the one that can be passed without resistance and without causing pain), and also the Hegar dilator that is the goal for that child based on the age:

1–4 months = Hegar # 12

4–8 months = Hegar # 13

8–12 months = Hegar # 14

1–3 years = Hegar # 15

3–12 years = Hegar # 16

More than 12 years = Hegar # 17

Every week the parents change the Hegar to the next size, until they reach the goal Hegar dilator. Once the goal number passes easily and without pain, twice a day, the parents can start tapering the frequency of dilatations: once a day for a month, every other day for a month, every third day for a month, once a week for a month, once a month for 3 months. Dilatations under anaesthesia at 1 week or more intervals will crack the anoplasty and lead to scarring and a fibrotic stricture.

## Further reading

Bischoff A, Levitt MA, Breech L, *et al*. Hydrocolpos in cloacal malformations. *J Pediatr Surg*. 2010; **45**(6): 1241–5.

Levitt MA, Peña A. Imperforate anus and cloacal malformations. In: Holcomb W, Murphy JP, editors. *Ashcraft's Pediatric Surgery*. 5th ed. Philadelphia, PA: Elsevier Saunders; 2010. pp. 468–90.

Torres R, Levitt MA, Tovilla JM, *et al*. Anorectal malformations and Down's syndrome. *J Pediatr Surg*. 1998; **33**(2): 194–7.

# SECTION IX

# Hepatobiliary disorders

# CHAPTER 48

# Biliary atresia

## ERIC JELIN, KELLY D GONZALES, HANMIN LEE

From the choices below each question, select the single best answer.

**Q1** What percentage of children who underwent successful Kasai's procedure (hepatoportoenterostomy) will have progressive liver disease that requires liver transplantation before adulthood?

  **A** 50%

  **B** 60%

  **C** 70%

  **D** 80%

  **E** 90%

**A1** **C** Kasai's procedure performed in the newborn is successful when bile flow is restored. Nonetheless, these patients still carry a risk of 70% or greater of developing cirrhosis that will require liver transplantation before adulthood.

**Q2** Biliary atresia liver histology is mimicked by all of the following diseases *except*:

  **A** total parental nutrition associated cholestasis

  **B** cystic fibrosis

  **C** Alagille's syndrome

  **D** choledochal cyst

  **E** hepatocellular carcinoma.

**A2** **E** The results of liver biopsy are critical in making the diagnosis of biliary atresia. The findings of a liver biopsy in biliary atresia include fibrosis, inflammation, and proliferation. These findings can also be seen with choledochal cysts, bile duct strictures and stones, total parenteral nutrition-associated cholestasis, alpha-1 antitrypsin deficiency, cystic fibrosis, multiple drug resistant 3 deficiency, North American Indian childhood cirrhosis (cirrhin deficiency) and Alagille's syndrome. The diagnosis of biliary atresia relies on multiple aspects of the patient history and examination rather than on a single test to make the diagnosis.

**Q3** Which of the following histological features can be seen with biliary atresia?
- **A** inflammatory cell infiltration
- **B** expansion of portal tracts with fibrosis
- **C** bile plugs in portal tracts
- **D** syncytial giant cell formation
- **E** all of the above

**A3** **E** Liver biopsies taken from a patient with biliary atresia usually show fibrosis, inflammation and proliferation. The characteristic features include expansion of portal tracts, infiltration of inflammatory cells, and portal tracts with bile plugs. The expansion of the portal tracts may carry varying degrees of fibrosis which may be predictive of long-term success of the Kasai procedure. There may also be parenchymal changes such as syncytial giant cell formation, lobular disarray and extramedullary haematopoiesis.

**Q4** All of these viral agents has been linked to biliary atresia *except*:
- **A** cytomegalovirus (CMV)
- **B** reovirus
- **C** rotavirus
- **D** human papilloma virus
- **E** hepatitis virus.

**A4** **D** There are three main viruses that are associated with biliary atresia. CMV was reportedly found in 24%–38% of affected patients while reovirus was seen in 55% of patients. An even higher percentage, 78%, of patients with both biliary atresia and choledochal cysts had identified reovirus infection. Although rotavirus has been identified in patients with biliary atresia, this has not been a consistent finding. In addition, mouse models have demonstrated that these viruses can cause inflammatory extra-hepatic biliary obstruction. Other viruses that have been reported with biliary atresia include respiratory syncitial virus, human papilloma virus and Epstein–Barr virus. Hepatotropic viruses such as hepatitis A, B and C have not been related to biliary atresia.

**Q5** Which of the following is considered non-controversial postoperative therapy after a Kasai procedure?
- **A** fat-soluble vitamins
- **B** ursodeoxycholic acid
- **C** steroids
- **D** all of the above
- **E** B and C

**A** The preoperative management of patients undergoing Kasai's procedure includes nutritional supplementation, fat-soluble vitamins and antibiotics. The postoperative management of patients following a Kasai procedure has brought forth various strategies that have not shown to be statistically beneficial and therefore remain controversial. The use of steroids is thought to improve bile flow following a Kasai procedure. When steroid use is implemented, the initial doses are given intravenously and then transitioned to oral steroids followed by a taper regimen. Ursodeoxycholic acid is another controversial therapy regimen which follows the administration of intravenous bile acids to also aid in bile flow following a Kasai procedure. The use of fat-soluble vitamins is a mainstay of both pre- and postoperative management and is not considered controversial.

**Q6** Postoperative cholangitis is characterised by which of the following?
  **A** fever
  **B** abnormal liver function tests
  **C** pale stools
  **D** jaundice
  **E** all of the above

**A6** **E** Cholangitis occurs in about 30%–50% of postoperative patients following a Kasai procedure. These patients usually present with fever and abnormal liver function tests. The patient may also develop signs and symptoms characteristic of their presentation prior to the Kasai such as jaundice and acholic stools. In this clinical scenario patients need to be evaluated for sepsis. In the case of recurrent cholangitis with resultant liver decompensation, the next treatment step is likely a liver transplant.

**Q7** Symptomatic portal hypertension may present with all of the following *except*:
  **A** variceal bleeding
  **B** ascites
  **C** splenomegaly
  **D** perianal hematoma
  **E** hepatic encephalopathy.

 **D** Portal hypertension has been documented to occur in almost two-thirds of patients following a Kasai procedure. The presenting symptoms are oesophageal varices, ascites, and splenomegaly. Portal hypertension is often accompanied by worsening jaundice and synthetic liver function, which in severe cases can lead to hepatic encephalopathy. Unlike hemorrhoids and anorectal varices, perianal hematoma is not associated with portal hypertension.

**Q**8 In children diagnosed with biliary atresia, improved outcome is mainly attributed to which of the following?

**A** early diagnosis

**B** referral to specialist centres

**C** steroid use postoperatively

**D** A and B only

**E** none of the above

**A**8 **D** Early Kasai and a multidisciplinary centre have both been shown to improve the success of Kasai's procedure, survival outcomes and patient quality of life. Performing Kasai's procedure within 60 days of life has shown significant benefit in patients and extended the number of years until liver transplantation. One study performed in France found that if the Kasai was performed before 45 days of life, 29% of children could live with their native liver for longer than 15 years. In addition, the preoperative and postoperative care of patients diagnosed with biliary atresia is best served by a team of specialists who are familiar with the disease, surgical procedure and postoperative complications.

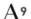**Q**9 The two main causes of cholestatic jaundice in early infancy are:

**A** idiopathic neonatal hepatitis and biliary atresia

**B** Gilbert's disease and biliary atresia

**C** haemolytic disease and biliary atresia

**D** haemolytic disease and Gilbert's disease

**E** none of the above.

**A**9 **A** The differential diagnosis for jaundice in early infancy is vast and requires a full workup. However, the two main causes of cholestatic jaundice are idiopathic neonatal hepatitis and biliary atresia. Causes of neonatal cholestatic jaundice can be divided into intrahepatic and extrahepatic causes. Extrahepatic causes include biliary atresia, choledochal cyst, bile duct stenosis, strictures and cholelithiasis, spontaneous perforation of the common bile duct, and tumours or masses. Intrahepatic causes are numerous and are generally divided into six possible categories: infectious, metabolic, genetic, toxic, cholangiopathies and others. Gilbert's disease is an inherited cause of unconjugated hyperbilirubinaemia. Although it is rare, Gilbert's disease is the most common genetic cause of unconjugated hyperbilirubinaemia. Haemolytic anaemia is caused by the destruction of premature erythrocytes and is also characterised by unconjugated hyperbilirubinaemia.

**Q10** What is the most reliable method to differentiate idiopathic neonatal hepatitis and biliary atresia?

   **A** magnetic resonance cholangiography (MRCP)

   **B** hepatobiliary scintigraphy (HBS)

   **C** abdominal ultrasound

   **D** liver biopsy

   **E** A and B

**A10**  **D** Radiation-sparing radiological studies are frequently employed in children because they are non-invasive. However, radiological studies cannot reliably differentiate causes of neonatal jaundice especially idiopathic neonatal hepatitis and biliary atresia. In one study, MRCP was shown to have a 85.29% sensitivity and 57.14% specificity for biliary atresia. HBS was documented to have a 88.24% sensitivity and 45.71% specificity while abdominal ultrasound had a 50% sensitivity and 82.85% specificity. Compared with liver biopsy (100% sensitivity, 94.29% specificity), these imaging modalities are less useful in making the diagnosis of biliary atresia.

**Q11** Biliary atresia is an obliterative cholangiopathy characterised by which of the following?

   **A** It can affect neonates and adults.

   **B** It should be treated primarily by liver transplant.

   **C** It always eventually requires transplant.

   **D** It can be effectively treated by the Kasai procedure.

   **E** It always involves obliteration of the extrahepatic bile duct.

**A11**  **D** Biliary atresia is an obliterative cholangiopathy that affects neonates. There is no similar process in adults. Liver transplant is reserved for those patients that deteriorate after primary therapy with Kasai's procedure. Some patients do well in the long term with only a Kasai and do not go on to need a liver transplant. Biliary atresia most commonly affects the extrahepatic bile ducts, but can occur in the intrahepatic bile ducts without affecting the extrahepatic duct.

**Q12** Which lab value is not helpful in making the diagnosis of biliary atresia?

   **A** elevated gamma-glutamyl transpeptidase (GGT)

   **B** elevated aspartate transaminase (AST)

   **C** decreased alanine transaminase (ALT)

   **D** decreased albumin

   **E** increased alkaline phosphatase

A12 **D** Biliary atresia is associated with an *increase* in AST, ALT, conjugated bilirubin, total bilirubin and GGT. It is also associated with malnutrition and a decrease an albumin.

Q13 Which of the following presentations is not consistent with biliary atresia?

    **A** A 22-day-old ex-34-weeker presents with jaundice, acholic stools, splenomegaly and indirect hyperbilirubinaemia.

    **B** A 15-day-old term male with jaundice and an elevated gamma-glutamyl transferase.

    **C** A 4-month-old term female with jaundice, tea-coloured urine, ascites and hepatomegaly.

    **D** A 20-day-old ex-34-weeker presents with jaundice and a normal liver biopsy.

    **E** A 1-month-old female term baby presents with acholic stools and a triangular cord sign on ultrasound.

A13 **A** The clinical presentation of biliary atresia is characterised by jaundice, acholic stools, splenomegaly in relationship to portal hypertension but NOT indirect hyperbilirubinaemia. There is no conjugation defect of bilirubin in biliary atresia and thus these patients have *direct* hyperbilirubinaemia. The most common abnormal liver function test in biliary atresia is an elevated gamma-glutamyl transferase. Patients who are diagnosed with biliary atresia late may present with ascites in addition to jaundice and tea-coloured urine. Liver biopsies taken before 6 weeks can sometimes lack the typical features of biliary atresia. The triangular cord sign or a hyperechogenic liver hilum on ultrasound is a specific finding for biliary atresia in most cases. It is, however, operator dependent and has varying sensitivity.

Q14 Post-surgical conditions associated with biliary atresia after Kasai's procedure include:

    **A** cholangitis, steatorrhoea, cholecystitis, biloma, afferent-loop syndrome

    **B** cholangitis, steatorrhoea, cholecystitis, biloma, sepsis

    **C** portal hypertension, cholangitis, afferent-loop syndrome, bile lake infection

    **D** afferent-loop syndrome, cholangitis, choledochal cyst, cholecystitis

    **E** cholangitis, steatorrhoea, oesophageal varices, dumping syndrome.

A14 **C** Kasai's procedure is largely palliative with the vast majority of patients going on to have progression of their disease including worsening progressive liver disease, portal hypertension, oesophageal varices and continued steatorrhoea.

Because the procedure directly connects the intestine to the biliary tree, recurrent cholangitis, bile lake infection and biliary sepsis are persistent postoperative risks. Biloma and afferent-loop syndromes can occur from technical complications at the portoenterostomy site. Cholecystitis, choledochal cyst and dumping syndrome are not associated with Kasai's procedure.

**Q15** Which of the following factors has not been shown to have prognostic value in determining the success of Kasai's procedure?

**A** surgeon experience

**B** presence of cirrhosis

**C** age of patient at the time of procedure

**D** biliary diversion

**E** polysplenia

**A15** **D** Biliary diversion has not been shown to have prognostic value in determining the success of Kasai's procedure. Improved outcomes are associated with increased surgeon experience and decreased patient age at the time of Kasai. Worse outcomes are associated with polysplenia and the presence of cirrhosis at the time of Kasai.

**Q16** In a case of diagnosed biliary atresia, what is the optimal timing of Kasai procedure?

**A** before 60 days of life

**B** before 50 days of life

**C** as soon as possible

**D** before 40 days of life

**E** none of the above

**A16** **C** Although timing is still controversial, the largest series of patients demonstrates that outcomes are improved the earlier a Kasai is performed. Thus the procedure should be performed as soon as possible after diagnosis.

**Q17** Which of the following is an indication for liver transplant after a successful Kasai procedure?

**A** refractory variceal bleeding

**B** elevated total bilirubin

**C** polysplenia

**D** recurrent cholangitis

**E** all of the above

**A17** **A** Refractory variceal bleeding is an indication of severe portal hypertension and cirrhosis. It is an indication to proceed to liver transplant. An elevated bilirubin, in and of itself, is not an indication for liver transplant. Polysplenia is associated with worse outcomes after Kasai but is not, by itself, an indication for liver transplant. Cholangitis in itself is not an indication for liver transplantation, and can be managed conservatively with antibiotics.

**Q18** At what age is liver transplant usually indicated for infants in whom the Kasai procedure is not technically successful and biliary drainage does not occur?

  **A** immediately

  **B** 2–4 years

  **C** 6 months to 2 years

  **D** 9 months to 1.5 years

  **E** none of the above

**A18** **C** The typical age of transplant in patients who have undergone a technically unsuccessful Kasai procedure is 6 months to 2 years.

**Q19** Which molecular marker has been shown to have a relationship with progression of disease after successful Kasai?

  **A** osteopontin

  **B** basic fibroblast growth factor

  **C** hepatocyte growth factor

  **D** transforming growth factor-β

  **E** all of the above

**A19** **E** Osteopontin, basic fibroblast growth factor and hepatocyte growth factor are associated with biliary atresia progression. A raised level of transforming growth factor-β is associated with improved biliary atresia outcomes.

## Further reading

Hartley JL, Davenport M, Kelly DA. Biliary atresia. *Lancet.* 2009; **374**(9702): 1704–13.

Khalil, BA, Perera MT, Mirza DF. Clinical practice: management of biliary atresia. *Eur J Pediatr.* 2010; **169**(4): 395–402.

Serinet M, Wildhaber BE, Brou P, *et al.* Impact of age at Kasai operation on its results in late childhood and adolescence: a rational basis for biliary atresia screening. *Pediatrics.* 2009; **123**(5): 1280–6.

Sokol RJ, Shepherd RW, Superina R, *et al.* Screening and outcomes in biliary atresia: summary of a National Institutes of Health workshop. *Hepatology.* 2007; **46**(2): 566–81.

Yang JG, Ma DQ, Peng Y, *et al.* Comparison of different diagnostic methods for differentiating biliary atresia from idiopathic neonatal hepatitis. *Clin Imaging.* 2009; **33**(6): 439–46.

# CHAPTER 49

# Choledochal cyst

## RICCARDO A SUPERINA, NIRAMOL TANTEMSAPYA

**From the choices below each question, select the single best answer.**

**Q1**  Possible aetiologic theories of choledochal cyst type I include all of the following *except*:

  **A**  Obstruction of the distal common bile duct including stenosis from biliary inflammation and inspissated bile syndrome.

  **B**  Disordered recanalisation of the biliary system leading to congenital weakness of the wall of the common bile duct.

  **C**  Local ischaemia during fetal hepatobiliary development resulting in abnormal vascular-ductal interactions.

  **D**  Abnormal innervation of the distal common bile duct resulting in functional obstruction and proximal dilatation.

  **E**  The pancreatic duct joining the common bile duct outside the ampulla of Vater resulting in reflux of pancreatic juice into common bile duct causing dilatation.

**A1**  **C**  During the course of normal biliary development the epithelial ductal plates induce vasculogenesis in the portal mesenchyme resulting in development of hepatic artery branches. These structures in turn influence development of the embryonic bile ducts. Arteriopathy resulting in abnormal vascular-ductal interactions is a possible mechanism in the development of biliary atresia and the focus of renewed interest. Other choices are possible aetiologies of choledochal cyst.

**Q2**  Which of the following is *not* true regarding choledochal cyst?

  **A**  Choledochal cyst type I fusiform is the most common type.

  **B**  Choledochal cyst is more common in females and Asians.

  **C**  More than two-thirds of cases are diagnosed in children less than 10 years of age.

  **D**  The majority of cases present with the classic triad of jaundice, right hypochondrial mass and pain.

  **E**  The malignancy risk is age related; malignancy mainly affects adults and may develop in the cyst wall or gallbladder.

**A2** **D** The classic triad of jaundice, pain and right hypochondrial mass is presented in less than 10% of patients. Infants typically present with obstructive jaundice, acholic stools with or without vomiting and an abdominal mass or hepatomegaly. Fever and failure to thrive may be noted. Recurrent abdominal pain is the dominant presenting feature in older children with or without intermittent jaundice. Occasionally signs of hepatic fibrosis are present even in young patients. The degree of histological damage and the rate of epithelial metaplasia and dysplasia is related to the age of the patient, and malignancy risk mainly affect adults. Other choices are true.

**Q3** Which of the following is true regarding the anatomy of the extrahepatic biliary system?

**A** Endangered structures while dissecting Calot's triangle include the right hepatic artery, aberrant right hepatic artery and accessory or replaced sectional ducts that join the common hepatic and the cystic duct.

**B** The hepatoduodenal ligament forms the anterior border of the foramen of Winslow and within the ligament are the common bile duct, hepatic artery and inferior vena cava.

**C** The proper hepatic artery divides into the right and left hepatic arteries at a variable level but at the hilum both arteries usually lie anterior to the bile ducts.

**D** The supraduodenal bile duct receives its blood supply from the hepatic and cystic arteries above and gastroduodenal and retroduodenal arteries below, forming a fine plexus with main arteries running longitudinally at the anterior and posterior aspects of the duct.

**E** Intramural resection of the posterior wall of the cyst may help to avoid damage to the pancreatic head and second part of the duodenum if there is dense inflammation or portal hypertension.

**A3** **A** The common hepatic duct and the cystic duct form the base and inferior margin of Calot's triangle. The superior border was formerly the cystic artery; however, the inferior surface of the right hemiliver is accepted as a better working definition. Dissection of this area, a crucial part of cholecystectomy, endangers the structures mentioned. The structures within the hepatoduodenal ligament are the common bile duct, hepatic artery and portal vein. The right and left hepatic arteries usually lie posterior to the bile ducts at the liver hilum. The common bile duct contains two main arteries running longitudinally at the medial and lateral aspects of the duct. Intramural resection of the posterior wall of the cyst may help to avoid damage to the portal vein and hepatic arteries if there is dense inflammation or portal hypertension.

**Q4** Which of the following is true regarding the clinical presentation of choledochal cyst?

   **A** Progressive hepatic fibrosis may develop in the infant and is reversible with surgical repair.

   **B** Infants typically present with obstructive jaundice and hyperamylasaemia.

   **C** Recurrent abdominal pain is the dominant presenting feature in older children with or without intermittent jaundice.

   **D** Portal hypertension may develop in older children because of portal vein obstruction from cyst compression or secondary biliary cirrhosis.

   **E** Spontaneous rupture may affect any part of the cyst and can be intraperitoneal or retroperitoneal.

**A4** **B** Even in the presence of pancreaticobiliary malunion, hyperamylasaemia is not found in infants with choledochal cyst. This is due to pancreatic immaturity and only reaches significant levels at about 1–2 years of age. However, biliary concentrations of pancreatic lipase, elastase and trypsin are significantly elevated in infants with a common channel. Other choices are true.

**Q5** In infants, choledochal cyst should be distinguished from:

   **A** duodenal atresia

   **B** duplication cyst

   **C** cystic biliary atresia

   **D** ovarian cyst

   **E** all of the above.

**A5** **E** In infants, choledochal cyst needs to be distinguished from cystic varieties of biliary atresia and other intra-abdominal cysts. Ovarian cysts are usually easily distinguishable by their location in the pelvis. In the rare instance that ovarian cysts reach the size that allows them to extend into the subhepatic space, clinical details allow differentiation from choledochal cysts.

**Q6** Which of these is not a complication of choledochal cyst?

   **A** sclerosing cholangitis

   **B** portal hypertension

   **C** cholelithiasis

   **D** pancreatitis

   **E** biliary cirrhosis

**A** Complications of choledochal cyst can occur at multiple levels from:
- pancreas – acute/chronic pancreatitis, pancreatolithiasis
- extrahepatic bile ducts – obstructive jaundice, cholangitis, cholelithiasis, cyst rupture and malignant transformation
- intrahepatic – biliary cirrhosis/hepatic fibrosis, portal hypertension, and liver abscess.

Sclerosing cholangitis is a chronic cholestatic liver disease, characterised by progressive inflammation and fibrosis of the bile ducts resulting in biliary cirrhosis and is associated with a high risk of cholangiocarcinoma. The majority of patients are young, male and have coexisting inflammatory bowel disease.

 Which of the following types of pathology can be associated with choledochal cyst?

**A** pancreaticobiliary malunion
**B** hepatic fibrosis
**C** inspissated bile plug syndrome
**D** ectopic pancreas
**E** all of the above

 **E** In more than 75% of cases, there is an anomalous junction between the distal common bile duct and the pancreatic duct, whereby they unite outside the duodenal wall proximal to the ampulla of Vater creating a long common channel. Consequently, pancreatic juice refluxes into the biliary tree producing chronic inflammation and is believed to be a potential cause of dilatation of the wall. Hepatic fibrosis may develop rapidly in prenatally detected cases with obstruction and is known to be reversible with surgical repair. Occasionally, in older patients, mild periportal fibrosis can be noted. Obstruction of the distal common bile duct has been a popular aetiologic theory for many years. Bile sludge may gather at the site of the stenosis or, less commonly, small stones. Whether the obstruction is congenital from a developmentally abnormal and stenotic bile duct or secondary to inflammation is not always clear. It may be difficult to differentiate congenital bile duct dilatation from dilatation secondary to an obstruction in cases where the dilatation of the duct is minimal or there is an absence of an anomalous junction. 'Forme fruste' is a term applied to cases believed to represent a choledochal cyst that has not yet reached a size that is easily detectable through ultrasonography and may require more invasive imaging such as magnetic resonance cholangio-pancreatography or endoscopic retrograde cholangio-pancreatography (ERCP) to detect subtle changes. Rarely, choledochal cyst can also be associated with ectopic and multiseptate gallbladder.

**Q8** Regarding investigations for choledochal cyst, which of the following is true?

**A** ERCP gives excellent visualisation of the pancreaticobiliary junction and is useful during episodes of acute pancreatitis.

**B** Intraoperative cholangiography is best performed by injection of contrast directly into the cyst.

**C** Ultrasonography can assess the size, contour and position of the cyst, the proximal ducts, vascular anatomy and hepatic echotexture.

**D** CT with contrast clearly demonstrates the cyst, intrahepatic bile ducts and associated pancreatitis, and is indicated in all cases of choledochal cyst.

**E** Hepatobiliary scintigraphy with technetium-99m is an excellent tool for detecting subtle biliary malformations in the liver.

**A8** **C** Ultrasonography is the initial investigation of choice not only to demonstrate the details of the cyst but also the vascular anatomy and hepatic echotexture as well. Stones or sludge in the ducts or extension of the cyst into the liver may be noted. Assessment of biliary anomalies in the liver may also be noted. ERCP and percutaneous transhepatic cholangiography give excellent visualisation of the duct anatomy. However, both invasive techniques carry a risk of iatrogenic pancreatitis and biliary sepsis, and should be avoided during and immediately after episodes of acute pancreatitis. Intraoperative cholangiography by injecting into the cyst itself is inefficient and awkward and may fail to fill the intrahepatic ducts. It is best performed through the cystic duct and may require large volumes of contrast to fill out the distal duct including the pancreatic duct and the ducts inside the liver. CT with intravenous and oral contrast may be used in patients in whom the ultrasound does not provide sufficiently detailed imaging, the cyst is not very dilated, or where an additional problem is suspected. In most patients a detailed ultrasonography supplemented by intraoperative cholangiography provides sufficient information. Hepatobiliary scintigraphy may be used after surgery to evaluate secretion of bile into the liver but serves almost no purpose in the preoperative workup.

**Q9** Which of the following is the treatment of choice for choledochal cyst type I?

**A** Cyst evacuation and Roux-en-Y cyst-jejunostomy leaving the distal bile duct draining into the duodenum.

**B** Cyst excision, cholecystectomy and Roux-en-Y hepaticojejunostomy.

**C** Cholecystectomy and transduodenal cyst excision.

**D** Cholecystectomy, excision of the cyst mucosa and choledochojejunostomy.

**E** Cholecystectomy and choledochoduodenostomy.

A9 **B** The optimum treatment for most types of choledochal cyst is complete cyst excision to the upper limit of the dilated portion of the common hepatic duct portion of the cyst and reconstruction by hepaticoenterostomy. Care must be taken not to injure any hepatic ducts that enter the cyst in an anomalous location, typically the posterior sectoral duct of the right lobe. Cholecystectomy should always be performed since the cystic duct is almost always involved in the cystic dilatation and empties into the cyst itself. Cystenterostomy is unacceptable due to the risk of long-term complications including cholangitis, cholelithiasis, pancreatolithiasis, anastomotic stricture, biliary cirrhosis and malignancy. Thus cyst excision, cholecystectomy and Roux-en-Y hepaticojejunostomy would be the treatment of choice and patients treated previously by cystenterostomy should undergo revisional surgery. Hepaticoduodenostomy may be an alternative technique, although it carries a risk of bilious gastric reflux, gastritis and oesophagitis; ulceration and malignant transformation such as hilar adenocarcinoma has been reported. Transduodenal cyst excision is the technique used for large cysts of type III choledochoceles.

Excision of the mucosa only is a technique that has been used when the cyst wall is extremely inflamed and very adherent to the underlying portal vein, but should not be utilised except under extreme circumstances.

Q10 Regarding prenatally diagnosed choledochal cyst, which of the following is *not* true?

**A** Early surgical treatment is recommended since biliary atresia presents the same way and may be hard to rule out except by surgery.

**B** Prompt surgical treatment can reverse associated hepatic fibrosis.

**C** Early surgical treatment can reduce the risk of cholangitis and perforation.

**D** Optimal timing for surgery is 3–6 months of age when the infant is stable.

**E** The results of early surgical treatment are generally excellent.

A10 **A** Progressive enlargement of a fetal choledochal cyst with a normal or distended gallbladder or hepatic ducts, or dilatation of the intrahepatic bile ducts demonstrated during pregnancy, favours choledochal pathology. Biliary atresia is not diagnosed prenatally and is rarely associated with large cysts in the hilum of the liver. In biliary atresia, the gallbladder is not typically enlarged and may be undetectable by ultrasound. Hepatic fibrosis may develop rapidly in prenatally detected cases and is known to be reversible with surgical repair. The optimal timing for surgical treatment of prenatally diagnosed choledochal cyst in infants who are otherwise well, is 3 months of age when the baby has established normal feeding patterns, has grown in size and has developed an established pulmonary circulation with resolution of fetal circulatory patterns. The results of surgical treatment at this age are generally excellent.

**Q11** Which of the following is *not* true regarding surgery of choledochal cyst?

   **A** Operative cholangiography is always indicated.

   **B** There has been a growing experience with laparoscopic excision of the choledochal cyst.

   **C** The common hepatic duct is transected just below the level of the confluence of the left and right hepatic ducts providing a single orifice that has not been involved in the cyst itself.

   **D** The common bile duct is dissected through the pancreas to its junction with pancreatic duct

   **E** Cholecystectomy should be performed even if cystic duct is normal in size.

**A11** **D** The distal common bile duct is divided just outside the pancreas and oversewn with absorbable suture. It is not followed down through the pancreas, to avoid injury to the pancreatic duct.

   Operative cholangiography is always advisable since it demonstrates the pancreaticobiliary junction, the anatomy of the intrahepatic ducts and provides a guide to the distal level of bile duct transection necessary. It also shows the position of the individual hepatic ducts in relation to the hepatic end of the cyst where the cyst must be transected without injuring anomalous hepatic ducts. The common hepatic duct is transected at the level of the bifurcation and cholecystectomy should always be performed despite the cystic duct being normal in size. Primary external T-tube drainage is helpful in patients with cyst rupture or uncontrolled cholangitis where cyst excision must be performed subsequently.

**Q12** Which of the following statements is *not* true regarding long-term complications of choledochal cyst excision and hepaticojejunostomy?

   **A** Malignancy not uncommonly affects residual extrahepatic or dilated intrahepatic ducts long after the surgery for type I cysts and lifelong follow-up is recommended.

   **B** Adenocarcinoma of the liver is the common form of cancer that arises in untreated cysts.

   **C** Pancreatitis may develop years after cyst excision especially in those with pre-existing dilated or complex common channel with protein plug.

   **D** Recurrent cholangitis years after surgical excision of the cyst may indicate an anastomotic stricture between the bowel and the bile duct remnant.

   **E** Type V disease with intrahepatic ductal dilatation may lead to progressive fibrosis and the need for liver transplantation.

A**12** **B** Cholangiocarcinoma is the type of cancer that develops in patients with poorly drained or untreated choledochal cysts. Long-term follow-up is indicated in all patients because of the sporadic reports of malignant degeneration in bile ducts near the anastomosis or even in ducts located in the liver.

Ultrasound of the liver and pancreas should be done annually or when necessary if patients become symptomatic particularly in those who had intrahepatic ductal dilatation preoperatively. Malignancy may affect residual extrahepatic or dilated intrahepatic ducts or residual intrahepatic cysts, and is more likely with associated chronic inflammation or bile stasis. Some surgeons advocate hepaticoduodenostomy in preference to hepaticojejunostomy because of a more physiological outcome, associated with a smaller risk of adhesive small bowel obstruction and late anastomotic stricture. However, good results can be achieved with hepaticojejunostomy provided that a wide anastomosis at the level of the common hepatic duct bifurcation is constructed. Hepaticoduodenostomy has been reported to have a higher risk of bile reflux gastritis. Pancreatitis is rare after cyst excision and Roux-en-Y hepaticojejunostomy, although it may develop many years after cyst excision in patients with a dilated or complex common channel containing protein plugs or calculi, or in those with a substantial segment of retained terminal common bile duct. Cholangitis may have preceding causes including anastomotic stricture, bile duct stricture, calculi or Roux-loop obstruction. Type IVa cysts are particularly prone to developing intrahepatic calculi. Thus appropriate follow-up with standard imaging methods is recommended to detect and correct these complications early.

Liver transplantation is necessary if cholestasis develops in patients with type V cysts in the liver because of the development of biliary cirrhosis in whom no drainage procedure can be done to improve biliary stasis.

## Further reading

Howard ER: Choledochal cysts. In: Howard ER, Stringer MD, Colombani PM, editors. *Surgery of Liver, Bile Ducts and Pancreas in Children*. 2nd ed. London: Hodder Arnold; 2002. pp. 149–68.

Howell CG, Templeton JM, Weiner S, *et al*. Antenatal diagnosis and early surgery for choledochal cyst. *J Pediatr Surg*. 1983; **18**(4): 387–93.

Miyano T, Yamataka A, Kato Y, *et al*. Hepaticoenterostomy after excision of choledochal cyst in children: a 30-year experience with 180 cases. *J Pediatr Surg*. 1996; **31**(10): 1417–21.

O'Neill JA. Choledochal cyst. In: Grosfeld JL, O'Neill JA, Fonkalsrud EW, *et al*., editors. *Pediatric Surgery. Vol 2*. 6th ed. St. Louis, MO: Mosby: 2006; pp. 1620–34.

Stringer MD, Dhawan A, Davenport M, *et al*. Choledochal cysts: lessons from a 20 year experience. *Arch Dis Child*. 1995; **73**(6): 528–31.

# CHAPTER 50

# Gallbladder disease

## N ALEXANDER JONES, ONYEBUCHI UKABIALA

From the choices below each question, select the single best answer.

**Q1** The most common aetiology of gallbladder disease in the paediatric population is:

   **A** congenital abnormality of the biliary tract
   **B** concurrent haematological disorder
   **C** primary cholelithiasis
   **D** prolonged total parenteral nutrition (TPN) use
   **E** history of ileal resection.

**A1**   **C**   Primary cholelithiasis is now the most common aetiology of gallbladder disease in the paediatric population. TPN use is commonly reported in association with cholelithiasis and contributes to the incidence of primary cholelithiasis. Haemolytic cholelithiasis secondary to disorders such as sickle-cell disease, spherocytosis, thalassaemia, and so forth. is the second most common cause of gallstones. Congenital abnormalities of the biliary tract are rarely associated with gallbladder disease. Ileal resection does contribute to the formation of pigment stones, but is not by itself the most common cause of gallbladder disease.

**Q2** Causes for the increased incidence of cholelithiasis and cholecystitis over the last 2 decades include all of the following *except*:

   **A** earlier pregnancy age
   **B** childhood obesity
   **C** increased use of TPN
   **D** increasingly deleterious high-calorie diet
   **E** decreased use of oral contraceptives.

**A2**   **E**   The incidence of cholelithiasis and resulting cholecystitis in the paediatric population has increased over the past 2 decades. This has been attributed to several factors including earlier pregnancy age, increased prevalence of childhood obesity, poor diet, increased use of prolonged TPN, and increased use of oral contraceptives. Ultrasound has aided in the increased sensitivity of detection.

**Q3** A dehydrated 6-year-old female is hospitalised with a diagnosis of mesenteric adenitis. She develops right upper quadrant discomfort and an ultrasound demonstrates distension of the gallbladder, some oedema of the gallbladder wall, absence of cholelithiasis, and a common bile duct measuring 3 mm. She is afebrile and her white blood cell (WBC) is 8.9. Which one of the following is the most appropriate initial treatment?

**A** continued supportive treatment

**B** antibiotics

**C** endoscopic retrograde cholangio-pancreatography (ERCP)

**D** cholecystectomy

**E** hepatobiliary iminodiacetic acid (HIDA) scan

**A3** **A** Hydrops of the gallbladder presents in conditions such as septic shock, severe diarrhoea and dehydration, hepatitis, Kawasaki's disease, and mesenteric adenitis. A palpable mass may be felt on physical exam. The gallbladder becomes acutely distended and develops wall oedema. Most cases will resolve spontaneously with supportive care. Antibiotics and cholecystectomy may become necessary if supportive care fails or cholecystitis develops.

**Q4** A 16-year-old slightly obese female presents with intermittent right upper quadrant pain. The episodes of pain seem to follow some meals by about 30–40 minutes, last for about an hour, and then resolve. Right upper quadrant ultrasound is normal. Laboratory workup reveals a WBC count of 9.3 and normal liver function tests. What is the most appropriate next step in management?

**A** CT of the abdomen and pelvis

**B** HIDA scan

**C** expectant management

**D** cholecystectomy

**E** ERCP

**A4** **B** This clinical scenario is consistent with biliary dyskinesia secondary to gallbladder dysmotility. Laboratory workup and ultrasound are typically unremarkable. The most appropriate next step is to order a HIDA scan. Studies have shown that using an ejection fraction less than 35% for a diagnosis of biliary dyskinesia and subsequent cholecystectomy, will achieve 80% or better success rates. ERCP and CT would be expected to be negative and would not be helpful in this workup. Expectant management may be appropriate pending the HIDA results, but would not be the appropriate next step in this case.

**Q5** Which of the following is not an indication to perform an intraoperative cholangiogram during a laparoscopic cholecystectomy?
A  acalculous cholecystitis
B  dilated common bile duct on preoperative ultrasound
C  elevated transaminases and gamma-glutamyl transpeptidase (GGT)
D  history of pancreatitis
E  unclear anatomy

**A5**  **A** This question demonstrates straightforward indications to perform an intraoperative cholangiogram. A dilated common bile duct, history of jaundice, history of pancreatitis, and elevated liver function tests and GGT are all preoperative findings that may represent choledocholithiasis. Unclear anatomy during a cholecystectomy may lead to iatrogenic damage to the common bile duct. Intraoperative cholangiogram should be performed in all of the above situations. Acalculous cholecystitis is not an indication to perform an intraoperative cholangiogram.

**Q6** A 13-year-old male presents with midgut volvulus. He requires extensive small-bowel resection due to bowel necrosis. He has been on TPN for 6 weeks during his prolonged recovery. He then develops a septic state and significant acute abdominal pain. A right upper quadrant ultrasound demonstrates gallbladder wall oedema and pericholecystic fluid. Sludge is seen within the gallbladder and the common bile duct diameter is 3 mm. Other workup is negative. What is the most logical next step in his management?
A  placement of a cholecystostomy tube
B  HIDA scan
C  medical management with antibiotics only
D  stopping the TPN and a trial enteral nutrition
E  cholecystectomy after resuscitation

**A6**  **E** The clinical scenario is an example of acalculous cholecystitis that develops as a result of an extensive bowel resection and prolonged TPN use. Prolonged TPN leads to decreased gallbladder contractibility, distension and stasis. These changes lead to an increased risk of infection and cholecystitis. The ultrasound findings of gallbladder-wall oedema, pericholecystic fluid, and sludge are all consistent with acalculous cholecystitis. After workup is completed for other causes for sepsis, cholecystectomy should be performed. A HIDA scan would not be needed after an ultrasound demonstrating findings consistent with acalculous cholecystitis. Antibiotics are an appropriate next step, but cholecystectomy should follow. Stopping the TPN and a trial of enteral nutrition is not appropriate in the setting of acute cholecystitis.

 **Q7** An asymptomatic 8-year-old male is having a right upper quadrant ultrasound to evaluate apparent hepatomegaly on pre-sports physical examination. During the ultrasound a 3 cm cystic mass is seen in the porta hepatis. The liver is normal in appearance. What should be the next step in management?

A ERCP

B exploratory laparoscopy

c HIDA scan

D endoscopic ultrasound

E repeat ultrasound of gallbladder only

 **A7** **A** In this question stem a cystic mass is diagnosed in the porta hepatis. The differential diagnosis includes choledochal cyst, cholangiocarcinoma, diverticulum of the biliary tree, other biliary anomalies and duodenal duplication and so forth. The ultrasound, while discovering the mass, cannot give a definitive diagnosis and does not give clear information regarding the association of the mass with the biliary tree. ERCP will be the best choice to give this information and is certainly less invasive than an operative diagnosis. Repeat ultrasound would not give additional information. Endoscopic ultrasound also will not give much additional information leading to a diagnosis. Likewise a HIDA scan would not be specific for any of the above conditions.

 **Q8** After further evaluation of the cystic mass discussed in question 7 a diagnosis of duplication of the gallbladder is made. Which of the following would be the next most appropriate step in management?

A CT of the abdomen and pelvis

B laparoscopic cholecystectomy

c open cholecystectomy

D reassurance and education

E MRI

 **A8** **D** Anomalies of the gallbladder and cystic duct are rare causes of gallbladder disease. These anomalies are usually diagnosed incidentally. Reassurance and education is the next most appropriate step in management. Cholecystectomy is not necessary without the presence of coexisting gallbladder disease. No further workup is needed for asymptomatic anomalies and additional imaging would not add more information.

Q9 Unconjugated calcium bilirubinate stones contribute to a significant incidence of gallbladder disease. Aetiology of these stones includes all of the following *except*:

  A prolonged TPN

  B high-fat diet

  C history of ileal resection

  D decreased gallbladder contractility

  E chronic haemolytic states.

A9 **B** The most common types of gallstones are cholesterol stones, especially in children without haematological diseases. Cholesterol stones are seen with increasing age, obesity and poor diet, oral contraceptive use and pregnancy. Approximately 10%–20% of gallstones are composed of calcium bilirubinate and are classified as pigment stones. These stones are mostly seen in patients with decreased gallbladder contractility, prolonged TPN use, history of significant ileal resection, or a chronic haemolytic state, e.g. hereditary spherocytosis and sickle-cell disease.

Q10 Prompt cholecystectomy is indicated in which one of the following clinical situations?

  A A 13-year-old boy with sickle-cell disease diagnosed with symptomatic cholelithiasis during a haemolytic crisis.

  B A markedly obese 12-year-old girl with a single episode of epigastric pain and an ejection fraction of 42% on HIDA scan.

  C An 8-year-old boy with spherocytosis diagnosed with cholelithiasis before undergoing splenectomy.

  D A 2-year-old male with recurrent intussusception requiring ileal resection due to a Meckel's diverticulum.

  E Prophylaxis in a 14-year-old female with cystic fibrosis.

A10 **C** Cholelithiasis occurs in 43%–63% of patients with hereditary spherocytosis. Ultrasound is therefore recommended before splenectomy. If cholelithiasis is documented, cholecystectomy should be performed at the time of splenectomy. Cholelithiasis is present in 10%–55% of patients with sickle-cell disease; however, cholecystectomy is not recommended unless the patient is symptomatic. Cholecystectomy should be performed electively and not during a haemolytic crisis. An ejection fraction of less than 35% is used most commonly to aid in the diagnosis of biliary dyskinesia. An ejection fraction of 42% should be considered normal and cholecystectomy should not be recommended based on the information given. Although an ileal resection can predispose to the development of gallbladder disease, a limited resection for Meckel's diverticulum should not. A cystic duct diverticulum is a rare anomaly of the biliary tree. The presence of this anomaly in an asymptomatic patient is not an indication for cholecystectomy.

**Q11** Principles of laparoscopic cholecystectomy include all of the following *except*:

    **A** retraction of the infundibulum laterally to expose the triangle of Calot

    **B** performing an intraoperative cholangiogram in the setting of unclear anatomy

    **C** attempting laparoscopic common-duct exploration if choledocholithiasis is diagnosed intraoperatively

    **D** conversion to an open cholecystectomy if the presence of adhesions prevents adequate visualisation

    **E** placing a drain in Morison's pouch before completion, when cholecystitis is present.

**A11** **E** There is currently no evidence to suggest that leaving a drain after cholecystectomy improves outcomes or prevents morbidity. Drain use should be selective and based on generally appropriate surgical considerations. The remainder of the answers are all principles of a laparoscopic cholecystectomy.

**Q12** With regard to ERCP in the paediatric population, which of the following is true?

    **A** Complication rates are higher in the paediatric population compared with adults.

    **B** Pancreatitis is the most common complication.

    **C** ERCP should not be performed in children less than 5 years of age.

    **D** Successful cannulation of the ampulla is significantly reduced when compared with the adult population.

    **E** ERCP should not be performed in a child with a history of pancreatitis.

**A12** **B** ERCP is effective in the paediatric population with documented success rates of 90% and greater by experienced practitioners. These success rates are similar to that in the adult population. Complication rates are similar or lower than those in the adult groups. Complications generally involve pancreatitis, haemorrhage, perforation and infection. Pancreatitis is the most common of these complications with a rate probably in the range of 3%–7%. Most of these cases of pancreatitis are mild. There is currently no age cutoff for the performance of ERCP. Success has been obtained safely in patients as young as 1 year of age. A history of pancreatitis is not a contraindication to ERCP; in fact, ERCP is a diagnostic tool for the evaluation of chronic or recurrent pancreatitis.

Q13 During a laparoscopic cholecystectomy on a 13-year-old female the common bile duct is nearly transected. Further inspection reveals a sharp injury of 80% on the duct diameter. The injury is 1 cm below the cystic duct. The most appropriate next step in management is:

A primary laparoscopic repair of the injury with a drain in Morison's pouch

B laparoscopic repair of the injury over a T-tube

C complete the transaction laparoscopically, clip the ends of the duct to prevent bile leak, complete the cholecystectomy, and leave a drain

D convert to an open operation and perform a choledochoduodenostomy

E convert to an open operation and perform a cholecystojejunostomy.

A13 D This question tests management of iatrogenic injury to the common bile duct during cholecystectomy. Limited injuries to the lateral aspect of the common bile duct can be repaired primarily with or without the use of a T-tube. Injuries involving greater than 50% of the duct diameter or involving electrocautery injury should be repaired with choledochojejunostomy or choledochoduodenoscopy, depending on the location of the injury. Repair of these more extensive injuries primarily leads to the development of significant biliary stricture and secondary morbidity.

## Further reading

Ashcraft KW, Holcomb GW, Murphy JP. *Pediatric Surgery*. 4th ed. Philadelphia, PA: Elsevier Saunders; 2005.

Grosfeld JL, O'Neill JA, Fonkalsrud EW, *et al.*, editors. *Pediatric Surgery*. Vol 2. 6th ed. Philadelphia, PA: Mosby Elsevier; 2006.

Halata MS, Berezin SH. Biliary dyskinesia in the pediatric patient. *Curr Gastroenterol Rep*. 2008; **10**(3): 332–8.

Paris C, Bejjani J, Beaunoyer M, *et al*. Endoscopic retrograde cholangiopancreatography is useful and safe in children. *J Pediatr Surg*. 2010; **45**(5): 938–42.

Ziegler MM, Azizkhan RG, Weber TR, editors. *Operative Pediatric Surgery*. New York, NY: McGraw-Hill Companies; 2003.

# CHAPTER 51

# Portal hypertension

## RICCARDO A SUPERINA, NIRAMOL TANTEMSAPYA

**From the choices below each question, select the single best answer.**

**Q1**   Which of the following is true regarding the development of the portal vein?

**A** The left and right omphalomesenteric veins drain the developing gut at the same time the umbilical veins transport blood from the placenta to the embryo.

**B** Blood from both the umbilical and omphalomesenteric veins drains through the hepatic sinusoids in developing liver.

**C** The right omphalomesenteric vein involutes and disappears by the sixth week.

**D** The left umbilical vein remains patent until shortly after birth, when it thromboses and becomes the ligamentum teres.

**E** Some of the blood from the umbilical vein drains through the ductus venosus, which develops into the permanent portal vein.

**A1**   **E**   The left and right omphalomesenteric veins drain the developing gut as it is formed from the yolk sac during the fourth to sixth weeks of gestation. At the same time, the umbilical veins transport blood from the placenta to the embryo. Blood from both the umbilical and the omphalomesenteric veins drains through the nascent hepatic sinusoids in the developing liver and into the hepatic veins back to the developing heart. Some of the blood from the umbilical veins bypasses the liver and drains directly into the inferior vena cava (IVC) through the ductus venosus, which normally closes during the first week of life in most full-term neonates. The right omphalomesenteric vein involutes and disappears by the sixth week of gestation. The left one develops into the permanent portal vein, which drains the mesenteric venous bed through the superior mesenteric vein and its branches. The right umbilical vein also involutes and the left remains patent until shortly after birth, when it thromboses and becomes the ligamentum teres.

**Which of the following is true regarding the anatomy of the portal and systemic venous systems?**

**A** The splenic and mesenteric veins normally drain into the coronary which then forms the main portal vein just behind the head of the pancreas.

**B** The portal vein normally sends large branches to the IVC just before bifurcating into left and right branches.

**C** As a consequence of portal hypertension, the haemorrhoidal plexus of the superior, middle and inferior rectal veins drain into the vein of Sappey.

**D** The left portal vein courses under segment IV of the liver then anteriorly in the recessus of Rex and ends into branches supplying segments II, III and IV.

**E** The recanalised umbilical veins drain the gastro-oesophageal area into the left portal vein producing prominent varicose veins known as caput medusae.

 **D** The portal vein is formed by the confluence of the splenic and superior mesenteric veins posterior to the head of the pancreas. The coronary vein drains the gastro-oesophageal venous bed into the portal vein just distal to the splenomesenteric confluence.

The portal vein does not normally communicate with the IVC in any fashion after birth. Communications between the portal vein and the IVC are known as the Abernethy malformation and deprive the liver of normal portal blood flow and may have significant harmful long-term side effects.

The extrahepatic portal vein divides into a left and a right branch. The left branch courses under segment IV of the liver, turns anteriorly in the recessus of Rex between segments II, III and IV, and ends by dividing into branches that supply those segments. The right branch divides into the posterior and anterior segmental branches at or just inside the liver plate at the capsule.

As a consequence of portal hypertension, blood from the superior mesenteric vein and its tributaries must find alternative routes back to the heart. The three most common collateral formations between the portal and systemic venous networks are in the rectum, periumbilical and gastro-oesophageal areas. In the rectum, a haemorrhoidal plexus forms between the superior haemorrhoidal vein and branches of inferior and middle haemorrhoidal veins. In the course of the ligamentum teres of the liver, small paraumbilical veins recanalises and establishes an anastomosis between the veins of the anterior abdominal wall and the portal, hypogastric and iliac veins. The gastric and oesophageal veins communicate through submucosal plexuses that empty in a direction away from the liver into the hemiazygos venous system. Other frequent shunts include the accessory portal system of Sappey with branches that course through the round and falciform ligaments to unite with the epigastric and internal mammary veins and through the diaphragmatic veins to unite with the azygos veins. Caput medusa refers to the cluster of prominent and visible collateral veins around the umbilicus on the anterior abdominal wall that results from the hepatofugal flow of blood through the recanalised umbilical and para-umbilical veins, that shunts blood into the systemic veins on the anterior abdominal wall. The caput medusa name alludes to the snake-like appearance of the venules radiating out from the umbilicus that reminded early anatomists of the snakes that emanated from the head of Medusa in Greek mythology.

The veins of Retzius connect the intestinal veins with the inferior mesenteric veins and the haemorrhoidal veins that open into the hypogastric veins.

 **3** Which of the following is *not* associated with prehepatic portal hypertension caused by obstruction at the extrahepatic portal vein?

**A** omphalitis

**B** enlarged hilar lymph nodes

**C** venous webs in hepatic veins

**D** sepsis and dehydration in infancy

**E** umbilical vein catheterisation

 **3** **C** Portal hypertension can be divided into two categories: (1) from hepatocellular injury and liver fibrosis, which are mainly intrahepatic causes and (2) from primary vascular causes, which can be classified into prehepatic, posthepatic and high flow or hyperkinetic.

Prehepatic portal hypertension is caused by obstruction at the level of the extrahepatic portal vein. Extrahepatic portal vein thrombosis may be a congenital lesion or acquired at a later time. Occlusion of the main trunk of the portal vein may lead to recanalisation of the vein and its transformation into a series of smaller collateral veins that appear as a venous cavernoma on ultrasonography. Thrombosis of the portal vein is associated with omphalitis, instrumentation and cannulation of the umbilical vein at birth, sepsis and dehydration in infancy and mass lesions that exert extrinsic compression on the vein. These lesions may be inflammatory or malignant such as reactive enlargement of the lymph nodes in the liver hilum, and malignancies such as pancreatic tumours or lymphoma involving the hilum of the liver. Portal vein obstruction may be termed as portal vein thrombosis, cavernous transformation of the portal vein, or extrahepatic portal vein occlusion.

Posthepatic portal hypertension is caused by occlusion of large or small hepatic veins draining blood from the liver into the IVC. Obstruction at this level leads to passive congestion of the liver and necrosis of the hepatocytes in the central areas of the hepatic lobule. Outflow occlusion causes include Budd–Chiari's syndrome or occlusion of the hepatic veins presenting with the classic triad of abdominal pain, ascites and hepatomegaly. Obstruction is primarily caused by thrombosis but can also be secondary to external compression from hepatic masses or surgical misadventure after hepatic resection. It is uncommon in children. Other causes of outflow occlusion are congenital venous webs in the hepatic veins, hydatid disease, myeloproliferative diseases, hypercoagulable states, veno-occlusive diseases from drug-induced phlebitis and thrombosis after liver transplantation.

A rare cause of portal hypertension is an abnormal communication between an artery and a vein of the mesenteric venous circulation. This kind of portal hypertension is termed hyperkinetic or high-flow because the elevation of portal pressure is due to the exposure of the portal vein and connecting mesenteric veins to arterial blood pressure and because of the high volume of blood that subsequently flows into the portal circulation. Bleeding from varices may be severe due to the exposure to arterial pressures. Causes can be congenital but more commonly they may be secondary to trauma that results in a breach of an arterial wall and a venous wall adjacent to each other.

 Which of the following is true of the clinical presentation of portal hypertension?

A Upper GI bleeding may be sudden and dramatic in a previously well child and is usually accompanied by signs of severe pain and peritonitis that may require urgent laparotomy.

B Upper GI bleeding most commonly originates from the lower oesophagus and the cardia of the stomach.

c Splenomegaly is usually a sign of advanced liver disease with synthetic failure, ascites, thrombocytopenia and leucopenia.

D Disorientation, memory loss and drowsiness commonly accompany episodes of bleeding from varices in children with accompanying hyperammonaemia.

E Hepatopulmonary syndrome occurring with cirrhotic portal hypertension is exacerbated by episodes of bleeding.

 B Unlike children with pre-existing liver disease, children with extrahepatic portal vein thrombosis are usually completely well before the sudden onset of symptoms.

GI bleeding is one of the most common clinical presentations of portal hypertension. Bleeding most commonly occurs from varices in the distal oesophagus and gastric cardia. It may take the form of haematemesis, haematochezia, melaena or chronic anaemia. Portal hypertensive gastropathy may cause less-acute bleeding; however, variceal bleeds are often dramatic and sudden and are usually not accompanied by abdominal pain. Although most patients with portal hypertension have varices, not all varices bleed. Rectal bleeding is less common and occurs from rectal and sigmoid varices. Melaena or the passage of gross blood through the rectum or accompanying a bowel movement may occur in the absence of haematemesis. Children with extrahepatic portal vein thrombosis have much less morbidity or mortality from bleeding than in those with liver disease, and bleeding in the former usually stops spontaneously and is generally well tolerated.

Silent splenomegaly without any other history suggestive of portal hypertension is often the first sign of a serious underlying disorder and can occur in children with extrahepatic portal vein obstruction and normal liver function or in children who have well-compensated cirrhosis with no outward manifestations of liver disease. It can easily be misinterpreted as a sign of haematological malignancy, particularly in children with extrahepatic portal vein thrombosis and no other stigmata of liver disease. In addition to splenic enlargement, patients may present with severe hypersplenism with thrombocytopenia and leucopenia from splenic sequestration of platelets and white blood cells.

Severe thrombocytopenia can lead to haematuria, menorrhagia in adolescent girls, epistaxis and haematochezia. In severe cases, spontaneous intracranial bleeding can also occur, with serious neurological consequences. Liver-dependent coagulation factor deficiencies also lead to bleeding, typically from the genitourinary tract or nose. In cases with advanced liver disease, haemorrhagic complications in the lungs may cause severe respiratory compromise.

Encephalopathy is extremely unusual in the absence of other signs of advanced liver disease, such as jaundice and synthetic failure causing disordered coagulation and hypoalbuminaemia. Learning disabilities and behavioural abnormalities are more subtle manifestations of encephalopathy in children, in contrast to the traditional signs of disorientation, memory loss and drowsiness commonly seen in adults. Hyperammonaemia can result from portosystemic shunting even in the absence of advanced liver disease but it may be exacerbated after a GI bleed.

Pulmonary hypertension can occur in children with both cirrhotic and non-cirrhotic forms of portal hypertension. It may be secondary to increased vasoactive substances that exert a vasoconstrictive or direct toxic effect on pulmonary vessels. Patients with both pulmonary and portal hypertension may develop pulmonary symptoms before there is any evidence of bleeding from portal hypertension. Symptoms may include exertional dyspnoea or chest pain, or no symptoms other than unheralded syncope or sudden death. Cirrhosis may be required, in addition to portal hypertension, for hepatopulmonary syndrome to become clinically apparent. Hepatopulmonary syndrome includes persistent hypoxaemia from arteriovenous shunting in the lungs, and may require liver transplantation whereas pulmonary hypertension from prehepatic portal hypertension may be reversed after eliminating portosystemic shunting.

**Q5** Which of the following clinical situations and physiological or physical changes are *not* correctly related?

A Small and non-palpable livers on physical examination are characteristic of patients with congenital hepatic fibrosis.

B Splenomegaly may occur in all pathophysiological conditions causing portal hypertension and is not helpful in arriving at a diagnosis.

C Jaundice, ascites and portal hypertension usually do not occur together unless there is advanced liver disease.

D Although encephalopathy may be exacerbated by acute GI bleeding, it usually signifies advanced hepatocellular disease that may require liver transplantation.

E Ascites may be accompanied by low serum albumin and increased renal tubular absorption of sodium in patients with decompensated cirrhosis or outflow obstruction.

**A5** A Hepatomegaly is often a sign of hepatocellular disease, although patients with cirrhosis may present with impalpable shrunken livers. A hard or nodular liver is evidence that the cause of portal hypertension is a diseased liver. Children with congenital hepatic fibrosis often present with very enlarged livers that may extend as far as the iliac crest on palpation. Children with outflow obstruction may also present with easily palpable liver enlargement.

Splenomegaly is a common finding in children with portal hypertension and often the first abnormality found on a routine physical examination before the onset of bleeding. Splenomegaly occurs in all forms of portal hypertension and is not helpful in diagnosing the cause.

Children with extrahepatic portal vein obstruction or well-compensated cirrhosis may have mild elevation of total bilirubin level, but jaundice is not a clinical feature. If jaundice is a prominent symptom in a child with portal hypertension and accompanied by ascites or coagulation disorder, then the liver disease is most probably quite advanced.

Clinically evident encephalopathy is a sign of advanced liver disease but also may be present in children with urea-cycle defects such as citrullinaemia that are associated with high ammonia levels but no other liver problem. Portal hypertension associated with encephalopathy exacerbated by blood in the gut may require evaluation for liver transplantation. Mild encephalopathy may be hard to quantify in young children who generally present with behavioural abnormalities that are different from adult clinical pictures of disorientation, memory loss and drowsiness.

Ascites may be associated with advanced liver disease with synthetic failure causing a low serum albumin level and decreased plasma oncotic pressure. Dilated lymphatics in the abdomen from increased hydrostatic pressure in all portal tributaries can lead to transudation of fluid across capillary membranes.

Occasionally, chylous ascites may develop. Additional mechanisms include increased nitric oxide production in capillaries causing vasodilatation, increase in renal tubular absorption of sodium in patients with decompensated cirrhosis, and can also occur in the setting of Budd–Chiari's syndrome or outflow obstruction. It is an alarming symptom that may herald the onset of liver decompensation.

 **Q6** Regarding laboratory investigations for portal hypertension, which of the following may be found?

**A** complete blood count: thrombocytopenia, leucopenia

**B** hepatic function panel: increased direct bilirubin fraction, low serum albumin

**C** coagulation panel: prolonged prothrombin time and INR (international normalised ratio)

**D** plasma ammonia level: hyperammonaemia

**E** all of the above

 **A6** **E** All of the laboratory investigations are helpful in the diagnostic evaluation of a patient suspected of having portal hypertension. Thrombocytopenia and/or leucopenia are indicative of hypersplenism. An increase in direct bilirubin fraction, a low serum albumin level and a prolonged prothrombin time all indicate significant hepatocellular disease and possible cirrhosis as the underlying cause of portal hypertension. Children with portal vein thrombosis may have laboratory evidence of a mildly disordered synthesis of liver-dependent coagulation factors in both procoagulant and plasminolytic pathways, but this is generally not evident clinically without detailed testing. An INR of more than 2 usually signifies a decrease in synthesis of the liver-dependent coagulation factors V and VII as long as the defect is not correctable by the administration of vitamin K. Giving vitamin K ensures that the abnormality in the INR is not due to a vitamin K deficiency that can be easily corrected. Additional laboratory investigations may be required to exclude a consumptive coagulopathy that can also cause an increase in INR.

A raised plasma ammonia level in the setting of portal hypertension signifies portosystemic shunting, and may occur with all forms of portal hypertension. Plasma ammonia levels do not necessarily correlate with degrees of encephalopathy, but an ammonia level greater than 100 in the absence of a urea-cycle defect probably indicates advanced liver disease and not only portosystemic shunting.

**Q7** Regarding investigations for portal hypertension, which of the following is incorrect?

    **A** Endoscopy done prior to the onset of bleeding provides valuable clues about the severity of portal hypertension and the likelihood of future bleeding.

    **B** Variceal diameter greater than 5 mm, the appearance of red wale markings on the varices, and clinically advanced liver disease indicate a greater probability for future bleeding and justify surgical treatment as a prophylactic measure against variceal haemorrhage.

    **C** Abdominal Doppler ultrasonography is a useful test in determining cavernous transformation or thrombosis of the portal vein; patency and flow direction of the splenic, superior mesenteric, hepatic veins and IVC at the same time; liver echogenicity; spleen size and kidney appearance.

    **D** Computed tomography (CT) and/or magnetic resonance (MR) angiography provide excellent detailed information of intra-abdominal vasculature and are useful adjunctive studies in planning operative strategies for portal hypertension surgery.

    **E** Transjugular hepatic venography is useful to measure pressures in the hepatic veins, and provides definitive imaging of the hepatic veins and their junction with the vena cava as well as patency of intrahepatic portal venous system.

 **A7**   **B** During episodes of bleeding, upper GI endoscopy provides direct confirmation of the bleeding source and the opportunity to intervene therapeutically and rule out other sources such as peptic ulcers and haemorrhagic gastritis. In cases of suspected portal hypertension, endoscopy is done before the onset of bleeding to evaluate the severity and likelihood of future bleeding. Variceal diameter greater than 5 mm, the appearance of red wale markings and more advanced liver disease indicate a greater chance for future bleeding and may justify the institution of prophylactic treatment with banding or sclerotherapy. In the absence of a previous GI bleed, surgical treatment cannot be justified under all circumstances. In selected patients, clinical conditions and the availability of experienced hepatobiliary surgery may justify early surgical intervention in patients with well-compensated cirrhosis. If the patient lives in a remote area where medical assistance may be relatively unavailable in the case of a severe GI bleed, prophylactic shunting may be considered. In patients who have poorly compensated cirrhosis or systemic symptoms of portal hypertension, surgery with a liver transplant may be necessary even in the absence of GI bleeding. Alternately, in patients with extrahepatic portal vein thrombosis, there are relative indications for surgical restoration of portal blood flow even in the absence of overt bleeding.

Abdominal Doppler ultrasonography can determine cavernous transformation and thrombosis of the portal vein with additional information of patency and flow directions of intra-abdominal vessels including the hepatic veins, splenic and superior mesenteric veins and the IVC. The liver parenchymal abnormalities, the size of the spleen and appearance of the kidneys can be obtained, which may yield useful diagnostic clues. For example, children with congenital hepatic fibrosis may also have autosomal dominant polycystic kidney disease that could easily be discerned by ultrasound.

In spite of Doppler ultrasonography being nearly 100% diagnostic, it is seldom sufficient for determining the patency of the intrahepatic portal vein. CT and/or MR angiography are often required in addition to Doppler ultrasonography in the initial workup for a detailed information of the intra-abdominal vessels especially the portal venous system for surgical planning. With the disadvantages of exposure to radiation, CT angiography can be done more quickly with less image degradation from motion artefact than MR angiography. In children, MR angiography should be done under general anaesthesia with ventilatory arrest to minimise motion artefact. Thus both CT and MR angiography are used as initial workup for definitive diagnosis, surgical evaluation and for assessment of postoperative complications in cases that underwent shunt procedures. Abdominal Doppler ultrasonography is used for routine annual postoperative follow-up cases.

Transjugular hepatic venography although invasive, is a very useful test to measure pressures in the hepatic veins and provides selective definitive imaging of the hepatic veins and their junction with the vena cava as well as of the portal venous system. This modality is operator dependent in selectively accessing veins and provides useful detailed information for decision-making and surgical planning. It can also be used therapeutically, for placement of a transjugular intrahepatic portosystemic shunt (TIPS) or dilatation of strictures causing venous outflow obstruction in older children.

Many children who present with portal hypertension undergo a liver biopsy. This can be done percutaneously in most cases provided that coagulopathies are corrected with vitamin K, fresh frozen plasma and platelets. Children with more profound coagulopathy manifested by a prothrombin time in excess of 20 seconds, should have a transjugular biopsy in the interventional radiology suite or an open biopsy in the operating room. Liver histology findings range from non-pathognomonic in cases of extrahepatic portal vein thrombosis to advanced fibrosis and cirrhosis in children with chronic liver disease.

**8** Which one of the following statements is true regarding the treatment of portal hypertension in both adults and children?

**A** The aetiology, of portal hypertension and the management and outcomes are the similar in adults and children.

**B** The 1-year mortality in adults who experience a severe GI bleed is higher than that in children who can tolerate the physiological consequence of hypovolaemia better than adults.

**C** Portal vein thrombosis is more easily correctable with the meso-Rex bypass in adults and adolescents than in smaller children because of the larger vessels available in larger patients.

**D** The main treatment goal is palliative in children, whereas in adults, corrective surgical intervention is often considered.

**E** Portal hypertension resulting from either parenchymal liver disease or vascular causes most likely will require liver transplantation in all age groups.

**A8** **B** The causes of portal hypertension in children are vastly different from those in adults. Whereas children are very often afflicted with congenital malformations, genetic disorders and primary vascular causes of the portal hypertension, adults more frequently have portal hypertension caused by hepatocellular diseases such as hepatitis C and B, and alcoholic liver disease. As such, children may more often undergo corrective surgery aimed at correcting the cause of the portal hypertension, whereas in adults, surgery is often palliative and aimed at temporising until liver transplantation can be achieved. In contrast, the medical management of portal hypertension in adults is much more evidence based and proven to be effective in decreasing the onset and frequency of GI bleeding.

The medical management of portal hypertension in children is empiric and further trials are necessary to prove benefit.

As a consequence of the higher incidence of advanced parenchymal disease in adults, once a GI bleed occurs, the outlook for long-term survival without a transplant is not good, with >50% mortality. In children, more than half of all oesophageal bleeding occurs as an isolated problem in a setting of normal liver. Even when portal hypertension has resulted from cirrhosis, the overall outcome in children is much better than that in adults.

Portal hypertension resulting from hepatocellular liver disease most likely will require liver transplantation in most instances in both age groups if the liver function deteriorates and cannot be actively treated. On the contrary, if patients are found to have good liver function, as in those with vascular causes, surgical intervention should always be considered.

Which of the following is true regarding management for variceal bleeding in portal hypertension?

**A** Continuous infusion of octreotide is effective in reducing acute bleeding.

**B** Sengstaken–Blakemore tube is more effective than Pharmacological therapy.

**C** Non-selective beta blockers replace the need for surveillance endoscopy.

**D** Variceal sclerotherapy is preferred to band ligation because of more effectiveness and fewer complications.

**E** All of the above.

 **A** Patients with acute variceal bleeding require intense resuscitation with blood and crystalloids, and replacement of coagulation factors with fresh frozen plasma. Factor VII replacement decreases the amount of sodium and fluid necessary to correct the liver-dependent factor deficiencies, although its use is limited by its cost. Close monitoring in the intensive care unit is mandatory including central venous and arterial pressures, hourly urine output and oxygen status. Mental status monitoring is essential in those with cirrhosis because bleeding into the GI tract may exacerbate encephalopathy.

Octreotide and other somatostatin analogues reduce hepatic blood flow and wedged hepatic vein pressure, and constrict splanchnic arterioles by a direct effect on arteriolar smooth muscle. They are very effective in reducing and temporarily stopping the bleeding from portal hypertension and can be used in the initial 24–72 hours while awaiting direct endoscopic management. Octreotide is started as a continuous infusion at 1–2 mcg/kg/hr up to a maximum of 100 mcg/hr and continued for as long as symptoms of bleeding persist. Pharmacological therapy has proved to be as effective as balloon tamponade in adults. The combination of improved Pharmacological and endoscopic therapies renders the role of balloon tamponade to almost obsolete.

Long-term medical management includes the use of non-selective beta blockers such as propanolol or nadolol, either alone or in combination with nitrate vasodilators, which is also the regimen for non-bleeding varices. For those who could not tolerate side effects of the regimen, endoscopic band ligation may be used as primary prophylaxis. Intervention of any kind before the onset of bleeding, is controversial. However, the benefit to the patient of preventing a first bleed may be considerable and may justify early prophylactic management. Studies in both adults and children have demonstrated that prophylactic treatment of varices by medication and endoscopic ligation reduces the frequency of bleeding; surgery for the prevention of an initial bleed is more controversial if there is no other primary goal, such as the treatment of severe hypersplenism.

Endoscopic sclerotherapy is associated with a fairly high incidence of complications in at least one-third of patients. Acute complications include chest pain, oesophageal ulceration and mediastinitis; chronic ones include oesophageal strictures from multiple injection sessions. Oesophageal band ligation was found to be a more effective and rapid method in bleeding cessation with fewer complications. Thus oesophageal banding and Pharmacological control has become the procedure of choice in the early therapy for bleeding oesophageal varices. Sclerotherapy is still necessary in babies since the instrumentation required for banding is too large to fit into the oesophagus of these small children.

**Q10** Which of the following is true regarding transjugular intrahepatic portosystemic shunts?

   **A** TIPS is the initial treatment for variceal bleeding with advanced liver disease.

   **B** Hepatic encephalopathy after TIPS is less common in adults than in children.

   **C** Its limitation of use in children is the high rate of shunt thrombosis.

   **D** TIPS facilitates the shunting of blood with hepatic clearance.

   **E** All of the above.

**A10**  **C**  TIPS or the percutaneous insertion of vascular stents to create channels between the portal vein and hepatic veins within the parenchyma of the liver is indicated in variceal bleeding difficult to control by other means. It should never be considered as the first line of defence. It is usually reserved for patients with advanced liver disease and serves as a bridge to transplantation. Other indications include refractory ascites, hepatic venous outflow obstruction in both transplant and non-transplant candidates and in patients with hepatorenal syndrome. TIPS facilitates the shunting of blood without the benefit of hepatic clearance. In some patients with compensated cirrhosis, TIPS may cause acute deterioration in liver function and precipitate severe encephalopathy and the need for urgent transplantation or at least the need to occlude the shunt.

    Its primary limitation in children is the high rate of shunt thrombosis and the aggravation of pre-existing encephalopathy as well as liver failure in patients whose livers are already borderline. Hepatic encephalopathy is less common after TIPS in children than in adults but the incidence of shunt occlusion is higher because of the smaller shunt diameter. In small infants, TIPS cannot be done due to size constraints.

**Q11** Examples of a non-selective shunt include all of the following *except*:

    **A** end-to-side portacaval shunt

    **B** side-to-side portacaval shunt

    **C** mesocaval shunt

    **D** proximal splenorenal shunt

    **E** distal splenorenal shunt.

**A11**   **E**   Non-selective shunts divert a large proportion of mesenteric blood flow away from the liver so that the entire GI tract, including the spleen and pancreas, is decompressed. Non-selective shunts can be further subdivided into total or partial portal diversions.

The end-to-side portacaval shunt completely redirects portal blood into the IVC below the liver oversewing the hepatic end of the portal vein, whereas the side-to-side portacaval shunt allows blood from the intestine and spleen to flow easily into the vena cava with the hepatic end of the portal vein changed into an outflow tract. The latter is effective for posthepatic portal hypertension such as cases with Budd–Chiari's syndrome, for it decompresses the liver and may result in long-term palliation of the disease with arrest or delay in the progression of liver fibrosis and ultimately failure.

The wide-diameter mesocaval shunt also completely diverts mesenteric blood away from the liver. The procedure can be done as a side-to-side anastomosis between the two veins or with the interposition of a short autologous vein graft or prosthetic graft. Exposure of both the superior mesenteric vein at the root of the bowel mesentery and the IVC below the duodenum is required.

The proximal splenorenal shunt is another example of a total diversion non-selective shunt. The splenic vein is divided close to the spleen and the mesenteric end sewn to the side of the left renal vein so that all the blood from the superior and inferior mesenteric veins is shunted into the systemic venous circulation through the left renal vein. The procedure almost invariably includes splenectomy and sometimes a direct attempt to ligate the gastro-oesophageal varices. Conversely, the distal splenorenal shunt is an example of a selective shunt. The splenic vein is divided close to the confluence with the superior mesenteric vein and anastomosed end to side with the left renal vein. The coronary vein and the gastroepiploic veins are ligated and divided. Hence blood flows from the gastric and oesophageal varices via the short gastric veins, across the spleen, and into the splenic vein. The spleen is also decompressed in this fashion while the portal flow to the liver is preserved.

## Further reading

Karrer FM. Portal hypertension. *Semin Pediatr Surg.* 1992; **1**(2): 134–44.

Miyano T. Biliary tract disorders and portal hypertension. In: Ashcraft KM, Holcomb GW, Murphy JP, editors. *Pediatric Surgery.* 4th ed. Philadelphia, PA: WB Saunders; 2005. pp. 586–608.

Superina R. Portal hypertension. In: Grosfeld JL, O'Neill JA, Fonkalsrud EW, et al: *Pediatric Surgery. Vol 2.* 6th ed. Philadelphia, PA: Mosby Elsevier; 2006. pp. 1651–70.

Superina R, Bambini DA, Lokar J, *et al.* Correction of extrahepatic portal vein thrombosis by the mesenteric to left portal vein bypass. *Ann Surg.* 2006; **243**(4): 515–21.

Superina R, Shneider B, Emre S, *et al.* Surgical guidelines for the management of extra-hepatic portal vein obstruction. *Pediatr Transplant.* 2006; **10**(8): 908–13.

Tagge EP, Thomas PB, Tagge DU. Portal hypertension and variceal bleeding. In: Oldham KT, Colombani PM, Foglia RP, *et al.*, editors. *Principles and Practice of Pediatric Surgery, Vol 2.* 1st ed. Philadelphia, PA: Lippincott Williams & Wilkins; 2005. pp. 1449–52.

# CHAPTER 52

# Pancreatic disorders in children

## CHRISTIAN J STRECK JR, ANDRE HEBRA

**From the choices below each question, select the single best answer.**

**Q1** Which of the following is true regarding pancreatic embryology?
  **A** The ventral pancreatic bud arises from the dorsum of the foregut just distal to the stomach.
  **B** The dorsal pancreas arises from the biliary diverticulum.
  **C** Fusion of the ducts of the two buds is typically complete by 7 weeks of gestation.
  **D** The islet cells make up 10% of the pancreas during fetal life but only 1% during adult life.
  **E** The major arterial blood supply to the pancreas is from the superior mesenteric artery (SMA) and inferior mesenteric artery.

**A1** **D** The dorsal pancreatic bud arises from the dorsum of the foregut just distal to the stomach and the ventral pancreas arises from the biliary diverticulum. Fusion of the parenchyma of the two buds is typically complete by 7 weeks' gestation but duct fusion is delayed until the perinatal period. The major arterial blood supply is from the coeliac axis and the SMA, which gives rise to the superior and inferior pancreaticoduodenal vessels.

**Q2** Which of the following is not associated with annular pancreas?
  **A** oesophageal atresia
  **B** hypertrophic pyloric stenosis
  **C** duodenal web
  **D** trisomy 21
  **E** complex congenital heart disease

**A2** **B** Duodenal atresia or stenosis is seen in as many as 50% of patients with annular pancreas. Trisomy 21 and malrotation occurs in about 20% of patients each. Complex congenital heart disease and tracheo-oesophageal fistula are also associated with annular pancreas.

**3** A 2-day-old male presents with bilious emesis and a 'double-bubble sign' on abdominal plain X-ray. Which of the following is the best surgical management for an intraoperative finding of annular pancreas?

**A** lateral duodenotomy with duodenal web excision

**B** division of the annular pancreatic segment anteriorly

**C** pancreaticoduodenectomy

**D** gastrojejunostomy

**E** duodenoduodenostomy

 **3** **E** In annular pancreas, frequently a thin, flat band of pancreatic tissue arising from the head of the pancreas surrounds the second portion of the duodenum. Typically there is coexisting duodenal stenosis or atresia and the pancreatic tissue may penetrate the duodenal muscularis. Bypass of the duodenal obstruction should be performed without mobilising the annular pancreas because injury to the pancreas could result in production of a chronic fistula.

 **4** Which of the following is true regarding pancreas divisum (PD)?

**A** The frequency of PD in the general population is less than 1%.

**B** PD results when the dorsal and ventral pancreatic ducts fail to fuse properly and there is inadequate drainage through a small dorsal duct (Santorini).

**C** The majority of patients with PD present with recurrent pancreatitis.

**D** Endoscopic sphincterotomy is the procedure of choice in children with symptomatic PD.

**E** CT scan is the diagnostic modality of choice to evaluate patients with suspected PD.

**4** **B** The frequency of PD in the general population is between 5% and 10%. The majority of patients with PD are asymptomatic. Endoscopic retrograde cholangio-pancreatography (ERCP) is the most helpful preoperative imaging study in patients with PD. For symptomatic patients, operative sphincteroplasty seems to have the greatest benefit. There is little data to support endoscopic sphincterotomy in children.

**Q5** Which of the following is true regarding patients with cystic fibrosis (CF)?

　**A** Results from a genetic defect in a cGMP-induced transmembrane sodium channel.

　**B** Rectal prolapse is the initial presenting symptom in 20% of patients.

　**C** Neonatal presentations include meconium cyst, meconium ileus, volvulus, atresia and diabetes.

　**D** At least two-thirds of patients have pancreatic insufficiency at birth.

　**E** All patients with CF are infertile.

**A5** **D** CF results from a defect in a cAMP-induced transmembrane chloride channel. Although rectal prolapse may be seen in up to 30% of patients with CF it is rarely the presenting symptom (<3%). Neonatal presentation rarely includes glucose intolerance. Male patients with CF are typically infertile and may have bilateral absence of the vas deferens noted at diagnostic laparoscopy. Fertility in women is reduced only slightly.

**Q6** One year after a male patient with CF is changed to high-dose pancreatic enzyme supplementation he develops intermittent abdominal pain with distension and bloody diarrhoea. Definitive therapy will most likely require which of the following?

　**A** transition to enteric-coated enzyme replacement

　**B** partial colectomy

　**C** Gastrograffin enema ± polyethylene glycol

　**D** discontinuation of pancreatic enzyme replacement

　**E** oral metronidazole and probiotic therapy

**A6** **B** Fibrosing colonopathy (FC) is a sequela of prolonged exposure to high-dose pancreatic exocrine supplementation. Fusiform segmental colonic narrowing with submucosal fibrosis presents with symptoms of distal colonic obstruction. Initial management includes reduction in supplemental enzyme dose. Most cases eventually require surgical therapy. Children should be maintained on less than 10 000 units/kg/day of pancreatic enzyme. The coating and manufacturer are not independently associated with the risk of FC. Gastrograffin enema and polyethylene glycol are effective therapies for distal intestinal obstruction syndrome.

**Q7** Which of the following is not a presenting feature of congenital hyperinsulinism?

   **A** hemihypertrophy and macroglossia

   **B** preprandial glucose <40 mg/dL (2.2 mmol/L)

   **C** frequent seizures, lethargy and hypotonia

   **D** fasting serum insulin level >5 mU/mL

   **E** glucose requirement exceeding 10 mg/kg/min

**A7**   **A** Congenital hyperinsulinism, or persistent hyperinsulinaemic hypoglycaemia of infancy (PHHI), is a rare disorder of glucose metabolism. Most patients have a disorder of the sulfonylurea receptor (SUR) gene or the *Kir6.2* gene regulating the associated potassium channel. Manifestations include severe hypoglycaemia with detectable insulin levels and maintenance glucose requirements greater than maximal hepatic production. Hypoglycaemia may occur in patients with Beckwith–Wiedemann's syndrome or in those with glycogen storage disease, which are separate disorders from PHHI.

**Q8** Which of the following is not an option for medical management of PHHI?

   **A** hydrochlorothiazide

   **B** octreotide

   **C** glucocorticoids

   **D** streptozotocin

   **E** nifedipine

**A8**   **A** Initial therapy of PHHI is directed at correcting hypoglycaemia including intravenous glucose administration, frequent oral feedings and medical therapy to control insulin secretion. First-line medications include diazoxide (activates potassium adenosine triphosphate channel through sulfonylurea receptor-1 to inhibit insulin secretion) and octreotide (activates beta-cell potassium channels to inhibit insulin secretion). Alternative therapies include glucocorticoids (promotes insulin resistance), streptozotocin (beta-cell toxin), nifedipine, and glucagon.

**Q9** The optimal initial surgical management for PHHI in a patient with a sulfonylurea receptor gene defect is?

   **A** pancreaticoduodenectomy

   **B** gastrostomy tube placement for continuous enteral feeding

   **C** near-total pancreatectomy with islet-cell preservation

   **D** limited pancreatic resection based on percutaneous transhepatic venous sampling preoperatively and intraoperative ultrasound

   **E** 95% pancreatectomy

**A⁹** **E** Because of the risk of brain injury, most clinicians believe pancreatic resection, rather than medical management and high-glucose diet, is necessary in patients with PHHI. Patients with a sulfonylurea receptor defect typically have a more severe, diffuse form of PHHI and require more extensive resection. Islet-cell preservation with autotransplantation is an evolving therapy which has not yet been tested in paediatric cases. Limited resection with image guidance is an excellent option in focal cases with a discrete pancreatic nodule.

**Q10** Which of the following is the most likely diagnosis in a 1-year-old patient with an incidentally discovered large, well-circumscribed, cystic mass involving the pancreatic body and tail?
  **A** pancreaticoblastoma
  **B** solid pseudopapillary tumour
  **C** intraductal papillary mucinous neoplasm
  **D** congenital pancreatic cyst
  **E** acquired pancreatic pseudocyst

**A10** **D** True congenital epithelium-lined cysts of the pancreas are rare and typically asymptomatic. When present they are typically found in infancy and are commonly seen in the body and tail of the pancreas. Pseudocysts account for more than 75% of cystic pancreatic lesions, are typically post-traumatic and are most commonly located in the lesser sac.

**Q11** A 4-year-old Asian female patient presents with vague abdominal discomfort. A CT scan demonstrates a large, well-marginated 10 cm mass in the pancreatic head. The lesion is multiloculated with enhancing septae. What is the most likely diagnosis?
  **A** solid pseudopapillary tumour
  **B** pancreaticoblastoma
  **C** ductal adenocarcinoma
  **D** lymphoma
  **E** acquired pancreatic pseudocyst

**A11** **B** Pancreaticoblastoma is the most common pancreatic tumour of small children with a mean age of presentation at 4.5 years. More than half of the reported cases are in Asians who typically present with an asymptomatic, large mass and non-specific abdominal complaints. These tumours are often very large at presentation, compressing adjacent structures without invasion, and often the organ of origin is unclear on preoperative imaging. In the majority of cases the mass is heterogeneous with internal cystic areas reflecting necrosis and the tumour is multiloculated with enhancing septa.

**Q12** A 14-year-old black female presents with nausea and vague abdominal discomfort. A CT scan demonstrates an 8 cm solid and cystic pancreatic mass, with intratumoural haemorrhage and a well-demarcated fibrous capsule, in the pancreatic body. What is the most likely diagnosis?

**A** solid pseudopapillary tumour

**B** pancreaticoblastoma

**C** intraductal papillary mucinous neoplasm

**D** congenital pancreatic cyst

**E** acquired pancreatic pseudocyst

**A12 A** Solid-pseudopapillary tumours most commonly affect females of reproductive age and have low malignant potential. The imaging features reflect the mixed cystic and solid nature of the lesion with encapsulation and intratumoural haemorrhage.

**Q13** The most common functioning pancreatic islet cell neoplasm is which of the following?

**A** insulinoma

**B** gastrinoma

**C** somatostatinoma

**D** VIPoma

**E** glucagonoma

**A13 A** Insulinoma is the most common endocrine tumour of the pancreas. Most patients have Whipple's triad of fasting hypoglycaemia, symptoms of hypoglycaemia, and resolution of symptoms with intravenous glucose administration. Gastrinoma is the second most common. All other functioning islet cell tumours are extremely rare in children.

**Q14** The most common pancreatic islet cell neoplasm seen in patients with multiple endocrine neoplasia 1 (MEN1) is which of the following?

**A** insulinoma

**B** gastrinoma

**C** somatostatinoma

**D** VIPoma

**E** glucagonoma

**A14 B** Gastrinoma is the most common islet cell tumour seen in MEN1 (seen in up to 50% of patients) and causes Zollinger–Ellison's (ZE) syndrome. Patients frequently have multiple or recurrent peptic ulcers, classically in uncommon locations. Approximately 75% of gastrinomas are sporadic and 25% are associated with MEN1. The mean age of presentation of ZE syndrome is 50 years old. Gastrinomas associated with MEN are more often benign, multicentric, and extrapancreatic. Insulinoma is seen in 10%–30% of patients with MEN1.

**Q15** What is the optimal surgical management for most patients with localised pancreatic insulinoma?
  A  distal pancreatectomy
  B  pancreaticoduodenectomy
  C  95% pancreatectomy
  D  total pancreatectomy
  E  tumour enucleation with intraoperative ultrasound guidance

**A15**  **E**  Insulinomas are typically benign (90%), solitary, and less than 2 cm in size. Insulinomas are found with relatively similar frequency in the head, body, and tail of the pancreas so intraoperative imaging is an important part of tumour localisation.

**Q16** The most reliable diagnostic method for detecting insulinoma is:
  A  blood glucose <50 mg/dL (2.8 mmol/L) following an overnight fast
  B  insulin/glucose ratio <0.3
  C  decreased serum C-peptide and proinsulin levels
  D  72-hour supervised fast with insulin >6 U/mL and glucose <60 mg/dL (3.3 mmol/L)
  E  positive secretin stimulation test.

**A16**  **D**  The most reliable method for diagnosing an insulinoma is the 72-hour supervised fast with blood glucose and insulin levels measured every 4–6 hours. The presence of hypoglycaemia with concurrent serum insulin elevation during a monitored fast is diagnostic. Insulin-to-glucose ratio of more than 0.3 is common; however, up to 20% of patients with insulinoma do not have an elevated insulin-to-glucose ratio. Measurement of C-peptide and proinsulin levels are helpful as these are typically increased in patients with insulinoma. Commercial insulin does not contain these products. Somatostatin receptor scintigraphy is of limited benefit in patients with insulinoma as they rarely have somatostatin receptors.

**Q17** What is the most common extrapancreatic site for a gastrinoma?
  A  gastric antrum
  B  proximal duodenum
  C  liver
  D  common bile duct
  E  ovary

$A$17   **B**   The classic description of gastrinoma location is within the 'gastrinoma triangle' which is bounded by the pancreatic body/neck, the third part of the duodenum and the cystic duct/common bile duct junction. Overall, 55% of gastrinomas are found in the pancreas, most commonly in the head. The most common extrapancreatic site is the proximal duodenum and these are typically microadenomas in the 2 mm size range. Oesophagogastroduodenoscopy and endoscopic ultrasound are important adjuncts to localising extrapancreatic gastrinomas. Evaluation of the liver and peripancreatic lymph nodes is an important part of the staging of pancreatic gastrinomas which are metastatic at least 50% of the time.

$Q$18   The best laboratory test to diagnose a gastrinoma is:
- **A**   fasting serum gastrin >200 pg/mL
- **B**   gastric pH >2.5
- **C**   positive urea breath test
- **D**   maximal acid output >10 mEq/L
- **E**   increase in serum gastrin >200 pg/mL over baseline level following intravenous secretin.

$A$18   **E**   A fasting serum gastrin level greater than 1000 pg/mL is usually diagnostic of gastrinoma. Most gastrinomas have more moderate gastrin level elevation. Gastric pH <2.5 excludes a physiologic response as the cause of hypergastrinaemia. Typically patients have a basal acid output of greater than 15 mEq/hr. Secretin provocative testing (administration of 2 U/kg of secretin following an overnight fast) showing paradoxical increase in serum gastrin levels by more than 200 pg/mL, is required to diagnose gastrinoma. The urea breath test is used to evaluate patients for *Helicobacter pylori* infection.

$Q$19   Which of the following is the most sensitive non-invasive study to localise a gastrinoma?
- **A**   abdominal ultrasound
- **B**   CT
- **C**   MRI
- **D**   hepatobiliary iminodiacetic acid scan
- **E**   somatostatin receptor scintigraphy

$A$19   **E**   Somatostatin receptor scintigraphy (SRS) is both sensitive and specific for localising gastrinomas, more so than other conventional modalities. Small duodenal gastrinomas may be missed and endoscopic ultrasound is an excellent complementary diagnostic tool to SRS.

**Q20** Following a motor vehicle collision, a 13-year-old intubated patient is haemodynamically stable, has a GCS of 6, and a seat-belt contusion over the mid-abdomen. What is the best way to evaluate the abdomen?

**A** FAST (focused assessment with sonography for trauma)

**B** diagnostic peritoneal lavage (DPL)

**C** serial abdominal exams

**D** CT scan of the abdomen and pelvis with intravenous contrast

**E** MRI of the lumbar spine

**A20** **D** CT scan is an excellent technique to evaluate stable paediatric trauma patients in whom a reliable physical examination cannot be performed and there is suspicion for significant abdominal trauma as in this patient with a seat-belt contusion. CT provides information relative to specific organ injury and extent and allows better evaluation of pelvic and retroperitoneal structures which are difficult to assess by physical exam, FAST scan, and DPL. Abdominal CT also provides information about the lower thoracic and lumbar spine which should be evaluated in this patient with a seat-belt contusion. Some gastrointestinal and pancreatic injuries may be missed on initial CT so close clinical follow-up is required.

**Q21** After falling from a bicycle an 11-year-old male has a 'handlebar contusion' in the epigastrium. A CT scan demonstrates a grade III pancreatic laceration with near-transection over L1, to the left of the superior mesenteric vein. What is the best management strategy for the injury to the pancreas?

**A** ICU admission with serial abdominal exams

**B** ERCP with stenting of the pancreatic duct

**C** distal pancreatectomy

**D** longitudinal pancreaticojejunostomy with Roux-en-Y reconstruction

**E** central pancreatectomy with pancreaticogastrostomy

**A21** **C** Management of traumatic injuries to the pancreas remains an area of controversy. Several studies have demonstrated that early operative intervention in a child with a major pancreatic ductal injury results in shorter hospitalisation, less total parenteral nutrition (TPN) dependence and fewer complications than in those initially managed non-operatively. Pseudocyst formation occurs in greater than 45% of patients managed non-operatively, many of whom require drainage procedures, resulting in a prolonged return to normal health. Early distal pancreatectomy avoids pancreatic fistula and pseudocyst formation.

**Q22** What is the most common cause of acute pancreatitis in children?

   **A** viral

   **B** drugs

   **C** familial/hereditary

   **D** gallstones

   **E** idiopathic

**A22** **E** In two large series evaluating the aetiology of acute pancreatitis in children, idiopathic and post-traumatic were the most commonly identified causes accounting for 34% and 14% of all cases, respectively, in the largest series.

**Q23** Eight weeks following an episode of acute pancreatitis a 14-year-old develops vague abdominal pain and nausea with a large, rim-enhancing 7 cm pseudocyst seen on abdominal CT. ERCP demonstrates communication between the pseudocyst and the pancreatic duct. What is the best management?

   **A** nil by mouth, TPN, repeat imaging in 4–6 weeks

   **B** percutaneous cyst aspiration by ultrasound guidance

   **C** external drainage by CT-guided drain placement

   **D** ERCP with pancreatic duct stenting

   **E** internal drainage by cyst-gastrostomy or cyst-jejunostomy

**A23** **E** Most pancreatic pseudocysts in children are the result of blunt abdominal trauma (60%–75%). Complications from untreated large pseudocysts can include mechanical obstruction, haemorrhage, perforation and infection. While more than 50% of acute peripancreatic fluid collections resolve, cysts larger than 4–6 cm with a well-defined thick wall and present for greater than 6 weeks are unlikely to resolve spontaneously. Internal drainage is the most effective option for large, persistent pseudocysts. Cysts which communicate with the main pancreatic duct have a high rate of recurrence following percutaneous aspiration. Endoscopic cyst-enteric drainage has been described in limited reports from a few experienced endoscopists.

**Q24** An ERCP performed on a 15-year-old male with chronic pancreatitis demonstrates a diffusely dilated, 6 mm pancreatic duct with stones. What is the best surgical management?

   **A** ERCP with stent placement

   **B** pancreaticoduodenectomy

   **C** distal pancreatectomy

   **D** longitudinal pancreaticojejunostomy with Roux-en-Y reconstruction

   **E** total pancreatectomy

$A$**24** **E** For symptomatic children with pancreatic duct obstruction with calculi, longitudinal pancreaticojejunostomy has demonstrated durable long-term results.

## Further reading

Chung EM, Travis MD, Conran RM. Pancreatic tumors in children: radiologic-pathologic correlation. *Radiographics*. 2006; **26**(4): 1211–38.

FitzSimmons SC, Burkhart GA, Borowitz D, *et al*. High-dose pancreatic-enzyme supplements and fibrosing colonopathy in children with cystic fibrosis. *N Engl J Med*. 1997; **336**(18): 1283–9.

Lenert JT, Bold RJ, Sussman JJ, *et al*. Pancreatic endocrine tumors and multiple endocrine neoplasia. In: Feig BW, Berger DH, Fuhrman GM, editors. *The M.D. Anderson Surgical Oncology Handbook*. Philadelphia, PA: Lippincott; 2003. pp. 324–51.

Mehta SS, Gittes GK. Pancreas. In: Oldham KT, Colombani PM, Foglia RP, *et al.*, editors. *Principles and Practice of Pediatric Surgery*. Philadelphia, PA: Lippincott; 2005. pp. 685–95.

Nakayama DK. Abdominal and genitourinary trauma. In: O'Neill JA, Grosfeld JL, Fonkalsrud EW, *et al.*, editors. *Principles of Pediatric Surgery*. St Louis, MO: Mosby; 2003. pp. 171–2.

O'Neill JA. Disorders of the pancreas. In: O'Neill JA, Grosfeld JL, Fonkalsrud EW, *et al.*, editors. *Principles of Pediatric Surgery*. St Louis, MO: Mosby; 2003. pp. 653–61.

Stringer MD. Pancreatitis and pancreatic trauma. *Semin Pediatr Surg*. 2005; **14**(4): 239–46.

Stylianos S, Hicks BA. Abdominal trauma. In: Oldham KT, Colombani PM, Foglia RP, *et al.*, editors. *Principles and Practice of Pediatric Surgery*. Philadelphia, PA: Lippincott; 2005. p. 441.

# CHAPTER 53

# Spleen

## ZACHARY KASTENBERG, SANJEEV DUTTA

**From the choices below each question, select the single best answer.**

1 Of the spleen's many peritoneal attachments, the only vascularised ligaments are:

   **A** the lienorenal ligament containing the splenic vessels and the lieno-phrenic ligament containing the short gastric vessels

   **B** the lienocolic ligament containing the splenic vessels and the lieno-renal ligament containing the short gastric vessels

   **C** the lienogastric ligament containing the splenic vessels and the lienorenal ligament containing the short gastric vessels

   **D** the lienorenal ligament containing the splenic vessels and the lie-nogastric ligament containing the short gastric vessels

   **E** the lienogastric ligament containing the splenic and short gastric vessels.

1   **D**  The spleen has up to six peritoneal attachments including the lienorenal liga-ment, which courses along the anterior surface of the left kidney and contains the splenic artery and the splenic vein, and the lienogastric ligament, which envelops the short gastric vessels. The avascular attachments of the spleen include the lienocolic, lienophrenic, lienopancreatic ligaments and the sometimes-present presplenic fold.

**2** Which of the following is not true regarding the development and basic physiology of the spleen?

**A** The splenic primordium originates in the dorsal mesogastrium at around 5 weeks' gestation.

**B** The spleen is the primary organ of haematopoiesis until approximately 1 year of age.

**C** The spleen consists of red pulp and white pulp. The red pulp is primarily responsible for haemofiltration and removal of damaged/senescent red blood cells and opsonised bacterial particles, while the white pulp contains lymphoid follicles and is a site of antigen presentation and initiation of the humoral immune response.

**D** The 'closed' circulatory theory describes a small portion of splenic blood flow that progresses directly from the arterial to the venous circulation through the splenic capillary bed.

**E** The 'open' circulatory theory describes the majority of the splenic blood that flows from the splenic arterioles into a sinusoidal network lined by the reticuloendothelial cells prior to entering the venous circulation.

 **2** **B** The spleen is the primary organ of haematopoiesis until approximately 5 months' gestation, at which point the bone marrow assumes the production of both red and white blood cells. With gastric rotation, the dorsal mesogastrium folds to situate the spleen in the left upper quadrant anterior to the left kidney. The dorsal aspect of the dorsal mesogastrium forms the lienorenal ligament while the more ventral portion forms the lienogastric ligament and extends caudad to form the greater omentum. The two major functions of the spleen are haematological ('pitting' and 'culling' of red blood cells) and immunologic (production of opsonins and complement, filtration of antigens, antibody production, and stimulation of the lymphoid proliferation). These functions primarily take place in the red and white pulp, respectively. A small percentage of the splenic blood flow bypasses the reticuloendothelial system through the 'closed' circulation while the majority flows through the reticuloendothelial meshwork and venous sinusoids of the 'open' circulation.

**Q3** During a routine prenatal ultrasound the diagnosis of transposition of the great vessels is made. The ultrasonographer has difficulty visualising the spleen. All of the following are associated with congenital asplenia except:

**A** right-sided stomach

**B** biliary atresia

**C** isomerism of the right atrial appendage

**D** Howell–Jolly bodies on postnatal peripheral blood smear

**E** increased rate of postnatal infection with encapsulated bacteria.

**A3** **B** The condition described is congenital asplenism, which is frequently associated with severe cyanotic heart disease, isomerism of the right atrial appendage, a right-sided stomach, central displacement of the liver and peripheral blood smear findings consistent with splenic insufficiency. Ivemark's syndrome or asplenia syndrome is the presence of visceral heterotaxy with bilateral right-sidedness. This syndrome is also associated with malrotation and increased frequency of midgut volvulus. Congenital polysplenism is associated with biliary atresia, situs inversus, absent inferior vena cava, preduodenal portal vein and aberrant hepatic artery.

**Q4** A 14-year-old female is struck by a car while riding her bicycle and sustains a grade 4 splenic laceration requiring an emergency splenectomy. Fifteen years later the patient presents again with an adhesive small-bowel obstruction requiring repeat laparotomy. The lysis of adhesions is carried out without difficulty; however, at the time of the operation she is found to have multiple 5 mm to 4 cm purple, fleshy nodules implanted on the surface of the liver, stomach and omentum. Which of the following statements is true about this patient's condition?

**A** The most common location for this tissue to be found is within the splenic hilum.

**B** The tissue is a congenital anomaly that occurs in 20%–30% of the general population.

**C** The nodules likely represent a malignant process and should be completely resected.

**D** This process occurs secondary to seeding of the peritoneum with splenic particles following splenic rupture and frequently provides adequate immunologic function to obviate the need for post-splenectomy vaccination.

**E** This tissue is likely to look similar to normal splenic tissue, histologically, with the exception of having a fibrotic capsule, multiple small vascular tributaries, and an incomplete or disorganised trabecular network.

**A4** **E** The condition described in this question is splenosis. It results from seeding of the peritoneum following splenic trauma and is most frequently found on the surface of the liver, stomach and omentum. It is a completely benign process and does not need to be resected unless it is causing a problem secondary to a mass effect. Histologically, the splenosis nodules appear similar to native spleen; however, they lack the dominant trabecular arterial inflow and structured splenic capsule. Splenosis often performs pitting and culling (i.e. removes deformed or senescent red blood cells), but for incompletely understood reasons, it does not provide the immunologic function of the native spleen. As a result, such individuals should be treated as asplenic. Options A and B refer to accessory spleens.

**Q5** A 12-year-old male with hereditary elliptocytosis is taken for a laparoscopic splenectomy. Intraoperatively, a 2 cm purple, fleshy nodule is visualised within the connective tissue of the splenic hilum. The spleen itself, while enlarged, appears otherwise normal. Which of the following is true regarding this finding?

**A** This nodule represents histologically normal, ectopic splenic tissue.

**B** The most common location to find this process is within the greater omentum.

**C** This tissue is non-functional and may be left in place at the time of elective splenectomy for the described condition.

**D** When present, this anomaly typically occurs in multiple locations.

**E** This condition is so rare that there is no need to actively assess for its presence during the initial operation.

**A5** **A** Accessory spleens are common, occurring in 20%–30% of the general population. They are most commonly located in the splenic hilum (~40%), lienorenal ligament (~20%), lienogastric (~15%), greater omentum, lienophrenic ligament, and very rarely in the scrotum. Accessory spleens are most frequently single (85%), occasionally double (10%), and rarely three or more (<5%). The tissue is histologically similar to normal spleen and provides typical immunologic and haematological functions of splenic tissue. As such, all accessory spleens should be removed at the time of splenectomy for any reason other than trauma.

**Q6** A 10-year-old male is referred by his primary care doctor with complaints of intermittent abdominal pain, a palpable mass in his left lower quadrant, and a computed tomography scan that shows a very low-lying spleen. He is currently asymptomatic. What is the appropriate next step in the management of this patient?

A Assure the patient and his parents that all is well and no further action is required.

B Advise the patient and his parents to return to the emergency room if the symptoms return.

C Administer splenectomy vaccines and schedule the patient for elective splenopexy.

D Proceed directly to the operating room for urgent splenectomy.

E Obtain further imaging and laboratory studies.

**A6** C This is a case of a wandering spleen with intermittent torsion. Wandering spleen is a rare condition in which the spleen is attached only to the hilar vessels and a small lienogastric ligament. The avascular peritoneal attachments are absent allowing the spleen to sit low in the abdomen and rotate around the narrow splenic pedicle. Wandering spleen occasionally presents as acute torsion and requires emergency operative intervention with splenectomy if infarction is present. In case of chronic, intermittent torsion, elective splenopexy may be performed, but vaccinations should be administered in case the patient has actually become functionally asplenic due to repeated partial infarction.

**Q7** A 5-week-old ex-36-week gestational age male is found to have only one testicle in his scrotum and a palpable mass in the left inguinal region. He is taken for a laparoscopic left herniorrhaphy and possible orchidopexy. Intraoperatively, the patient is found to have an indirect left inguinal hernia and an undescended left testis sitting in the left inguinal canal with an associated nodule of purple, fleshy tissue that appears to be attached to the native spleen by a fibrous band of connective tissue. Which of the following statements is false regarding this patient's condition?

A These findings likely represent *in utero* testicular torsion.

B This is one of two typical presentations for this rare congenital anomaly.

C This condition is thought to result from the close proximity of the left mesonephros and spleen during early organogenesis.

D The appropriate next step in management is transection of the fibrous band, resection of the ectopic tissue, herniorrhaphy and orchidopexy if possible.

E The ectopic tissue in this condition is histologically normal spleen.

**A7**  **A** The congenital anomaly described in this question is splenogonadal fusion. It occurs in two forms, one being the 'continuous' form with an associated band of fibrous connective tissue, the other being the 'discontinuous' form without any connection to the native spleen. The continuous form is often associated with other congenital anomalies, while the discontinuous form is usually isolated and sometimes considered simply an ectopic or accessory spleen. The testis is often normal. Management consists of resection of the ectopic tissue, salvage or removal of the left testis, and repair of any concomitant hernia defect.

**Q8** In which of the following patients is splenectomy indicated?

   **A** A 6-year-old female with a recent history of cough and rhinorrhoea who presents with petechiae. She has a palpable spleen and a platelet count of $30 \times 10^9/L$.

   **B** A 6-year-old male with splenomegaly, jaundice, anaemia requiring increasingly frequent transfusions and spherocytes on peripheral blood smear.

   **C** A 2-year-old male with β-thalassaemia, stable transfusion requirements, and no splenomegaly.

   **D** A 10-year-old black female with sickle-cell disease and multiple repeated attacks of extremity pain requiring admission to the hospital for pain control and hydration.

   **E** A 17-year-old male recently diagnosed with Hodgkin's lymphoma.

**A8**  **B** There are very few absolute indications for splenectomy in children. Symptomatic hereditary spherocytosis in a child over the age of 5 is an indication for splenectomy given that there is no medical management for this disease and the patient is old enough to receive pre-splenectomy vaccinations with relative success. The patient in option A is presenting with findings characteristic of idiopathic thrombocytopenic purpura. Spontaneous resolution or resolution with medical management (steroids or intravenous immunoglobulin) occurs in greater than 90% of affected children and should be attempted prior to splenectomy. Indications for splenectomy in β-thalassaemia include increasing transfusion requirements or symptomatic splenomegaly and one should attempt to avoid splenectomy until the patient reaches the age of 5 years to increase the efficacy of preoperative vaccination. Splenectomy is indicated in the setting of sickle-cell anaemia when acute splenic sequestration is encountered. Typically, sickle-cell anaemia leads to repeated episodes of microinfarction and eventual autosplenectomy. Historically, Hodgkin's lymphoma was staged by laparotomy with concomitant splenectomy. This is rarely indicated today with the available imaging options (CT, MRI, PET) and systemic therapies (combined chemo/radiation therapy).

Q9 Which of the following statements is true regarding blunt splenic trauma in children?

**A** Splenectomy is indicated in a haemodynamically stable patient with free fluid in the pelvis and an isolated grade 3 splenic laceration on computed tomography scan.

**B** Non-operative management of splenic trauma has led to increased hospital lengths-of-stay.

**C** Non-operative management of splenic trauma has resulted in increased rates of transfusion.

**D** Non-operative management of isolated splenic injuries is associated with decreased mortality compared with patients with isolated splenic injuries undergoing splenectomy.

**E** There is a relatively high rate of overwhelming post-splenectomy infection in children who undergo splenectomy for trauma relative to those undergoing splenectomy for one of the haemoglobinopathies.

A9 **D** Non-operative management of isolated splenic injuries is associated with a lower mortality rate than splenectomy (0.7% vs. 8%, respectively). There is no grade of injury or imaging finding that is a definite indication for splenectomy. A patient that is haemodynamically unstable after receiving adequate crystalloid resuscitation and two units of packed red blood cells or requires continued transfusions to maintain a haematocrit >25 should be considered for splenectomy. Both rates of transfusions and length of stay have decreased as non-operative management of paediatric splenic trauma has become ubiquitous. Children undergoing splenectomy for trauma have a lower rate of overwhelming post-splenectomy infection when compared with children who undergo splenectomy for haemoglobinopathies. For reasons that are not entirely understood, patients undergoing splenectomy for β-thalassaemia have the highest rate of post-splenectomy infection.

Q10 An 8-year-old female with hereditary spherocytosis has required more frequent transfusions over the past year, has experienced increasing splenomegaly, and has been found to have gallstones on right upper quadrant ultrasound. What is the most appropriate next step in the management of this patient?

**A** preoperative vaccines followed by open splenectomy

**B** open splenectomy without preoperative vaccines

**C** preoperative vaccines followed by open partial splenectomy

**D** open partial splenectomy without preoperative vaccines

**E** preoperative vaccines followed by laparoscopic partial or total splenectomy with combined cholecystectomy

**A10  E**  Partial splenectomy has been proven to provide good long-term haematological outcomes with prolonged elevation in haemoglobin levels and decreased
reticulocyte counts in patients with hereditary spherocytosis. In the appropriate
hands, laparoscopic partial splenectomy can be performed safely with retained
immunologic function when 10%–30% of the original splenic mass is preserved.
It is important to always vaccinate patients undergoing both total and partial
splenectomy, as there is always the chance that the patient will be left functionally asplenic. Finally, when gallstones are found preoperatively, it is necessary
to perform a cholecystectomy given the high rate of future biliary colic in these
patients. Of note, performing a total splenectomy with cholecystectomy would be
an acceptable management strategy in this patient.

**Q11**  All of the following are true of laparoscopic splenectomy *except*:

   **A**  there is a higher rate of complications associated with laparoscopic
   splenectomy in patients with sickle-cell disease relative to other
   haemoglobinopathies

   **B**  compared with the open procedure, there is a higher rate of postoperative pancreatitis associated with laparoscopic splenectomy

   **C**  laparoscopic splenectomy leads to extensive left upper quadrant
   adhesions and makes it impossible to undergo future laparoscopic
   procedures

   **D**  laparoscopic splenectomy is associated with a negligible rate of
   surgical site infection

   **E**  laparoscopy is safe and efficacious and is now considered the procedure of choice for most splenic operations in children.

**A11  C**  Current literature reports multiple cases of reoperation performed laparoscopically for completion splenectomy following partial splenectomy as well as
repeat laparoscopy for missed accessory spleens. A recent report cites an overall
complication rate of 22% in patients with sickle-cell disease compared with 11%
for all patients undergoing laparoscopic splenectomy. The same report noted a
zero incidence of both pancreatitis and surgical site infection for laparoscopic
splenectomy.

Q12 Whether performing an open or laparoscopic splenectomy the basic steps of the operation remain the same. Which of the following statements is incorrect regarding the technical aspects of paediatric splenectomy?

   A  Right-side down or partial right-side down facilitates suspension of the spleen from its superolateral attachments.
   B  By first dividing the lienocolic and gastrocolic ligaments one frees the splenic flexure of the colon and gains access to the lesser sac.
   C  Leaving the lienophrenic ligament intact allows for continued suspension of the spleen while carrying out the dissection and ligation of the short gastric and hilar vessels.
   D  Division of the lienogastric ligament with ligation of the short gastric vessels exposes the lienorenal ligament.
   E  The final stage of the operation includes division of the lienophrenic ligament followed by ligation of the splenic vessels near the hilum of the spleen.

A12  E  The final stage of the operation involves ligation of the splenic vessels followed by division of the remaining avascular superolateral attachments. One of the keys to the operation is to leave these attachments intact until the ligation of all the splenic vessels is complete to avoid having the spleen fall into the field of dissection.

Q13 Which of the following statements is true regarding overwhelming post-splenectomy infection (OPSI)?

   A  In vaccinated patients, most cases of OPSI occur within 1 month of splenectomy.
   B  Patients at the highest risk for OPSI are 6–10 years old at the time of splenectomy.
   C  The most common pathogen in all age groups is *Haemophilus influenzae*.
   D  The incidence of OPSI drops dramatically if splenectomy is performed after the age of 5 years.
   E  Early recognition and initiation of broad-spectrum antibiotic therapy does not improve outcomes.

A13  D  Existing data show a dramatic increase in the incidence of OPSI when splenectomy is performed in patients <5 years old compared with patients >5 years old (as high as 5% in some studies compared with <1%). Mortality in documented cases of OPSI approach 50% in paediatric populations. In non-vaccinated patients OPSI frequently occurs within the first few weeks following splenectomy. In vaccinated individuals, however, OPSI most frequently occurs 2–3 years postoperatively. The most common pathogen is *Streptococcus pneumoniae* in all age groups (50%–90% of all cases of OPSI). *H. influenzae* and *Neisseria meningitidis* are the two other encapsulated organisms most commonly associated with OPSI. Patient and parent education to seek medical attention at the first signs of infection, followed by prompt initiation of broad-spectrum antibiotics, is the most effective management strategy. The most common signs of OPSI include fever, chills, general malaise and rigors leading to rapid deterioration with or without the overt signs of meningitis and or pneumonia.

**Q14** Which of the following is false regarding immunisation in splenectomised patients?

**A** Current guidelines recommend giving the following vaccines up to 1 month prior to elective splenectomy: 23-valent pneumococcal vaccine, *H. influenzae* type b conjugate vaccine, and the meningococcal polysaccharide vaccine.

**B** The majority of OPSI cases today occur in patients who were not vaccinated postoperatively.

**C** Recent data shows that in splenectomies performed for trauma, postoperative vaccines are given to patients 95% of the time before they leave the hospital.

**D** Most immunocompetent splenectomy patients will show a greater than twofold rise in antibody titres within 2 weeks of vaccination.

**E** There are no strong data to support or refute the need for revaccination.

**A14  C** Studies suggest that patients undergoing urgent/emergency splenectomy receive their recommended postoperative vaccinations approximately 10%–75% of the time and that the majority of contemporary cases of OPSI occur in individuals who have not been properly vaccinated. There are no strong data to support revaccination; however, given the relatively high risk of developing OPSI in young children many healthcare providers recommend revaccination after 5 years in children 10 years or younger.

Q15 Which of the following statements is true regarding the use of antibiotic prophylaxis in children following splenectomy?

   A There is no strong evidence to support or refute the use of prophylactic antibiotics in splenectomised patients.

   B There is strong evidence to support the use of lifelong daily antibiotic prophylaxis in all children following splenectomy.

   C There is strong evidence to support the use of 'as needed' penicillin, to be taken by the patient at the first sign of infection.

   D There is strong evidence to support the use of daily antibiotic prophylaxis for 2 years following splenectomy in all children and for 5 years in children with sickle-cell disease.

   E There are strong data to support the use of daily antibiotic prophylaxis for 6 months followed by 'as needed' penicillin thereafter in all children undergoing splenectomy.

A15 A There are no definitive evidence to support or oppose the use of prophylactic antibiotics in splenectomised children. Given that all children are at relatively high risk for developing OPSI, most haematologists and surgeons recommend at least a 6-month to 2-year course of daily penicillin prophylaxis.

## Further reading

Davies DA, Pearl RH, Ein SH, *et al*. Management of blunt splenic injury in children: evolution of the nonoperative approach. *J Pediatr Surg*. 2009; **44**(5): 1005–8.

Jugenburg M, Haddock G, Freedman MH, *et al*. The morbidity and mortality of pediatric splenectomy: does prophylaxis make a difference? *J Pediatr Surg*. 1999; **34**(7): 1064–7.

Lane PA. The spleen in children. *Curr Opin Pediatr*. 1995; **7**(1): 36–41.

Rescorla FJ, West KW, Engum SA, *et al*. Laparoscopic splenic procedures in children: experience in 231 children. *Ann Surg*. 2007; **246**(4): 683–7, discussion 687–8.

Slater BJ, Chan FP, Davis K, *et al*. Institutional experience with laparoscopic partial splenectomy for hereditary spherocytosis. *J Pediatr Surg*. 2010; **45**(8): 1682–6.

# SECTION X

# Genitourinary disorders

# CHAPTER 54

# Renal diseases in children

## STEPHEN D MARKS

From the choices below each question, select the single best answer.

**Q1** A 4-year-old boy presents with severe abdominal pain with right lower quadrant tenderness and guarding. A clinical diagnosis is made of appendicitis and he proceeds to appendicectomy, with normal findings at operation and on histology. He is making a good postoperative recovery the following day but is noted to have purpuric lesions surrounding his incision. What further test/investigation is *not* required?

   **A** blood pressure measurement
   **B** blood test for urea, creatinine, electrolytes and serum albumin
   **C** lumbar puncture
   **D** urine dipstick
   **E** wound swab

**A1** **C** This patient has presented with severe abdominal pain with right lower quadrant tenderness and guarding with a clinical diagnosis of appendicitis, but no evidence of this at time of appendicectomy. He has a rash around his wound postoperatively, which is not typical for a wound infection but a wound swab is worthwhile. However, all the clinical symptoms and signs together may suggest a vasculitis for which all the investigations are warranted, except that lumbar puncture is not required to check for meningitis at this stage (if severe sepsis was evident with him being unwell, then blood cultures and commencing intravenous antibiotics would be the first step).

**Q2** What is the most likely diagnosis for the child in question 1?
   **A** candida infection
   **B** Henoch–Schönlein's purpura (HSP)
   **C** idiopathic thrombocytopenic purpura
   **D** meningococcal disease
   **E** pneumococcal sepsis

**A2**  **B**  This presentation does not fit for an infectious rash caused by candida, meningococcal or pneumococcal infections, although petechial and purpuric lesions are characteristic of meningococcaemia. Although purpuric rashes occur with idiopathic thrombocytopenic purpura, the constellation of features correspond to the most common childhood vasculitis of HSP. The classification criteria for HSP is palpable purpura with at least one of the following four features: diffuse abdominal pain, any biopsy showing Immunoglobulin A deposition, arthritis and/or arthralgia, and haematuria and/or proteinuria.

**Q3**  A 4-week-old baby is referred for assessment of bilateral hydroceles. On examination, he is also found to have ascites, and massive scrotal and peripheral oedema. What further test and investigation is *not* required?

  **A**  blood pressure measurement
  **B**  blood test for urea, creatinine and electrolytes
  **C**  blood test for serum albumin
  **D**  urine culture
  **E**  urine dipstick for proteinuria and haematuria

**A3**  **D**  Although surgical consideration of ligation of patent processus vaginalis should be sought for hydroceles, the fact that this neonate has evidence of oedema should alert the clinician for paediatric review to consider hypoalbuminaemia, which could result from kidney, liver, gastrointestinal or metabolic conditions. Therefore, all tests are warranted, apart from urine culture, as there is no evidence of urinary tract infection.

**Q4**  What is the most likely diagnosis for the child in question 3?
  **A**  congenital nephrotic syndrome
  **B**  neonatal lymphoedema
  **C**  neonatal lymphoma
  **D**  neonatal systemic lupus erythematosus
  **E**  postinfectious glomerulonephritis

**A4**  **A**  In view of the age and presentation, the most likely diagnosis from the choices is congenital nephrotic syndrome, where this neonate has significant proteinuria resulting in hypoalbuminaemia and subsequent oedema.

**Q5** A healthy term baby is born weighing 3.5 kg after having antenatal diagnosis of bilateral hydroureteronephrosis. What further test and investigation is required?
- **A** blood pressure measurement
- **B** blood test for urea, creatinine and electrolytes
- **C** urine tests with dipstick and culture/sensitivity
- **D** renal ultrasound
- **E** all of the above

**A5** **E** There is no information regarding how much dilatation was present at different gestational ages. A renal ultrasound is the most important investigation but can be falsely reassuring within the first 48 hours because of relative dehydration, and the degree of hydronephrosis may not be become prominent until a few days later. In view of bilateral involvement, all of the tests are warranted to exclude hypertension, renal failure (although initial plasma creatinine will reflect maternal renal function) and urinary tract infection.

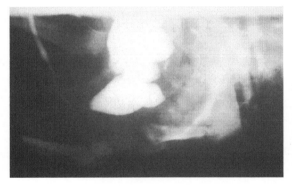

**FIGURE 54.1 Micturating cystourethrogram of this term baby with an antenatal diagnosis of bilateral hydroureteronephrosis**

**Q6** He had a micturating cystourethrogram, as shown in Figure 54.1. Which of the following is the most likely diagnosis for the baby in question 5?
- **A** bilateral pelviureteric junction obstruction
- **B** bilateral vesicoureteric reflux
- **C** bilateral vesicoureteric junction obstruction
- **D** posterior urethral valves
- **E** ureterocele

**A6** **D** This micturating cystourethrogram shows a dilated posterior urethra with trabeculated bladder consistent with posterior urethral valves.

**Q7** What treatment option should be considered for the baby in question 5?

   **A** deflux procedure

   **B** intravenous antibiotics

   **C** oral prophylactic antibiotics

   **D** re-implantation of ureters

   **E** watchful expectancy

**A7** **C** He requires insertion of urinary catheter, commencing on prophylactic antibiotics, and paediatric surgical/urological referral. If there is significant renal impairment due to bilateral renal dysplasia, then referral to a paediatric nephro-urological unit is required.

**Q8** A 2-month-old boy presents with acute pyelonephritis as he is clinically unwell with history of fever, lethargy and loin tenderness. He has a proven pseudomonas urinary tract infection. Which investigation should be performed during his follow-up?

   **A** DMSA nuclear medicine scan

   **B** micturating cystourethrogram

   **C** renal ultrasound

   **D** all of the above

   **E** only A and C

**A8** **D** This is a high-risk scenario because of an unusual pathogen with pseudomonas pyelonephritis in a 2-month-old infant. Therefore, he requires all investigations with renal ultrasound, micturating cystourethrogram and DMSA nuclear medicine scan.

**Q9** Which of the following is a possible diagnosis for the infant in question 8?

   **A** posterior urethral valves

   **B** renal calculi

   **C** renal dysplasia

   **D** vesicoureteric reflux

   **E** all of the above

**A9** **E** The clinical information makes the underlying diagnosis difficult to establish but pseudomonas pyelonephritis may occur because of an underlying congenital abnormality of the kidney and/or urinary tract or renal calculi, so all of the suggestions are 'possible'.

Q10 A 1-year-old boy is referred for bilateral inguinal herniotomies. He is ready to go to theatre and is found to have an automated blood pressure reading of 140/96 mmHg. What would be your plan?

A Arrange a paediatric outpatient appointment.

B Perform serial manual blood pressure measurements.

C Proceed to theatre to undergo bilateral inguinal herniotomies.

D Commence antihypertensive medications.

E Perform an urgent electrocardiogram.

A10 B This is significant hypertension in a 1-year-old until proven otherwise. The operation should be postponed and the patient should be monitored on the ward with serial manual blood pressure measurements using an appropriately sized cuff. If hypertension is evident, investigations should be carried out to determine the underlying cause as well to check that there is no evidence of target organ damage (such as renal dysfunction, proteinuria, left ventricular hypertrophy and hypertensive retinopathy).

Q11 His medical notes state that he was seen by the general paediatricians recently for failure to thrive, and a blood test was performed, as he looked pale. His plasma creatinine is within the normal range for the laboratory. What would be a normal plasma creatinine for a 1-year-old boy?

A 40 μmol/L

B 50 μmol/L

C 60 μmol/L

D 70 μmol/L

E 80 μmol/L

A11 A Creatinine comes from muscle so the fact that this child is failing to thrive means that the plasma creatinine should be low if he has normal renal function. The normal plasma creatinine is 40 μmol/L and values of 50–80 μmol/L are evidence of renal dysfunction.

Q12 What is the most likely diagnosis for the child in question 10?

A coarctation of the aorta

B congenital adrenal hyperplasia

C essential hypertension

D obesity-related hypertension

E renovascular hypertension

$A$12  **A**  The most likely reason, assuming that the blood pressure has been checked manually using the correct cuff is coarctation of the aorta. However, other causes occur and renovascular hypertension could be due to fibromuscular dysplasia in this child.

$Q$13  A 4-year-old girl with known chronic kidney disease has been referred for adenotonsillectomy and insertion of grommets. Her preoperative management should include which of the following?

    **A**  blood pressure measurement

    **B**  blood tests for urea, creatinine and electrolytes

    **C**  priority on surgical list

    **D**  intravenous fluids

    **E**  all of the above

$A$13  **E**  Due to the fact that this child has chronic kidney disease, it is important that correct preoperative checks, including blood pressure and renal function are made so that the anaesthetist is happy to proceed. In addition, the patient should not be fasted for a long period of time so being first on the surgical list with intravenous fluids is safe management. All of the suggested answers are correct in this question.

$Q$14  What postoperative check should be considered for the child in question 13?

    **A**  blood pressure measurement

    **B**  blood tests for urea, creatinine and electrolytes

    **C**  fluid balance

    **D**  intravenous fluids

    **E**  all of the above

$A$14  **E**  The question does not state the degree of chronic kidney disease, but it would be reasonable to continue intravenous fluids and checking fluid balance carefully while monitoring blood pressure and renal function postoperatively.

$Q$15  A 14-year-old boy has been hit by a car while riding his bicycle and has presented with macroscopic haematuria. Which of the following is first priority in his initial management?

    **A**  assessment of airway

    **B**  assessment of breathing

    **C**  assessment of circulation

    **D**  intravenous fluids

    **E**  oxygen therapy

A**15** **A** This question is regarding the correct management of an adolescent who has sustained traumatic injuries. The correct answer is A, as assessment of the airway should be carried out first, prior to assessment of breathing and circulation.

Q**16** With respect to the patient in question 15, which of the following tests should be undertaken most urgently?
**A** CT abdomen
**B** cystoscopy
**C** diagnostic peritoneal lavage
**D** Doppler renal ultrasound
**E** MRI abdomen

A**16** **D** In view of this patient having macroscopic haematuria, the initial and easiest assessment would be Doppler renal ultrasound to look for renal and/or bladder injury, haemorrhage and clots, although depending on the degree of injury, an abdominal CT (or MRI) scan could be undertaken.

## Further reading

Marks SD, Geary DF. Nephrology. In: Laxer RM, Ford-Jones EL, Friedman J, *et al*. *The Hospital for Sick Children: atlas of pediatrics*. Philadelphia, PA: Current Medicine LLC; 2005. pp. 319–38.

Marks SD, Lehnhardt A. Nephrology and urology. In: Gardiner M, Eisen S, Murphy C, editors. *Oxford Specialty Training: training in paediatrics*. Oxford: Oxford University Press; 2009. pp. 119–42.

Marks SD, Trompeter RS. Common renal problems. In: Bannon MJ, Carter YH. *Practical Paediatric Problems in Primary Care*. Oxford: Oxford University Press; 2007. pp. 41–9.

Marks SD, Winyard PJD. Pediatric nephrology. In: Godbole P, Gearhart JP, Wilcox DT, editors. *Clinical Problems in Pediatric Urology*. Oxford: Blackwell Publishing Limited; 2006. pp. 1–8.

Strobel S, Smith PK, El Habbal MH, *et al*. *The Great Ormond Street Colour Handbook of Paediatrics and Child Health*. London: Manson Publishing; 2007.

## CHAPTER 55

# Developmental and positional anomalies of the kidney

### IAN E WILLETTS

**From the choices below each question, select the single best answer.**

 **Q1** Which one of the following is *not* thought to be aetiologically associated with renal ectopia?

- **A** abnormalities of the ureteric bud
- **B** genetic abnormalities
- **C** abnormalities of the metanephros
- **D** abnormalities of the vascular supply
- **E** abnormalities of the pronephros

 **A1** **E** All the abnormalities listed are associated with renal ectopia except those of the pronephros. The fetal kidney develops from the metanephros. The ureteric bud develops from the mesonephros, and its cranial section merges with the developing metanephros anteriorly. In the ensuing month, this fused mass migrates cephalically, undergoing a final medial rotation of 90 degrees. During ascent, the cephalic end of the ureteric bud divides to form the pelvicalyceal system. During ascent, the blood supply of the kidney is drawn from local vessels. Any deviation from this process will lead to anomalies of renal position and fusion.

 **Q2** With regard to simple ectopic kidneys, which of the following statements is true?

- **A** Patients rarely require intervention unless they develop a complication.
- **B** The most common problem associated is vesicoureteric junction obstruction.
- **C** Renal ectopia occurs in ~1 : 100 persons in a screened population.
- **D** Vesicoureteric (VU) reflux is rarely associated with abnormally positioned kidneys.
- **E** Ectopic kidneys are usually anatomically normal.

**A2**  **A**  Failure to achieve full migration of the kidney to the normal anatomical position occurs in ~1 : 1000 persons. Screened populations have an incidence of 1 : 5000 persons. Only 50% of ectopic kidneys are recognised clinically. Ectopic kidneys, although often asymptomatic, are rarely anatomically normal – they tend to be small, lobulated, abnormally rotated, with extrarenal calyces and abnormal vascularity.

**Q3**  The following are more commonly found in patients with an ectopic kidney *except*:

   **A**  malformations of the contralateral kidney
   **B**  genital tract anomalies
   **C**  malformations of the skull, ribs and vertebrae
   **D**  nephrolithiasis
   **E**  reduced life expectancy.

**A3**  **E**  Fifteen per cent of males with an ectopic kidney have genital anomalies (hypospadias, undescended testes); 75% of females have genital anomalies (duplications, septations of the genitourinary-tract). These may cause problems during female reproductive function. Impaired drainage at the pelviureteric junction and nephrolithiasis are more commonly seen, possibly due to the anatomical arrangement. Life-expectancy is normal.

**Q4**  What is the most common site for renal ectopia?

   **A**  immediately inferior to the aortic bifurcation
   **B**  at the level of L2 vertebral body
   **C**  within the thoracic cavity
   **D**  on the opposite side (crossed ectopia)
   **E**  half of the patients have bilateral renal ectopia

**A4**  **A**  10% of patients have bilateral renal ectopia.

**Q5**  Which of the following is true about horseshoe kidney?

   **A**  It occurs twice as commonly in females than males.
   **B**  In 95% of cases the fusion occurs at the upper poles.
   **C**  The inferior mesenteric vessels pass posterior to the renal isthmus.
   **D**  The ureters pass anterior to the renal isthmus.
   **E**  The superior mesenteric vessels pass anterior to the renal isthmus.

**A5**  **D**  Horseshoe kidney is the most common abnormality of renal fusion. It occurs twice as commonly in males. Incidence 1 : 500–1000. Inherited renal diseases (polycystic kidney disease) occur with the same frequency as in normal kidneys.

Ninety-five per cent of fusion occurs at the lower poles, the inferior mesenteric vessels and the ureters passing anteriorly over the renal isthmus joining the two moieties.

 **Q6** Which of the following is true regarding horseshoe kidneys?

    **A** Associated anomalies of the skeletal, cardiovascular and genitourinary systems are rare.

    **B** The incidence of Wilms's tumour is similar to that seen in normal kidneys.

    **C** There is an association between horseshoe kidneys and development of abdominal aortic aneurysms later in life.

    **D** The majority of horseshoe kidneys have normal anatomical blood supplies.

    **E** The renal isthmus rarely impairs the drainage of the renal pelves.

**A6**   **C** Associated anomalies occur in almost 80% patients reported with horseshoe kidneys. Wilms's tumour occurs with a 1.5- to 8-fold increased risk in a horseshoe kidney. Impaired drainage of the pelviureteric junction is the most common problem seen in a horseshoe kidney, particularly on the left side. Blood supply to the horseshoe kidney is highly variable – 70% are supplied by combinations of vessels entering from the aorta, or the renal, mesenteric, iliac or sacral arteries. The isthmus may have its own blood supply, which may on occasion represent the whole renal supply.

**Q7** Which of the following is not true with regard to horseshoe kidneys?

    **A** The renal isthmus may be fibrotic, dysplastic or normal renal tissue.

    **B** The isthmus frequently has a separate blood supply to the rest of the horseshoe kidney.

    **C** 70% of horseshoe kidneys are supplied with blood from the aortic, renal, mesenteric, iliac or sacral arteries rather than the normal anatomical arrangement.

    **D** Reconstruction of the pelviureteric junction may require ureterocalicostomy.

    **E** Radiological imaging (MRU/IVU) will often identify bilateral renal malrotation with calyces lateral to the renal pelvis and with a vertical axis.

**A7**   **E** The calyces on imaging lie medial to the vertically orientated renal pelvis. The ureters are often in a more lateral position.

**Q8** In pelviureteric junction impaired drainage (PUJO) associated with horseshoe kidney, which of the following is not true?

**A** PUJO is more commonly seen in the left-sided renal moiety.

**B** The PUJO can be approached through an extraperitoneal flank incision.

**C** Bilateral PUJO may be best approached transperitoneally.

**D** Ureterocalicostomy utilising the upper pole calyces has been described with good success.

**E** Stone disease is treated as that occurring with a normal kidney

**A8** **D** Ureterocalicostomy utilising the lower pole calyces has been described with good success. Stone disease in the presence of hydronephrosis may require pyeloplasty.

**Q9** With regard to crossed renal ectopia, which of the following is *not* true?

**A** It occurs with an incidence of 1 : 7000 at autopsy.

**B** More commonly the renal moieties are not fused.

**C** There is a 2 : 1 male predominance.

**D** The left kidney migrates more commonly than the right.

**E** There is an increased incidence of coexistent malformations in other organ systems.

**A9** **B** Eighty-five per cent of crossed ectopic kidneys are fused. The left kidney migrates three times more commonly than the right. Coexistent malformations are frequently described (VACTORL), especially if there is a single ureter.

**Q10** Which of the following is *not* true of crossed ectopic kidneys?

**A** The blood supply is variable and may cross the midline.

**B** Urinary drainage is usually by two ureters entering the bladder on one side.

**C** Most fused kidneys are undetected during life.

**D** CT/MRI imaging may allow better definition of the exact anatomy.

**E** Renal function rather than position or anatomy dictate management.

**A10** **B** Ureters usually enter the bladder on either side of the trigone. The blood supply is variable and may cross the midline.

Q11 Which of the following statements is true with regard to the solitary kidney?

    A The incidence in the normal population on screening is ~10%.

    B Mutations in the *RET*, *PAX2* and *WT1* genes result in renal agenesis in animal models.

    C Branchio-oto-renal syndrome is associated with renal agenesis and is autosomal recessive in inheritance.

    D Progressive glomerular damage is not associated with the congenital solitary kidney.

    E More commonly the solitary kidney lies on the left side of the abdomen.

A11 **B** Radiological screening studies have identified renal agenesis in 0.3% of a control population. In animal models, mutations of the *WT1* gene result in renal agenesis because of failure of induction of the renal mesenchyme. *RET* and *PAX2* mutations lead to failure of the ureteric bud to develop from the mesonephric duct. Branchio-oto-renal syndrome is an autosomal dominant condition; affected individuals have ear, neck and renal anomalies. While controversial, studies suggest that progressive glomerular damage (focal segmental glomerulosclerosis) with proteinuria can develop in the congenitally solitary kidney.

Q12 Which of these statements is not true with regard to renal tract ultrasonography?

    A It provides a good and accurate measure of the degree of hydronephrosis or hydroureter.

    B It provides some estimation of renal parenchyma but can miss significant renal scars.

    C It can accurately evaluate bladder emptying and bladder wall anatomy.

    D It can detect the presence of VU reflux.

    E It is largely risk free.

A12 **D** While modifications of ultrasonography are improving its ability to identify VU reflux, grading necessitates micturating cystourethrogram studies. Some studies suggest that up to 50% of renal scars are missed on ultrasonography when compared with technetium-99m ($^{99m}$Tc)-DMSA scanning.

**Q13** Which of the following statements is true regarding renal scintigraphy?

**A** $^{99m}$Tc-DMSA scanning provides better evaluation of renal parenchymal function than $^{99m}$Tc-MAG3 studies.

**B** $^{99m}$Tc-DMSA scanning can accurately separate acute from chronic renal parenchymal defects.

**c** MAG3-indirect radionuclide cystography (MAG3+IRC) is as sensitive as micturating cystourethrography in detecting vesicoureteric reflux in potty-trained infants.

**D** The radiation dose of a typical $^{99m}$Tc-DMSA study is 7.0 mSv, equivalent to 10 abdominal X-rays.

**E** MAG3+IRC provides good anatomical images for grading of vesicoureteric reflux.

**A13** **A** The radiation dose of a typical $^{99m}$Tc-DMSA study is approximately 0.7mSv; equivalent to one abdominal X-ray film.

**Q14** In a child with a significant urinary tract infection (UTI), which of the following is less likely to lead to the identification of an important anatomical anomaly in the urinary tract?

**A** palpable abdominal mass present

**B** impaired urine flow

**c** elevated serum creatinine concentration

**D** rapid clinical response to treatment (<48 hours)

**E** infection with a non-coliform bacterium

**A14** **D**

**Q15** Risk factors for recurrent UTI and/or renal scarring include all *except*:

**A** recurrent episodes of acute pyelonephritis

**B** delay in treatment

**c** severity of coexistent VU reflux (grades III–V)

**D** coexistent voiding/bowel dysfunction

**E** female child.

**A15** **E**

**Q16** Which of the following statements is *not* true with regard to UTI/renal scars?

**A** Renal scars can occur in a child with or without VU reflux.

**B** Renal scarring is rare with lower grades of VU reflux.

**C** Most cases of severe 'reflux nephropathy' are congenital.

**D** There is *good* evidence that antibiotic prophylaxis reduces recurrent UTI and renal scarring.

**E** In spite of the treatment of VU reflux, transplant registries have not shown a reduction in the proportion of end-stage renal disease attributable to VU-reflux.

**A16** **D** This is controversial. While the evidence may suggest a benefit of prophylaxis, it is not good evidence. Indeed, the UK Dept of Health has suggested there may be no role for prophylactic urinary tract antibiotics in a considerable number of children (NICE, 2009).

## Further reading

Driss M, Boukadi A, Charfi L, *et al.* Renal cell carcinoma associated with Xp11.2 translocation arising in a horseshoe kidney. *Pathology.* 2009; **41**(6): 587–90.

Glodny B, Petersen J, Hofmann KJ, *et al.* Kidney fusion anomalies revisited: clinical and radiological analysis of 209 cases of crossed fused ectopia and horseshoe kidney. *BJU Int.* 2009; **103**(2): 224–35.

Guarino N, Tadini B, Camardi P, *et al.* The incidence of associated urological abnormalities in children with renal ectopia. *J Urol.* 2004; **172**(4 Pt. 2): 1757–9.

Rinat C, Farkas A, Frishberg Y. Familial inheritance of crossed fused renal ectopia. *Pediatr Nephrol.* 2001; **16**(3): 269–70.

Sundararajan L, Mohan PV, Chandran H. Horseshoe kidney: retroperitoneoscopic nephrectomy. *J Pedriatr Urol.* 2007; **3**(2): 159–61.

Symons SJ, Ramachandran A, Kurien A, *et al.* Urolithiasis in the horseshoe kidney: a single-centre experience. *BJU Int.* 2008; **102**(11): 1676–80.

# CHAPTER 56

# Cystic disease of the kidneys

## HARISH CHANDRAN

**From the choices below each question, select the single best answer.**

**Q1** The most common type of renal cystic disease is:
  A developmental
  B malignant
  C simple cyst
  D genetic
  E acquired.

**A1**  **C**  The most common cystic lesions of the kidneys overall are simple cysts, which occur in 25%–33% of the population over 50 years of age. Autosomal dominant polycystic kidney disease (ADPKD), a genetically determined disease, with an incidence of 1 in 1250 live births, is the most common genetic cystic disease. Malignant cysts are rare. Developmental cysts such as multicystic dysplastic kidneys (MCDKs) are uncommon and sporadic. Acquired renal cysts are usually seen in patients on dialysis.

**Q2** Inherited cystic renal disease is seen in which of the following?
  A adult polycystic kidney disease
  B MCDKs
  C simple cysts
  D medullary sponge kidney
  E cystic renal carcinoma

**A2**  **A**  ADPKD is also known as adult polycystic kidney disease and is inherited by a gene defect on chromosome 16 or 4. MCDKs occur sporadically due to ureteric atresia or dysfunction of the nephrogenic blastema. Simple cysts increase in frequency with age and are not inherited.

**Q3** Acquired cystic renal disease is seen in which of the following?
  **A** adult polycystic kidney disease
  **B** MCDKs
  **C** medullary cystic kidney disease
  **D** patients on dialysis
  **E** glomerulocystic disease

**A3** **D** Patients on either haemo- or peritoneal dialysis develop renal cysts and this is thought to be related to the uraemic state. After 10 years of dialysis >90% of patients will have developed renal cysts, bilaterally. ADPKD and medullary cystic kidney disease are genetic in origin; MCDK is caused by a developmental error.

**Q4** Regarding MCDK aetiology, which of the following is true?
  **A** It is genetic.
  **B** It is acquired.
  **C** It is associated with urethral atresia.
  **D** It is associated with ureteric atresia.
  **E** It is associated with tuberous sclerosis.

**A4** **D** MCDKs are thought to be due to dysfunction of the nephrogenic blastema and associated with ureteric obstruction or atresia. The pelviureteric system is absent. There is no genetic basis and it is not associated with systemic disease.

**Q5** Regarding simple renal cysts, which of the following is true? They are typically:
  **A** familial
  **B** present in over 80% of the population
  **C** multiloculated
  **D** large, unilocular cysts
  **E** tiny, multiple cysts.

**A5** **D** Simple renal cysts are usually large by the time they are detected. Typically they are unilocular and unilateral. They are not familial. Simple renal cysts are present in about 25% of people over the age of 50 years.

**Q6** Regarding autosomal recessive polycystic kidney disease (ARPKD), which of the following is *not* true?

**A** ARPKD is usually bilateral.

**B** Most present in late childhood.

**C** The genetic defect is on chromosome 6.

**D** It is associated with respiratory disease.

**E** The kidneys are usually large.

**A6** **B** ARPKD is a genetic disease with a defect on chromosome 6. The disease is always bilateral and most present in the neonatal period or with antenatal diagnosis. Most of these children will have significant respiratory compromise. Respiratory failure, rather than renal failure, is the cause of death in the neonatal period.

**Q7** In ARPKD, which of the following is *not* true?

**A** Patients have very enlarged kidneys.

**B** 75% present in the neonatal period.

**C** Respiratory failure is the usual cause of death in the neonatal period.

**D** Renal failure is the usual cause of death in the neonatal period.

**E** The child may be hypertensive.

**A7** **C** Neonates with ARPKD often have huge, visible abdominal masses and most will present in the first few weeks of life. Renal failure may take many years to develop. Respiratory failure is the usual cause of death in the newborn period. Hypertension is present in 80%.

**Q8** Which of the following statements regarding ARPKD is true?

**A** It can be transmitted in an autosomal dominant fashion.

**B** The kidneys continue to grow in size as the child grows.

**C** The gene defect is located on chromosome 6.

**D** Respiratory disease is not usually a feature.

**E** Hypertension is uncommon.

**A8** **A** In ARPKD, the inheritance is by a recessive pattern and the kidneys usually become smaller as the child grows. The gene defect is located on the short arm of chromosome 6. Most neonates (80%) with ARPKD have hypertension and significant respiratory compromise.

**Q9** Which of the following statements about ADPKD is *not* true?

   **A** It presents in the first decade of life.

   **B** It is the most common form of inherited cystic renal disease.

   **C** It is caused by a gene defect on chromosome 16.

   **D** It is associated with cysts on other organs.

   **E** Hypertension occurs late.

**A9**   **A**   ADPKD is a genetic disease that presents in the third or fourth decades of life and is due to a gene defect on chromosome 16. It is the most common form of genetic cystic disease and is frequently associated with cysts on other organs, especially the liver.

**Q10** In patients with ADPKD, which of the following is *not* true?

   **A** Men are more likely to have massive renal enlargement.

   **B** It is associated with intracranial aneurysms.

   **C** They may have hypertension.

   **D** They do not usually have pain as a presenting feature.

   **E** Renal failure is a late feature.

**A10**   **D**   Pain as a presenting feature occurs in 60% of patients with ADPKD. Men have a tendency towards massive renal enlargement. In ADPKD, there is a well-recognised association with intracranial aneurysms. Hypertension occurs in about 60% in the fifth or sixth decade of life. Progression to end-stage renal failure usually is a slow process.

**Q11** With regard to the genetics of ADPKD, which of the following is *not* true?

   **A** There is a 50% chance of inheritance.

   **B** 25% of patients do not have a family history of ADPKD.

   **C** Homozygous ADPKD is common.

   **D** The gene defect is on the short arm of chromosome 16.

   **E** Both *PKD1* and *PKD4* are implicated.

**A11**   **C**   The homozygous state has not been described. ADPKD is transferred in a dominant pattern and with a 50% chance of inheritance. Twenty-five per cent will not have a positive family history because affected relatives may die of other causes before diagnosis, or may not yet be aware of their disease; or because of non-paternity and spontaneous mutations. The genetic defect is in *PKD1* on the short arm of chromosome 16 and the *PKD4* locus on chromosome 4.

Q12 In ADPKD, which of the following statements is true?
  A Renal function decreases rapidly.
  B There is a greater risk of renal failure in women.
  C Symptomatic urinary tract infections are uncommon.
  D There is an inability to concentrate urine.
  E It is usually present in the first decade of life.

A12 D Of the choices given the only true statement is that there is an inability to concentrate urine. It is usually the first sign of renal failure, later followed by a decrease in glomerular filtration rate, proteinuria and raised creatinine. The risk of renal failure is greater the younger the age at diagnosis, in males, with urinary tract infections, with more severe proteinuria, and in those of African descent. Presentation is typically in the third or fourth decade of life.

## Further reading

Holcomb GW, Murphy JP. *Ashcraft's Pediatric Surgery*. 5th ed. Philadelphia, PA: Saunders/Elsevier; 2010.

Lippert MC. Renal cystic disease. In: Gillenwater J, Howards SS, Grayhack JT, *et al. Adult and Pediatric Urology*. 4th ed. St Louis, MO: Elsevier Health Sciences; 2002. pp. 829–78.

Stringer MD, Oldham KT, Mouriquand PDE, editors. *Pediatric Surgery and Urology: long-term outcomes*. 2nd ed. Cambridge: Cambridge University Press; 2006.

# CHAPTER 57

# Obstructive uropathies

## JULIAN ROBERTS

**From the choices below each question, select the single best answer.**

 **1** Regarding MAG3 mercaptoacetyltriglycine renogram, which of the following is true?

   **A** It is a reliable investigation for renal scarring.

   **B** MAG3 is labelled with $^{90m}$Tc.

   **C** MAG3 stands for mercapto adenosine triglycine.

   **D** It relies on tubular extraction of the MAG3 from the blood to urine.

   **E** It is usually performed after administration of intravenous furosemide.

 **1** **D** Intravenous injection of MAG3 labelled with technetium-99m ($^{99m}$Tc) (a meta-stable nuclear isomer with a half-life of 6 hours) produces a dynamic renal scan. High extraction rates and lack of reliance on glomerular filtration results in better kidney-to-background activity. $^{99m}$Tc-MAG3 is useful for evaluating the degree of obstruction. $^{99m}$Tc-DMSA (dimercaptosuccinic acid) on the other hand is taken up and fixed in functional proximal renal tubular tissue. Only around 10% appears in the urine. This makes $^{99m}$Tc-DMSA the most reliable way to estimate differential function and diagnose renal scarring.

Furosemide is used to promote diuresis, and may be injected at the beginning of the $^{99m}$Tc-MAG3 study or at varying times during the study (individual protocols vary). This needs to be taken into account when interpreting the scan.

**Q2** Which of the following is true for antenatal renal dilatation detected by ultrasound?

   **A** Antenatal ultrasound correctly diagnoses the cause of renal dilatation in 80% of cases.

   **B** It should be confirmed by postnatal ultrasound at 2 weeks of age.

   **C** If there is severe dilatation on the postnatal scan a $^{99m}$Tc-MAG3 scan should be performed by the age of 3 weeks.

   **D** Oligohydramnios associated with upper tract dilatation is an indicator of poor outcome.

   **E** Diagnosis of unilateral upper tract dilatation before 32 weeks is associated with poor function in that kidney postnatally.

**A2**   **D** Antenatal diagnosis is now the commonest presentation of upper tract renal dilatation. Diagnosis is constantly improving but the correlation with postnatal findings is still only around 60%. It is essential, therefore, to confirm the dilatation postnatally with ultrasound. Antenatal prognostic indicators for poor outcome with upper tract obstruction are gestational age at diagnosis (particularly <24 weeks), oligohydramnios (indicator of poor urine production and affects lung development) and 'bright kidneys' (indicates poor differentiation of renal tissue).

**Q3** Which of the following is true in the postnatal management of antenatally diagnosed upper tract dilatation?

   **A** Renal ultrasonography (USG) should not be performed in the first 48 hours, as urine production is reduced in the first few days of life.

   **B** A micturating cystourethrogram (MCUG) is the first investigation if the renal pelvis dilatation is 20 mm on a postnatal ultrasound.

   **C** $^{99m}$Tc-MAG3 renogram is the first investigation if the renal pelvis dilatation is 12 mm on a postnatal ultrasound.

   **D** If a day 2 renal USG is normal the baby does not need further investigation.

   **E** $^{99m}$Tc-MAG3 renogram is the first investigation if the renal pelvis dilatation is 25 mm on a postnatal ultrasound.

**A3**   **E** Local protocols for management of antenatally diagnosed upper tract dilatation vary, including the need for antibiotic prophylaxis, but usually renal ultrasound is performed within the first 24–48 hours (if posterior urethral valves (PUVs) suspected, should be within 12–24 hours). Urine production is low in this period so the USG may underestimate the degree of dilatation. For unilateral hydronephrosis a USG is repeated at 4–6 weeks, irrespective of the findings on the early postnatal scan.

In general terms, the more severe the dilatation the more likely the kidney is to be obstructed. The normal anteroposterior (AP) diameter of the renal pelvis is 5–7 mm. Mild dilatation (AP diameter of the pelvis of <12–15 mm) is more likely to be reflux than obstruction so an MCUG is usually requested first. With dilatation more than this, ureteropelvic junction (UPJ) obstruction is most common and a $^{99m}$Tc-MAG3 renogram is more likely to yield a positive result.

**Q4** Which of the following is *not* associated with upper tract obstruction?
  **A** Bardet–Biedl's syndrome
  **B** PUVs
  **C** hypospadias surgery
  **D** neurogenic bladder
  **E** ureterovesical junction obstruction

**A4**   **A** Bardet–Biedl's syndrome is one of many syndromes associated with renal anomalies and renal failure but not with overt upper tract obstruction. Chronic urethral narrowing following hypospadias surgery has rarely caused obstruction and renal failure so that postoperative flow rates on such children are necessary.

**Q5** The most appropriate investigation suggested by this ultrasound finding would be (*see* Figure 57.1):

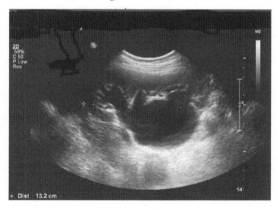

**FIGURE 57.1** Renal ultrasound scan

  **A** $^{99m}$Tc-DMSA renogram
  **B** micturating cystourethrogram
  **C** intravenous urogram
  **D** $^{99m}$Tc-MAG3 renogram
  **E** magnetic resonance (MR) urogram

**A5**  **D**  The ultrasound suggests ureteropelvic junction (UPJ) obstruction (significant pelvicalyceal dilatation without ureteric dilatation). $^{99m}$Tc-MAG3 is the investigation of choice. Intravenous urography would confirm the anatomical obstruction but would give no indication of renal function (pictures in babies are also often poor). $^{99m}$Tc-DMSA would give differential function but no indication of renal drainage. MR urogram gives excellent anatomical definition but no good indication of renal function.

**Q6**  In Figures 57.2, what do the ultrasound appearances suggest?

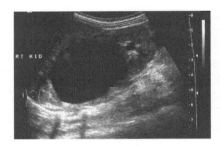
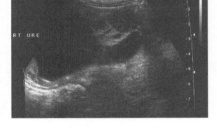

FIGURE 57.2A  Renal ultrasound scan    FIGURE 57.2B  Renal ultrasound scan

A  hydronephrosis due to UPJ obstruction
B  severe reflux into a single system
C  severe reflux into a duplex system
D  obstructed upper moiety (with or without ureterocele)
E  hydroureteronephrosis due to vesicoureteric junction obstruction

**A6**  **D**  The ultrasounds show a clear duplex with dilated upper moiety collecting system and upper ureter with a non-dilated lower moiety collecting system. Generally in duplex systems the upper moiety is affected by obstruction, due to ectopic insertion of the ureter with or without a ureterocele. The lower moiety is more likely to suffer dilatation arising from vesicoureteric reflux (and rarely UPJ obstruction).

**Q7**  Which of these conditions does not often present with evidence of bladder outlet obstruction?
A  PUV
B  sphincter dyssynergia
C  posterior urethritis
D  prolapsing ureterocele
E  syringocele

**A**7   **C**   Posterior urethritis usually presents in peripubertal boys and is character-ised by dysuria and terminal haematuria. It may be confirmed by cystoscopy and will often respond to anti-inflammatory drugs. It is important to remember other common causes of urethral obstruction such as balanitis xerotica oblit-erans (BXO) and postoperative meatal stenosis. BXO is unusual under the age of 5 years. It typically presents with increasing phimosis often associated with dysuria. Obstruction can arise from the severity of the phimosis or narrowing of the urethra when this is also affected. Treatment is traditionally by circumcision (meatotomy may be required if the glans meatus is affected), but more recently prepucioplasty and steroid injection has been used as an alternative. Other causes of urethral obstruction are rare but include syringoceles (dilatation of the Cowper's gland ducts), anterior urethral valves and trauma.

**Q**8   Which of the following is true regarding PUVs?

    **A**  When detected before 32 weeks' gestation they are best treated with intra-amniotic shunt.

    **B**  Valve ablation should be performed immediately after the diagnosis is made.

    **C**  Bilateral hydronephrosis in a baby male should always be investi-gated with urgent micturating cystogram.

    **D**  They always present with bilateral upper tract dilatation.

    **E**  Antenatal ultrasound has high sensitivity and specificity for dia-gnosis of PUVs.

**A**8   **C**   PUV is now commonly diagnosed antenatally, with the findings of persisting upper tract dilatation and non-emptying bladder. However, diagnosis by ultra-sound is not always reliable. Prenatal management is still controversial but currently there does not appear to be any advantage (in terms of renal outcome or lung function) in intra-amniotic shunting unless it is done for poor prognostic indicators (such as diagnosis before 24 weeks, thick-walled bladder, oligohy-dramnios and 'bright kidneys', which suggests poor renal tissue differentiation). PUVs will classically, on postnatal ultrasound, show bilateral hydronephrosis with thick-walled bladder and sometimes dilatation of the posterior urethra, but the appearances can vary widely. Occasionally there is severe unilateral dilatation and little or no dilatation on the other side (so-called blow-off situation, where preferential reflux into one system results in sparing of the other side). Certainly any male child born with bilateral hydronephrosis (particularly if the ureter is involved) should have an early cystogram to exclude PUV. Although primary valve ablation is standard definitive treatment the initial treatment is bladder drainage (by catheter) until the baby is stabilised.

**Q⁹** Which of the following is *not* associated with neurogenic bladder?

    **A** myelomeningocele

    **B** anorectal anomalies

    **C** sacrococcygeal teratoma

    **D** cerebral palsy

    **E** prune belly syndrome

**A⁹**   **E** Neurogenic bladder is an important cause of chronic upper tract obstruction and deterioration in renal function. Spina bifida has in the past been the commonest cause of neurogenic bladder. In prune belly syndrome the abnormality lies in the abdominal muscle and ganglion cells, and pelvic innervation is normal. Neurogenic bladder can also result from spinal cord injuries or infection and various types of pelvic tumours.

**Q10** Which of the following is the most common management of a high-pressure neurogenic bladder?

    **A** bladder expression (Credé's manoeuvre)

    **B** regular assessment with ultrasound and urodynamics

    **C** bladder augmentation

    **D** clean intermittent catheterisation (CIC)

    **E** vesicostomy

**A10**   **D** Persisting high pressure (usually regarded as greater than 30 cm $H_2O$) can lead to renal damage because of back pressure on the kidney. Management has been revolutionised by CIC, which is easily taught in boys and girls especially with an insensate urethra. The majority of neuropathic bladders can be managed with CIC with or without medication such as oxybutynin (used to reduce associated bladder overactivity).

    Bladder enlargement (augmentation) is indicated to allow low-pressure storage of urine when other therapies fail or when the outlet pressure of the bladder needs to be increased to stop persisting incontinence. Augmentation can be performed with various tissues such as small or large bowel, stomach or occasionally a very dilated ureter.

**Q11** Which of the following is true for ureteroceles in infants?

    **A** They are associated with obstruction of the lower moiety of a duplex kidney.

    **B** The primary treatment is usually cystoscopic incision.

    **C** They are not associated with single systems.

    **D** They always cause significant obstruction.

    **E** The primary standard treatment is usually excision and ureteric reimplantation.

**A11**  **B**  A ureterocele is a localised dilated section of the ureter within the wall of the bladder. On scanning it appears similar to the balloon of a catheter. The most common type of ureterocele is 'ectopic', associated with the upper moiety of duplex kidneys. 'Orthotopic' ureteroceles can occur with single systems and these may be asymptomatic without significant obstruction (MAG3 is indicated). In infants with significantly dilated upper moiety and ureterocele the primary treatment is usually incision of the ureterocele to relieve the obstruction. The function of the upper moiety may then be assessed with $^{99m}$Tc-DMSA to decide what, if any, further treatment is required.

**Q12**  Which of the following is true for ureterovesical junction (UVJ) obstruction in an infant?

    **A**  It may resolve after temporary stenting of the UVJ with a double-J stent.

    **B**  It is more common in females.

    **C**  The ureteric orifice inserts laterally to the trigone.

    **D**  It is commonly bilateral.

    **E**  It is best treated by early reimplantation of the dilated ureter.

**A12**  **A**  UVJ obstruction is due to an abnormality of the muscle or increased collagen in the distal ureter. It is seen more commonly in males and on the left side. As a cause of megaureter it needs to be differentiated from a refluxing megaureter (by micturating cystourethrogram). Occasionally some megaureters are both obstructed and refluxing.

    There are many reports of UVJ obstruction improving spontaneously after stenting. Those that do not resolve may be treated with ureteric reimplantation. This is not recommended under 1 year of age due to technical difficulties reimplanting a large ureter into a small bladder.

**Q13**  Which of the following is true for UPJ obstruction?

    **A**  It is commonly symptomatic in young children.

    **B**  It may be due to intrinsic and/or extrinsic obstruction.

    **C**  It is commoner on the right side.

    **D**  Endopyelotomy has a high success rate in treatment of UPJ obstruction.

    **E**  Pyelopexy is a standard treatment of UPJ obstruction.

**A13**  **B**  Most UPJ obstruction is asymptomatic in infancy and is commonly found as a result of antenatal ultrasound screening. UPJ may present with infection, pain (especially in older children), abdominal mass and occasionally haematuria. Two-thirds occur on the left side. The cause can be intrinsic (abnormality of the muscular wall of the UPJ), extrinsic (such as kinking of the ureter, obstruction by lower pole vessels) or a combination of both. Dismembered (Hynes–Anderson) pyeloplasty is the standard procedure, with a high success rate. Endopyelotomy (incision of the UPJ) has been used in children but with much lower success. Pyelopexy (hitching the UPJ away from obstructing lower pole vessels) may be used if the obstruction is solely caused by lower pole vessels.

**Q14** Which of the following is an indication for urgent percutaneous nephrostomy?

   **A** gross hydronephrosis with a pelvic AP diameter of 4.0 cm

   **B** obstructed upper moiety of duplex kidney with a large ureterocele

   **C** a baby with UVJ obstruction, when a retrograde pigtailed stent cannot be passed

   **D** child with a urinary tract infection and hydroureteronephrosis on ultrasound

   **E** pyonephrosis

**A14** **E** Percutaneous nephrostomy is a useful temporising procedure for relieving renal obstruction, particularly where retrograde drainage (double-J stent) is not possible. It does, however, come with complications, especially displacement and infection. The combination of obstruction and infection (not quickly responsive to antibiotics, debris in the kidney on ultrasound) can cause rapid renal damage, and is an indication for nephrostomy. There is usually time for investigation and more definitive treatment in other circumstances.

## Further reading

Belman AB, King LR, Kramer SA. *Guide to Clinical Pediatric Urology*. London: Martin Dunitz; 2002.

Godbole P, Gearhart J, Wilcox DT. *Clinical Problems in Pediatric Urology*. Oxford: Blackwell; 2006.

Thomas DFM, Duffy PG, Rickwood AMK. *Essentials of Paediatric Urology*. 2nd ed. London: Informa Healthcare; 2008.

# CHAPTER 58

# Vesicoureteric reflux and urinary tract infection

## FRANCESCA CASTILLO, IAN E WILLETTS

From the choices below each question, select the single best answer.

**Q1** Regarding urinary tract infection in the *neonatal* period, which one of the following is true?

    **A** The incidence is greater in boys.

    **B** The incidence is greater in girls.

    **C** The rate in uncircumcised boys equals the rate in circumcised boys.

    **D** Cystitis occurs as frequently as pyelonephritis.

    **E** *Escherichia coli* and *Proteus* spp. are the dominant organisms in female urethral flora.

**A1**   **A** Urinary tract infection occurs more commonly in males in the neonatal period. From 1 year of age onwards, the incidence of recurrent and first-time urinary tract infection is greater in females. Most episodes of urinary tract infection in the first year of life are pyelonephritis. Uncircumcised male infants under 1 year have a 10 times greater risk of urinary tract infection than those who have been circumcised. The female urethra is colonised predominantly with *E. coli*, and the male urethra with *E. coli* and *Proteus* spp. These normal bacterial flora usually decrease over the first year of life.

**Q2** Which of the following is true regarding the incidence of urinary tract infection?

    **A** It is about 2% in all children by the age of 2 years.

    **B** It is more common in girls of all ages.

    **C** It decreases with age.

    **D** Under the age of 1 year is *not* associated with an increased likelihood of future urinary tract infections.

    **E** It is not related to the presence of vesicoureteric reflux (VUR).

**A2**  **A** Studies have shown that at least 2.2% of boys and 2.1% of girls have suffered from a urinary tract infection by the age of 2 years. Under the age of 6 months, boys are more commonly affected by urinary tract infection than girls. After this age, girls are more commonly affected. By the age of 16, over 11% of girls will have suffered a urinary tract infection. Seventy-eight per cent of girls (71% of boys) who had a urinary tract infection under the age of 1 had a recurrence, compared with 45% of girls (39% of boys) who presented with their first urinary tract infection after the age of 1. VUR is present in up to 40% of patients presenting with urinary tract infection.

**Q3** Which of the following is true with regard to the investigation of suspected urinary tract infections?

  **A** Microscopy is not required if dipstick testing is positive for leucocyte esterase but negative for nitrites.

  **B** Cotton wool balls can reliably be used to collect urine samples.

  **C** Suprapubic aspiration should not be used for urine sampling because of risks involved with the procedure.

  **D** Unexplained fever should be investigated by urine sampling.

  **E** Microscopy is not required if dipstick is positive for leucocyte esterase *and* nitrites.

**A3** **D** Infants and children presenting with unexplained fever should have a urine sample checked within 24 hours of presentation. Urine should be sent for culture in all infants with either positive leucocyte esterase or nitrites. Antibiotics should only be commenced where there is clear clinical evidence or suspicion of urinary tract infection. Cotton wool balls are not a reliable method of urine sampling. Suprapubic aspiration is recommended where a clean sample cannot otherwise be obtained. Dipstick positive for leucocyte esterase and nitrites is highly indicative of urinary tract infection and urine should therefore be cultured to confirm this and provide evidence about the causative bacteria. In the context of clinical suspicion or urinary tract infection, this dipstick result should be treated with antibiotics while culture and sensitivities are awaited. Unexplained fever in a neonate, infant or child should be investigated thoroughly and this should include urine sampling as urinary tract infection and pyelonephritis can present insidiously and in a variety of ways. Not all bacteria are capable of reducing nitrates to nitrites, therefore a urine sample positive for leucocyte esterase and negative for nitrites should still be sent for microscopy and culture.

Q4  The most appropriate imaging for a 3-year-old boy with a first episode of uncomplicated culture-proven urinary tract infection is:

A  a renal tract ultrasound scan

B  a renal tract ultrasound scan and a micturating cystourethrogram

C  a renal tract ultrasound scan and a technetium-99m ($^{99m}$Tc)-DMSA scan

D  a renal tract ultrasound scan and a $^{99m}$Tc-MAG3 renogram study

E  an intravenous urogram.

A4  **A**  In the UK, NICE (National Institute for Health and Clinical Excellence) guidelines suggest that in an infant/child over the age of 6 months, an uncomplicated urinary tract infection that responds to treatment within 48 hours does not require any imaging; however, in practice a renal tract ultrasound would be performed. A recurrent or atypical urinary tract infection requires a DMSA. If the ultrasound scan showed any dilatation or if there was poor urinary flow or a family history of VUR then a micturating cystourethrogram (MCUG) should be performed. Intravenous urogram has limited and specific uses in clinical practice.

Q5  Antibiotic urinary tract prophylaxis would be most appropriately commenced in which one of the following?

A  An infant under the age of 1 year with a first episode of urinary tract infection.

B  An infant under the age of 6 months with a single episode of pyelonephritis.

C  A child with asymptomatic bacteriuria.

D  An infant under the age of 1 year with VUR and renal scarring.

E  A child with recurrent urinary tract infections and normal renal radiological imaging.

A5  **D**  Antibiotic prophylaxis is useful in certain situations. The infant under the age of 1 year with VUR and mild scarring may benefit from prophylactic antibiotics. An infant under the age of 6 months with pyelonephritis will need imaging, and if there is evidence of VUR/scarring will require prophylaxis. There is no evidence to show that prophylactic antibiotics prevent new renal scarring in patients with asymptomatic bacteriuria or those with a normal renal tract.

Q**6** In a child with symptomatic bacteriuria, which of the following is true?
   **A** The presence of loin pain does not confirm pyelonephritis.
   **B** Treatment should always commence with intravenous antibiotics.
   **C** The presence of a fever of 38°C suggests pyelonephritis.
   **D** Absence of systemic symptoms is common in those under 3 months of age.
   **E** Treatment rarely involves intravenous antibiotics.

A**6**   **C**  An infant or child with bacteriuria and a fever of 38 °C or with loin pain or tenderness should be considered to have pyelonephritis. Treatment in those under 3 months of age should be with intravenous antibiotics, and those older than 3 months should initially be treated with oral antibiotics if tolerated. Infants under 3 months are most likely to present with systemic features, and more commonly suffer from pyelonephritis.

Q**7** Regarding urine dipstick and culture results, which of the following is true?
   **A** Urine dipstick positive for leucocyte esterase but negative for nitrites should be treated with antibiotics.
   **B** Urine dipstick positive for nitrites but negative for leucocyte esterase should be treated with antibiotics.
   **C** Pyuria positive on microscopy and culture, but bacteriuria negative should always be treated with antibiotics.
   **D** Bacteriuria in the absence of pyuria is never a clinical infection.
   **E** In the absence of symptoms, pyuria and bacteriuria do not imply urinary tract infection.

A**7**   **B**  Dipstick positive for nitrites but negative for leucocyte esterase is likely to be caused by urinary tract infection, in the absence of other likely diagnoses. Antibiotics should be commenced while microscopy results are awaited. Leucocyte esterase may be indicative of infection outside of the urinary tract. Microscopy and culture that is pyuria positive but bacteriuria negative should be treated with antibiotics only if there is clinical evidence of urinary tract infection. If symptomatic, bacteriuria confirms urinary tract infection, even in the absence of pyuria. The presence of white cells and the growth of bacteria in the urine confirm urinary tract infection.

**Q8** Which of the following is indicative of a urinary tract infection?

    **A** $>10^5$ colony-forming units (CFU)/mL of a single urinary pathogen confirms diagnosis.

    **B** $>10^7$ CFU/mL of mixed urinary pathogens confirms diagnosis.

    **C** $>10^4$ CFU/mL of a single urinary pathogen confirms diagnosis.

    **D** $>10^3$ CFU/mL of a single urinary pathogen confirms diagnosis.

    **E** None of the above.

**A8**   **A** A mid-stream, clean catch urine that cultures $>10^5$ CFU/mL of a single urinary pathogen confirms diagnosis of a urinary tract infection.

**Q9** Regarding radiological grading of VUR, which one of the following is not true?

    **A** Grade I refers to reflux of contrast into a dilated ureter.

    **B** Grade II refers to reflux into the renal pelvis and calyces without dilatation.

    **C** Grade III refers to mild/moderate dilatation of the ureter, renal pelvis and calyces.

    **D** Grade IV refers to dilatation of the renal pelvis and calyces with moderate ureteral tortuosity.

    **E** Grade V refers to gross dilatation and tortuosity of the ureter, pelvis and calyces.

**A9**   **A** Grade I refers to reflux of contrast into a non-dilated ureter.

**Q10** Which of the following is *not* a characteristic of the normal anatomical vesicoureteric junction?

    **A** Oblique entry of the ureter into the bladder.

    **B** Length of submucosal ureter.

    **C** A high ratio of ureteric submucosal tunnel length to ureteral diameter.

    **D** A low ratio of ureteric submucosal tunnel length to ureteral diameter.

    **E** Low bladder pressure.

$A$10   **D**   The oblique entry of the ureter into the bladder and the length of submucosal ureter combine to create a high ratio of tunnel length to ureteral diameter. As the bladder fills, the pressure increases thus compressing the ureteral tunnel and aiding in the prevention of retrograde reflux of urine from the bladder into the ureters.

$Q$11   Which of the following is true regarding the incidence of VUR?

**A**   Estimated at 5% in otherwise normal children.

**B**   Estimated at 3% in otherwise normal children.

**C**   Estimated between 30% and 40% in children undergoing investigation for urinary tract infection.

**D**   Estimated between 20% and 30% in children undergoing investigation for urinary tract infection.

**E**   None of the above.

$A$11   **C**   The incidence of VUR is estimated at 1% in otherwise normal children, but rises to 30%–40% in children under investigation for urinary tract infection.

$Q$12   Which of the following is true regarding reflux nephropathy?

**A**   Reflux of urine (sterile or otherwise) causes scarring.

**B**   Asymptomatic bacteriuria can cause scarring.

**C**   Scarring is maximal with second and subsequent urinary tract infections.

**D**   Scarring visible on $^{99m}$Tc-DMSA imaging is more likely a result of infective damage than congenital dysplasia.

**E**   The radiological grade of reflux does not correlate with the degree of renal scarring.

$A$12   **D**   Scarring visible on DMSA is more likely a result of infective damage than congenital dysplasia. The higher the grade of reflux the greater the risk of scarring, and although sterile urine may cause scarring, it is much more commonly a result of reflux of infected urine. Recurrent infections combined with reflux will lead to progressive scarring but one widely held theory states that the greatest degree of scarring occurs with the first episode of infection (Ransley's 'big bang' theory). Asymptomatic bacteriuria in the absence of reflux does not cause scarring.

**Q13** Which one of the following treatment options for urinary tract infection (UTI) is correct?

    **A** Antibiotic prophylaxis should be commenced on all infants under the age of 1 year with first episode.

    **B** Intravenous antibiotics should be used for all infants under the age of 3 months with suspected UTI.

    **C** Children developing a UTI while on prophylaxis should be prescribed therapeutic doses of the same antibiotic.

    **D** Asymptomatic bacteriuria should be treated with antibiotics.

    **E** Antibiotic prophylaxis should be prescribed for all patients with recurrent UTI.

**A13**   **B**   Infants under the age of 3 months with possible urinary tract infection should be treated with intravenous antibiotics in accordance with guidelines on the management of febrile illness in children. Antibiotic prophylaxis should not routinely be started for first-time urinary tract infection. Children on prophylactic antibiotics who develop a urinary tract infection should not be treated with a higher dose of the same antibiotics. Asymptomatic bacteriuria should not be treated with antibiotics. Antibiotic prophylaxis should be considered for all infants and children with recurrent urinary tract infection.

**Q14** Which of the following is true regarding the incidence and inheritance of VUR?

    **A** Offspring of parents with VUR have a 50% incidence of VUR.

    **B** Daughters of parents with VUR have a greater chance of having VUR than male offspring.

    **C** Siblings of children with VUR have a 50% risk of having VUR.

    **D** Siblings of children with VUR have a 15% risk of having VUR.

    **E** Sons of parents with VUR have a greater chance of having VUR than female offspring.

**A14**   **B**   Offspring of parents with VUR have a 66% incidence of also having VUR – higher in female offspring than male offspring. Siblings of children with VUR have a 25%–33% risk of having VUR. The exact mode of inheritance is as yet unclear.

**Q15** Which of the following is *not* associated with VUR?

    **A** neurovesical dysfunction (secondary reflux)

    **B** bladder-outlet obstruction (secondary reflux)

    **C** incompetent vesicoureteric junction

    **D** reduced bladder pressure

    **E** ureterocele

A15 **D** VUR is more commonly associated with a high-pressure bladder, and therefore conditions that give rise to an increased bladder pressure can also potentiate reflux, e.g. neurovesical dysfunction and bladder-outlet obstruction. Primary VUR occurs where there is incompetence of the valve mechanism at the vesicoureteric junction, e.g. inadequate length of submucosal tunnel, or inadequate musculature of submucosal tunnel.

Q16 Regarding VUR, which of the following is true?
  **A** It rarely presents with antenatally diagnosed hydronephrosis.
  **B** It is found in most infants and children presenting with urinary tract infection.
  **C** It may present with advanced reflux nephropathy.
  **D** It is always picked up on antenatal anomaly scans.
  **E** None of the above.

A16 **C** Though rare these days, advanced reflux nephropathy (with signs of hypertension or renal failure) can be the presenting manifestation of VUR. VUR is more commonly found in patients being investigated for antenatal hydronephrosis or in infants or children being investigated for urinary tract infection. The incidence of VUR in normal children is 1%, and this increases to 30%–40% in patients undergoing evaluation for urinary tract infection. Antenatal ultrasounds scans do not see the reflux itself – only the resultant hydronephrosis if present.

Q17 Regarding investigation for VUR which of the following is true?
  **A** Normal $^{99m}$Tc-DMSA isotope scan suggests that clinically significant VUR is not present.
  **B** All children with recurrent urinary tract infection need a MCUG to exclude the presence of VUR.
  **C** $^{99m}$Tc-MAG3 renogram with indirect voiding radioisotope cystography is unhelpful in the diagnosis of VUR.
  **D** MCUG should be performed under general anaesthetic.
  **E** Ultrasound scan is of little value in the investigation of VUR.

A17 **A** A normal DMSA in a child over the age of 2 years suggests that clinically significant VUR is unlikely to be present as scarring is not seen. Under this age scarring may still be in progress and prophylactic antibiotics are likely to be indicated. Asymptomatic children with a sibling affected by VUR need to be investigated and a normal DMSA scan in this situation is a non-invasive method of doing this. Infants and children over the age of 6 months with recurrent urinary tract infections need an ultrasound scan first, then a DMSA. If both are normal, MCUG is not indicated. MCUG should be performed on an awake child using a small catheter and physiological filling rates where possible, to simulate normal conditions. Ultrasound scan of the renal tract is useful in assessing renal parenchymal thickness, size of kidneys and presence/degree of dilatation.

**Q18** Regarding treatment for VUR which of the following is true?

    **A** It is rarely managed non-operatively.

    **B** Antireflux surgery is more beneficial in patients with secondary VUR than primary VUR.

    **C** Indications for surgery include progressive renal injury.

    **D** It is rarely managed operatively.

    **E** Treatment is rarely required as up to 85% of patients with grade I–III VUR will undergo spontaneous resolution.

**A18** **C** Indications for surgery for VUR include progressive renal injury, documented failure of renal growth, breakthrough pyelonephritis, severe VUR, and persistent VUR in a female approaching puberty. VUR is more commonly treated non-operatively and surgery for secondary VUR is less likely to be beneficial and the underlying cause should be investigated and treated fully first. Up to 85% of infants and children with grade I–III VUR will undergo spontaneous resolution, and medical management therefore spares these children the morbidity and risks associated with operative management.

**Q19** Regarding surgical management options for VUR, which of the following is true?

    **A** The Politano–Leadbetter ureteric reimplantation procedure is performed via an extravesical approach.

    **B** The Cohen technique of ureteric reimplantation involves pulling the ureter across the trigone through a submucosal tunnel.

    **C** The aim in ureteric reimplantation is to achieve a length of ureteric submucosal tunnel to ureteric diameter ratio of 1 : 5.

    **D** Endoscopic treatment (STING procedure) is more effective in high-grade reflux.

    **E** Success rates of endoscopic treatment with a bulking agent to the ureteric orifice are around 90%.

**A19** **B** The Cohen technique is performed via an intravesical approach. The aim is to dissect the ureter from its attachments and pull it across the trigone through a submucosal tunnel. The meatus is sutured into a new position at the end of the tunnel. Success rates range from 97% to 99%. The Politano-Leadbetter technique is also performed via an intravesical approach. It involves separating the ureters from their attachments to the bladder muscle and connective tissue and passing them through a new muscular hiatus created higher on the bladder wall. The ureter is then passed through a submucosal tunnel and the orifice sutured to the mucosa at its original meatal position. The idea is to create the necessary 5 : 1 length-to-diameter ratio. Endoscopic treatment with bulking agents such as Deflux (dextranomer/hyaluronic acid copolymer) has gained popularity recently because of low surgical morbidity and preservation of future possibility of open surgical correction. However, success rates are lower: 74% for first injection, 85% after successive injections and success rates are lower for higher-grade reflux.

Q20 Which of the following is *not* associated with persistent VUR in the pregnant female?

A no increased incidence of pre-term spontaneous labour

B an increased incidence of maternal pyelonephritis

C a reduced incidence of maternal pre-eclampsia

D no increased risk of instrumental delivery

E no increased risk of late stillbirth

A20 C Recent surveys in Scandinavia have suggested that the presence of VUR in the pregnant female has little deleterious effect on the outcome of pregnancy. The incidence of pre-eclampsia is similar in women with or without VUR.

Q21 Which of the following is not a useful technique in the management of UTI in children?

A circumcision in the male child

B strict adherence to a continence protocol

C oral intake of cranberry juice

D cycling urinary tract prophylactic antibiotics

E restricting oral fluid intake during the day

A21 E Adherence to a continence protocol, which reinforces the establishment of complete, regular voiding patterns for the child is essential. A 3- to 4-hourly regular voiding pattern should be established. Constipation should be avoided and good volume oral fluid intake should be promoted. The avoidance of bladder irritants (caffeine and so forth) may be of benefit, and oral intake of cranberry juice has been shown to be beneficial in reducing the incidence of urine infection by acidification of the urine. The assessment of the child in the clinic should include the completion of fluid input/output charts, uroflow assessments and the assessment of post-void residual urine volume by ultrasound. Significant residual urine volumes after voiding can be managed by asking the child to utilise double-voiding techniques. Reverse voiding (sitting the opposite way around on the toilet) may be helpful for girls, as it lessens the degree of vaginal reflux of urine. Circumcision can significantly reduce the risk of recurrent UTI in boys who have an abnormal urinary tract.

**Q22** Which of the following is *not* useful in the management of a child with high grade VUR and breakthrough UTI?

**A** clean intermittent urethral catheterisation

**B** cystoscopic injection of 'Deflux' to the bladder neck

**C** cystoscopic injection of 'Deflux' to the submucosal area of the ureteric orifice (STING procedure)

**D** cystoscopic injection of 'Deflux' to the distal ureteric wall under ureteric hydrodistension (HIT procedure)

**E** unilateral loop refluxing ureterostomy

**A22** **B** The STING and HIT procedures are both good at reducing the incidence of VUR in the affected child. It has been reported that HIT has better outcomes, although others have reported similar incidences of persistent VUR with both techniques. The longevity of both techniques in successfully preventing VUR is awaited. Deflux appears to be a safe material to use, and does not migrate, as did Teflon when used in early animal models of VUR. However, whether treating VUR has an impact on subsequent renal scarring developing is controversial. Clean intermittent catheterisation ensures complete bladder emptying and is sometimes valuable in the child with bladder dysfunction – indeed, these children may well have a form of 'secondary' VUR, i.e. the bladder function is the primary pathology. A unilateral loop refluxing ureterostomy may be a valuable option in the septic infant with high-grade VUR, in whom formal operation on the bladder (reimplantation) is to be avoided (under the age of 2 years) for fear of worsening subsequent bladder function.

**Q23** Which of the following is true with regard to the treatment of UTI/VUR in childhood?

**A** The risk of recurrent VUR after operative ureteric reimplantation is >10%.

**B** The STING procedure prevents VUR in >90% boys with grade V VUR.

**C** Prophylactic urinary tract antibiotics reduce the risk of recurrent urinary tract infection.

**D** Prophylactic urinary tract antibiotics reduce the risk of renal scarring.

**E** Assessment of bladder function is clinically important in management of the child.

**A23** **C** Smellie's original work published in the *Lancet* in the 1970s identified a cohort of children in whom prophylactic urinary tract antibiotics reduced the risk of a subsequent UTI following an initial infection. However, subsequent population studies have failed to identify a reduction in the rate of renal scarring with any particular treatment mode (antibiotics, surgical intervention) in a child known to have VUR. Indeed, it has even been voiced that no clinician has ever prevented a new renal scar developing, and that apparent new scars seen on DMSA merely represent differential renal growth in an area of previous scar that becomes more apparent with time. It is vital to ensure normal bladder function in the clinic; formal invasive urodynamic studies may be warranted in a small group of children, although a complete clinical assessment in conjunction with fluid-volume charts and assessment of bladder emptying by ultrasound are extremely valuable, and frequently abrogate the necessity for invasive studies with their attendant morbidity. The failure rate of the ureteric reimplantation is ~1% in reported series. The STING procedure is not that effective in the high-grade refluxing male infant.

 **24** Which of the following is true in an infant with unilateral pyelonephritis?

   **A** $^{99m}$Tc-DMSA isotope scan in the acute period may help to define the 'kidney at risk'.

   **B** Immediate nephrectomy is often necessary.

   **C** Antibiotic therapy should be avoided until urine culture results are available.

   **D** Immediate circumcision should be performed in males.

   **E** None of the above.

A**24** **A** It has been suggested that a $^{99m}$Tc-DMSA scan performed during the acute phase of urine infection could help in identifying the renal moiety at risk for subsequent renal injury. It is suggested by some that an apparently normal $^{99m}$Tc-DMSA scan in the presence of active urine infection excludes the need for MCUG in this group of children. While circumcision and nephrectomy may have a role in subsequent management, they are certainly rarely, if ever, required immediately.

## Further reading

Chertin B, Kocherov S. Long-term results of endoscopic treatment of vesicoureteric reflux with different tissue-augmenting substances. *J Pediatr Urol*. 2010; **6**(3): 251–6.

Craig JC, Simpson JM, Williams GJ, *et al*. Antibiotic prophylaxis and recurrent urinary tract infection in children. *N Engl J Med*. 2009; **361**(18): 1748–59.

Demirbag S, Atabek C, Caliskan B, *et al*. Bladder dysfunction in infants with primary vesicoureteric reflux. *J Int Med Res*. 2009; **37**(6): 1877–81.

Sholtmeijer RJ, Nijman RJ. Vesicoureteric reflux and videourodynamic studies: results of a prospective study after three years of follow-up. *Urology*. 1994; **43**(5): 714–18.

Smellie JM, Poulton A, Prescod NP. Retrospective study of children with renal scarring associated with reflux and urinary infection. *BMJ*. 1994; **308**(6938): 1193–6.

Williams GJ, Sureshkumar P, Wheeler D, *et al*. Paediatrician's responses to an evidence summary about renal tract imaging tests in children after urinary tract infection. *Arch Dis Child*. 2009; **95**(4): 271–5.

# CHAPTER 59

# Urinary incontinence

## ASHOK RAJIMWALE

**From the choices below each question, select the single best answer.**

$Q^1$    Which of the following statement is true?
- A   Children with diurnal urinary incontinence without any anatomical abnormality, are those who have never been potty-trained.
- B   Diurnal incontinence affects nearly 20% children between 4 and 6 years of age.
- C   The infant bladder functions under the influence of supraspinal centres.
- D   It is not possible to estimate bladder capacity in infants or children.
- E   Dysfunctional voiding is a congenital problem.

$A^1$    **B**   Incontinence of urine may be either daytime or nocturnal or both. Patients with diurnal incontinence often begin having symptoms 3–6 months after achieving urinary control.

     In infants, the bladder functions by a simple sacral reflex arc without input from the supraspinal centre. In the absence of an anatomical obstruction, this reflex arc allows the bladder to empty at low pressure without any resistance to urine flow. The adult pattern of urinary control evolves over time and continence is first achieved by voluntary contraction of the external striated sphincter and later by supraspinal inhibition of the voiding reflex. Over time, bladder capacity increases to allow the bladder to function as an adequately sized reservoir. Bladder capacity can be calculated within the first 2 years of life by multiplying the patient's weight in kilograms by 8, while after 2 years of age bladder capacity can be estimated in milliliters using the following equation – age in years + 2 × 30. Most children achieve day- and night-time control by 4 years of age and the sequence of events is as follows: bowel control at night-time followed by bowel control during the daytime, which is followed by urinary control during the day and lastly urinary control at night-time. Daytime incontinence affects approximately 20% of children between the ages of 4 and 6 years and 3% of these children usually wet more than twice per week. As children get older, the incidence of enuresis declines;

however, those children who fail to grow out of these problems require further evaluation and management.

 Which of these statements is *not* true?

A Staccato or fractionated voiding is a learned behaviour leading to incoordination between bladder and external sphincter.

B The consequences of bladder sphincter discoordination are increased bladder wall thickness, large post-void residual urine (PVR) volumes and recurrent urinary tract infection (UTI).

C Urge syndrome is a congenital condition in children.

D Giggle incontinence is an involuntary loss of urine induced by laughter.

E The majority with giggle incontinence have associated dysfunctional voiding symptoms.

 C After the child is potty-trained, daytime incontinence usually begins a few months after achieving control and these children, who are not yet able to inhibit their voiding reflex, try to stay dry by voluntarily contracting their external sphincter during uninhibited bladder contractions. In these children, the persistence of this learned behaviour leads to voiding dysfunction and is due to incoordination between the bladder and external sphincter. These patients often void in staccato or fractionated patterns. Instability of the bladder, increased bladder-wall thickness, high post-void residual volumes and recurrent infections, are often the consequences of this discoordination between bladder and sphincter. Urinary frequency and small voided volumes are mostly secondary to detrusor overactivity that is either primary or secondary. Primary instability (sometimes referred to as urge syndrome) is commonly seen after a viral or bacterial infection. These children experience the urge to void several times per hour and symptoms resolve spontaneously. Secondary urinary incontinence is due to discoordination between bladder and external striated sphincter.

Giggle incontinence (enuresis risoria) is the involuntary loss of urine induced by laughter. It has been documented that in 95% of children with giggle incontinence, dysfunctional voiding symptoms and detrusor instability contribute to the wetting. These children achieved nearly 90% remission rate within 10 weeks of being treated with timed voiding, anticholinergic medication and a bowel management programme. Others have reported success with the use of methylphenidate (Ritalin) for the treatment of giggle incontinence.

Enuresis can be associated with other complex voiding dysfunctions including frequency, urgency, urge-associated incontinence and other lower urinary tract symptoms (LUTS). Additionally some patients may have voiding dysfunction associated with constipation or bowel dysfunction, and they are classed as having dysfunctional elimination syndrome.

**Q3** Which of the following statements regarding dysfunctional elimination syndrome is true?

**A** Lower urinary tract symptoms are never associated with constipation.

**B** Acute bladder instability does not resolve spontaneously.

**C** Treatment of constipation resolves day and night incontinence in most children.

**D** Normally, children void more than 10 times per day.

**E** High post-void residual does not contribute towards UTI.

 **A3** **C** It has been well documented that until proven otherwise, all patients with lower urinary tract dysfunction have constipation. Constipation is defined by passing hard stool, painful defaecation and failure to pass three stools per week. Encopresis or faecal soiling occurs when the child is constipated or avoids defaecation through fear of painful defaecation, and they leak soft stools. When the rectum is full with impacted stool, this can cause bladder instability and impedes bladder filling because of its proximity to the bladder; successful treatment of constipation has been shown to resolve daytime incontinence in up to 89% of children, night-time incontinence in 65%, and resolution of UTI in 100% of patients. Evaluation of dysfunctional elimination syndrome includes taking a detailed history, examination and investigation.

A detailed history of dysfunctional elimination is important and it helps to rule out the most common anatomical or neurological cause of the symptoms. Acute onset of bladder instability often resolves spontaneously shortly after the onset of symptoms and does not require intervention. Dampness is often secondary to patients pulling up their underwear before they have completed the voiding process. These children simply need coaching to encourage spending an extra few minutes to empty their bladder before getting dressed. We urge boys to shake their penis after voiding to prevent dripping of urine and girls are encouraged to spread their legs and to pause an extra moment to allow for emptying of the urine that sometimes pools in the vagina.

The normal frequency of voiding in a child is between 4–7 times per day or approximately every 2–3 hours. Increased frequency of voiding exists if a child is passing more than eight times per day or more frequently than every 1½ hours. Infrequent voiding also contributes to recurrent bladder infections and lower urinary tract symptoms. It is important to take detailed history about the bladder dysfunction and associated UTI. In some cases, the high PVR volume of urine and/or high-pressure voiding with turbulent flow can precipitate a UTI. It is also important to note the flow pattern, whether it is staccato or slow and also whether the child is straining to pass urine to empty their bladder completely. In such cases it is important to rule out any anatomical bladder outlet obstructions such as posterior urethral valves, meatal stenosis or urethral stricture. It is also pertinent to know the fluid consumption over a 24-hour period as both dehydration and overhydration may result in abnormal patterns and occasional wetting. Similarly it is important to know if diurnal incontinence is associated with any lower urinary tract symptoms such as urge incontinence, and to know how the child tries to stay dry – as girls often either squat or sit on their heel on one foot (Vincent's curtsey) or cross their legs, to stay dry or prevent the urge to pass urine.

It has been suggested that a dysfunctional-voiding scoring-system questionnaire is a helpful tool for diagnosing and monitoring the treatment of children with dysfunctional elimination syndrome. The scoring system includes whether they have wet clothes or underwear during the day or at night; how severe is the wetting (soaking or just damp); whether the child crosses his/her legs or squats on their heel to hold their urine; whether they have an urge to void that they cannot resist; whether they have to push to pass urine, or whether is there any dysuria.

The history should include information about bowel habits, such as how often the child has a bowel movement, its consistency, and whether there is any difficulty with defaecation.

**Q4** Which statement is *not* true regarding evaluation of dysfunctional voiding?

A Examination of the abdomen, back and genitalia is not important.

B Inspection of the back includes skin discolouration, dimple, patch of hair and so forth.

C Uroflowmetry is an important tool to diagnose dysfunctional voiding.

D Renal ultrasound is important to identify bladder-wall thickness, dilated ureter and PVR volumes.

E Primary bladder-neck dysfunction (PBND) can lead to diurnal incontinence.

**A4** **A** Examination of the abdomen, genitalia and back is important in children with urinary incontinence. Inspection of the back includes checking for any skin discolouration, dimples, hair patches or subcutaneous lipomas; spinal defects, asymmetry of buttocks or a gluteal cleft may suggest the presence of a neurological disease including sacral agenesis. It is also important to examine the lower extremities including strength, sensation, reflexes and gait and also to note a high-arched foot or hammer toes. Examination of the external genitalia in boys includes checking for meatal stenosis, which may present with LUTS such as urinary hesitancy, incontinence and decreased or deflected urinary stream. In girls, labial synechiae may present with dysuria, dribbling or incontinence and occasionally the vaginal introitus examination may reveal a ureterocele or an ectopic ureteric opening may present with continuous incontinence between normal voiding of urine. Rash on the genital area or the inner thigh may indicate constant exposure of the skin to urine, which may be an indication of an ectopic ureteric opening in girls. It is important to inspect the child's undergarments, as some parents believe that their child is always wet and yet when the child is examined in the clinic, their clothing is dry. This inconsistency of findings may be because of the fact that he/she was going to the toilet several times per day to keep their undergarments dry, which proves to both child and parent, that by going to the bathroom at regular intervals, the child can stay dry.

Urine analysis should be carried out to rule out any UTI, proteinuria or glycosuria. Uroflowmetry is a non-invasive tool to assess voiding disorders in paediatric patients. It measures peak flow rate, average flow rate, volume of urine voided and also assesses the shape of the voiding curve. Children with significant detrusor instability void very small amounts and this can lead to underestimating their true flow rates. When uroflowmetry is combined with pelvic floor EMG tracings, it should show a normal smooth bell-shaped curve in the absence of pelvic floor activity, but a staccato or interrupted voiding curve when they void with simultaneous pelvic floor contractions.

Bladder US is valuable for documenting PVR volumes and bladder-wall thickness, and to identify whether there is any distal ureteric dilatation. When upper tract changes are identified such as hydronephrosis, it should be documented whether there is any change, resolution or improvement between pre-voiding and post-voiding images.

Micturating cystourethrogram (MCUG) is important to detect any vesicoureteric reflux with a UTI or any anatomical cause such as bladder-outlet obstruction due to posterior urethral valves or urethral stricture. Irregular bladder wall, elongated bladder or filling of the posterior urethra on MCUG is a sign of bladder instability. Filling of the posterior urethra while the bladder is overactive is due to simultaneous contraction of the external sphincter and some take it as a typical and a constant sign of bladder instability. Normally pelvic floor relaxation occurs 1–4 seconds prior to the commencement of voluntary detrusor contraction at the time of micturition; urine flow that occurs simultaneously with, or even before, relaxation of the pelvic floor, indicates instability on EMG. Some have even measured the internal diameter of external urethral sphincter on cystogram and found that this is a sensitive predictor of detrusor and sphincter incoordination when the diameter is less than 3 mm.

PBND is a new entity that has received much attention recently. Videourodynamic study shows prolonged opening times (time between bladder contractions and the start of urine flow), incomplete bladder-neck funnelling, prolonged pelvic floor EMG lag time during voiding, and abnormal pressure–flow parameters. These children have high voiding pressures and low flow rates with an obstructive pattern. They also show detrusor instability and a long history of LUTS.

**5** Which of the following statements regarding treatment of diurnal urinary incontinence is *not* true?

**A** Timed voiding and dietary restrictions can alleviate symptoms of urinary incontinence.

**B** Behavioural therapy improves daytime incontinence in up to 60% of cases.

**C** Biofeedback therapy and computer-assisted feedback therapy helps to improve PVR and urinary flow patterns.

**D** Combination therapy including biofeedback and pharmacotherapy has no role in treatment of urinary incontinence.

**E** Peripheral nerve stimulation (sacral, tibial) has been shown to improve LUTS.

**5** **D** The treatment options for children with diurnal urinary incontinence include conservative measures such as timed voiding, behavioural therapy, biofeedback, computer-assisted pelvic-floor-muscle retraining, direct sacral or tibial nerve stimulation, pharmacotherapy including anticholinergics and alpha-1 adrenergic receptor blocking drugs and clean intermittent catheterisation (CIC).

Timed voiding requires a great deal of cooperation from parent, teacher and child, and in addition to timed voiding, the child must spend at least 30–60 seconds voiding and must relax to ensure efficient emptying of their bladder. Girls are advised to pull their pants or skirts down to their ankles and sit with their legs apart to help bladder emptying and avoid vaginal pooling. Timed voiding also plays an important role in curing or preventing diurnal incontinence and patients should be advised to avoid the four Cs (caffeine, chocolate, carbonated drinks and citrus beverages), as they are known to cause urgency and frequency or incontinence. Behavioural therapy has long-term efficacy for simple daytime wetting in up to 60% of patients and improvement in lower urinary tract symptoms, such as frequency and urgency, in up to half of the patients. Biofeedback is an important technique to help children perceive their specific physiologic process of bladder storage and emptying. It teaches the patient how to relax their pelvic floor muscles during voiding thereby improving flow parameters and decreasing PVR volumes. It is important that the patient is both attentive and motivated, as they need to learn how to isolate the pelvic floor muscles while passing urine. Biofeedback therapy is very successful in treating children with voiding dysfunction either used alone or in combination with other treatment modalities; however, it is time-consuming for the clinician and the child and families alike and sometimes this may lead to problems with compliance. In one study, bio feedback made one-third of children dry, half of the children improved, and the remaining 20% had no change after treatment. In a study of computer-assisted pelvic floor muscle retraining, there was over 95% compliance and subjective improvement was seen in 87% of these children with lower urinary tract dysfunction. Computer-assisted pelvic floor muscle retraining may fail if the bladder capacity is less than 60% of the predicted volume or if the patient is non-compliant. However, the efficacy of this treatment can be improved in up to 83% of non-responders by adding anticholinergic medications.

Sacral nerve stimulation has been used to treat refractory lower urinary tract dysfunction in adults, but has fallen into disrepute in children because of its invasive nature. However, there are other methods, which are also invasive, for treating children with diurnal incontinence: by genital, anal, intravesical and percutaneous tibial nerve stimulation. Percutaneous tibial nerve stimulation in children is found to be minimally invasive and has shown an improvement in micturition symptoms, flow rates, PVR volumes and incontinence.

Patients with LUTS sometimes require drug therapy in addition to conservative treatment measures. Medical therapy includes anticholinergics, which act by blocking the muscarinic receptors on the detrusor muscle during bladder filling, and by decreasing the urge to void, they effectively increase the bladder capacity.

Recently, children with voiding dysfunction have been treated with alpha-1 adrenergic receptor blocking agents, which have been shown to improve bladder emptying and reduce the PVR. When combined with biofeedback treatment, 82% of children have significant reduction in PVR and improvement in peak flow rates.

Children who fail to respond to the above forms of treatment should be taught CIC to treat incontinence and reduce PVR and thereby UTI. The last resort is surgical intervention in form of augmentation cystoplasty with catheterisable channel for CIC.

 Which statement is true regarding primary nocturnal enuresis (PNE)?
  A The incidence of bedwetting in children at 5 years of age is 3%–5%.
  B The majority continue to wet their beds during teen years.
  C Monosymptomatic PNE refers to nocturia without lower tract symptoms.
  D PNE does not resolve spontaneously.
  E The prevalence of PNE increases with age.

 C Nocturnal enuresis (NE) is defined as the leakage of urine while sleeping, in children over the age at which bladder control is supposed to be present. The term is usually applicable to children who are 5 years of age or older. Typically children with NE are neither woken up by the urge to void nor by the wetting incident itself. It is initially more common in boys but evens out between the sexes by early adolescence. Its frequency is 15%–20% in 5-year-old children, decreasing to 7% by the age of 10 years. Only 2%–3% of affected children with NE will continue to wet the bed during their late teens and early adulthood if they do not receive active treatment for their condition during childhood. Many of these children will probably have a lifelong problem with NE estimated to affect approximately 0.5%–2% of adults particularly males aged 16–64 years. The term PNE should be used only for children who have never been dry at night or for an uninterrupted period of at least 6 months; secondary NE is a term reserved for patients who have had a previous dry period for at least 6 months. This group of patients are further subdivided into monosymptomatic or non-monosymptomatic NE. Monosymptomatic NE refers to bedwetting in children who lack other urinary symptoms except for nocturia (defined as waking at night to void in patients aged 5 years or older) and who have no previous history of bladder dysfunction. The term non-monosymptomatic NE refers to the presence of other urinary symptoms such as increased or decreased voiding frequency, daytime incontinence, urgency, postmicturition dribble and genital pain. Persisting NE can be associated with abnormal urodynamics. Bedwetting can resolve spontaneously (14%–16% of cases annually), but some cases persist into adulthood.

 **Q7** Which statement is *not* true regarding the psychological impact of PNE?

**A** PNE has a negative effect on a patient's life and is distressing for the whole family.

**B** Boys with PNE have low self-esteem.

**C** Children with PNE are more aggressive in behaviour and have problems with attention.

**D** Children and parents do not worry about PNE at all.

**E** PNE places a financial burden on the family.

 **A7** **D** PNE has a negative effect on a patient's quality of life. Although common, PNE is a misunderstood condition that is often trivialised and is distressing for the whole family. The disorder can be particularly upsetting to the individual, such as feeling cold upon waking in a damp bed, needing to shower or bathe immediately upon waking, needing to regularly change the bedclothes and coping with the smell that permeates the bedroom. The majority of young people are sad and ashamed about their bedwetting and it can be psychologically upsetting. Children with enuresis, especially boys, are susceptible to low self-esteem, particularly when from a lower social economic background. Children whose enuresis has been unsuccessfully treated and children who wet during the daytime are also particularly susceptible to low self-esteem. One survey of children with PNE showed that 65% were unhappy and older children in particular felt humiliated and guilty and experienced a sense of victimisation due to their condition. Children and adolescents may avoid certain social situations such as camping, and trips that require an overnight stay, and at times they also go to great lengths to avoid having friends in their rooms. Children with PNE feel socially isolated and have more attention problems and aggressive behaviour. Children may feel punished by having to wear pull-ups, and sometimes siblings and other family members ridicule them, which may further aggravate the child's poor self-esteem and the nocturnal enuresis. They may also perform less well at school and be less socially competent.

PNE also affects the patient's family. In a population-based analysis of NE it was found that 17% of parents worry a great deal about their child's condition, and 46% worried some or a little. Mothers worry about the emotional impact on the child, the child's social relationships, the smell and the extra washing involved, and the financial burden of NE resulting from the cost of nappies and medical treatment and the expense of washing and drying bedding and clothing.

**Q8** Which of these statements is true regarding aetiology of PNE?

  **A** Environmental factors have no role in the aetiology of PNE.
  **B** Several loci on different genes have been identified in causing PNE.
  **C** A family history of enuresis has no bearing in the causation of PNE.
  **D** The common mode of transmission is autosomal recessive.
  **E** The risk of developing PNE is very low if one or both parents were bedwetters.

**A8**  **B** PNE is a genetically complex disorder; however, environmental factors such as the mother smoking at home, mother's age at the time of the child's birth, and whether the child is the first, second or third born, play a major part in the phenotypical expression of nocturnal enuresis. The risk of childhood enuresis is 40% if one parent, and 70% if both parents, had been enuretic. Earlier studies report that 2% of fathers and nearly a quarter of mothers of children with enuresis were themselves enuretic as children. Based on some studies, the most common mode of transmission is autosomal dominant with high penetrance; approximately 45% of patients with PNE were found to have an autosomal dominant mode of inheritance. The defective genes are found on several different loci – for example, chromosomes 12, 13 and 22 – but no clear genotype–phenotype relationship exists for the disorder.

**Q9** Which statement is *not* true regarding the pathophysiology of PNE?

  **A** Nocturnal polyuria is the principal mechanism of causing PNE.
  **B** High arousal threshold is a factor for PNE.
  **C** Reduced functional bladder capacity can lead to PNE.
  **D** Antidiuretic hormone (ADH) circadian rhythm is normal.
  **E** Hormones such as angiotensin II, aldosterone and atrial natriuretic peptide are implicated in the causation of PNE.

**A⁹**  **D**  There are several pathophysiological mechanisms of PNE such as:
- nocturnal polyuria
- reduced nocturnal functional bladder capacity (FBC)
- high arousal thresholds.

Unusually large urine production at night or nocturnal polyuria is considered one of the principal pathophysiological factors in PNE. Studies have demonstrated abnormalities in the circadian rhythm of antidiuretic hormone secretion in bedwetters. These children usually wet in large quantities soon after going to sleep; however, nocturnal urine production may vary considerably from night to night and urine volume is significantly larger on wet nights compared with dry nights in enuretics. In children under 12 years of age, nocturnal polyuria is defined as nocturnal urine output exceeding 130% of the expected bladder capacity. In children over 12 years of age, the expected bladder capacity is 390 mL and in adults the nocturnal polyuria is defined as a nocturnal urine volume exceeding 20%–30% of the 24-hour urine volume. The nocturnal urine volume excludes the last void prior to sleep but include the first void in the morning. Using desmopressin, response rates of achieving night-time dryness of approximately 7% have been reported. Other factors that may contribute to excessive urine production at night include an increase in nocturnal release of other hormones that regulate solute secretion (for example, angiotensin II, aldosterone and atrial natriuretic peptide), abnormalities of renal function, hypercalciuria, prostaglandin production, aquaporin II dysfunction and sleep apnoea. Nocturnal urine production is approximately 50% of daytime production in early childhood, and children with PNE due to nocturnal polyuria generally have normal functional bladder capacity. These children respond favourably to the treatment with desmopressin (DDAVP).

Enuretic boys are more difficult to arouse from sleep than age-matched controls and this can be secondary to brainstem dysfunction.

Studies have shown that non-enuretic children have a night-time FBC 1.6–2.1 times larger than children with enuresis. Small functional bladder capacity and detrusor overactivity may play an important role in pathophysiology of PNE. Approximately 30% of enuretic patients studied at night with simultaneous sleep EEG and cystometric monitoring showed detrusor instability while sleeping. One study showed that patients with PNE who are refractory to treatment were found to have a small functional bladder capacity. Additionally, up to 70% of adult patients with persistent PNE have been found to have detrusor instability and reduced functional bladder capacity. The incidence of significant anatomical and functional bladder abnormalities is low in primary PNE; however, patients with severe, treatment-resistant enuresis and adults with new-onset NE may have an underlying abnormality that should be thoroughly investigated.

In children with PNE, the normal waking-to-void reaction to bladder distension is absent. In the past this led to the conclusion that enuretics are unusually deep sleepers. However, the majority of studies indicate that sleep patterns are similar between enuretics and controls.

**Q10** Which one of the following statements is true regarding evaluation of PNE?

**A** Keeping a voiding diary is not important.

**B** Underlying voiding dysfunction is not important in PNE evaluation.

**C** Neuropathic causes of bladder dysfunction should be evaluated.

**D** Abdominal examination for palpable bladder and stool is not important in evaluation of PNE.

**E** Genital examination is not necessary.

**A10  C**  A clinical history is important to determine whether the enuresis is primary or secondary. It is important to know whether bedwetting is the result of nocturnal polyuria or is caused by reduction in nocturnal functional bladder capacity. It is also important to rule out an underlying voiding dysfunction by asking questions regarding daytime incontinence, urgency, frequency, infrequent voiding and difficulty in voiding. Despite day-to-day variation, a voiding diary is important for helping to determine the aetiology of PNE, for devising a treatment plan, and for monitoring the response to this treatment. In children with secondary enuresis, the social and psychological history is important such as family situation, school environment and other changes in a child's daily life.

It is important to rule out any anatomical and behavioural causes for enuresis. Significant neurologic signs should be sought such as abnormal gait, spinal deformities, foot abnormalities (including asymmetry or high-arched feet or hammer toes), and evidence of occult spinal dysraphism including sacral dimple, tuft of hair, skin discolouration, lipoma, or asymmetrical buttocks or gluteal clefts. It is also important to assess anal sphincter tone and perineal sensation and reflexes.

The abdomen should be palpated to identify a distended bladder and stools. If the colon is impacted with stool, the possibility of dysfunctional elimination syndrome should be considered. In boys, a genital examination may reveal an abnormal meatus – stenosis, hypospadias or epispadias – and in girls, abnormal female perineum such as the presence of labial adhesions, a urogenital sinus, ectopic ureteral orifice or a hypospadic urethral meatus. For a healthy child with monosymptomatic PNE, laboratory tests are rarely necessary; however, urine analysis and urine culture may be considered to screen for UTI, diabetes mellitus and diabetes insipidus. Ultrasonography examination of the urinary tract or urodynamic evaluation is necessary only when there is suspicion of neurological dysfunction.

Q11 Which statement is *not* true regarding treatment of PNE with alarm?

A A small percentage of children will experience resolution of PNE following simple lifestyle measures.

B The exact mechanism of alarm therapy is not known but it works by negative reinforcement or avoidance.

C Alarm therapy is not successful in treating PNE.

D For lasting benefit, alarm therapy should be continued for some time after resolution of PNE.

E Successful alarm therapy implies no relapse for 2 years following initial success.

A11 C The attitudes, the experiences, and the compliance of parents can have a decisive influence on the success of PNE treatment; therefore, full communication between the PHYSICIAN and family is to be encouraged, to help overcome the problem. It is essential for the physician to explain to parents and the child the importance of regular eating, drinking and voiding throughout the day and the importance of fluid restriction and relaxed bedtime routine in the evening to complement any treatment modality. A very small percentage of children will experience spontaneous resolution of their bedwetting within 8 weeks of following simple lifestyle advice, without further treatment. PNE can have a profound effect on the child's quality of life, therefore early identification and treatment of children with enuresis is important to raise the child's self-esteem, independence and quality of life. When the child gains sufficient maturity and motivation to cooperate, other treatment strategies for PNE can be offered. There are two main approaches to the active treatment of bedwetting: (1) conditioning devices and (2) pharmacological treatment.

Alarm therapy requires a motivated child and family and a significant effort and time. The alarm may not only interrupt the affected child's sleep but also the parents and other siblings. Once the alarm is activated, parents will often need to get out of bed to assist the child in going to the bathroom to finish voiding, change the sheets and pyjamas, and return the child to bed and reset the alarm. Parental fatigue and intolerance may lead to discontinuation or early withdrawal of alarm therapy.

Although highly effective, the exact mechanism by which alarm treatment works is not known. It is thought that the alarm works by negative reinforcement or avoidance. Alarm therapy is successful for bedwetting with initial and long-term success rates of 70%–90% and 50%–70%, respectively. The child should continue to use the alarm for at least 1 month after a period of sustained dryness. Although up to 70% of children may relapse this does not preclude repeated use of the alarm. To define outcomes, the evaluation of the effectiveness of alarm therapy includes (a) initial success means the minimum of 14 consecutive dry nights within 16 weeks of alarm therapy (b) continued success implies no relapse within 6 months of the initial success, and (c) complete success means no relapse within 2 years after initial success; a relapse following alarm therapy is defined by two wet nights in 2 weeks. Predictors of poor response with an enuresis alarm include parental intolerance and annoyance, children with low self-esteem, behavioural problems, lack of motivation, a family history of bedwetting, associated daytime wetting, lack of supervision, inconsistent use, psychiatric disorder in the child and failure to awaken in response to the alarm. Conditioning treatment with an alarm has been shown to provide a lasting response without relapse in approximately 40% of patients, and 45% of children may relapse 6–12 months after initial response to enuresis alarm. Not all children treated with an enuresis alarm have a positive experience to this approach and one analysis showed that 44% of children had a negative opinion of alarms despite successful treatment.

 **12** Which statement is *not* true regarding desmopressin treatment?

    **A** Vasopressin is effective in treating PNE.

    **B** Vasopressin acts on V1 receptors.

    **C** Vasopressin acts on V2 receptors.

    **D** It can cause hyponatraemia and water intoxication.

    **E** Permanent cure is expected in over 75% cases when it is gradually withdrawn.

**A12**   **B**   Three types of pharmacological agents have been evaluated in the treatment of PNE; namely, antidiuretic therapy, antimuscarinics and tricyclic antidepressants.

    Antidiuretic therapy is effective in treating PNE that is secondary to polyuria or nocturia where reducing urine output at night is beneficial. This therapy works by decreasing tubular filtrate in the kidneys and reducing urine production leading to a reduced rate of bladder filling and postponement of voiding. Arginine vasopressin is a polypeptide synthesised in the hypothalamus and stored in the pituitary gland. This polypeptide has an effect on V2 receptors of the collecting ducts and distal tubules to enhance water resorption. It also acts on the V1 receptor, a potent vasopressor. Desmopressin is an analogue of vasopressin and has a half-life of 1.5–3.5 hours. It is commercially available in an oral and intranasal form and the usual dose is 0.2–0.6 mg orally or 10–40 mcg intranasally at bedtime with immediate clinical effects. Fluid intake should be limited when the drug is used. A simple suggestion is to avoid drinking for 2 hours prior to bedtime. The risk of water intoxication should be discussed with parents before initiating desmopressin therapy and fluid intake during the evening meal and before bedtime should be limited, to prevent the occurrence of hyponatraemia. In children who do not respond to treatment with desmopressin, nocturnal hypercalciuria and hypernatriuria should be suspected. Factors that can predict good outcome include, large bladder capacity, fewer wet nights at presentation, enuretic episode occurring in first 2 hours of sleep, family history of NE, and initial good response to the smallest dose of DDAVP.

Patients treated with DDAVP are 4–5 times more likely to achieve dryness than with placebo. Positive response with DDAVP, defined as >50% reduction of wet nights, has been reported in 60%–70% of patients. The Swedish Enuresis Trial (SWEET) evaluated the long-term effect in children aged 6–12 years over a 12-month period showed 69% of children either halved the number of wet nights or were free of PNE. Permanent cure may increase to 75% by gradually discontinuing the drug and positively reinforcing dry nights. DDAVP therapy is also useful in children that have failed alarm therapy.

**Q13** Which statement is true regarding other therapy in PNE treatment?

  **A** Oxybutynin has some role in treatment of NE when associated with daytime incontinence.

  **B** Nearly 30% of non-responders to DDAVP with detrusor overactivity may respond to combined therapy.

  **C** Tricyclic antidepressants have a high success rate in treating PNE.

  **D** Behavioural therapy and acupuncture have a role to play in PNE treatment.

  **E** Low-calcium diet coupled with desmopressin is important in treating children with refractory PNE who excrete excess calcium in urine.

**A13** **C** Antimuscarinic (oxybutynin) therapy acts by decreasing the involuntary bladder contractions and increasing the bladder capacity. Yeung *et al.* has found that 30% or more of children with refractory enuresis have detrusor overactivity and in these children the success rate is between 67% and 90%. Oxybutynin therapy should also be considered in children with day and night wetting and in DDAVP non-responders.

Tricyclic antidepressants (imipramine) act by reducing detrusor overactivity and increasing bladder capacity, and may have an effect on the arousal mechanism (suppress REM sleep) and an antidiuretic action. Treatment provides a lasting response in only 17% of children and is associated with serious and sometimes fatal adverse effects, including psychomotor and cognitive impairment, sedation and cardiotoxicity.

Combined therapy such as DDAVP with alarm therapy, is useful in children where NE is due to lack of arginine vasopressin and poor arousal response, and children with behavioural problems.

Behavioural therapy includes arousal training (waking and toileting in response to alarm's trigger). This normalises voiding, increases their fluid intake and increases their cognitive control over voiding. Dry-bed training uses an enuretic alarm that encourages the child to take responsibility of removing wet sheets and remaking the bed. It also includes two waking schedules to ease arousability from sleep. Alternative therapy includes Chinese or laser acupuncture therapy and is found in some cases to be as effective as DDAVP.

Absorptive hypercalciuria may be responsible for DDAVP treatment resistance; however, these children become responders (80%) once they are treated with low-calcium diet. Abnormalities in aquaporin (AQP2) and hypercalciuria urinary levels correlated with severity of NE.

**Q14** Which statement is true regarding incontinence and functional bladder disorder?

**A** Night-time urinary control is achieved before daytime and 10% may have nocturnal enuresis beyond puberty.

**B** Intermittent voiding and recurrent UTI are uncommon findings in small capacity hypertonic bladder.

**C** Detrusor overactivity is common in children with attention deficit disorder, poor writing abilities, learning difficulties and constipation.

**D** Lazy-bladder syndrome has a small bladder that is non-compliant.

**E** Hinman's syndrome is due to an isolated neurological lesion.

**A14** **C** Urinary incontinence has been defined by the National Children's Society as uncontrolled leakage of urine, which can be continuous or intermittent, occurring during day- or at night-time. Continuous incontinence particularly in girls where there is constant dampness with normal voiding may indicate an ectopic ureter. Diurnal incontinence may be associated with stress activity such as coughing or running or in girls can occur just after voiding due to vaginal trapping of urine.

Girls tend to become toilet trained before boys and daytime continence is achieved before night-time urinary control. Urinary control is rarely achieved prior to 18 months of age and thereafter approximately 20% of children gain control each year for 2½ years of life. By the age of 10 years, approximately 5% of children will have some nocturnal wetting. This diminishes to 2% after puberty. Recent studies have shown that there may be a genetic basis for the development of urinary control. Evaluation of an incontinent child begins with taking a detailed family history of enuresis, details of mother's pregnancy including the presence of maternal insulin dependent diabetes, gestational age of the child, APGAR scores at birth, developmental milestones (fine and gross motor coordination), interaction with other siblings and social settings. The diagnosis of urge incontinence should be considered in boys beyond the age of 5 years if they suffer from urinary urgency. Indications for urodynamics study include suspicion of any neurological condition, diurnal incontinence with no associated pathology, faecal and urinary incontinence at any age, persistent voiding difficulties long after urinary infection has been treated, and recurrent UTI despite continuous antibiotics and bladder trabeculations and/or 'sphincter spasms' on MCUG.

A spectrum of voiding disorders has been identified on urodynamic findings including: a small-capacity bladder, detrusor overactivity, infrequent voider – lazy-bladder syndrome and psychological non-neuropathic bladder (Hinman syndrome).

### Small capacity hypertonic bladder

Inflammation of the bladder wall secondary to recurrent UTIs can cause detrusor irritability. This may be responsible for symptoms such as urgency and increased frequency of urination, staccato or intermittent voiding, nocturia (increased urine production at night) or even enuresis. Children sometimes attempt to hold back urination by tightening or partially/intermittently relaxing their external sphincter during voiding, either because it is painful because of recurrent UTIs or because it is inappropriate to void. This 'stop and start' voiding is a prominent dysfunction in girls leading to recurrent infection, due to 'milk-back' phenomena occurring within the urethra, which cause bacteria to be carried back into the bladder from the meatus.

Investigations include renal ultrasonogram, which is usually normal. MCUG will show thickened and trabeculated bladder wall and varying degrees of dilated urethra during the voiding phase, with narrowing towards the external sphincter. This sign is called 'spinning top deformity'. In boys this can be mistaken for posterior urethral valve, which is due to failure of complete relaxation of external sphincter.

Urodynamic studies can show elevated detrusor pressure during filling associated with uncontrolled urge to void. Bladder contractions are usually sustained but emptying may not always be complete. EMG recording of external sphincter activity may show complex repetitive discharges (pseudomyotonia) or even periodic relaxation of external sphincter during filling, contributing to the sense of urgency or an actual incontinent episode.

Treatment of this condition includes long-term prophylactic antibiotics for recurrent UTIs. Antispasmodic/anticholinergic should be continued for at least 6–9 months. Children should be advised to take showers instead of baths and taught to completely relax when they are voiding so that they have a steady stream of urine. They should also be taught biofeedback techniques to relax their sphincter during voiding in order to empty their bladder completely.

### Detrusor overactivity

Symptoms of detrusor overactivity in children include: daytime urgency and frequency, sudden incontinence, nocturia and/or enuresis, and Vincent's curtsey (a characteristic posturing by these children in an attempt to prevent voiding) is a commonly described behaviour pattern. Other family members often have a history of delayed control over micturition and those affected may have continued daytime frequency or nocturia, or both. Physical examination in these children is usually normal; however, the deep tendon reflexes are sometimes exaggerated, more commonly in lower extremities but also in the upper extremities. Ankle clonus or difficulty with tandem walking, and mirror movements (similar motion in the contralateral hand when the individual is asked rapidly to pronate and supinate on one hand) may be evident. Attention deficit disorder, poor writing abilities and/or incoordination and learning difficulties are more commonly found in these children. Detrusor overactivity can also be found in children who have had cerebral insult, however mild, in the neonatal (or even prenatal) period, but they are linked more commonly to delayed maturation of central pathways and inhibitory centres in the midbrain and cerebral cortex. On occasion, children with intractable profound constipation can develop detrusor overactivity leading to urinary incontinence. The aetiology of this condition is not very well understood but the treatment of constipation has resulted in a dramatic improvement in bladder dysfunction. Sometimes repeated urinary infection may produce symptoms of detrusor overactivity, which can be explained by 'milk-back' phenomena, as these children tighten their external sphincters to avoid any inappropriate voiding or incontinence.

X-ray evaluation is usually normal except for mild trabeculation or a thick-walled bladder on ultrasonography examination. Urodynamic studies may show premature contraction of the bladder and filling capacity may be reached sooner than expected. Sometimes detrusor overactivity may only be demonstrated following a cough or strain or even when the child assumes a different posture.

Treatment includes anticholinergic medication (either alone or in combination such as oxybutynin and tolterodine) and biofeedback training of the bladder using a computer. If there is a history of recurrent infection, the child should be treated with the appropriate antibiotic followed by long-term prophylaxis.

## Infrequent voiding – lazy-bladder syndrome

Most children urinate four or five times per day and defaecate daily or every other day but these children, perhaps due to a fear of strange bathrooms or to a fetish for cleanliness, void infrequently or void just enough to relieve the pressure. The infrequent voiding and incomplete emptying produces an ever-increasing bladder capacity and diminished stimulus to urinate, and the chronically distended bladder is at risk for recurrent UTIs, overflow, and stress incontinence. Ultrasonography investigation is normal, but MCUG shows a larger-than-normal capacity bladder and high residual urinary volumes following micturition. Urodynamic study will demonstrate a very-large-capacity highly compliant bladder with either normal or unsustained detrusor contractions. Urinary flow rate may fluctuate with sudden peaks coinciding with straining, or it may be normal but short-lived secondary to an unsustained detrusor contraction. Treatment of these children involves changing voiding habits, having a rigid schedule of toileting, encouraging children to empty to completion each time they void, and behavioural therapy techniques to encourage compliance. Rarely, intermittent catheterisation is necessary to allow the detrusor muscle to regain its contractility. Antibiotics are required when these children are suffering from recurrent UTIs.

## Psychological non-neuropathic bladder (Hinman's syndrome)

This bladder voiding dysfunction mimics neurogenic bladder. At first it was believed to be caused by an isolated neurological lesion, but it is now thought to be an acquired abnormality. Two explanations have been proposed: (1) that it may be due to persistence of the transitional phase of gaining control in which the child learns to prevent voiding by voluntarily contracting the external urethral sphincter and (2) that it may be the child's normal response to uninhibited contractions of the bladder, the behaviour becoming habitual because of the child's inability to distinguish between voluntary and involuntary voiding, and as a consequence, inappropriate sphincter activity occurs all the time. Observing the family dynamics is important as it has been found that parents especially the father, tend to be domineering, unyielding and intolerant of weaknesses or failures. Divorce and alcoholism are common, and in these families wetting is perceived as immature, defiant or even purposeful behaviour and these children often subjected to punishments. These children are often confused, depressed and tend to withdraw into themselves, which may aggravate the undesirable voiding behaviour by increasing contraction of their sphincter muscles. Hinman's bladder should be diagnosed only when many of the following features are present: day- and night-time wetting, encopresis, constipation and impaction, recurrent UTIs, and parental characteristics as described above. Radiological investigations will show hydronephrosis with or without pyelonephritis, usually a high degree of VUR, a large and trabeculated bladder, increased PVR volume, dilated posterior urethra with narrowing at the external sphincter, and a heavily loaded colon. Urodynamic studies demonstrate a large-capacity bladder with poor compliance, and overactive detrusor with high pressure or ineffective detrusor contractions during voiding. They also show a high resting sphincteric EMG, unsustained sphincter relaxation during voiding and large urinary residual volume.

The treatment of these children should be individualised and can be divided into (1) bladder retraining, (2) medication and (3) bowel regulation programme. ladder retraining includes behavioural modification, double voiding, and biofeedback techniques for sphincteric relaxation, and sometimes even intermittent catheterisation to empty the bladder completely and prevent recurrent episodes of UTI. Medication to treat Hinman's syndrome includes anticholinergics (oxybutynin and tolterodine), antispasmodics (including flavoxate and glycopyrrolate) and medications such as prazocin, diazepam and alpha blockers to relax the external sphincter during voiding. The bowel regulation programme includes stool softeners, stool bulking agents, and laxatives. Enemas and psychotherapy may be an integral part of the rehabilitative process to re-educate both the child and parents in appropriate voiding habits. Punishments should be stopped and a reward system initiated in order to improve the child's self-image and confidence. This comprehensive approach provides the best means to rehabilitate the child as well as to preserve and maintain good renal health in these children.

## Further reading

*Clinical Pediatric Urology.* 4th ed. 2002.

Joseph DB. This month in pediatric urology. *J Urol.* 2010; **183**(2): 414–15.

Yeung CK, Chiu HN, Sit FK. Bladder dysfunction in children with refractory monosymptomatic primary nocturnal enuresis. *J Urol.* 1999; **162**: 1049–54.

## CHAPTER 60

# Neurogenic bladder

## ASHOK RAJIMWALE

**From the choices below each question, select the single best answer.**

 **1** Which of the following statements is true?
- **A** Dysfunctional voiding is not included in bladder dysfunction.
- **B** Assessment of bladder dysfunction should be thorough including detailed history, physical examination and radiological investigations.
- **C** Irritative or obstructive symptoms are not important in evaluation of a child with bladder dysfunction.
- **D** Examination of the back in these children is not necessary.
- **E** MRI of spine is not indicated in children with skin stigmata and asymmetrical gluteal crease with bladder problem.

**A1** **B** Disorders of the bladder can range from the most common problems such as dysfunctional voiding to very complex neuropathic bladder dysfunction.

All children with overt or suspected bladder dysfunction should undergo a thorough evaluation including history and physical examination followed by laboratory tests.

Taking a detailed history is of paramount importance in the workup of children with bladder dysfunction, including prenatal health and complications, birth and development. Evaluation of bladder dysfunction in any child should begin with establishing both day and night voiding symptoms. These can be classified into (1) irritative symptoms such as urgency, urge incontinence, frequency and dysuria, while (2) obstructive symptoms include urinary retention, hesitancy, staccato voiding (starting and stopping), straining to void, and the feeling of incomplete emptying of the bladder. It is important to enquire about bladder and bowel habits and pattern of incontinence. If the child suffers from constipation, it may reflect a form of retentive behaviour as seen in dysfunctional elimination syndrome or neuropathic bowel dysfunction.

The physical examination of a child with bladder dysfunction should include an examination of the abdomen, back, genitalia and lower extremities. While examining the abdomen, it is important to look for any palpable faeces and/ or bladder. Examination of the back is critical and important findings include a hair tuft, naevus overlying the lumbar spine (a sign of abnormal migration of neuroectoderm signifies abnormal lumbosacral spinal cord), a dimple over the lumbosacral spine and asymmetrical gluteal crease (suggests impaired innervation of two groups of gluteal muscles). Reflexes of lower extremities, muscle mass and strength, gait and perineal sensation/tone, gross and fine motor coordination should be included in the physical examination. If the patient has any of these cutaneous findings they should undergo MRI of the lumbosacral spine. They should also have lab tests such as urine analysis, culture, urine specific gravity, serum creatinine level. Children should have X-ray of spine, ultrasonography (US) of urinary tract, micturating cystourethrogram (MCUG), and urodynamics.

**Q2** Which of the following statements is *not* true regarding neurogenic bladder?

**A** Lower urinary tract components such as detrusor muscle, bladder neck and urethra work in unison.

**B** Detrusor function is altered due to loss of elasticity, central nervous system (CNS) lesion or overactivity of detrusor muscle.

**C** Incomplete evacuation of urine may be due to hypoactive or areflexic detrusor or inadequate urethral closure mechanism.

**D** Detrusor myogenic failure is the end result of persistent bladder outflow obstruction.

**E** Neuropathic bladder can result from spinal or supraspinal lesion.

**A2** **A** Bladder dysfunctional disorders can be divided into (1) neuropathic bladder and (2) functional voiding disorders, the latter including (a) small capacity bladder, (b) detrusor overactivity, (c) lazy-bladder syndrome, and d) psychological non-neuropathic bladder (Hinman's syndrome).

Causes for neurogenic bladder can be at the supraspinal, spinal cord or peripheral level. Spinal and supraspinal lesions can be traumatic or secondary to neoplastic, infective, vascular, or degenerative causes. Non-neurogenic causes can be classified into anatomical (such as posterior urethral valves), myopathic, psychological or secondary to endocrine disturbance. Occasionally bladder dysfunction can be seen in conjunction with other neurological lesions such as cerebral palsy.

The function of the bladder is to store urine at low pressure and to empty efficiently at a socially acceptable time. Under normal conditions all portions of lower urinary tract (detrusor, bladder neck and external sphincter mechanism) function as a coordinated unit for adequate storage and efficient evacuation of urine. When a neurological lesion exists these components usually fail to act in unison; therefore, classification is based on dysfunction of a specific area of the vesicourethral unit rather than on a specific aetiology. Alteration in detrusor function or an inadequate urethral closure mechanism may be responsible for problems in urine storage.

The bladder may have increased tone because of loss of detrusor muscle elasticity. Detrusor overactivity may be due to excessive and unopposed sympathetic discharges, or hyperreflexic due to a CNS lesion that prevents normal inhibitory centres from influencing the sacral reflex arc. Incontinence may occur when bladder neck and urethra do not provide adequate resistance or fail to increase the outflow resistance during filling of the bladder.

Incomplete evacuation of the bladder may be due to hypoactive or an areflexic detrusor muscle, secondary to a CNS lesion affecting the parasympathetic efferents. However, detrusor sphincter dyssynergia can also result from a CNS lesion in the pontine micturition centre. Myogenic failure occurs as the detrusor muscle hypertrophies and then decompensates owing to the persistent bladder outflow resistance, which eventually leads to overflow incontinence. In short therefore, it can be divided into two categories:

- Storage
  — Detrusor tone – which can be normal or increased (non-elastic overactive, hyperreflexic) or decreased.
  — Urethral closing mechanism – incompetence of either the bladder neck or external sphincter.
- Evacuation
  — Detrusor contraction – normally active or underactive (areflexic or hypoactive).
  — Urethral closing mechanism (non-synchronous bladder neck or at external sphincter level).

 **Q3** Which of the following statements is true regarding myelodysplasia (spina bifida)?

**A** The incidence of myelodysplasia is increasing.

**B** Folic acid supplementation during pregnancy has no role in preventing spina bifida.

**C** There is 2%–5% chance of myelodysplasia occurring in a family with one child with similar condition.

**D** Myelomeningocele is common over the cervical and thoracic spine area.

**E** Arnold–Chiari's malformation is uncommon with myelodysplasia.

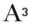 **A3** **C** The most common aetiology of bladder dysfunction in children is abnormal development of the spinal canal and spinal cord.

The incidence of spina bifida is one or two cases per 1000 live births; however, there is a marked geographic variation in the incidence; for example, the highest rates (three to four cases per 1000) occur in parts of the British Isles mainly Ireland and Wales. The prevalence is declining for two reasons including the widespread perinatal supplementation of folic acid (a metabolite important for spinal cord formation) and termination of pregnancy. Dietary supplementation with folic acid can reduce the incidence of myelodysplasia by approximately 50%. In contrast, the incidence in African Americans is 0.1–0.4 per 1000 live births vs. 1 in 1000 live births in the white population. A family with one child with myelodysplasia has a 2%–5% chance of each subsequent sibling suffering from the same condition; however, this risk doubles if more than one family member has a neurospinal dysraphism.

Myelomeningocele accounts for more than 90% of all open spinal dysraphism and most spinal defects occur at the level of the lumbar vertebrae with sacral, thoracic, and cervical areas being affected in decreasing order of frequency. Almost all meningoceles are directed posteriorly but on rare occasions the meningocele may protrude anteriorly, particularly in the sacral areas as a part of Currarino's syndrome. In children with spinal dysraphism 85% of the affected children may have an associated Arnold–Chiari's malformation (herniation of cerebellar tonsils through the foramen magnum) causing obstruction to the fourth ventricle.

The neurological lesion produced by myelodysplasia is quite variable. The bony vertebral level often gives little or no clue to the exact neurological level or deficits it may produce. The bony level and the highest extent of the neurologic lesions may vary from one to three vertebrae and there may be a difference in the function from one body part to the other at the same neurologic levels. In addition 20% of affected children may have a vertebral bony or intraspinal abnormality more cranially from the vertebral defect. Children with thoracic and upper lumbar meningocele (with no myelocele component) often have intact sacral reflex arc and no demonstrable loss of function.

 **Q4** Which of the following statements is true regarding assessment of myelodysplasia in the newborn?

A Detailed assessment in early life is not important, as it is not necessary in management of these children.

B Upper tract dilatation and vesicoureteric reflux (VUR) are rare in neonates with spinal dysraphism.

C The development of new VUR is uncommon with detrusor sphincter dyssynergia.

D Clean intermittent catheterisation (CIC) has no role in the management of myelodysplasia in newborn period.

E Urodynamic evaluation, CIC and anticholinergic medication are not necessary in the management of spina bifida.

**A4**   **B** Assessment includes renal US, voiding cystourethrography and random CIC on multiple occasions to determine whether the child is retaining excess amounts of urine. Approximately 15% of affected neonates will be found by renal US to have an abnormal urinary tract or hydroureteronephrosis secondary to spinal shock from the closure procedure, and less than 5% of children experience a change in their neurologic status as a result of spinal canal closure. Renal fusion anomalies and other upper urinary tract abnormalities found in 10% of children usually denote *in utero* abnormal lower urinary tract function in the form of outlet obstruction.

Vesicouretric reflux is present in only 3%–5% of newborns with myelodysplasia on MCUG. Reflux is usually seen in children with detrusor hyperreflexia or detrusor sphincter dyssynergia. By 5 years of age new VUR can develop in approximately 30%–40% of children with unfavourably high-pressure bladder dynamics if proper treatment is not undertaken.

Children with a mild to moderate degree of reflux (grade 1–3) who void spontaneously or who have complete lesions with little or no outlet resistance require antibiotic prophylaxis to prevent recurrent UTI. When these children have high-grade reflux (grade 4 or 5) intermittent catheterisation is recommended to ensure complete bladder emptying. Children with detrusor hypertonicity with or without hydroureteronephrosis are treated with oxybutynin to reduce intravesical pressure and decompress the upper tract. When managed with these measures, reflux resolves in 30%–55% and renal function remains stable. Credés manoeuvre is to be avoided in children with reflux and reactive external sphincter as it reflexly increases urethral resistance and aggravates the degree of reflux, causing further upper tract dilatation.

A vesicostomy in these children is reserved for (1) infants who have such severe reflux that intermittent catheterisation and anticholinergic medication fail to improve the upper tract drainage and (2) children whose parents cannot adapt to a catheterisation programme. Antireflux surgery can be successful in children with neuropathic bladder dysfunction as long as it is combined with measures to ensure complete bladder emptying.

Parents are taught to carry out CIC three times a day after discharge home if the urine volumes obtained are in excess of predicted capacity for age on random CIC.

Infants who have high outlet obstruction in the form of detrusor sphincter dyssynergy or denervation fibrosis are at increased risk of urinary tract deterioration; therefore these children should be prophylactically treated with CIC. When CIC is commenced in the newborn period, it becomes easy for parents to master and for children to accept, as they grow older. CIC alone or in combination with anticholinergic agents has resulted in only 8%–10% incidence of urinary tract deterioration in children whose detrusor filling pressures are more than 40 cm $H_2O$ and voiding pressures of more than 80–100 cm $H_2O$. Edelstein *et al.* demonstrated that if one aggressively and proactively treats high-risk patients (those with high outlet resistance or detrusor sphincter dyssynergy or hyperreflexic bladder, so called hostile bladder) with CIC and anticholinergic medication, the rate of upper tract injury could be substantially reduced. The incidence of bladder augmentation in these proactively treated children has been substantially reduced to 17% compared with 41% in children followed expectantly (a 2.5-fold reduction).

Urodynamic evaluation should be carried out at 3 months of age. Performing urodynamic studies earlier than 3 months of age is discouraged due to the fact that the spinal shock following spinal closure may last for up to 2 months. Early urodynamic assessment serves two purposes: first, a baseline against which all future urodynamic evaluation can be compared. Changes in the urodynamic profile may the first indication (often before functional changes in the lower extremity) that spinal cord tethering has occurred after myelomeningocele closure and that surgical intervention will be required. This can happen in 3%–5% of cases. The second purpose of urodynamic evaluation is to determine the overall storage characteristic of the bladder, and sphincter function.

Studies in the newborn period have shown that 57% of infants with myelomeningocele display three types of lower urinary tract dynamics including synergy, dyssynergia, with and without detrusor hypertonicity, and complete denervation. Bauer et al. found that 19% of patients will demonstrate synergic voiding, 45% will have dyssynergic voiding and the remaining 36% will suffer from complete denervation. They found that within the first 3 years of life, 71% of newborns with detrusor sphincter dyssynergia had urinary tract deterioration on initial assessment or subsequent studies, whereas only 17% of synergic children and 23% of completely denervated individuals have shown similar changes. Infants in the synergic group who developed upper urinary tract deterioration due to dyssynergic pattern conversion, and infants with complete denervation who showed upper tract changes, elevated levels of urethral resistance were presumably secondary to fibrosis of the skeletal muscle component of the external sphincter. It appears that outlet obstruction is a major contributor to the development of the upper urinary tract deterioration in these children. Bladder tonicity and outlet resistance plays a critical role in bladder compliance. Poor detrusor compliance can cause upper tract changes; therefore, these children may benefit from botulinium toxin injection into the detrusor muscle.

Sequential urodynamic testing on an annual basis commencing in the newborn period and continuing until 5 years of age, provides the means for carefully following these children to detect any signs of changes to the upper tracts.

## Continence

Urinary and faecal continence is becoming increasingly important to deal with at an early age as parents try to mainstream handicapped children. Urinary continence can be initially managed by CIC, and pharmacotherapy to maintain low intravesical pressure if there is a reasonable level of urethral resistance. If urodynamic study showed urethral resistance is inadequate to maintain continence, alpha-sympathomimetic agents can be added to the regime. If medical management fails, endoscopic treatment using bulking agents to increase the bladder outlet resistance, is also used. Faecal continence can be achieved in children by dietary manoeuvres and more recently with antegrade continence enema (ACE) procedure.

### Sexuality

A few studies are available that look critically at sexual function in these patients. In one study it was shown in men that 72% had erections and 66% had ejaculations while a different study revealed that 70% women with minor spinal dysplasia were able to become pregnant and had an uneventful pregnancy and delivery. It is more likely for males to have problems with erectile and ejaculatory function due to frequent neurologic involvement of the sacral spinal cord whereas reproductive function in females, which is under hormonal control, is not affected.

Boys reach puberty at an age similar to that of normal males whereas female breast development and menarche tend to start as much as 2 years earlier – possibly related to pituitary function changes in girls secondary to their hydrocephalus.

 **Q5** Which of the following is true regarding occult spinal dysraphism, and effects of spina bifida?

- **A** Urinary and faecal incontinence is difficult to manage with CIC, drugs and ACE procedure.
- **B** Reproductive function is affected in both males and females with spina bifida.
- **C** Occult spinal dysraphism can be identified by the presence of cutaneous stigmata.
- **D** It is not necessary to investigate children with spina bifida occulta with bladder/bowel problems.
- **E** Abnormal urodynamic findings cannot revert to normal following untethering of the spinal cord.

**A5** **C** Occult dysraphism, which affects the development of the spinal column but does not result in open vertebral canal, occurs in approximately 1 in 4000 live births. The lesions may result in no obvious neurological signs. However many have a cutaneous abnormality overlying the affected part of the spine such as a very small dimple or skin tag or tuft of hair or dermal vascular malformation. Occasionally this may be associated with a very noticeable subcutaneous lipoma. In such cases, on careful inspection one may/may not find high-arched feet or claw/hammer digits. In older children absent perineal sensation and back pain are not uncommon. Lower urinary tract function is abnormal in up to 40% of affected individuals and they may present with urinary incontinence (especially during the pubertal growth spurt) or retention of urine and recurrent urinary infections. These children may or may not present with faecal soiling.

If the child is younger than 4–6 months of age, before the vertebral bones ossify, US may be useful to image the spinal canal as at this age there is good correlation between the US and MRI findings. However, the MRI gives a much better definition of the lesion affecting the spinal cord.

Urodynamic examination in these children is essential, as it will reveal lower urinary tract function abnormality. In approximately one-third of babies younger than 18 months of age, upper motor neurone lesion is the most likely abnormality on urodynamic study, characterised by detrusor hyperreflexia and some form of detrusor sphincter dyssynergia. Lower motor neurone signs are present only in 10% of very young children. However, 92% of children older than 3 years of age who have not been operated upon will have either an upper or lower motor neurone lesion on urodynamic testing.

The reason for this difference in neurologic findings may be related to (1) compression of the cauda equina or sacral nerve roots due to lipoma or lipomeningocele or (2) tension of the cord from tethering secondary to differential growth rates between the bony and neural elements. Under normal circumstances the conus medullaris ends just below the L2 vertebra at birth and proceeds upwards to T12 by adulthood. If the cord does not rise because of tethering or compressive lesions ischaemic injury may occur. Overstretching can also cause injury to the nerve tracts when there is a forcible flexion or extension.

Abnormal urodynamic findings due to tethering of the cord can revert to normal in 60% of babies postoperatively, while improvement may be noted in 30%. The remaining 10% children worsen with time. However, in older children 27% each become normal, improve or stabilise while the remaining 19% worsen with time. Older individuals with hyperreflexia tend to improve whereas those with areflexic bladder do not. Less than 5% of children operated on in early childhood develop secondary tethering when they are observed for several years, which is suggestive of beneficial affects of early surgery.

It is extremely important to follow up these children with both MRI and urodynamic testing, as subsequent tethering can occur in up to 10%–20% of children.

**Q6** Which of the following statements is *not* true regarding sacral agenesis?

    **A** Neurogenic bladder is common when more than two sacral pieces are missing.

    **B** Children with sacral agenesis are more likely to have diabetic mothers than normal children.

    **C** Diagnosis of agenesis is often delayed until attempts at toilet training have failed.

    **D** More than 50% of children with sacral agenesis will have normal bladder function on urodynamic examination.

    **E** Upper and lower motor neurone lesions are found in almost equal numbers of children with sacral agenesis.

**A6**   **D** Sacral agenesis has been defined as absence of part or all of the two or more lower vertebral bodies. Patients with sacral agenesis frequently suffer from neuropathic bladder dysfunction. Aetiology of sacral agenesis is still uncertain; however, insulin dependent mothers have a 1% chance of giving birth to a child with sacral agenesis and 16% of children with sacral agenesis have a diabetic mother. Drug exposure (minoxidil) has also been reported to cause sacral agenesis. Familial cases of sacral agenesis associated with Currarino's syndrome (presacral mass, sacral agenesis and anorectal formation) may have a deletion in chromosome 7, which is responsible for neural plate infolding.

Diagnosis is often delayed as there is little or no orthopaedic deformity in the lower extremities and these children have near-normal sensation. Diagnosis is often made when there are failed attempts at toilet training, which brings the child to the attention of the physicians. High-arched feet and/or claw toes may be present; however, the underlying lesion is often overlooked and in up to 20% of children these lesions are not detected until the age of 3–4 years. Occasionally the only clue is flattened buttocks with a low short gluteal cleft. The lateral film of lower spine mostly confirms the diagnosis. MRI has shown a consistent finding of a sharp cut-off of the conus medullaris opposite T12 vertebra. Urodynamic testing shows that an almost equal number of individuals manifest upper motor neurone lesion (35%) or a lower motor neurone lesion (40%) (atonic areflexic bladder), whereas 25% will have no signs of bladder dysfunction. VUR occurs almost exclusively in children with hyperreflexia with or without dyssynergia.

Management depends on the specific type of neurological dysfunction seen on urodynamic investigation. Anticholinergic agents should be given to those children with an upper motor neurone lesion, and CIC and alpha sympathomimetics may be helpful in individuals with lower motor neurone lesions. When anticholinergic medication is ineffective in controlling detrusor hyperreflexia, intravesical botox may be helpful in severe cases and in some patients augmentation cystoplasty may be required. In children with lower motor neurone lesions who do not respond to alpha sympathomimetic medication, endoscopic injection of bulking agents or even artificial urinary sphincter (AUS) implantation to increase the bladder outlet resistance, is recommended.

 **Q7** Which of the following statements is true regarding neurogenic bladder in anorectal malformation?

**A** Neurogenic bladder is common in this condition because of the anatomy of the malformation and associated spinal cord defects.

**B** Neurogenic bladder in males with high anomaly is uncommon.

**C** Cloacal and non-cloacal female patients have a high incidence of upper motor neurone lesion.

**D** Associated vertebral anomalies and spinal cord tethering have no effects on bladder and bowel functions.

**E** Patients who have a normal number of sacral vertebral segments but a very abnormal short sacrum will be continent for faeces and urine.

 **A7** **A** A neurogenic bladder occurs in a significant number of children who are born with anorectal malformation for two reasons: (1) most cases have the rectum connected to the genitourinary tract through a fistulous communication and repair of this malformation requires a mandatory step to separate the rectum from the genitourinary tract, which can cause damage to these structures or the nerves that innervate them; (2) anorectal malformations can have associated spinal cord defects including hemivertebrae, tethered cord, different degrees of sacral anomalies and myelomeningocele. Neurogenic bladder in anorectal malformation in children can be split into two categories: (1) males with or without spinal cord anomalies and (2) females with anorectal malformations other than cloacal malformations. The repair of anorectal malformation using the posterior sagittal approach, even when performed in a meticulous manner, may have some sort of temporary or permanent affect on the innervation of the bladder. These changes can be demonstrated on urodynamic studies. Evidence is clear that up to 26% of children who suffer from faecal and urinary incontinence have varying degrees of neuropathic bladder. Peña (Levitt and Penã, 2010) believes that this is because of inadequate delineation of the termination of the rectum either at the prostatic urethra or at the bladder neck. This can cause inadvertent injury to nerves over the genitourinary tract when looking for the rectal communication with the bladder neck (through posterior sagittal approach), as the rectum is high up in the abdomen.

Non-cloacal patients with normal spine and cord should not suffer from neurogenic bladder and according to Marc Levitt (Levitt and Peña, 2010) this group may suffer from neurogenic bladder secondary to iatrogenic cause.

Cloacal patients, on the other hand, present a completely different spectrum of problems, which vary according to the length of the common channel. Of babies born with a common channel less than 3 cm long, which is repaired through the posterior sagittal route, only 20% require intermittent catheterisation to empty the bladder. However, when the common channel is longer than 3 cm, 80% of patients require intermittent catheterisation to empty the bladder. However, Peña has found that bladder malfunction seen in patients with cloaca is different from the one seen in spina bifida and meningocele patients. Peña's series have shown that a combination of very efficient bladder neck and hypotonic large bladder may require intermittent catheterisation. On the other hand, babies with cloaca and separate pubic bones (spectrum of cloacal exstrophy) have small bladder and incompetent bladder neck. These children have a different degree of short colon, which is an important factor for the final functional prognosis for bowel control.

Regarding associated spinal cord problems with anorectal malformation, a number of patients with anorectal malformations may have a hemivertebra, but hemivertebra itself has very little negative influence on the final functional prognosis of bowel or bladder control.

Twenty-five per cent of patients with anorectal malformation have tethering of the cord, which can affect bladder and bowel function adversely.

Regarding sacral anomalies, traditionally the sacrum was evaluated by counting the number of the vertebrae and in the past it was proposed that fewer than three sacral vertebrae would result in faecal and urinary incontinence in all children; however, it was observed that many patients who had a normal number of vertebrae but an abnormally short sacrum were incontinent for faeces and urine. Therefore, Peña came up with an idea of sacral ratio and suggested that a sacral ratio of less than 0.4 is likely to be associated with bowel and bladder incontinence.

**8** Which of these statements is true regarding bladder dysfunction in cerebral palsy and spinal trauma?

**A** Bladder control in cerebral palsy children develops in a similar way to that in normal children.

**B** Progressive urinary tract deterioration is common in cerebral palsy.

**C** Spinal cord injury in neonates and children can be iatrogenic or secondary to hyperextension injury.

**D** Sacral cord and upper spinal cord injuries produce upper and lower motor neurone type lesions respectively on urodynamic study.

**E** Identifying a hostile bladder in spinal cord injury is unimportant as it does not cause upper tract deterioration.

A8 **C** Cerebral palsy is due to a hypoxic non-progressive injury occurring in the perinatal period that results in neuromuscular disability. The incidence is approximately 1 in 1000 births; however, it seems to be increasing as smaller premature infants survive in intensive care units. Bladder control in cerebral palsy children is usually delayed,but is similar to that in normal children; diurnal dryness occurs first and nocturnal dryness is achieved in the majority of cases some years later. It has also been found that children with spastic tetraplegia and/or low intellectual capacity achieve continence in 42%–60% of cases, and 92% of those with high mental capacity achieve continence by the age of 8 years.

It has been reported in the literature that 86% will show upper motor neurone type of injury and 11% of children's electromyographic findings suggest an incomplete lower motor neurone sphincter injury. Urodynamic study has shown reduced compliance in 91% of children with cerebral palsy and in 70% of children an increased leak point pressure. Progressive urinary tract deterioration remains uncommon.

The treatment usually centres on abolishing the uninhibited bladder contractions with anticholinergic medication and using intermittent catheterisation for those children who cannot empty their bladders effectively. Selective dorsal sacral rhizotomy has helped with spasticity and incontinence in over 95% of children with only less than 5% children developing incontinence.

Traumatic spinal cord injury affects over 200000 people in the United States with nearly 10000 new injuries annually. Children comprise 2%–5% of all patients with spinal cord injuries. Newborns are particularly prone to hyperextension injuries during a high forceps delivery; infants are more prone to an injury from a motor vehicle accident (71%), and adolescent spinal trauma is usually secondary to a fall or a sport-related injury (48% and 29%, respectively), Spinal cord injury can also occur iatrogenically following surgery to correct scoliosis, kyphosis or other intraspinal problems as well as correction of congenital aortic arch anomalies or even repair of patent ductus arteriosus. Children with neurological injury sometimes may not reveal any bony abnormality on radiological investigations because of the high elasticity of vertebral ligaments. This is called spinal cord injury without radiological abnormality or SCIWORA and can account for up to 38% of spinal cord injuries in children. Spinal cord injury can present temporarily with urinary retention requiring indwelling urinary catheter or intermittent catheterisation. Those children who show no improvement in the urinary tract function after 4–6 weeks should have urodynamic studies to determine whether the condition is the result of spinal shock or as a result of spinal cord injury.

Most traumatic injuries involve either the upper thoracic or cervical spinal cord and some may affect the cauda equina region. The sacral cord injury most likely produces a lower motor neurone deficit of the striated sphincter, which usually leads to low-pressure bladder emptying. On the other hand, upper spinal cord injuries produce an upper motor neurone type of lesion with detrusor hyperreflexia and detrusor sphincter dyssynergia. Even if the child is continent and voiding to completion or requires CIC, it is important to measure detrusor compliance, the presence of detrusor hyperreflexia and actual voiding pressures to rule out a hostile bladder, as this can put the upper tract at risk of hydroureteronephrosis or the development of VUR. Therefore, early identification and the institution of proper management may prevent the effects of bladder outlet obstruction before it becomes permanent.

 **Which statement is *not* true regarding surgical treatment of neurogenic bladder?**

A It is important to achieve nappy-free state as early as possible in life by teaching CIC, and increasing bladder outlet resistance by procedures such as AUS.

B Bladder neck tubularisation procedures are easy to perform with excellent outcome.

C AUS has a higher rate of success in achieving continence when implanted in a virgin bladder neck.

D Seromuscular colocystoplasty has the advantage of reducing mucus production and electrolyte disturbances and reduction in the incidence of postoperative spontaneous perforations.

E Revision of continent catheterisable stoma is less common when appendix is used.

 **B** Urinary incontinence in patients with a neurogenic bladder is often multifactorial. A 1994 survey in the UK found that about 29% had some form of diversion and 62% of those who were not operated on were incontinent of urine and half of these patients had faecal incontinence. The study suggested that non-surgical measures such as CIC and anticholinergics could make only one-third of patients reliably dry. It is therefore important that we address the concept of dryness to these families by discussing the optimum timing of surgery to achieve continence, the chances of continence following surgery, methods to increase the outlet resistance and also ways and means of doing bladder augmentation.

It is important that we achieve nappy-free state at the beginning of primary school. In the past this was delayed until puberty on the assumption that continence will improve with time and that an older child can participate in the choice of treatment. These delays have significant consequences as adolescents are still on nappies; they refuse treatment out of fear and they believe that urinary and faecal incontinence are not important factors that contribute to their social isolation. On the contrary children who grow up dry and clean will not tolerate the need to wear protection and will seek prompt treatment if complications occur. It is therefore, imperative to offer parental counselling on sphincteric control at their first encounter. Ideally this counselling should be shortly after the birth of the child, which will help parents to accept early intervention. Initiation of CIC at an early age is indicated to orient the child and family to this procedure. Over time, intermittent catheterisation becomes integrated into the daily routine both at home and at school. Those children who fail to achieve continence on CIC plus anticholinergic medication, should be given information about the various surgical procedures so that the family can make an informed choice.

Alpha-adrenergic agents may help a few children with a mild degree of incontinence by prolonging the dry interval, but the low efficacy and potential side effects make prolonged use ill-advised. Other surgical methods to increase outlet resistance include slings, AUS and injection of bulking agents to the bladder neck, and bladder neck tubularisation procedures. Injection of bulking agents at the bladder neck have mixed results and in the past it has shown that Teflon-based injection at the bladder neck can adversely affect the subsequent attempts at bladder neck surgery. However, it is not known if the bladder neck or the periurethral injection of Deflux will later compromise the outcome of more effective bladder beck procedures.

Bladder neck tubularisation procedures such as Pippi Salle's or Kropp's onlay procedures are cumbersome to perform, of uncertain outcome and almost invariably require bladder augmentation with ureteral reimplantation and always a continence stoma for catheterisation. These procedures are unreliable in the majority of cases in males and yield no better results than in females with a much simpler procedure such as periurethral sling.

Urethral slings can be effective in females if performed in conjunction with a bladder augmentation. In males, the experience has been mixed. Urethral slings can be in the form of cadaveric fascia lata, autologous rectus fascia or off-the-shelf material such as submucosal intestinal sling. Females with bladder augmentation and sling should also have a catheterisable stoma as it is not uncommon to find difficulty with urethral catheterisation following a sling procedure.

In some centres, AUSs continue to be the first choice of treatment to increase the outlet resistance. Literature suggests that 80% of these AUS devices will continue to function without requiring any revision for up to 10 years after implantation. The chance of infection can be minimised with good preoperative preparation even when it is performed in conjunction with bladder augmentation. AUS can be implanted prior to puberty though some reports have suggested that this can incur major complications. Literature has also suggested that AUS yields the best result when implanted on a virgin bladder neck as this can minimise tissue erosions, infection and revision. On the other hand, when an AUS is used as a salvage procedure after failed bladder neck surgery, the chance of cuff erosion is high.

Whenever the bladder requires augmentation, enterocystoplasty should be performed. Ureterocystoplasty is rarely necessary in this day and age in a well-managed child with neurogenic bladder, as regular surveillance should have prevented ureteral dilatation to a degree required for ureterocystoplasty.

Partial detrusorectomy (auto augmentation) has yielded inconsistent urodynamic improvement and is not widely practised.

Enterocystoplasty with either the ileum or colon can be used depending upon the surgeon's preference. It is advisable not to use an ileocaecal segment in children with neurogenic bowel as it can decrease intestinal transit time due to loss of ileocaecal valve and can make subsequent efforts to achieve faecal continence more difficult. Some centres use sigmoid colon as it is anatomically convenient and achieves a good capacity and compliance. It usually has no nutritional or digestive consequences. Earlier studies suggested a lower incidence of postoperative small-bowel obstruction when the sigmoid colon is used.

Seromuscular colocystoplasty lined with urothelium is another option to produce rewarding results in selected patients. Seromuscular colocystoplasty has the advantage of reducing mucus production and electrolyte disturbances and reduction in the incidence of postoperative spontaneous perforations.

Catheterisable channels are essential in many patients to have urinary and faecal continence. Sometimes it is difficult to use native urethra because of pain, tortuosity or the impossibility of the patients to reach the meatus, as is frequently the case in wheelchair bound females or in obese males. When only one stoma is to be constructed, the preferred site is at the umbilicus, which is totally concealed and sufficiently high in the abdomen to be accessible by wheelchair-bound and obese patients. Revision is less common; in one survey approximately 15% of cases required revision when the appendix was used but the revision rate was higher if non-appendiceal conduits were used. The preferred organ for catheterisable channel is appendix and long appendix to be divided into two channels for bladder and bowel. If the appendix is not available or not long enough for use then the transverse tubularised ileum (Yang–Monti) technique is second choice of catheterisable conduits. The site of implantation of the conduit can be the native bladder or augmented segment. Reimplantation of the conduit into the augmented segment is effective when the colon is used as a simple submucosal tunnel and can be achieved easily.

When urinary continence surgery is undertaken, ACE procedure can be undertaken at the same time as achievement of urinary and faecal continence. The real goal for these operations is to render these patients more independent and the construction and planning for the stoma conduits is best achieved in the same surgical setting.

## Further reading

Bauer SB, Hallett M, Khoshbin S, *et al.* Predictive value of urodynamic evaluation in new-borns with myelodysplasia. *J Am Med Assoc.* 1984; **252**: 650–2.

Edelstein RA, Bauer SB, Kelly MD, *et al.* The long-term urological response of neonates with myelodysplasia treated proactively with intermittent catheterisation and anticholinergic therapy. *J Urol.* 1995; **154**: 1500–4.

Esposito C, Guys JM, Gough D, *et al.*, editors. *Pediatric Neurogenic Bladder Dysfunction: diagnosis, treatment, long-term follow-up.* Berlin: Springer-Verlag; 2006.

Grosfeld JL, O'Neill JA, Fonkalsrud EW, *et al.*, editors. *Pediatric Surgery. Vol 2.* 6th ed. Philadelphia, PA: Mosby; 2006.

Homsy YL, Austin PF. Dysfunctional voiding disorders and nocturnal enuresis. In: Belman AB, King LR, Kramer SA, editors. *Clinical Pediatric Urology.* 4th ed. Florence, KY: Dunitz; 2002. pp. 345–70.

Levitt MA, Peña A. Cloacal malformations: lessons learned from 490 cases. *Semin Pediatr Surg.* 2010. 19: 128–38.

Stringer MD, Oldham KT, Mouriquand PDE, editors. *Pediatric Surgery and Urology: long-term outcomes.* 2nd ed. Cambridge: Cambridge University Press; 2006.

## CHAPTER 61

# Posterior urethral valves

### BRICE ANTAO, GEORGE NINAN

**From the choices below each question, select the single best answer.**

1 Which of the following is true regarding posterior urethral valves (PUVs)?
- **A** Type I valves are non-obstructive.
- **B** Type II valves are most common.
- **C** Type III valves are due to a congenital obstructing posterior urethral membrane (COPUM).
- **D** It is an autosomal dominant disorder.
- **E** The incidence is between 1 in 2000 to 1 in 3000 live births.

A1  **C**  PUVs are the most common congenital anomaly causing bladder outlet obstruction in boys, with an incidence of 1 in 5000 to 1 in 8000 male births. At 5–6 weeks' gestation, the orifice of the mesonephric duct normally migrates from an anterolateral position in the cloaca to Müller's tubercle on the posterior wall of the urogenital sinus. The remnants of the mesonephric duct remain as small distinct paired lateral folds termed plicae colliculi. When the insertion of the mesonephric ducts into the cloaca is anomalous or too anterior, the ducts fuse anteriorly resulting in the formation of abnormal ridges called PUVs. Hugh Hampton Young classified posterior urethral valves into three types: Type I are the most common and present in 95% of cases. They are an obstructing membrane that originates at the verumontanum and travels distally to insert in the anterior proximal membranous urethra with an opening present posteriorly at the verumontanum. Type III valves make up the remaining 5% and appear as a membranous diaphragm with a central aperture at the verumontanum, also described as COPUM. Type II valves are non-obstructive and clinically insignificant prominent longitudinal folds of hypertrophied smooth muscle that radiate cranially from the verumontanum to the posterolateral bladder neck. This condition occurs sporadically without any genetic inheritance.

Q2 On antenatal ultrasonography, PUVs have similar resemblance to which one of the following?

  A  prune belly syndrome
  B  urethral atresia
  C  megacystis–megaureter syndrome
  D  bilateral high-grade vesicourethral reflux
  E  all of the above

A2  E  PUVs make up 10% of prenatally diagnosed obstructive uropathy, and two-thirds of cases of PUV are diagnosed antenatally. Typical findings include bilateral hydroureteronephrosis, a distended bladder, and a dilated prostatic urethra, called a 'keyhole' sign. Prenatally, PUV, prune belly syndrome, urethral atresia, and bilateral high-grade vesicourethral reflux (megacystis–megaureter syndrome) all have similar appearances. The presumptive diagnosis of PUV cannot be confirmed until postpartum radiological studies are performed.

Q3 Which of the following is *not* associated with a poor prognosis for PUV on antenatal ultrasonography?

  A  echogenic kidney
  B  renal cyst
  C  polyhydramnios
  D  increased beta-2 microglobulin
  E  increased fetal urine electrolytes

A3  C  Discrete focal renal cysts in the renal parenchyma are diagnostic of renal dysplasia. Oligohydramnios, and not polyhydramnios is suggestive of significant obstructive uropathy and/or renal dysplasia and is associate with a poor prognosis. Prenatal diagnosis prior to 24 weeks' gestation has been associated with a worse prognosis. Normally fetal urine is hypotonic, with sodium level <100 mEq/L, chloride level <90 mEq/L and osmolality <210 mOsm/L. Elevated fetal urine electrolytes and beta-2 microglobulin levels are an indication of irreversible renal dysfunction. Likewise, bright echogenic kidneys in suspected cases of PUV, are suggestive of renal dysplasia and associated with a poorer prognosis.

Q4 Which of the following is true regarding fetal intervention in PUV?

  A  It is indicated in cases with polyhydramnios.
  B  It is indicated in cases with hypotonic fetal urine.
  C  It is associated with 5% procedure-related fetal loss.
  D  Early fetal intervention improves bladder and renal function.
  E  It is performed in fetuses >32 weeks' gestation.

**A4** **C** In suspected cases of PUV, fetal intervention is indicated if the fetal urine is hypotonic and associated with oligohydramnios, with the goal of preventing life-threatening pulmonary hypoplasia. In fetuses with gestational age >32 weeks, early delivery is advisable, while in fetuses<32 weeks' gestation, vesicoamniotic shunts can be used. Other fetal interventions which have been performed include *in utero* cutaneous vesicostomy or ureterostomy and percutaneous *in utero* endoscopic ablation of PUV. Vesicoamniotic shunt, which is the most common fetal intervention in suspected cases of PUV, is associated with a 5% procedure-related rate of fetal loss and can be obstructed or displaced in 25% of cases. Currently, no evidence exists that drainage of fetal bladder obstructed by PUV will improve renal or bladder function. In an attempt to answer question 4, a multicentre randomised control study (PLUTO – Percutaneous shunting in Lower Urinary Tract Obstruction) is being conducted by the Birmingham Clinical Trials Unit, UK. Their primary goal is to determine if intrauterine vesicoamniotic shunting for fetal bladder outflow obstruction, compared with conservative, non-interventional care improves prenatal and perinatal mortality and renal function.

**Q5** The clinical presentation of PUV includes which of the following?

 **A** respiratory distress

 **B** ascites

 **C** urosepsis

 **D** abdominal mass

 **E** all of the above

 **A5** **E** Two-thirds of cases of PUV are diagnosed antenatally. Those that are not may present postnatally with delayed voiding or a poor urinary stream. Severe cases can present with respiratory distress secondary to pulmonary hypoplasia. Other common presentations include a palpable abdominal mass, failure to thrive, lethargy, poor feeding, urosepsis and urinary ascites. Infants can present with urinary tract infections. Older boys may have persistent diurnal incontinence or abdominal distension as their only manifestation.

**Q6** Posterior urethral valves can be reliably diagnosed with which of the following techniques?

 **A** antenatal ultrasonography

 **B** postnatal ultrasonography

 **C** micturating cystourethrogram

 **D** technetium-99m ($^{99m}$Tc)-labelled dimercaptosuccinic acid scan ($^{99m}$Tc-DMSA)

 **E** all of the above

**A6**   **C**   The diagnosis of PUV is suspected *in utero* when a male fetus is seen with bilateral hydroureteronephrosis and a thick-walled bladder that does not empty. Typical findings include bilateral hydroureteronephrosis, a distended bladder, and a dilated prostatic urethra, called a 'keyhole' sign. However, other causes of lower urinary tract obstruction such as urethral atresia, prune belly syndrome and megacystis–megaureter syndrome may have similar appearances on antenatal ultrasonography. Postnatal ultrasonography may demonstrate a thick-walled bladder with a dilated prostatic urethra, which is pathognomonic for PUV. However a micturating cystourethrogram (MCUG) remains the only radiographic study that definitively establishes the diagnosis of PUV. The valves appear as a sharply defined perpendicular or oblique lucency in the distal prostatic urethra. The posterior urethra is dilated and elongated and has the appearance of a shield. The bladder is trabeculated with a prominent bladder neck. Renal nuclear scintigraphy with $^{99m}$Tc-labelled dimercaptosuccinic acid ($^{99m}$Tc-DMSA) or mercaptoacetyltriglycine ($^{99m}$Tc-MAG3) scan is useful in demonstrating baseline differential renal function, but not for the diagnosis of PUV. Likewise, contrast-enhanced magnetic resonance urography can provide a good assessment of differential renal function.

**Q7**   Which of the following is *not* a favourable postnatal factor for PUV?
  **A**   VURD syndrome
  **B**   bilateral hydronephrosis
  **C**   urinary ascites
  **D**   perinephric urinoma
  **E**   bladder diverticulum

**A7**   **B**   The prognosis for satisfactory renal function may be predicted from several factors. A serum creatinine concentration of less than 0.8 mg/dL one month after initial treatment or at one year of age is associated with favourable renal function. Other favourable factors are visualisation of corticomedullary junction on renal ultrasonography, normal appearance of contralateral kidney, absence of reflux on initial MCUG, diurnal continence by age of 5 years and presence of pop-off phenomenon. These pop-off mechanisms include massive reflux into a non-functioning kidney (VURD syndrome: valves, unilateral reflux, dysplasia), urinary leak (urinary ascites or urinoma) and large bladder diverticulum. The pop-off mechanism acts to protect the other normal kidney by dissipating the high intravesical pressure.

Q8   The initial management of suspected cases of PUV is:
   **A** decompression of urinary tract with feeding tube
   **B** decompression of urinary tract with a Foley catheter
   **C** serum creatinine levels measured at birth
   **D** endoscopic valve ablation
   **E** cutaneous pyelostomy.

A8   **A**   The initial management of neonates with suspected PUV is to decompress the urinary tract with a 5 or 8Fr feeding tube passed transurethrally. At times the catheter is difficult to pass because of significant dilatation of the prostatic urethra and hypertrophy of the bladder neck. If there is difficulty in passing the feeding tube transurethrally, either a suprapubic route or a vesicostomy can be performed. A Foley catheter should be avoided because the inflated balloon can obstruct the ureteral orifices when the thick-walled bladder is decompressed. Prophylactic antibiotics should be commenced. The next step is to assess the renal tract with renal ultrasonography and to confirm the diagnosis with an MCUG. The renal function and electrolytes should be carefully monitored and patients adequately resuscitated before definitive valve ablation is done. The serum creatinine concentration at birth reflects maternal renal function. A vesicostomy is also an option in premature neonates, as the urethra may be too small to accept a standard cystoscope (8 or 9Fr). Although a small cystoscope (6.9Fr) can be used, the visualisation of PUV may be suboptimal. Once the bladder is decompressed with a vesicostomy these neonates can have the valves incised when they are big enough to accept 8 or 9Fr cystoscope. The valves can be incised with a Bugbee electrode, resectoscope or using neodymium : yttrium-aluminium-garnet (YAG) laser at the 5 and 7 o'clock positions. Some surgeons also like to incise the valves at the 12 o'clock position, where the valves fuse. Other temporary diversion procedures like cutaneous pyelostomy or ureterostomy can also be used. Circumcision is commonly performed as well to reduce the risk of urinary tract infection.

Q9   The aetiopathogenesis for urinary incontinence in boys with PUV is:
   **A** poor compliance of bladder
   **B** overflow incontinence
   **C** diabetes insipidus
   **D** incomplete valve ablation
   **E** all of the above.

A9   **E**   About 50% of boys with PUV have ongoing daytime incontinence into late childhood. In a small proportion of patients this could be secondary to injury to the bladder neck during valve ablation. In most other cases, urinary incontinence in boys with PUV is related to the following potential causes.

- Detrusor abnormalities such as an overactive bladder, overflow incontinence, poor compliance and myogenic failure.
- High-pressure voiding secondary to incomplete valve ablation.
- Detrusor sphincter dyssynergia.
- Polyuria secondary to a concentrating defect as a result of renal tubular damage.
- Valve bladder: this is a bladder with poor compliance resulting from fibrosis secondary to long-standing obstruction. The obstructed renal tract develops an irreversible urinary concentrating defect secondary to renal tubular damage. This polyuria causes decompensation of the bladder, incontinence, and persistent backpressure on the upper urinary tracts, with persistent hydroureteronephrosis.

**Q10** The management of bladder dysfunction due to PUV includes all of the following *except*:

- **A** timed voiding
- **B** overnight bladder drainage
- **C** intermittent catheterisation
- **D** antidiuretic hormone
- **E** anticholinergics.

**A10** **D** Close follow-up is important in PUV after valve ablation, ideally under the joint care of a paediatric surgeon and a nephrologist as a third of them can end up with end-stage renal failure. In patients with bladder dysfunction after valve ablation, an MCUG should be performed to document that bladder outlet obstruction has been relieved. The polyuria seen in cases of PUV is due to renal tubular damage, and is unresponsive to vasopressin. These cases may benefit from timed voiding, double or triple voiding. Urodynamics should be performed to assess bladder function. If detrusor instability is demonstrated, anticholinergics might be beneficial. If bladder hypocontractility is present, clean intermittent catheterisation is necessary. This is usually difficult as these patients have a sensate urethra. Such cases may need Mitrofanoff's procedure to allow intermittent catheterisation. In valve bladder syndrome, it has been shown that overnight bladder drainage results in significant improvement in hydroureteronephrosis and improved voiding dynamics during the day. If urodynamics demonstrate a poorly compliant or small-capacity bladder, augmentation cystoplasty is indicated. If a dilated ureter is present, ureterocystoplasty is a good option, and can be done in conjunction with removal of a non-functioning kidney.

**Q11** Which of the following is true regarding the long-term outcome of PUV?

**A** End-stage renal failure develops in 30%–40% of cases.

**B** Vesicoureteric reflux is present in 50% of boys with PUV.

**C** It can cause infertility in men.

**D** It is associated with a higher incidence of cryptorchidism compared with the general population.

**E** All of the above.

**A11** **E** The prognosis for boys with PUV depends on the status of the kidneys and bladder at the time of diagnosis, and subsequent bladder management. In 30%–40% of cases end-stage renal disease or chronic renal failure develops. Vesicoureteral reflux is present in approximately 50% of boys, often bilaterally. Infertility in cases of PUV is related to a number of factors. It is postulated that prostate function might be affected because of elevated urethral pressure during embryonic development and ongoing voiding dysfunction. Also cryptorchidism is present in 13% of PUV cases, 5% of which are bilateral, in contrast with the general population where the incidence is 0.7%–0.8% and 10% bilaterally. This in itself, or as a result of orchidopexy, could be a cause of infertility.

**Q12** Which of the following is true regarding anterior urethral valves?

**A** Their incidence is similar to PUVs.

**B** They are more common in the bulbar urethra.

**C** They can be treated conservatively.

**D** They have minimal impact on the urinary tract compared with PUVs.

**E** They share a common aetiology with PUVs.

**A12** **B** Anterior urethral valves are rare anomalies, occurring 7–8 times less frequently than PUVs, but their overall presentation and consequences are just as devastating as PUV. These lesions can occur anywhere in the anterior urethra, with a slight predominance in the bulbar urethra. The valve mechanism is usually formed by an associated diverticulum; isolated valves formed by cusps or iris-like diaphragms have also been reported. The diverticulum has been postulated to arise from incomplete formation of the ventral corpus spongiosum, an incomplete urethral duplication, or a congenital cystic dilatation of a periurethral gland. However, these lesions are embryologically distinct from the much more common PUV and occur distal to the urinary sphincter. The diagnosis is made with a micturating cystourethrogram and the valves are treated by endoscopic incision.

## Further reading

Elder J, Shapiro E. Posterior urethral valves. In: Holcomb GW, Murphy JP. *Aschraft's Pediatric Surgery*. 5th ed. Philadelphia, PA: Elsevier; 2010. pp. 744–54.

Koff SA, Mutabagani KH, Jayanthi VR. The valve bladder syndrome: pathophysiology and treatment with nocturnal bladder emptying. *J Urol*. 2002; **167**(1): 291–7.

Morris RK, Kilby MD. An overview of the literature on congenital lower urinary tract obstruction and introduction to the PLUTO trial: percutaneous shunting in lower urinary tract obstruction. *Aust N Z J Obstet Gynaecol*. 2009; **49**(1): 6–10.

# CHAPTER 62

# Hypospadias

## ASHOK RAJIMWALE

**From the choices below each question, select the single best answer.**

**1** Which of the following is true regarding hypospadias?

   **A** Hypospadias is an uncommon congenital anomaly in boys.

   **B** Caucasian mothers appear to be at a higher risk of having offspring with hypospadias than non-Caucasian mothers.

   **c** Hypospadias is uncommon in babies whose birthweight is low.

   **D** Hypospadias has not been found to be associated with twin birth.

   **E** Maternal vegetarian diet has not been found to be associated with higher incidence of occurrence of hypospadias.

**A1**   **B** The word ' hypospadias' is derived from Greek 'hypo' meaning 'under', and 'spadon', meaning rent or fissure. Hypospadias is one of the most common congenital anomalies found in up to 1 : 200 boys. The urethral meatus in hypospadias is found proximal to its normal glanular position to anywhere along the penile shaft, scrotum or even perineum.

   Eighty per cent of hypospadias is minor, involving glanular and penile hypospadias forms, whereas only 20% are classified as scrotal or perineal. These latter forms frequently occur in association with other genital anomalies such as micropenis, bifid scrotum, penoscrotal transposition, cryptorchidism, partial or complete androgen insensitivity syndrome and may also occur in association with malformations of other organs.

   Caucasian mothers appear to be at a higher risk of having offspring with hypospadias than non-Caucasian mothers. Low birthweight, small head circumference and birth length are also associated with an increased risk of hypospadias. It has been found that low maternal age, low parity, gravidity and also mothers over 35 years of age with low parity are associated with a higher risk of hypospadias, and studies have shown that late menarche or previous stillbirth are also risk factors. Several studies have shown an increased risk of hypospadias after *in vitro* fertilisation, particularly when intracytoplasmic sperm injection is used. Hypospadias is nearly 10 times more frequent when the placenta weight is lower than normal. Pre-eclampsia is associated with an increased risk of hypospadias and this could be the cause of placental growth retardation.

Hypospadias has long been found to be associated with twin birth. The incidence of hypospadias in male/male pairs is nearly twice that of male/female pairs. Hypospadias is more common in the first born and inversely related to the maternal parity. Maternal ill health has also been implicated as a cause of hypospadias, including maternal diabetes, epilepsy, renal failure, asthma and influenza during the first trimester. Maternal vegetarian diet has also been found to be associated with hypospadias, possibly due to an increased amount of phyto-oestrogens.

**Q2** Which of the following statement is not true about hypospadias?

   **A** Idiopathic hypospadias is *not* caused by multiple factors.

   **B** Isolated hypospadias of unknown cause accounts for 70% of all cases and chromosomal causes account for the remaining 30% of cases.

   **C** In approximately10% of cases first- or second-degree relatives are affected.

   **D** The risk of hypospadias in subsequent siblings is about 15%.

   **E** The risk is higher in subsequent siblings if the hypospadias is of severe degree in index patient.

**A2**   **A** Isolated hypospadias of unknown cause accounts for 70% of all cases whereas monogenic or chromosomal causes account for remaining 30% of cases.

One or more first-, second- or third-degree relatives affected with hypospadias, is seen in about 10% of cases. The risk of hypospadias in subsequent siblings of affected patients is about 15%, whereas 7% of fathers of a child with hypospadias are also affected. It has also been found that the more severe the malformation of the index patient, the higher the risk of hypospadias in subsequent male siblings.

It is widely accepted that idiopathic hypospadias is caused by multiple factors whereby the cumulative effects of minor genes and environmental factors result in the malformation. Genetic factors play an important role in the occurrence of hypospadias in either non-syndromic or syndromic forms.

**Q3** Which of the following is *not* true about genetics causing hypospadias?

**A** Autosomal dominant forms of syndromic hypospadias are caused by mutations in genes involved in early genital development.

**B** The recessive form is caused by mutation in the genes affecting the actions and metabolism of androgens.

**C** Early atrophy of the Leydig cells of the fetal testes does not cause hypospadias.

**D** Chromosomal anomalies are found in about 7% of children with hypospadias.

**E** Mutations in androgen receptor (AR) gene can cause severe forms of hypospadias.

 **A3** **C** Gender is genetically determined at conception. The urogenital sinus is formed at the sixth week of gestation and the whole process of sex differentiation, which involves tubularisation of the urogenital sinus, is completed by week 16.

Early genital development is controlled by the genetic programme operating prior to the production of steroid hormones, whereas the second phase of penile development requires exposure to an androgen, either testosterone or dihydrotestosterone. Testosterone is synthesised by Leydig cells of the testes and is first seen just prior to the second phase of penile development. Hypospadias probably results from factors such as abnormal androgen production by the fetal testes, altered sensitivity to androgen in the developing genitalia, or secondary to early atrophy of the Leydig cells of the testes.

Autosomal dominant forms of syndromic hypospadias are caused by mutations in the genes involved in early genital development, whereas the recessive form is caused by mutations in genes affecting the actions and metabolism of androgens such as mutations of the 5-alpha reductase gene (*SRD5A2*). Mutations in the AR gene have also been found in patients with penoscrotal or perineal hypospadias and hypospadias associated with cryptorchidism, micropenis, and partial and complete androgen insensitivity syndromes.

Nearly 198 syndromes have been identified with hypospadias, and about 7% of patients with hypospadias have chromosomal anomalies of widely varying type including Klinefelter's syndrome and mixed gonadal dysgenesis. Autosomal abnormalities, such as translocations, deletions (Wilms's tumour, aniridia, genitourinary anomalies, and mental retardation (WAGR) syndrome, *WT1* gene, chromosome 11p13), or duplications have also been associated with syndromic hypospadias.

Sonic hedgehog gene (Shh) is expressed in the endodermal epithelium of the developing urethral plate, which is essential for outgrowth and patterning of the genital tubercle. It has been found that targeted deletion of Shh gene in mice results in penile and clitoral agenesis.

Q4 Which of the following is *not* true regarding endocrine factors, actions of proteins, or environmental factors, contributing to hypospadias?

A Endocrine factors causing hypospadias include disorders of Leydig cell differentiation or androgen biosynthesis.

B Hypospadias may be due to defects in dihydrotestosterone synthesis and its action.

C The fine balance between structuring proteins (growth factors) and de-structuring proteins (proteases) is not necessary for penile development.

D Environmental pollutants have both oestrogenic and antiandrogenic action.

E Environmental factors compete with natural androgens for the ligand binding domain of the AR and cause hypospadias.

A4 C **Endocrine causes of hypospadias**

Endocrine causes of hypospadias may be secondary to either (1) disorders of testes development, subsequent to Leydig cell differentiation; (2) disorders of androgen biosynthesis; (3) defects in dihydrotestosterone synthesis and its action; or (4) an intrinsic defect in phallic growth.

a) Complete gonadal dysgenesis (Swyer's syndrome) is characterised by severe abnormalities of testes development with marked under-androgenisation and persistent müllerian structures due to reduced müllerian inhibiting substance secretions from Sertoli cells of the testes. However, partial forms of gonadal dysgenesis with regression of müllerian structures (e.g. uterus) are associated with various degrees of testicular descent and genital ambiguity/hypospadias. The milder mutations affecting testes-developing or promoting factors – such as the Wilms's tumour 1 (*WT1*) gene and steroidogenic factor 1 (*SF1*) gene – can present with various degrees of hypospadias.

b) Partial loss of luteinising-hormone-receptor function, which is secondary to Leydig cell hypoplasia, has been found to be associated with hypospadias or even micropenis. It has also been found that defects in steroidogenic protein such as CYP11E, p450 and 3β-hydroxysteroid dehydrogenase deficiency can cause salt-losing adrenal insufficiency and under-androgenisation and hypospadias. It has also been found that combined 17α-hydroxylase/17,20-lyase deficiency can present with varying degrees of hypospadias or micropenis associated with hypertension or skeletal abnormalities.

c) Complete or partial androgen insensitivity syndrome can occur with 5α-reductase gene polymorphism, causing defects in the androgen receptor leading to various forms of hypospadias.

## Proteins and hypospadias

Several types of proteins including transcription factors, growth factors and their receptors, apoptotic and antiapoptotic factors, and proteases are found to be essential in penile development.

There is a fine balance between structuring proteins (such as growth factors, antiproteases, transcription factors, tight-junction proteins and so forth) and de-structuring proteins such as proteases, and apoptotic factors in penile development.

Failure of this protein balance could lead to hypospadias.

Transcription factors (homeobox proteins) are expressed along the axis of the urogenital tract. These homeobox proteins are essential for normal expression of fibroblast growth factor (FGF) in the genital tubercle and essential for penile development. Defects in this FGF expression can lead to hypospadias.

Growth factors such as epidermal growth factor (EGF) along with FGF play an important role in genital development. Androgen receptor mediates the role of EGF in male differentiation, and deficiency of these growth factors could lead to variable forms of hypospadias.

Proteases and antiproteases are regulators of differentiation, remodelling, apoptosis and wound healing, and are expressed in reproductive organs. Increased metallo-protease (MMT) activities have been found on the ventral aspects of a hypospadiac penis compared with the preputial hood of the same patient, suggesting that an excess of MMTs can induce an excessive tissue loss leading to hypospadias.

## Environmental factors

There is a long list of substances found in the environment that may potentially interfere with male genital development because of their similarity with hormones. These substances are contained in herbicides, fungicides, insecticides and industrial by-products or end-products. They enter the body either by ingestion, inhalation, and absorption, or maybe conveyed through the placenta. They are also found in breast milk and the amniotic fluid. As most of these chemicals use the same pathways as natural hormones, they are known as xeno-oestrogens or environmental disrupting chemicals. These xeno-oestrogens have both oestrogenic and antiandrogenic action, and they compete with natural androgens for the ligand binding domain of the AR. Because of this competition the conformation of ligand binding domain is changed. The nuclear transfer of AR is also altered, leading to the alteration of the transcriptional factors and expression of androgen-specific genes causing endocrine dysfunction leading to hypospadias.

**Q5** Which of the following is true regarding testicular dysgenetic syndrome (TDS) and hypospadias?

   **A** TDS does not include poor semen quality, testicular cancer or cryptorchidism.

   **B** TDS includes abnormal development of germ cells, Leydig cells and Sertoli cells.

   **C** Leydig cell dysfunction does not cause androgen deficiency in TDS.

   **D** Sertoli cell dysfunction in testicular maldescent can lead to testicular cancer.

   **E** Germ cell dysfunction in TDS can cause poor semen quality.

**A5**   **B** The term testicular dysgenesis includes reproductive problems such as low semen quality, testicular cancer and cryptorchidism along with hypospadias. These disorders are believed to be secondary to abnormal pre- and perinatal development of the testes, involving germ cells, Sertoli cells and Leydig cells, caused by environmental factors such as xeno-oestrogens. When there is Leydig cell dysfunction this can lead to androgen insufficiency causing hypospadias and testicular maldescent, and also impaired germ-cell differentiation, whereas Sertoli cell dysfunction can lead to poor semen quality and to testicular cancer. The exact role of genetic mutation and environmental factors (endocrine disrupters for the development of TDS and hypospadias) is not known; however, in the last few decades environmental factors have been found to play an important role in TDS and hypospadias association.

**Q6** Regarding the initial evaluation of hypospadias, which of the following is *not* true?

   **A** Distal hypospadias (85% of cases) does not require any investigation.

   **B** Twenty per cent of cases of distal hypospadias may have testicular dysfunction or end-organ dysfunction.

   **C** Hormonal or genetic workup is not necessary in posterior hypospadias associated with cryptorchidism.

   **D** Preoperative hormonal stimulation does not influence the result of hypospadias.

   **E** The only accepted treatment testosteronein 5α-reductase deficiency is local treatment with dihydrotestosterone cream.

**A6**   **C** Most hypospadias is of mild degree (almost 85%) with the meatus at the distal shaft or in the glans. Therefore, such children do not require any preoperative evaluation. But hormonal and genetic workup should be performed in cases of posterior hypospadias associated with cryptorchidism when one or both testes are undescended, to evaluate testicular function and also to define the type of disorder of sexual differentiation. This work should be performed during the neonatal period, especially when the gender identity is in doubt. The routine workup for isolated posterior hypospadias is still questionable although we are aware that approximately 20% of such children may have either testicular dysfunction or anomalies of the end organ, such as androgen insensitivity syndrome or 5α-reductase deficiency. It is therefore obvious that simply carrying out karyotype evaluation in children with isolated posterior hypospadias is not adequate.

The role of preoperative hormonal manipulation in the form of topical testosterone cream or intramuscular testosterone or β-hCG injection is either to improve the penile length or to facilitate posterior penile hypospadias reconstruction. However, there is no evidence to suggest that preoperative hormonal manipulation influences the results for hypospadias repair nor that it decreases the morbidity. It is commonly believed that exogenous androgen exposure compromises adult penile length possibly through the down-regulation of androgen receptors. However, this has not been supported by Baskin's work on humans. The local treatment with dihydrotestosterone in the 5α-reductase deficiency has been the only universally accepted indication for the treatment.

 **7** Which of the following is *not* an aim of hypospadias repair?
  **A** to move the urethral meatus to the tip
  **B** to have a straight penis
  **C** to have a penis adequate for sexual function
  **D** to void urine with a normal stream
  **E** to make any residual curvature acceptable

**A7** **E** The goals of the hypospadias repair are to provide a straight penis adequate for sexual function and to move the urethral meatus to the tip of the penis to allow the boy to void with a normal urinary stream. The factors that can determine the choice of hypospadias repair include glans size, degree of chordee, the meatal location and also the quality of foreskin.

 **8** Which of the following is true regarding hypospadias repair?
  **A** Distal hypospadias repair is not amenable to meatal advancement and glanuloplasty or tubularised incised plate technique.
  **B** Treating posterior hypospadias in stages depends on factors such as quality of urethral plate, severity of chordee and available preputial skin.
  **C** Residual chordee of more than 15 degrees does not require any treatment.
  **D** Urethral plate transaction is not required even if the chordee is more than 45 degrees following dorsal midline albuginea plication.
  **E** Urethral plate substitution is not necessary in severe chordee.

**B** Eighty-five per cent of hypospadias is of the distal variety and is amenable to repair using Snodgrass's procedure called tubularised incised plate urethroplasty. Meatal advancement and glanuloplasty technique is suitable for hypospadias where the meatus is located at a glanular or occasionally at a coronal location. In the remaining 15% of patients where the urethral meatus is located posteriorly and the urethral plate is hypoplastic, staged urethroplasty is indicated.

Most cases of posterior hypospadias can be treated in a single stage, but a decision to perform the repair in stages is often made at surgery. The decision to treat posterior hypospadias in a single stage or in two stages depends on a variety of factors including the quality of the urethral plate, the amount of preputial skin available and also the severity of the penile curvature (chordee). If the chordee is severe and cannot be corrected or residual chordee is more than 15 degrees after a complete skin degloving, dorsal tunica albuginea plication and subsequent ure-thral plate transection should be carried out. However, when the chordee is more than 45 degrees even after transecting the urethral plate, a substitution in the form of tunica vaginalis flap, free skin graft or SIS (small intestinal submucosal graft) is used after cutting the tunica albuginea on the ventral aspect.

Urethral plate substitution is usually achieved by covering the ventral aspect with the prepuce (when available) as a free graft (Bracka's procedure) or Byar's flaps rotated ventrally.

 **9** The following complications after hypospadias repair can occur except:
**A** megaprepuce
**B** urethral stricture
**C** urethral diverticulum and glans dehiscence
**D** recurrent penile curvature
**E** meatal stenosis.

**A9** **A** Early complications of hypospadias repair include infection, loss of skin flap, haemorrhage, retrusive meatus (more common in older types of hypospadias repair), bladder spasms (when a catheter is left inside the bladder postoperatively for urinary drainage; this is successfully treated with anticholinergic medicine, e.g. oxybutynin), and catheter blockage (this is usually troublesome, and requires removal of the catheter and insertion of a suprapubic catheter). Wound infection is a rare problem in hypospadias repair nowadays. However, wound infection in postpubertal patients is common and therefore it is advisable to do a skin pre-paration several days prior to surgery in the form of skin cleansing two to three times a day. Megaprepuce is a congenital disorder, where the prepuce from birth presents a very extensive and redundant mucosa accompanied by scarce and thickened preputial skin totally covering the glans, over a penis that otherwise appears normal in aspect and size.

## Meatal stenosis

Meatal stenosis can result from technical error in making the new meatus or be secondary to balanitis xerotica obliterans. Meatal stenosis can also occur if the urethral plate is flat and narrow and is not incised prior to tubularisation, or if the incision onto the urethral plate has been extended beyond the limits of the urethral plate. The other reason for meatal stenosis is secondary to suturing the neo-urethra too far distally.

## Urethral cutaneous fistula

This is the most common complication following hypospadias surgery. Several factors have been implicated such as apposing suture lines between new urethra and skin closure, distal obstruction secondary to meatal stenosis, turbulent urine flow (such as with a diverticulum), or secondary to impaired vascularity. Urethral cutaneous fistulas are usually apparent within the first few months of surgery but occasionally can develop several years later. Some close spontaneously but most require surgical correction.

Covering the urethroplasty using a dorsal dartos barrier layer can reduce this complication. It has been found that a barrier layer alone is not adequate to prevent fistula formation (20% incidence) and occurrence can be further reduced if subcuticular stitches are employed for urethroplasty. Fistula can also be secondary to rough handling of tissues; to the use of poorly vascularised tissue such as when the urethral plate is very thin or fibrotic, and also to the type of suture material used (e.g. PDS inside the urethra or using a non-absorbable suture material). Additionally, using fine instruments with magnification helps prevent fistula occurrence.

Fistula repairis usually performed 6 months after the primary repair to allow postoperative oedema and tissue inflammation to resolve. Fistulas at the coronal margin or on the proximal glans require repeat hypospadias surgery. Immediate repair of fistulas has been reported in a small series of patients in whom topical corticosteroids was applied for a few days to reduce the tissue reaction and then tissue glue such as cyanoacrylate was applied to the fistula following insertion of the catheter. Larger and multiple fistulas have a higher recurrence rate which may indicate impaired local vascularity.

## Urethral stricture

Urethral strictures have been found to be more common in procedures that involve end-to-end circumferential anastomosis or when pedicle flaps are used to reconstruct the urethra. It is recommended that end-to-end circumferential anastomosis be carried out after spatulation or triangulation of the hypospadic meatus. It is important to avoid devascularisation when pedicle flaps are used for the reconstruction. It has also been found that meatus-based flaps and onlay flap urethroplasties have a low risk of stricture formation.

Short strictures that are detected fairly soon after hypospadias repair are amenable to treatment by dilatation or by optical urethrotomy. However, strictures that develop late often require open repair.

## Diverticulum

Diverticulum is suspected when there is a ballooning of the new urethra while voiding. Common causes for diverticulum formation include distal obstruction, turbulent urine flow or creation of a large new urethra. The incidence is as high as 21% in preputial flap urethroplasty but is not known to occur following buccal mucosal graft urethroplasty. It is believed that this variation in diverticulum formation may be secondary to the elasticity of the tissue used for urethroplasty.

## Dehiscence

Partial or complete dehiscence of the glans is more common than meatal stenosis or urethral stricture but is under-reported. It is secondary to infection, poor vascularity, technique, inappropriate suture usage or when the glans repair is under tension.

## Recurrent penile curvature

In one study, a group of 12- to 18-year-old adolescent males who had had their chordee corrected, were found to have recurrence of chordee. It is important to know whether straightening of the penis was achieved during the repair of hypospadias and maintained during puberty. Data are lacking about the long-term results of dorsal tunica albuginea plication or other forms of ventral corporal grafting. In a minority of cases recurrence of chordee has been associated with the incorporation of unhealthy urethral plate in the initial urethroplasty, particularly when the chordee is more than 45 degrees. It has been found that the recurrence of chordee is more common when tunica vaginalis or SIS was used for corporal grafting to correct penile curvature. Corporal dermal grafting is successful in 90% of cases to correct penile chordee.

Contracture of the new urethra, tubed urethroplasty for proximal hypospadias repair, and tubularisation of unhealthy urethral plate, can all lead to recurrence of chordee.

## Skin complications

Fistulisation of suture tracks can occur and therefore subepithelial sutures are recommended to close penile shaft skin.

Secondary phimosis or wound dehiscence occurs in up to 15% of cases following foreskin reconstruction of hypospadias repair. To prevent this, manipulation of the foreskin should be carried out 3 months after hypospadias repair.

**Q10** Which of the following is *not* true regarding long-term outcomes after hypospadias repair?

**A** Poor urinary stream and flow rate occur following severe hypospadias repair.

**B** Sexual dysfunction may be due to soft glans, poor ejaculation, pain or poor penile appearance.

**C** Poor semen ejaculation is common in posterior hypospadias repair due to stricture or diverticulum.

**D** Boys with uncomplicated hypospadias repair are all infertile.

**E** Adolescent boys who have previously had severe hypospadias tend to have low self-esteem and can be poor achievers in life.

**A10 D Appearance**

The Hypospadias Objective Scoring Evaluation has been developed to obtain a more objective assessment of hypospadias repair. The outcome of an adolescent male survey suggests that up to 80% were dissatisfied with their penile appearance but only 30%–45% were sufficiently displeased to want further surgery to improve the appearance. The other scoring system – genital perception score – assesses the opinions of the surgeons and the patients regarding the outcome of the hypospadias repair with respect to correctable features (glans shape, position of meatus, scars, scrotum, and general appearance), and non-correctable features (penile size, penile thickness and glans size). The eight features are given scores from 1 to 4 each, making a possible total of 32 points – the best result.

**Voiding**

The aim of hypospadias repair is that the child should be able to stand and void and the stream should be directable, which can be achieved by creating an oval meatus. In severe degrees of hypospadias, e.g. penoscrotal hypospadias, the urinary stream is poor and the flow rate is on the lower side of normal, which can be secondary to urethral narrowing of the new urethra.

**Sexual function**

Physical causes of sexual dysfunction have been ascribed to soft glans, poor ejaculation, tight foreskin, pain, small penile size and poor penile appearance. Emotional causes are reported to be secondary to erection problems. Hypospadiac men are found to be more sexually inhibited. Disorders of sexual differentiation can be a part of the severe hypospadias anomaly and another reason for these patients having sexual dysfunction.

## Ejaculation

Normally, a bolus of semen is formed in the prostatic urethra and forcefully expelled by contraction of the prostatic urethral muscle while the bladder neck is closed. This process is hampered if there is an associated anomaly of the prostatic urethra/prostatic utricle, which is found in intersex disorders. In posterior hypospadias repair patients it was found that 63% of these patients had poor ejaculation secondary to diverticulum or stricture.

## Fertility

Boys with uncomplicated hypospadias repair are fertile; however, some patients with severe hypospadias were found to have a lower sperm count and more than 50% of these children have associated problems such as undescended testicle or intersex anomaly. It has also been found that in intersex patients, the hypothalamo–gonadal axis is abnormal.

## Psychological consequences

Adolescents who had undergone severe hypospadias repair were found to have a tendency to low self-esteem, were underachievers in academic life, and made poor use of mental resources. Frustration anxiety is higher in these patients. As children they are timid and isolated, and as adults they are more neurotic than the general population and have less-rewarding and less-demanding jobs.

# Further reading

Hayashi Y, Kojima Y. Current concepts in hypospadias surgery. *Int J Urol.* 2008; **15**(8): 651–64. Epub 2008 Jun 3.

Holland AJ, Smith GH, Ross FI, *et al*. HOSE: an objective scoring system for evaluating the results of hypospadias surgery. *BJU Int.* 2001; **88**(3): 255–8.

Retik AB, Atala A. Complications of hypospadias repair. *Urol Clin North Am.* 2002; **29**(2): 329–39.

## CHAPTER 63

# Circumcision and disorders of penis

### ASHOK RAJIMWALE

**From the choices below each question, select the single best answer.**

1 Which of the following is true regarding circumcision in children?

   **A** The incidence of circumcision in the United States has gone up since 1960.

   **B** Circumcision is uncommon in Muslims, Jews and some tribes in Africa.

   **C** It is believed that 6%–7% children in the UK are circumcised by the time they are 15 years old.

   **D** Europeans have the highest incidence of circumcision in the world.

   **E** Among Europeans, Sweden has the highest annual rate of circumcision.

**A**1   **C** Circumcision is the most commonly performed operation in males. It was initially performed for religious, ritual or cultural reasons and did not become 'medicalised' until the nineteenth century. Ritual circumcision is practised in Jews, Muslims, Aboriginals and certain tribes in Africa. The prevalence of routine neonatal circumcision in the United States has dropped from close to 90% in the mid-1960s to an estimated 64% in 1995. The American Academy of Pediatrics task force report on circumcision (1999) supports a growing trend away from neonatal circumcision. This task force report acknowledges potential medical benefits to neonatal circumcision; however, it concludes that routine circumcision in neonates is not necessary.

    Currently in England, approximately 21 000 childhood circumcisions are performed annually for medical reasons (compared with 1.2 million in the United States). It is estimated that 6%–7% of boys are circumcised before their 15th birthday, which is significantly less than the 24% reported in the 1950s. In Scandinavian countries, particularly Sweden, the circumcision rate is the lowest among Western cultures.

Q2 Regarding the development and retraction of prepuce:
  A the developing prepuce cannot be identified until late in gestation
  B preputial development is independent of glans development
  C the foreskin is retractile in 80% of the boys at birth
  D nearly 10% boys can retract their foreskin by 3 years of age
  E the prepuce grows over developing glans more quickly on the ventral aspect than on the dorsum side.

A2 C By 8 weeks of gestation, there is a thickened ridge of epidermis proximal to the glans, which is prepuce that grows forwards over the developing glans penis more quickly on the dorsum than on the ventral side. The circumferential full development is dependent upon final formation of the glanular urethra. The epithelium on the inner surface of the prepuce fuses with the developing glans and full separation takes place only later in life. Four per cent of foreskins are retractile at birth and 10% of boys can retract their foreskin by the age of 3 years. Spontaneous separation of the prepuce from the glans penis usually proceeds proximally due to desquamation of cells at a variable rate and only 1% of the foreskin remains non-retractile at 16 years of age.

Q3 Which of the following is *not* true for balanitis xerotica obliterans (BXO)?
  A Pathological phimosis due to BXO is uncommon before 5 years of age.
  B BXO is a contraindication for circumcision.
  C The aetiology of BXO is not known.
  D BXO can occur simultaneously to glans and meatus.
  E Histologically BXO is similar to vulval lichen sclerosis.

A3 B When the foreskin is non-retractile, it may be long and during attempted retraction it may exhibit 'flowering', and there may be blanching of the preputial skin proximal to the preputial orifice. It is called 'physiological phimosis'.

When the preputial orifice itself is abnormal and scarred, it is known as pathological phimosis. The scarring is called BXO. The incidence peaks in early adolescence and is approximately 1.5% at the age of 17 years. It is rare before the age of 5 years.

**Q4** Regarding indications for circumcision, which of the following is true?

    **A** Recurrent balanoposthitis and paraphimosis are not the indications for circumcision.

    **B** Circumcision can provide protection against diseases, e.g. penile cancer, sexually transmitted diseases.

    **C** AIDS is less common in uncircumcised males as the AIDS virus attaches to Langerhans's cells, which are deficient in foreskin.

    **D** Circumcision is indicated in boys with hypospadias/severe chordee.

    **E** Circumcision is indicated in buried penis or penoscrotal web.

 **A4**   **B** Medical indications for circumcisions are few and can be divided into absolute and relative. The absolute indication for circumcision is phimosis secondary to BXO, which is identical to vulval lichen sclerosis et atrophicus. The aetiology of BXO is unknown but it has some resemblance to autoimmune collagenosis. BXO may simultaneously affect the glans penis and urethral meatus much more commonly in adult men than boys. Meatal disease (BXO) can occasionally occur *de novo* after a circumcision; however, it has been suggested, with no proof, that BXO never follows neonatal circumcision.

    Relative indications include balanoposthitis (erythema and oedema of the prepuce, purulent discharge from the preputial orifice, dysuria in older children, with 20% incidence of recurrence) and paraphimosis (tight preputial ring proximal to the coronal sulcus resulting in oedema and swelling of the distal penis). Prevention of penile and cervical cancer, prevention of sexually transmitted disease (particularly HIV/AIDS), and prevention of urinary tract infection (UTI) are also relative indications. Circumcision has been found to be directly related to reducing the risk of HIV acquisition by reducing the ability of the virus to attach to and enter the Langerhans's cells. (The inner layer of the foreskin contains a high density of these cells, a target cell for HIV infection.) As the foreskin is more susceptible to trauma, this may predispose to HIV infection during sexual activity. A systematic review summarising studies from sub-Saharan Africa, has shown an adjusted relative risk of HIV acquisition of 0.42 (95% confidence interval) in circumcised, compared with uncircumcised male subjects.

    Tears, zip injury or pressure injuries usually heal well with some scarring and in such cases a circumcision is necessary only when the foreskin becomes scarred and non-retractile.

    Circumcision is contraindicated in hypospadias, chordee, penoscrotal fusion, buried penis, micropenis, bleeding disorders, and megameatus intact prepuce variant of hypospadias.

**Q5** Which of the following statement is true regarding the protective effect of circumcision on UTI?

   **A** Circumcision does not provide protection against UTI.

   **B** Circumcised infant boys are 3–10 times less likely to get a UTI than uncircumcised infants.

   **C** Neonatal circumcision offers no reduction of renal scarring in children with vesicoureteric reflux.

   **D** Circumcision has no role in reducing UTI in children with posterior urethral valves or neuropathic bladder.

   **E** UTI in male infants is less common in uncircumcised boys.

**A5**  **B** Circumcision reduces the risk of UTI. The risk of UTI in normal boys is approximately 1%. Almost 20 years ago Wisewell *et al.* found that uncircumcised infant boys were 3–10 times more likely to develop UTI than circumcised male infants, secondary to an increased rate of periurethral and inner preputial skin colonisation with bacteria. This association has also been shown in a report published in Sweden (Jakobsson *et al.*, 1999), which showed a preponderance of UTI in male infants where newborn circumcision is unusual.

   In boys with high-grade vesicoureteric reflux (VUR) the risk of UTI recurrence in uncircumcised and uncircumcised boys is 10% and 30%, respectively. It is a common practice by urologists to offer a circumcision to a boy with recurrent UTI, or a boy who develops a UTI despite conservative treatment in the presence of serious underlying urinary tract abnormality including VUR, posterior urethral valves, neuropathic bladder and so forth. It is also interesting to note that a controlled trial by Kwak *et al.* could find no benefit for circumcision when it was done at the same time as antireflux surgery for severe VUR, irrespective of age. One randomised controlled study showed (Nayir, 2001) significant reduction of renal scarring on DMSA scan following neonatal circumcision.

 **Q6** Regarding complications following circumcision, which of the following is true?

   **A** Bleeding following circumcision is an uncommon complication.

   **B** Necrotising fasciitis, Fournier's gangrene are common following circumcision.

   **C** Meatal ulceration can be found in 20%–30% of infants following circumcision and can cause meatal stenosis.

   **D** There is a high incidence of amputation of glans during circumcision

   **E** Penile lymphoedema is commonly seen following circumcision.

A6   **C**   The risk of complication following circumcision is 0.2%–5%. The most common complication following circumcision is bleeding (occurring in 0.1%), which is usually self-limiting, but some studies have suggested that haemorrhage requiring readmission and operation varies from 1.4% to 20%. Infection usually responds to local care and rarely requires antibiotics; however, such infections can occasionally cause necrotising fasciitis, Fournier's gangrene and tetanus. Such severe sepsis is quite rare following circumcision but when it occurs it usually results in death. Other complications include recurrent phimosis or buried penis, which may require a re-circumcision when too much skin is left behind. Macarthur reported 1% revision of skin complications following freehand circumcision.

Excessive loss of skin can either be due to local infection or secondary to diathermy injury. In smaller children these usually heal well while in older children it may require skin grafting. Other complications include glanular adhesions (adhesions of circumcision scar to the traumatised ulcerated glans), epidermal inclusion cysts, and penile lymphoedema – rarely seen and of unknown aetiology.

Amputation of part or all of the glans is rare but can happen if it is caught within the jaws of the circumcision clamp. Pressure necrosis of the glans is also rare but is usually seen with Plastibell circumcision especially when the bell of the Plastibell is too small. Injury to the urethra can be caused by overzealous haemostasis with diathermy on the ventral surface of the penis in the region of frenular artery. This can also be secondary to circumcision performed with a Gomco or Plastibell clamp. These techniques can cause subcoronal fistula, which requires a secondary repair. Meatal ulceration has been documented in 20%–30% of infants within 2–3 weeks following circumcision. This is thought to be due to chemical and physical irritation within the wet nappy. The incidence is lower (4%) when the circumcision is performed in older boys. The meatal ulcer will usually heal without sequel but chronic irritation or scarring can lead to meatal stenosis, which is reported in 2%–12% of patients following circumcision. The other proposed theory for meatal stenosis is relative ischaemia to the meatus following division of the frenular artery. Berry Croft studied the urethral meatus in children and adults and found that 60% of circumcised men had a meatus of 20Fr or less compared with only 25% of uncircumcised men. Rarely the bladder and upper tracts are secondarily affected by meatal stenosis causing bladder hypertrophy and upper tract dilatation.

Which of the following is true regarding concealed penis?

  A  Concealed penis is because of congenitally short penis.

  B  Concealed penis is due to inadequate attachment of the dartos layer and Buck's fascia.

  C  Concealed penis is a self-limiting condition and gets better as the child gets older.

  D  Concealed penis is secondary to childhood obesity.

  E  Balanitis, psychological stress and poor self-esteem are contraindications for surgical correction.

A7  B  Concealed or buried penis appears small; it is secondary to inadequate attachment of the dartos or spermatic fascia to the deeper Buck's fascia. The diameter and stretched penile length are normal. Earlier thinking was that this condition was due to childhood obesity (prominent prepubic fat) or inadequate or overzealous circumcision. It was believed that it would correct itself over time with growth; however, experience has suggested that this retrussive penile appearance cannot and does not correct itself.

Balanitis, urinary tract infections, skin adhesions, deflected urinary stream, psychological stress about the appearance of the penis, and boys who have poor self-esteem and are socially withdrawn are indications for correction.

Various surgical techniques have been described to correct this penile abnormality. They include attaching dartos layer to Buck's fascia after degloving the penis. Dorsally Scarpa's fascia superficial to the pubis is pulled down and attached to the Buck's fascia with non-absorbable sutures, safeguarding dorsal penile nerves.

Other techniques described are prepubic liposuction and lipectomy with Z-plasty for penoscrotal webbing to correct concealment.

 Regarding micropenis, which of the following is true?

  A  Stretched penile length less than 2 cm in newborns is normal.

  B  Micropenis may be secondary to panhypopituitarism or due to syndromes such as Klinefelter's or Prader–Willi's syndrome.

  C  Micropenis can not be associated with testicular dysgenesis or 5α-reductase deficiency.

  D  Evaluation of testicular function is not necessary in the management of micropenis.

  E  Gender reassignment should be offered to those who respond to androgen stimulation.

A8  B  Micropenis is defined as a normally formed penis with a stretched penile length >2–2.5 standard deviations below the mean length for age. In a newborn, stretched penile length less than 2 cm is considered abnormal. It may be associated with undescended testes.

Aetiology of micropenis includes idiopathic, gonadotropin deficiency with/ without pan hypopituitarism deficiency of growth hormone, testicular dysgenesis, 5α-reductase deficiency and partial androgen insensitivity syndrome. It may be present in conditions such as Klinefelter's syndrome, Laurence–Moon–Biedl's syndrome, Prader–Willi's syndrome and Robinow's syndrome.

Evaluation of these children includes karyotyping, and measurement of serum glucose, electrolytes, cortisol, growth hormone and thyroid function tests.

Testicular dysfunction as a cause of micropenis should be ruled out by measuring serum luteinising hormone, follicle-stimulating hormone, and measurement of testosterone before and after human chorionic gonadotropin stimulation (hCG) – 500–1500 IU of hCG is given alternate days for 5–7 days and testosterone is measured 24–48 hours after the last dose.

Androgen stimulation therapy is the treatment of choice. Testosterone 25 mg is given by intramuscular injection every month for several months in infants to assess the penile growth. Palpable testes and significant response to hCG stimulation test suggest there will be long-term penile growth. It has been shown that in peripubertal boys in whom testosterone therapy has failed, dihydrotestosterone cream can be an effective alternative.

Gender reassignment was advised in the past with failed response to testosterone but this has been questioned in genetic males with functioning testes. Adequate sexual function and clear male identity has been reported in some patients raised as males with persistent small penis; therefore, reassignment of gender should be performed with caution and should be accompanied by expert, patient and family counselling.

 **9** Regarding priapism, which of the following statements is true?

**A** Priapism is an involuntary, prolonged and painful erection not resulting from sexual desire.

**B** Priapism is uncommon in children with sickle-cell disease.

**C** Tricorporeal priapism does not involve tumescence of the spongiosum.

**D** Priapism may not be secondary to perineal trauma or haematological diseases.

**E** Ischaemic (veno-occlusive) priapism is secondary to perineal trauma.

 **9** **A** The term is derived from the Greek god Priapus, son of Aphrodite. He became famous for his giant phallus. Priapism is defined as an involuntary, prolonged, painful erection that does not result from sexual desire. It has been classified into primary or idiopathic, and secondary. Haemodynamically, it can be classified as veno-occlusive (ischaemic) and arterial (non-ischaemic). Non-ischaemic priapism is secondary to trauma and rarely is seen in sickle-cell disease. The ischaemic (low-flow) variety of priapism is commonly seen in children with sickle-cell disease. The reported incidence of priapism in sickle-cell disease varies from 2% to 35%. Stuttering episodes of priapism in patients with sickle-cell disease are common and usually these episodes last for less than 24 hours. Commonly tumescence involves only the corpora cavernosa but occasionally it may also involve the corpus spongiosum and is then known as tricorporeal priapism.

There is a long list of causes of priapism. Although demographically the incidence of priapism varies, nearly one-third of cases are idiopathic, 21% are caused by alcohol abuse or drug therapy, 12% following perineal trauma and 11% are due to sickle-cell disease. The secondary causes for priapism include haematological disorders (sickle-cell disease), drugs (anticoagulant, antihypertensive, drugs acting on central nervous system and so forth), metabolic disorders (amyloidosis, gout, diabetes, nephrotic syndrome and so forth), trauma, malignancy (leukaemia) and Kawasaki's disease.

It has been suggested that ischaemic priapism is due to failure of the detumescence mechanism from causes including excessive release of neurotransmitters, blockage of draining venules and prolonged relaxation of the intracavernous smooth muscle. In sickle-cell disease, intravascular thrombosis and haemolysis is caused by hypoxia. This in turn causes release of haemoglobin and L-arginase in the extracellular space. The free arginase consumes L-arginine, which is a substrate for the endothelial synthesis of nitric oxide. Nitric oxide is consumed in the oxidation of haemoglobin to methaemoglobin and in the neutralisation of heme and ferrous ions. This process leads to deficiency of nitric oxide along with release and activation of inflammatory and thrombogenic factors and a tendency to vasoconstriction. Nitric oxide is the main physiologic mediator of the detumescence mechanism; hence its deficiency in sickle-cell disease may cause priapism.

**Q10** Which of the following statements is true regarding priapism?

**A** Arterial priapism is due to excessive release of neurotransmitters.

**B** Ischaemic priapism is due to intracavernosal thrombosis and haemolysis due to hypoxia.

**C** Low-flow priapism is characterised by alkalosis, hypocarbia on penile blood.

**D** Surgical treatment is never required for priapism.

**E** Hydration and blood transfusion to decrease haemoglobin S concentration below 30% is not indicated for the treatment of priapism due to sickle-cell disease.

**A10** **B** Electron microscopic studies have shown that interstitial oedema with destruction of sinusoidal endothelium causing exposure of the basement membrane, occurs with 12 hours of priapism. Thrombocytes then adhere to basement membrane within 24 hours. By 48 hours, thrombi have been shown in the sinusoidal spaces along with some degree of smooth muscle cell necrosis.

It is an interesting fact that even after many days of low-flow priapism, there is a lack of thrombosis of penile blood. This is probably due to ×3 increase in activity of fibrinolysis locally in the cavernosal blood compared with peripheral blood.

In low-flow priapism, penile blood gas analysis is characterised by acidosis, hypercarbia and hypoxaemia. The usefulness and reliability of penile nuclear scans and Doppler studies in children remains unclear.

Treatment of low-flow priapism lasting for more than 4 hours in sickle-cell disease includes intracavernosal aspiration of blood and irrigation with sympathomimetic drugs. This treatment should be carried out concurrently with hydration and blood transfusion to achieve the haemoglobin S concentration of less than 30%. Exchange transfusion has been associated with acute neurologic events termed ASPEN syndrome (Association of Sickle cell disease, Priapism, Exchange transfusion and Neurologic events). The morbidity of ASPEN can be reduced by gradual or partial exchange transfusion, close monitoring and recognising the early prodromal symptoms such as headache.

Surgical intervention is required when medical and intracavernosal therapies fail.

For low-flow priapism, distal shunt procedures are recommended. These include Ebbehoj's, Winter's and Al Ghorab's procedures.

Ebbehoj's shunt is the simplest, between glans spongiosum and the corpora cavernosa. Winter described a similar technique using a Trucut biopsy needle instead of the knife, obtaining a core from the tunica albuginea of the corpora cavernosa. Al Ghorab's procedure is a modification of Winter's procedure. In this technique the glans is incised on the dorsum at corona level to expose bulging cavernosal bodies. A 5 × 5 mm segment of tunica albuginea is excised from the tip to create a cavernous–glanular shunt. The glans incision is then closed.

In long-standing priapism, distal shunts do not work very well and more proximal shunts such as Quackles's (cavernospongiosum) and Grayhack's (cavernosaphenous) shunts should be created.

In arterial priapism (non-ischaemic), which is secondary to perineal trauma, the tumescence is compressible because of open venous channels. Pain in this condition is less, as it is not ischaemic.

For high-flow priapism, initial treatment involves ice packs and site-specific compression. If this fails then selective arterial embolisation of the ruptured artery is indicated.

$Q$11 Which of the following statements is true about penile torsion?

    **A** Penile torsion can be associated with functional abnormality.

    **B** Penile torsion is common in the general population.

    **C** Penile torsion is almost always counterclockwise and can be associated with hypospadias and chordee.

    **D** Surgical correction of penile torsion is not advised even when it is more than 60–90 degrees.

    **E** Deviation of ventral penile raphae is always associated with penile torsion.

$A$11 **C** Penile torsion is a congenital rotational abnormality of the penis. It is almost always in counterclockwise direction. It is often an isolated abnormality or can be associated with hypospadias or chordee. The true incidence in normal males is 1.5% and with torsion of more than 90 degrees has been seen in 0.7%. Deviation of ventral midline raphe was noted in 10% of newborns without any rotational deformity.

    There is no functional abnormality associated with this condition and correction is indicated if the deformity is 60–90 degrees or more or the parents want it corrected. There are various techniques described to correct the anticlockwise rotation of penis including, penile skin degloving and realignment of penile skin, dorsal dartos flap counter-rotation, suturing penile tunica albuginea to pubic periosteum, and by removing angular ellipses of corporal tissue and plication.

## Further reading

American Academy of Pediatrics. Task force on circumcision. Circumcision policy statement. *Pediatrics.* 1999; **103**(3): 686–93.

Das S, Tunuguntla HS. Balanitis xerotica obliterans: a review. *World J Urol.* 2000; **18**(6): 382–7.

Jakobsson B, Esbjorner E, Hansson S. Minimum incidence and diagnostic rate of first urinary tract infection. *Pediatrics.* 1999; **104**: 222–6.

Kwak C, Oh SJ, Lee A, Choi H. Effect of circumcision on urinary tract infection after successful antireflux surgery. *BJU Int.* 2004; **94**: 627–9.

Nayir A. Circumcision for the prevention of significant bacteriuria in boys. *Pediatr Nephrol.* 2001; **16**: 1129–34.

Redman JF. Buried penis: congenital syndrome of a short penile shaft and a paucity of penile shaft skin. *J Urol.* 2005; **173**(5): 1714–17.

Weiss HA, Larke N, Halperin D, *et al.* Complications of circumcision in male neonates, infants and children: a systematic review. *BMC Urol.* 2010; **10**: 2.

Wiswell TE, Smith FR, Bass JW. Decreased incidence of urinary tract infections in circumcised male infants. *Pediatrics.* 1985; **75**: 901–3.

## CHAPTER 64

# Testicular problems and varicoceles

### JULIAN ROBERTS

**From the choices below each question, select the single best answer.**

 **1** Which of the following is true of testicular torsion?
- **A** It is the most likely cause of acute scrotum in an 8-year-old boy.
- **B** In children it can be reliably diagnosed by Doppler ultrasound.
- **C** In neonates it is due to intravaginal torsion.
- **D** Scrotal inflammatory change is a late sign associated with necrosis.
- **E** Bilateral fixation (after de-rotation) of the testes is best performed with dissolving sutures.

 **1**   **D**   Testicular torsion can occur at any age but it is the most common cause of acute scrotum at puberty. There is a second peak of incidence in infancy. The aetiology in this age group is different as the torsion is extravaginal. At puberty the torsion is intravaginal due to an abnormally high insertion of the tunica vaginalis. Typically torsion presents with acute onset of scrotal pain, often accompanied by nausea and vomiting. Early examination reveals a hard tender testicle, which may be lying high in the scrotum. The cord is often tender and the cremasteric reflex is absent. The overlying scrotum is of a normal appearance until late when inflammation, secondary to testicular necrosis, causes swelling and redness. Diagnosis is essentially clinical. While Doppler ultrasound can be helpful in postpubertal testicular torsion it is unreliable in younger children. Bilateral fixation is essential although the exact technique of doing this remains controversial, including whether to use permanent or dissolving sutures. In general the fixation should be at multiple points with the tunica everted.

Q2   Which of the following is true of idiopathic scrotal oedema?
   A   Pain is more severe than expected from the physical findings.
   B   Redness extends beyond the hemiscrotum, often into the perineum.
   C   It does not recur.
   D   The testes are enlarged and tender.
   E   Scrotal exploration is indicated to confirm the diagnosis.

A2   B   Once seen, idiopathic scrotal oedema is easily recognised and rarely confused
   with other causes of the acute scrotum. The history is of rapid onset of swelling
   and redness of the scrotum. This commonly occurs bilaterally and spreads to the
   inguinal or perineal regions. The appearance is florid but the signs minor. The
   testes are normal with only mild tenderness. Treatment is symptomatic and the
   condition resolves in a few days. It may recur.

Q3   Which of the following is true for torsion of the appendix testis?
   A   Most of the appendices are situated on the lower pole of the testis.
   B   It always requires operative intervention.
   C   During operation the contralateral testis should be explored.
   D   A tender 'blue spot' is pathognomonic but not common.
   E   The onset of pain is acute and severe.

A3   D   Torsion of the appendix testis is the commonest cause of an acute scrotum
   in prepubescent boys. In general the pain is less severe and of slower onset
   than with testicular torsion. They often present with a red, swollen scrotum and
   the appearance may then be undistinguishable from a late testicular torsion.
   Occasionally examination reveals a tender blue spot at the upper pole of the
   testis (where most appendices are located) with little testicular tenderness. This
   is pathognomonic of the condition. If the condition is not severe and the diagnosis
   is not in doubt then the patient can be managed symptomatically. If in doubt or
   if pain is severe, exploration and excision will ease symptoms quickly. Although
   there are often appendices on the contralateral testis, exploration is not indicated.

Q4   When considering epididymo-orchitis, which of the following is true?
   A   Postpubertal boys should be investigated for underlying urinary
       abnormalities.
   B   It is always associated with dysuria.
   C   It is more common than acute torsion in pubertal boys.
   D   In infants, urinary investigations should be performed.
   E   It is rare in the first 6 months of life.

**A4** **D** Occurrence of epididymo-orchitis has a bimodal distribution like testicular torsion. In infancy it may be associated with anatomical abnormalities of the urinary tract so should be further investigated. Epididymo-orchitis then becomes common again after puberty where it is associated with sexually transmitted infections or blood-borne infections (e.g. mumps). Clinically there is rapid onset of swelling, redness and tenderness of the scrotum sometimes associated with dysuria. Ultrasound may demonstrate an enlarged epididymis with fluid and debris and normal/increased blood flow. Treatment is with analgesia and antibiotics.

**Q5** Which of the following is true for testicular tumours?
  **A** Teratoma is the commonest tumour in the paediatric age range.
  **B** The incidence is increased 25-fold with intra-abdominal testes.
  **C** Teratoma is associated with raised levels of alpha-fetoprotein.
  **D** Dysgenetic testes are associated with granulosa cell tumours.
  **E** All should be explored through an inguinal approach.

**A5** **E** Testicular tumours can be divided into those arising from germ cells (yolk-sac tumours and teratomas in children) and those arising from gonadal stroma (Leydig cell, Sertoli cell or granulosa cell tumours). Yolk-sac tumours are the commonest tumour in childhood and are usually associated with raised levels of alpha-fetoprotein. The β-hCG levels are rarely raised in paediatric testicular tumours. The incidence of tumours is increased with intra-abdominal testes but in the order of 5–10 times normal. Gonadoblastoma is a rare testicular tumour (1% of all tumours), which occurs almost exclusively in dysgenetic gonads usually associated with intersex disorders. It frequently develops into seminoma. While there is a lower incidence of malignancy in childhood, all tumours should be treated as such and explored via an inguinal incision.

**Q6** Which of the following is true for testicular tumours?
  **A** They should always be treated with inguinal orchidectomy.
  **B** They can be the presenting feature of Burkitt's lymphoma.
  **C** The cord should be clamped and divided before the testis is mobilised.
  **D** They metastasise to the inguinal lymph nodes.
  **E** 80% have an associated hydrocele.

**A6** **B** Testicular tumours in prepubertal boys tend to be more benign than those occurring in adults. Certain benign tumours such as teratoma and Leydig cell tumours can be treated with testicle-sparing surgery, using an inguinal approach and frozen section. The inguinal approach involves opening the canal and mobilising the vessels. These are then occluded with a soft clamp. The testis is mobilised and biopsied if required before ligation and division of the vessels. The lymphatic drainage of the testis is to the retroperitoneal nodes along the iliac vessels. It is important therefore not to approach the testicle via the scrotum as lymphatic spread may also occur to the superficial inguinal nodes. Most testicular tumours present with increase in size of the testicle and sometimes discomfort. A hydrocele is present in 10%–20%. The testes can also be a site of secondary tumours particularly T-cell leukaemia.

 **Q7** Which of the following is true for testicular maldescent?

  **A** The commonest position for an 'ectopic' testis is in the perineum.

  **B** The gubernaculum is important in the intra-abdominal phase of testicular descent.

  **C** Testes may descend spontaneously in term babies at up to 7 months of life.

  **D** Undescended testes are associated with abnormally fused epididymis.

  **E** Normal descent of the testes is dependent on testosterone.

**A7**  **D** Descent of the testes occurs in two phases: intra-abdominal descent, controlled by müllerian inhibiting substance, and inguinoscrotal descent which depends on the gubernaculum. Testes in the line of descent but which are not fully descended have been called 'arrested' testes and those which are outside the line of descent, 'obstructed' or 'ectopic'. The commonest position of these is the superficial inguinal pouch (a space between tissue planes superficial to the external oblique). Other positions include perineal, femoral or pubopenile. The testes may not be fully descended at birth, but in the term baby they should have fully descended by 4 months (later in pre-term babies). At orchidopexy for undescended testes, abnormalities of fusion between the testis and epididymis are not uncommon and may be related to later fertility.

 **Q8** Which of the following is not associated with cryptorchidism?

  **A** Peutz–Jeghers's syndrome

  **B** cloacal exstrophy

  **C** Klinefelter's syndrome

  **D** prune belly syndrome

  **E** myelomeningocele

**A8**  **A** Peutz–Jeghers's syndrome is an autosomal dominant condition characterised by mucocutaneous pigmentation and hamartomatous intestinal polyps. It is associated with some types of testicular tumour. The others are just some of the associations of cryptorchidism, and also include posterior urethral valves and cerebral palsy.

**Q9** When examining for an undescended testis, which of the following manoeuvres is not required?

  **A** 'milking' the inguinal canal towards scrotum, gently grasping testicle between fingers of other hand

  **B** examining the other testicle

  **C** examining the perineum, femoral area and base of penis

  **D** releasing the testis if it can be manipulated into the scrotum

  **E** eliciting the cremasteric reflex by stroking the inside of the thigh

**A9** **E** Examination normally begins by looking at and palpating the scrotum. If the scrotum is empty palpate the inguinal area. If a testicle is palpable 'milk' the testicle to the external ring by firmly running fingers from the anterior superior iliac spine to the pubic tubercle. The testis can be gently grasped between the forefinger and thumb of the other hand and put under traction to find the lowest point of descent. If a testicle is not palpable in the inguinal area, other positions of an ectopic testis are palpated. In younger children, gentle abdominal pressure can sometimes force a testis lying just inside the internal ring, into the canal. If the testis is still impalpable, measuring the contralateral testis may indicate the likely presence of the impalpable testis (if absent there is often compensatory hypertrophy). The cremasteric reflex may be helpful to indicate to parents the mechanism of a retractile testis, but is not useful clinically.

**Q10** Which of the following is true for retractile testis?

  **A** The cremasteric reflex is mediated by the ilioinguinal nerve.

  **B** It is often smaller than 'normally descended' testes.

  **C** It is easily manipulated into the scrotum where it will stay (at least temporarily) when released.

  **D** It should be kept under review, as almost 50% may reascend during childhood.

  **E** It is uncommon.

**A10** **C** The retractile testicle is probably the commonest diagnosis in patients referred with undescended testes. It is characteristically a normal-sized testis that can be manipulated to a normal position in the scrotum and will remain there without immediately springing back into the groin (suggesting tension of the cord). These patients usually have a very noticeable cremasteric reflex whereby stimulation of the medial aspect of the thigh results in contraction of the dartos and cremasteric muscles pulling the testis from the scrotum. This reflex is mediated by the genitofemoral nerve. There is an incidence (~15%) of later ascent of the testes.

**Q11** Which of the following is true for intra-abdominal testis?

**A** MRI is the best investigation to locate an intra-abdominal testis.

**B** It can be effectively treated with intranasal luteinising hormone-releasing hormone.

**C** Ultrasound is useful in locating an intra-abdominal testis.

**D** At laparoscopy the appearance of the vas going through the internal ring indicates the testis is outside the abdomen.

**E** It is associated with an increased risk of seminoma.

**A11** **E** Laparoscopy is generally considered the most effective investigation for intra-abdominal testes. In children who are difficult to examine, ultrasound can be helpful if the testis is within the canal. MRI can detect intra-abdominal testes but is unreliable (relatively high false-negative rate). At laparoscopy the testis can be assessed in terms of position (whether a single-stage or two-stage procedure is preferable) and size (some small testes may be best removed). It is essential to see both blind-ending vas and vessels before concluding the testis in not in the abdomen.

**Q12** Which of the following is true for orchidopexy?

**A** It should be performed in all boys by the age of 2 years.

**B** Depending on position it may be performed by an inguinal or scrotal approach.

**C** It has no effect on the subsequent testicular cancer rate of the undescended testis.

**D** Fowler–Stephens's two-stage orchidopexy has a testicular atrophy rate of less than 5%.

**E** The testicle should be left within the tunica vaginalis.

**A12** **B** Orchidopexy is usually planned for between 12 and 18 months, although some will perform as early as 6 months. There is an incidence of late (after the age of 2 years) orchidopexy because of the phenomenon of the ascending testis (an initially descended testes that gradually retracts from the scrotum as the child grows). Orchidopexy can be performed by the inguinal or scrotal route. For the latter the testis should be able to be manipulated into the scrotum under anaesthetic. The operation then consists of dissecting the coverings from the cord, dissecting and dividing any associated patent processus vaginalis, dividing the gubernaculum and fixing the testis in a subdartos pouch. The tunica is everted and the testicle delivered (this allows inspection of the testis, the removal of any hydatids/appendices, and promotes fixation). The specific complications of the procedure are damage to the vas, re-ascent and testicular atrophy. With a standard orchidopexy the risks of atrophy are around 2%–5%, depending on the position of the testis. Atrophy rates are higher than this for two-stage procedures (10%–20%).

It appears that prepubertal orchidopexy reduces the rate of subsequent testicular tumour compared with later orchidopexy. In addition, orchidopexy reduces the risk of seminoma (which accounts for two-thirds of malignant tumours that develop in undescended testes).

Q13 Following testicular trauma which of the following is true?

    **A** An avulsed testis can be reimplanted up to 24 hours if kept in saline slush.

    **B** Doppler ultrasound is indicated to ensure adequate blood flow in the testis.

    **C** The management of all blunt testicular trauma is rest, elevation and analgesia.

    **D** A large scrotal haematoma should be explored and drained.

    **E** Operative exploration is indicated if the tunica albuginea is ruptured.

A13 **E** Testicular trauma is not common in children and is usually due to blunt trauma. It is important to distinguish between a scrotal haematoma (best managed conservatively) and haematocele secondary to rupture of the tunica albuginea (best managed by operative drainage, debridement of the seminiferous tubules and closure of the tunica). The distinction may be difficult clinically, in which case ultrasound is useful to detect damage to the tunica (but not to indicate blood flow). In the very rare instance where a testicle is avulsed, it needs to be reimplanted within 4–6 hours to ensure viability.

Q14 Which of the following is true for varicoceles?

    **A** They occur with equal frequency on the right and left sides.

    **B** They do not occur before puberty.

    **C** They always require surgical management.

    **D** They may be uncomfortable and interfere with testicular growth.

    **E** They are best managed by radiologically controlled embolisation.

A14 **D** A varicocele is an abnormal dilatation of the pampiniform plexus of veins in the scrotum. Ninety per cent occur on the left side and they become increasingly prevalent around puberty, although they have been reported in the under-10 age group. Many small varicoceles are asymptomatic; they may, however, cause discomfort. There is evidence that larger varicoceles can impair testicular growth and may lead to reduced fertility. Surgery is usually reserved for symptomatic larger varicoceles particularly if there is evidence of poor testicular growth. There are several possible treatment options, including retrograde or antegrade embolisation or sclerotherapy, microsurgical inguinal ligation, open or laparo-scopic ligation. There are advantages and disadvantages to each technique and none has been proven superior to the others.

**Q15** Which of the following is a common complication of varicocele surgery?

**A** hydrocele formation

**B** renal vein thrombosis

**C** testicular atrophy

**D** sigmoid injury with the laparoscopic approach

**E** focal testicular necrosis.

**A15** **A** These are all described complications following varicocele surgery. The com-monest complications are recurrence (around 5%–10%) and hydrocele formation (5%–20%). The incidence and type of complications vary according to technique. Focal testicular necrosis is specific to antegrade scrotal sclerotherapy for example.

## Further reading

Gatti JM, Patrick Murphy J. Current management of the acute scrotum. *Semin Pediatr Surg.* 2007; **16**(1): 58–63.

Hutson JM, Clarke MC. Current management of the undescended testicle. *Semin Pediatr Surg.* 2007; **16**(1): 64–70.

Ross JH. Prepubertal testicular tumors. *Urology.* 2009; **74**(1): 94–9.

Wood HM, Elder JS. Cryptorchidism and testicular cancer: separating fact from fiction. *J Urol.* 2009; **181**(2): 452–61.

# CHAPTER 65

# Disorders of sexual differentiation

## SARAH M LAMBERT, HOWARD M SNYDER III

From the choices below each question, select the single best answer.

**Q1** The *SRY* gene that encodes the testis determining factor is located at which of the following locations?

  **A** long arm of the X chromosome
  **B** long arm of the Y chromosome
  **C** short arm of chromosome 3
  **D** short arm of the Y chromosome
  **E** chromosome 11p13

**A1** **D** The *SRY* or sex-determining region of the Y chromosome contains the testis determining factor and is located on its short arm. Chromosome 3p contains the gene that is associated with von Hippel–Lindau's syndrome. Chromosome 11p13 is the locus for the *WT1* gene.

**Q2** The first sign of male phenotypic differentiation is which of the following events?

  **A** The distal wolffian ducts join the immature rete testes.
  **B** The müllerian ducts degenerate because of secretion of müllerian inhibiting substance by the Sertoli cells.
  **C** The wolffian ducts organise to form the epididymis by secretion of testosterone from the Leydig cells.
  **D** The müllerian ducts degenerate because of secretion of müllerian inhibiting substance by the Leydig cells.
  **E** Wolffian ducts organise to form the epididymis by secretion of dihydrotestosterone from the Leydig cells.

**A2** **B** The first sign of male phenotypic differentiation is the degeneration of the müllerian ducts adjacent to the testes. This degeneration results from the secretion of müllerian-inhibiting substance by the Sertoli cells. This process begins between the seventh and eighth weeks of gestation.

**Q3** A chromosomal complement of 47,XXY is most commonly associated with which of the following characteristics?

**A** shield-shaped chest

**B** cardiac defects

**C** electrolyte abnormalities

**D** azoospermia

**E** renal agenesis

 **A3** **D** The chromosomal complement 47,XXY results from non-disjunction during meiosis and is the classic chromosomal complement of Klinefelter's syndrome. The syndrome is characterised by eunuchoid body habitus, gynaecomastia, increased gonadotropin levels, small firm testes and azoospermia. Shield-shaped chest, coarctation of the aorta, and renal anomalies are associated with Turner's syndrome (45,XO). Unilateral renal agenesis is a component of Mayer–Rokitansky–Küster–Hauser's syndrome. Electrolyte abnormalities, specifically salt wasting, are present in 75% of patients with congenital adrenal hyperplasia secondary to 21-hydroxylase deficiency.

 **Q4** In the newborn period, the most common aetiology of ambiguous genitalia is which of the following conditions?

**A** congenital adrenal hyperplasia

**B** complete androgen insensitivity syndrome

**C** mixed gonadal dysgenesis

**D** persistent müllerian duct syndrome

**E** partial androgen insensitivity

 **A4** **A** Congenital adrenal hyperplasia is the most common cause of ambiguous genitalia in the newborn period. Mixed gonadal dysgenesis is the second most common cause of ambiguous genitalia in the newborn period. Complete androgen insensitivity syndrome and persistent müllerian duct syndrome do not typically present in the newborn period. Partial androgen insensitivity is a rare condition that manifests with varying degrees of feminisation phenotypically.

 **Q5** Which of the following is *not* a presenting symptom in male neonates with 21-hydroxylase deficiency?

**A** failure to thrive

**B** dehydration

**C** emesis

**D** death

**E** ambiguous genitalia

A5   E   Male neonates with congenital adrenal hyperplasia do not present with ambiguous genitalia. Female neonates present with varying degrees of virilisation due to excess androgen production. Because of the absence of phenotypic changes, male neonates with congenital adrenal hyperplasia often present with symptoms of salt wasting including failure to thrive, dehydration, emesis and even death.

Q6   The diagnosis of 11β-hydroxylase deficiency can be confirmed by increased plasma levels of which of the following?
   A   17-hydroxyprogesterone
   B   deoxycorticosterone
   C   17-hydroxypregnenolone
   D   dehydroepiandrosterone
   E   androstenedione

A6   B   The diagnosis of 11β-hydroxylase deficiency is confirmed by the identification of increased serum levels of deoxycorticosterone and 11-deoxycortisol. The diagnosis of 21-hydroxylase deficiency is confirmed by the identification of increased serum levels of 17-hydroxyprogesterone. The diagnosis of 3β-hydroxysteroid dehydrogenase deficiency is confirmed by the identification of increased serum levels of 17-hydroxypregnenolone and dehydroepiandrosterone.

Q7   The strongest indication for surgical removal of the streak gonad in patients with mixed gonadal dysgenesis is which of the following?
   A   the risk of gonadal torsion
   B   to obviate the need for orchidopexy
   C   the risk of malignancy
   D   the risk of inguinal hernia
   E   for histological evaluation

A7   C   The strongest indication for surgical removal of the streak gonad in patients with mixed gonadal dysgenesis is the risk of malignancy. Presence of Y chromosome material in patients with a streak gonad significantly increases this risk. Gonadoblastoma has been described in children as young as 26 months and prophylactic excision of the streak gonad should be strongly considered if Y chromosomal material is present.

**Q8**  In the repair of a urogenital sinus, the difference between a total urogenital mobilisation and partial urogenital mobilisation is which of the following?

   **A**  Partial urogenital mobilisation mobilises only the posterior vagina.

   **B**  Total urogenital mobilisation includes amputation of the redundant mobilised sinus.

   **C**  Partial urogenital mobilisation utilises the redundant mobilised sinus tissue to complete the reconstruction but total urogenital mobilisation does not use this tissue.

   **D**  Total urogenital mobilisation includes transection of the pubourethral ligament.

   **E**  Total urogenital mobilisation is used exclusively for patients with cloacal abnormalities.

**A8**  **D**  The anterior dissection performed during partial urogenital mobilisation stops at the pubourethral ligament. Both total and partial urogenital mobilisation include mobilisation of the posterior vaginal wall and utilise the redundant mobilised sinus tissue to complete the reconstruction. Total urogenital mobilisation can be used for all high urogenital sinus repairs.

**Q9**  Initial evaluation of a neonate with ambiguous genitalia should include all of the following tests *except*:

   **A**  karyotype

   **B**  serum electrolytes

   **C**  testosterone, dihydrotestosterone levels

   **D**  17-hydroxyprogesterone, 11-deoxycortisol, deoxycorticosterone levels

   **E**  exogenous hCG stimulation test.

**A9**  **E**  During the first 60–90 days of life, a normal gonadotropin surge occurs with a resultant increase in the testosterone level and its precursors. In the initial evaluation, exogenous hCG stimulation for androgen evaluation can be postponed. All the other tests should be performed in the immediate neonatal period.

**Q10** In a male neonate with distal hypospadias and a unilateral undescended testis, which of the following statements is true?

   **A** No further evaluation is needed if one testis is descended and normal to palpation.

   **B** Evaluation is indicated if the hypospadias is at the midshaft or more proximal.

   **C** No further evaluation is needed if the undescended testis is in the inguinal canal.

   **D** Evaluation is recommended.

   **E** Evaluation is indicated if a family history of disorders of sexual differentiation (DSD) exists.

**A10** **D** An evaluation including a karyotype is recommended in a neonate with hypospadias and a unilateral undescended testis, even if the genitalia appear unambiguous. With hypospadias and a unilateral undescended testis, the incidence of DSD is 30% overall in some patient series. The incidence increases to 50% if the undescended testis is non-palpable and decreases to 15% if the undescended testis is palpable.

**Q11** Which statement below is *false* regarding the use of ultrasonography in children with DSD?

   **A** Pelvic ultrasound is the first radiographic test obtained.

   **B** Pelvic ultrasound reliably detects intra-abdominal testes.

   **C** Scrotal ultrasound reliably detects testes in the superficial inguinal pouch.

   **D** Pelvic ultrasound documents the presence of müllerian structures.

   **E** Magnetic resonance imaging can be utilised to further delineate pelvic anatomy.

**A11** **B** Although scrotal ultrasound can provide visualisation of testes distal to the external inguinal ring and müllerian structures, ultrasound is only 50% accurate in detecting intra-abdominal testes. Pelvic ultrasound should be the first radiographic study obtained. Questionable anatomy can be further delineated with magnetic resonance imaging.

**Q12** Postnatal treatment of girls with congenital adrenal hyperplasia includes which of the following?

   **A** oestrogen supplementation

   **B** glucocorticoid replacement

   **C** mineralocorticoid replacement

   **D** all of the above

   **E** B and C only

A12 **E** Girls with congenital adrenal hyperplasia present with ambiguous genitalia because of the production of excess adrenal androgens. Defective synthesis of cortisol from cholesterol diverts its precursors to androgen pathways. Oestrogen production by the ovaries is not affected.

Q13 Primary amenorrhoea in association with normal ovarian function is present in which of the following conditions?

  **A** Turner's syndrome
  **B** complete androgen insensitivity syndrome
  **C** Mayer–Rokitansky–Küster–Hauser's syndrome
  **D** hypopituitarism
  **E** Swyer's syndrome

A13 **C** Girls with Mayer-Rokitansky-Kuster-Hauser's syndrome often present with primary amenorrhoea because of congenital absence of the vagina and often uterus. Although this syndrome is associated with renal anomalies, ovarian development is normal. Complete androgen insensitivity syndrome and Swyer's syndrome are associated with XY karyotype. The classic 45,XO karyotype of Turner's syndrome results in bilateral streak ovaries. Hypopituitarism results in abnormal ovarian function and a low oestrogen state.

Q14 A neonate is noted to have female external genitalia, cortisol and aldosterone deficiency, and large, lipid-laden adrenal glands on computed tomography of the abdomen. What is the most likely diagnosis?

  **A** congenital adrenal hyperplasia
  **B** pure gonadal dysgenesis
  **C** Leydig cell aplasia
  **D** StAR deficiency
  **E** partial androgen insensitivity syndrome

A14 **D** A neonate with female external genitalia, cortisol and aldosterone deficiency, and large, lipid-laden adrenal glands on computed tomography of the abdomen is likely to have a StAR deficiency. The steroidogenic acute regulatory protein (StAR) stimulates cholesterol transport from the outer to the inner mitochondrial membrance. This transport is the rate-limiting step in acute steroid synthesis. Affected 46,XY neonates require glucocorticoid and mineralocorticoid replacement therapy.

Q15 An abnormally elevated testosterone to dihydrotestosterone ratio is characteristic of which of the following conditions?

  A persistent müllerian duct syndrome

  B 5α-reductase deficiency

  C partial androgen insensitivity syndrome

  D complete androgen insensitivity syndrome

  E mixed gonadal dysgenesis

A15 B An abnormally elevated testosterone to dihydrotestosterone level is characteristic of 5α-reductase deficiency. The 5α-reductase catalyses the conversion of testosterone to dihydrotestosterone. This is an autosomal recessive condition. 46,XY male neonates present with ambiguous genitalia and virilisation at puberty.

## Further reading

Diamond DA. Sexual differentiation: normal and abnormal. In: Wein AJ, Kavoussi LR, Novick AC, *et al. Campbell-Walsh Urology.* 9th ed. Philadelphia, PA: Saunders Elsevier; 2007.

Lambert SM, Vilain EJN, Kolon TF. A practical approach to ambiguous genitalia in the newborn period. *Urol Clin North Am.* 2010; **37**(2): 195–205.

Rink RC, Cain MP. Urogenital mobilization for urogenital sinus repair. *BJU Int.* 2008; **102**(9): 1182–97.

# CHAPTER 66

# Prune belly syndrome, bladder and cloacal exstrophy

## KATE H KRAFT, HOWARD M SNYDER III

**From the choices below each question, select the single best answer.**

**Q1** The classic triad found in prune belly syndrome (PBS) comprises which of the following?

   **A** hypospadias, bilateral intra-abdominal testes, deficiency of abdominal wall musculature

   **B** deficiency of abdominal musculature, ventricular septal defect, bilateral intra-abdominal testes

   **C** bilateral intra-abdominal testes, prostatic hypoplasia, renal dysplasia

   **D** deficiency of abdominal musculature, bilateral intra-abdominal testes, anomalous urinary tract

   **E** deficiency of abdominal musculature, renal dysplasia, unilateral undescended testis

**A1** **D** The classic triad found in PBS, also known as the triad syndrome or Eagle–Barrett's syndrome, is deficiency of the abdominal musculature, bilateral intra-abdominal testes and an anomalous urinary tract. Urinary tract abnormalities may include variable degrees of hydronephrosis, renal dysplasia, dilated tortuous ureters, an enlarged bladder and a dilated prostatic urethra. Patients do not typically present with unilateral cryptorchidism and rarely have palpable testes. Additional associated anomalies may involve the respiratory tract, gastrointestinal tract, cardiac system and musculoskeletal system.

**Q2** The incidence of PBS is:

   **A** 1 : 900 to 1 : 2000 live births

   **B** 1 : 9000 to 1 : 20 000 live births

   **C** 1 : 19 000 to 1 : 30 000 live births

   **D** 1 : 29 000 to 1 : 40 000 live births

   **E** 1 : 39 000 to 1 : 50 000 live births.

**A2**   **D**  The incidence of PBS has been reported as 1 : 29 000 to 1 : 40 000. This is similar to the reported incidence of bladder exstrophy. Males comprise 95% of cases. Female cases have abdominal musculature deficiency and urinary tract anomalies but do not carry the gonadal component of the triad. The incidence of PBS has declined over the last several decades.

**Q3**   Which of the following is *not* true of the clinical features of PBS?

   **A**  Severely dysplastic kidneys are usually associated with bladder outlet obstruction.

   **B**  Vesicoureteral reflux is present in approximately 25% of patients.

   **C**  The bladder usually appears massively enlarged with a pseudodiverticulum at the urachus.

   **D**  The dilatation of the posterior urethra is likely due to prostatic hypoplasia.

   **E**  Both testes are typically found overlying the ureters at the pelvic brim near the sacroiliac level.

**A3**   **B**  Vesicoureteral reflux is present in up to 75% of patients with PBS. Approximately 25%–30% of patients will have a patent urachus, allowing decompression of bladder outlet obstruction associated with PBS. In those patients without a patent urachus, severe renal dysplasia may result. Dysplasia may present in up to 50% of cases, but laterality and severity is variable. The bladder usually appears enlarged with a urachal pseudodiverticulum. Unlike other cases of bladder outlet obstruction, the bladder in PBS is smooth walled. However, smooth muscle hypertrophy is present. Urodynamic evaluation generally demonstrates normal compliance with delayed first sensation to void, a very large capacity, and variable bladder emptying. Prostatic hypoplasia is likely related to abnormal mesenchymal-epithelial development and results in posterior urethral dilatation. One of the hallmarks of PBS is bilateral intra-abdominal testes, which are usually found overlying the iliac vessels. Mechanical features such as intra-abdominal pressure and bladder distension have been implicated in testicular maldescent, although some patients may present with descended testes, suggesting that other factors may play a role.

**Q4**   Prenatal intervention for suspected PBS is most strongly indicated in:

   **A**  urethral atresia with progressive oligohydramnios

   **B**  pulmonary hypoplasia

   **C**  hydroureteronephrosis

   **D**  renal dysplasia

   **E**  bladder distension.

A4    **A**   In suspected PBS, hydroureteronephrosis and bladder distension are usually well-tolerated entities. Pulmonary hypoplasia and renal dysplasia do not necessitate immediate prenatal intervention. If urethral atresia results in worsening oligohydramnios and subsequent pulmonary hypoplasia, this condition may be reversed with decompression of the urinary tract *in utero*.

Q5    Initial management of the PBS patient in the newborn period should include:

     **A**   assessment of pulmonary status, suprapubic tube placement

     **B**   assessment of pulmonary status, vesicostomy creation

     **C**   assessment of pulmonary status, renal and bladder ultrasound

     **D**   stabilisation, bilateral percutaneous upper tract urinary diversion

     **E**   voiding cystourethrogram to rule out posterior urethral valves.

A5    **C**   Initial evaluation of the newborn with PBS requires a multidisciplinary approach involving specialists from neonatology, nephrology and urology. Pulmonary status must be assessed immediately, usually with a chest radiograph to rule out pulmonary abnormalities as sequelae of oligohydramnios. Initial evaluation of renal function should include serum electrolytes, blood urea nitrogen and creatinine, as well as a renal and bladder ultrasound. Creatinine may reflect maternal renal function, and this must be taken into account in the first few days of life. If renal insufficiency or bladder outlet obstruction is evident, voiding cystourethrogram is indicated to assess the bladder outlet and bladder emptying. Bladder outlet obstruction may be relieved with bladder diversion in the form of a percutaneous suprapubic tube. If this cannot be performed in the neonatal intensive care unit, vesicostomy may be performed if the infant is stabilised, has bladder outlet obstruction, and has salvageable renal function. Supravesical urinary diversion is warranted in rare instances of ureteropelvic or ureterovesical junction obstruction.

Q6    The incidence of bladder exstrophy is estimated as:

     **A**   1 : 100 to 1 : 500 live births

     **B**   1 : 1000 to 1 : 5000 live births

     **C**   1 : 10 000 to 1 : 50 000 live births

     **D**   1 : 100 000 to 1 : 500 000 live births

     **E**   1 : 1 million to 1 : 5 million live births.

A6    **C**   The incidence of bladder exstrophy has been estimated between 1 in 10 000 and 1 in 50 000 live births. The male to female ratio is 2.3 : 1, although some series report a slightly higher incidence in males. The risk of recurrence of bladder exstrophy within the same family is approximately 1 in 100. The risk of bladder exstrophy in the offspring of individuals with bladder exstrophy and epispadias is 1 in 70 live births.

 **Q7** The primary embryonic theory for the development of exstrophy is:

    **A** abnormal caudal insertion of the body stalk, resulting in failure of interposition of the mesenchymal tissue in the midline

    **B** maldevelopment of the bony pelvis with lack of rotation of the pelvic ring primordium

    **C** invasion of endoderm into the cloacal membrane

    **D** abnormal underdevelopment of the cloacal membrane, inhibiting the medial migration of mesenchyme towards the midline and disrupting normal lower abdominal wall development

    **E** abnormal overdevelopment of the cloacal membrane, inhibiting the medial migration of mesenchyme towards the midline and disrupting normal lower abdominal wall development.

 **A7** **E** The primary embryonic theory for development of exstrophy as held by Marshall and Muecke suggests that the basic defect is an abnormal over-development of the cloacal membrane, which prevents medial migration of the mesenchymal tissue and proper lower abdominal wall development. The timing of the rupture of the cloacal membrane determines where on the spectrum of epispadias to cloacal exstrophy the patient's phenotype will fall. Another theory proposes an abnormal caudal insertion of the body stalk, resulting in failure of interposition of the mesenchyme in the midline. As a result, translocation of the cloaca into the abdominal cavity does not occur. This explanation remains controversial. The traditional theory does not account for the bowel anomalies, particularly the absence of the ileocaecal region, seen in exstrophy. Therefore, additional theories involving absence of migration, ascent, or alignment of the allantois with the yolk sac with persistence at the dome of the cloaca, have also been described. Another recent hypothesis suggests that maldevelopment of the bony pelvis with lack of rotation of the pelvic ring primordium could account for exstrophy, although additional work has demonstrated that the anatomical structure of the pelvic ring in exstrophy is similar to that in age-matched controls. The most universally accepted theory to date remains that of Marshall and Muecke.

**Q8** Which of the following statements is *true* regarding the male genital defects in exstrophy?

**A** The posterior corporal length in exstrophy patients is almost 50% shorter than that of normal controls.

**B** The anterior corporal length in exstrophy patients is almost 50% shorter than that of normal controls.

**C** The pubic diastasis does not affect the intercorporal distance but does change the angle between the corpora cavernosa.

**D** The autonomic nerves innervating the corpora cavernosa are displaced medially.

**E** Testes are most commonly found in an intra-abdominal position bilaterally.

**A8** **B** MRI has been used to measure the corpora in men with a history of bladder exstrophy, who were compared with age- and race-matched controls. Results showed that the anterior corporal length of male patients with bladder exstrophy is almost 50% shorter than that of controls. Posterior length is the same as that of controls. Pubic diastasis increases the intrasymphyseal and intercorporeal distances but the angle between the corpora is unchanged. The autonomic nerves are displaced laterally. Testes appear undescended secondary to the pubic diastasis but are usually retractile and can easily be brought into the scrotum. Bilateral intra-abdominal testes are a hallmark of PBS.

**Q9** Which of the following statements is *false* regarding the bladder in classic exstrophy?

**A** Muscarinic cholinergic receptor density and binding affinity is similar in both exstrophy patients and normal controls.

**B** There is a significant decrease in the number of myelinated nerves per field in the exstrophy bladder compared with that of controls.

**C** Functional repair should not be attempted when the bladder is small, fibrotic or covered in polyps.

**D** There is no significant difference in the amount of type I and type III collagen between the bladders of exstrophy patients and normal controls.

**E** In exstrophy patients who gain adequate bladder capacities after bladder neck closure, the ratio of collagen to smooth muscle decreases.

**A9** **D** Evaluation of the collagen-to-smooth-muscle ratio in bladder biopsies from newborns with classic exstrophy, demonstrated a similar amount of type I collagen but a threefold increase in type III collagen compared with controls. Patients with adequate bladder capacity following closure have a marked decrease in the ratio of collagen to smooth muscle, provided the bladder remained infection free. Experimental studies show similar muscarinic cholinergic receptor density and binding affinity in exstrophy patients and controls. Examination of myelinated nerves per field, in exstrophied bladders and controls, has revealed a significant decrease in the exstrophy patients. If the exstrophied bladder is small and covered in polyps, closure should be delayed until the patient has grown. The bladder mucosa should be frequently irrigated and covered in a protective dressing such as Saran™ Wrap.

**Q10** Which of the following is not a prenatal ultrasound characteristic of bladder exstrophy?

**A** high-set umbilicus

**B** absence of bladder filling

**C** widening of the pubic rami

**D** diminutive genitalia

**E** lower abdominal mass that increases in size over time

**A10** **A** Bladder exstrophy is difficult to distinguish on prenatal ultrasound and can be confused with omphalocele or gastroschisis. Several reviews have identified prenatal ultrasound criteria that corroborate the diagnosis of bladder exstrophy, including a low-set umbilicus, absence of bladder filling, widening of the pubic rami, diminutive genitalia, and a lower abdominal mass that increases in size over the course of the pregnancy.

**Q11** Advantages in performing pelvic osteotomies at the time of initial closure include:

**A** easy closure of the pubic symphysis

**B** decreased tension on the abdominal wall closure

**C** placement of urethra deep within pelvic ring

**D** bringing pelvic floor muscles near the midline for increased bladder neck support

**E** all of the above.

**A11** **E** Pelvic osteotomy at the time of initial bladder-exstrophy closure offers a number of advantages including easy approximation of the pubic symphysis with decreased tension on the abdominal wall closure and elimination of the need for fascial flaps; placement of the urethra deep within the pelvis, which enhances bladder outlet resistance; and bringing the pelvic floor muscles near the midline where they can support the bladder neck and potentiate urinary control.

**Q12** The most important criterion for selecting a patient for immediate exstrophy closure in the newborn period is:

    **A** an adequate phallic size

    **B** a narrow pubic diastasis

    **C** a large potential bladder capacity

    **D** the position of the anus in relation to the bladder

    **E** the presence of vesicoureteral reflux on preoperative imaging.

**A12** **C** The potential functional capacity of the bladder is probably the most important consideration for successful closure. The bladder plate itself may appear small but will demonstrate adequate capacity by bulging when the child cries or by indenting when touched under general anaesthesia. While the other criteria listed are important considerations when reconstructing an exstrophy patient, they do not dictate whether a patient should be closed in the newborn period.

**Q13** Which of the following is not true of the modern staged reconstruction of bladder exstrophy?

    **A** early bladder, posterior urethral, and abdominal wall closure

    **B** bladder neck repair at the time of bladder closure

    **C** early epispadias repair at 6–12 months of age

    **D** conversion of the bladder exstrophy to a complete epispadias with the initial closure

    **E** creation of pelvic osteotomies at the time of intial closure

**A13** **B** Many modifications have been made to the surgical approach to exstrophy closure over the past decades. The primary principles associated with the modern staged repair include early closure of the bladder and abdominal wall, essentially converting the male patient into a complete epispadias, and delaying the epispadias repair until 6–12 months of age to allow for adequate phallic growth. Bladder neck repair may be delayed to as late as 4 or 5 years of age when the patient can participate in toilet training, although reconstruction of the bladder neck is typically attempted earlier in life to allow for bladder cycling. Ureteral reimplantation is usually performed at the time of bladder neck reconstruction.

**Q14** Reconstruction of epispadias includes which of the following goals?

    **A** chordee correction

    **B** urethral reconstruction

    **C** penile lengthening

    **D** glans reconstruction

    **E** all of the above

**A14** **E** Various repairs for reconstructing epispadias have been described, including Cantwell–Ransley's repair, the modified Cantwell–Ransley repair and the penile disassembly technique. Regardless of which method is used, the primary principles of epispadias closure remain the same: correction of dorsal chordee, urethral reconstruction, glanular reconstruction, penile lengthening and penile skin closure.

**Q15** Which of the following is not a presentation of cloacal exstrophy?
    **A** exstrophy of the bladder halves
    **B** exstrophy of the caecum
    **C** complete phallis/clitoral separation
    **D** imperforate anus
    **E** omphalocele

**A15** **B** Like bladder exstrophy, cloacal exstrophy is an anterior abdominal wall defect but presents with a more severe spectrum of abnormalities. The incidence is much rarer, with 1 : 200 000 to 1 : 400 000 live births. The hallmark anomalies associated with this entity include: exstrophy of the bladder as two separate halves, complete phallic or clitoral separation, a wide pubic diastasis, exstrophy of the terminal ileum with a separate rudimentary hindgut, imperforate anus and omphalocele. Patients may have additional associated neurospinal and lower extremity defects.

## Further reading

Caldamone AA, Woodard JR. Prune belly syndrome. In: Wein AJ, Kavoussi LR, Novick AC, *et al*. *Campbell-Walsh Urology*. 9th ed. Philadelphia, PA: Saunders Elsevier; 2007.

Ebert AK, Reutter H, Ludwig M, *et al*. The exstrophy-epispadias complex. *Orphanet J Rare Dis*. 2009; **4**: 23.

Gearhart JP, Mathews R. Exstrophy-epispadias complex. In: Wein AJ, Kavoussi LR, Novick AC, *et al. Campbell-Walsh Urology*. 9th ed. Philadelphia, PA: Saunders Elsevier; 2007. pp. 3497–553.

Grady RW, Mitchell ME. Surgical techniques for one-stage reconstruction of the exstrophy-epispadias complex. In: Wein AJ, Kavoussi LR, Novick AC, *et al. Campbell-Walsh Urology*. 9th ed. Philadelphia, PA: Saunders Elsevier; 2007. pp. 3554–72.

Marshall VF, Muecke EC. Variation in exstrophy of the bladder. *J Urol*. 1962; **88**: 766–96.

Routh JC, Huang L, Retik AB, *et al*. Contemporary epidemiology and characterization of newborn males with prune belly syndrome. *Urology*. 2010; **76**(1): 44–8.

# CHAPTER 67

# Gynaecological disorders in children

## LISA M ALLEN, RACHEL F SPITZER

From the choices below each question, select the single best answer.

**Q1** Which of the following is true regarding labial adhesions?
- **A** The incidence of labial adhesions is 2%–7%.
- **B** Labial adhesions are an indication of previous sexual abuse.
- **C** Labial adhesions occur as frequently in postpubertal girls as in prepubertal girls.
- **D** Labial adhesions occur congenitally.
- **E** The peak incidence of labial adhesions is at 5–6 years of age.

**A1** **A** Labial adhesions (also known as labial agglutination) occur in prepubertal girls with a peak incidence at 13–23 months of age, but can occur as early as 3 months and up to 6 years of age. The overall incidence of labial adhesions in prepubertal girls is 1.8%–7% but may be higher in select populations. The pathophysiology of labial adhesions may involve poorly regulated wound-healing, with re-epithelialisation resulting in an avascular adhesion, essentially cross healing areas of denuded epithelium and fusing the labia minora which are naturally in close apposition. Labial adhesions are associated with any condition that traumatises, irritates or inflames the unoestrogenised prepubertal labia; for example, vulvovaginitis, dermatological conditions, local irritants and recurrent diarrhoea. Labial agglutination is a non-specific vulvovaginal condition and therefore is not a definite indicator of sexual abuse. Labial adhesions that occur after puberty are much less common; they are usually a result of trauma or a surgical procedure to the labia and are hence of a different pathophysiology.

**Q2** Which of the following is true regarding the treatment of labial adhesions?

**A** Manual separation of labial adhesions has a lower recurrence rate than topical oestrogen therapy.

**B** Treatment is uniformly applied to all children presenting with labial adhesions.

**C** Children presenting at older ages are more likely to fail topical oestrogen therapy

**D** Topical oestrogen therapy is successful in 10%–20% of children.

**E** Topical oestrogen therapy is poorly tolerated with a high incidence of side effects.

**A2** **C** Treatment of labial adhesions is generally reserved for patients who are symptomatic, i.e. with urinary tract infections, altered voiding such as urinary dribbling or incontinence, or almost complete occlusion. It is not clear if treatment of labial adhesions prevents the development of asymptomatic bacteruria and subsequent development of urinary tract infections. When adhesions involve almost the entire labia, treatment is often offered to avoid the development of symptoms. Occasionally treatment will be initiated to allay parental concerns and allow demonstration of normal genital anatomy. Adhesions may resolve spontaneously with correction of vulvar hygiene, and application of a bland emollient to act as a barrier cream. Treatment of persistent or symptomatic adhesions includes either parental application of topical oestrogen cream daily or twice daily over 2–6 weeks or surgical separation of the adhesions under anaesthesia. Resolution rates with medical therapy range from 47% to 91%. Topical oestrogen therapy is well tolerated with minimal local side effects of vulvar irritation and/or pigmentation or with systemic absorption. Breast budding occurs in 5% of patients. Both medical and surgical therapy have high rates of recurrence: 19%–33% for medical therapy and 17%–40% after manual separation. Post-separation use of topical oestrogen may decrease recurrence rates. Risk factors for failure of medical therapy are related to thicker and longer duration of adhesions (age greater than 6, thickness >3–4 mm) or associated with persistent irritating factors.

**Q3** A 4-year-old presents with a history of recurrent brown vaginal discharge, associated with odour. It has recurred despite multiple courses of oral antibiotic therapy with amoxicillin. What is the next most appropriate step?

**A** Consult child protective services.

**B** Perform a vulvar biopsy.

**C** Flush or irrigate the vagina.

**D** Prescribe an antifungal cream.

**E** Prescribe a course of trimethoprim and sulfamethoxazole.

**A3**   **C**   Foreign bodies often are diagnosed after a prolonged period (up to a year or more) of persistent or recurrent vaginal discharge. The discharge is typically either brown or bloody. Eighty per cent of vaginal foreign bodies are small pieces of toilet paper. Toilet paper can be flushed from the vagina successfully in cooperative patients. Older children (mean age of 7 years) tend to be more compliant with office vaginal irrigation performed with a paediatric catheter or feeding tube and a syringe. Foreign bodies should be suspected: if discharge is refractory to implementation of appropriate hygiene measures and antibiotic therapy, if discharge is bloody or if there is a history of previous foreign body placement. A foreign body will be recovered in up to 10% of girls taken for vaginoscopy under anaesthesia with symptoms suspicious for one.

The differential diagnosis of a patient with vaginal discharge includes non-specific vulvitis, infectious vaginitis, lichen sclerosis, atopic dermatitis and other dermatoses. Recurrent discharge that is specifically bloody suggests a foreign body. Prepubertal girls with unoestrogenised genitalia rarely have yeast vaginitis, unless they have a predisposing factor such as immunocompromisation, diabetes or are still wearing nappies. Non-specific vulvitis generally responds well to improved vulvar hygiene measures.

In regard to specific vaginal infections, shigella can cause an acute vaginitis associated with bloody vaginal discharge. Shigella is more common in communities where infection is endemic. Transmitted by the faecal–oral route it may also produce severe diarrhoea and fever associated with either a mesenteric adenitis or acute terminal ileitis. Shigella is treated with sulfa antibiotics. The most common causes of infectious vaginitis are the upper respiratory tract pathogens: streptococcccus group A and *Haemophilus influenzae*; both usually present with an acute course, with profuse vaginal discharge and associated severe vulvar and vaginal erythema. Chlamydia and gonorrhoea do produce vaginitis in prepubertal girls, and may present with vaginal discharge. The prevalence of sexually transmitted infections in sexually abused children is low; chlamydia rectovaginal infection rates range from 4% to 17% of abused children. If a sexually transmitted infection is suspected, culture remains the preferred method of documentation of infection to limit the risk of false positive tests in a low prevalence population. Cultures should be obtained from any suspected site of penetration (oral, genital, rectal). If a nucleic acid amplification test (NAAT) is performed, a positive result should be confirmed by a second different NAAT test.

Q4  The following image represents the findings in a 5-year-old girl who presents to the emergency department with a history of genital trauma. In taking a history, which of the following mechanisms of injury would not be consistent with the pattern of injuries seen?

A  fall on an upturned chair leg

B  fall straddling a cross bar on a bicycle

C  penetrating water injury from a jet of water

D  fall on a toy with a sharp narrow edge

E  a motor vehicle accident with pelvic fracture

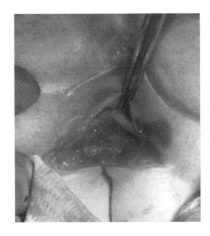

FIGURE 67.1 Penetrating injury to vagina

A4  **B**  The most common mechanism of genital trauma is a straddle injury. A straddle injury causes perineal trauma as a result of falling or striking an object or surface with the force of one's body, crushing the soft tissue between the object and the bony margins of the pelvic outlet. In a straddle or blunt injury the object is not capable of penetrating above the pelvic floor. Straddle injuries are the most common mechanism of injury in the 5- to 9-year-old age group of girls. Penetrating injuries can be accidental or intentional (i.e. related to sexual abuse). Penetrating injuries comprise only 3%–20% of accidental genital injuries. The pattern of injuries seen with a straddle injury and a penetrating injury of the vagina vary. Either type of injury can involve the posterior fourchette. Straddle injuries tend to demonstrate ecchymosis, linear abrasions or lacerations and haematomas from extravasation of blood into the loose areolar tissues of the mons, clitoris and labia. Hymenal and vaginal injuries are far more common with penetrating injuries, with hymenal involvement in 40%–80% of penetrating injuries. In the image above, a laceration extending into and involving the hymen is evident. Hence the mechanism of injury is likely penetrating. The mechanism of genital injury taken on history from either a verbal child or their caretaker should be plausible, timely and most importantly consistent with the findings evident on physical examination. As a fall straddling a crossbar of a bicycle would be of a straddle-injury type without a mechanism for penetration, and as the examination reveals a laceration of the hymen extending into the vaginal mucosa, the history and examination would be inconsistent. A lack of correlation between the history and physical findings is an indication to consider a sexual abuse evaluation. Each of the other options listed above could result in hymenal and vaginal lacerations.

**Q5** Surgical management of genital trauma is more likely if:
  A  the child is less than 5 years old
  B  the patient presents within an hour of the injury
  C  the size of the laceration is equal to or more than 1 cm
  D  the size of the laceration is equal to or more than 2.5 cm
  E  the mechanism of injury is a straddle type.

**A5**  D  Surgical management of genital trauma is required in 5%–37% of all cases. The severity of injury varies with the mechanism of the injury and not the age of the patient. More severe trauma occurs from motor vehicle injuries, followed by abuse or assault, with the least severe injuries being those from straddle mechanisms. A review of the factors associated with surgical repair in a tertiary care centre demonstrated that surgical repair was significantly associated with injuries that were of a penetrating type and hence involved the hymen. In addition, the mean size of lacerations that required surgical repair was 2.88 cm, compared with a mean size of 0.9 cm for those who were managed with secondary healing.

**Q6** A 5-year-old is referred for assessment of vaginal bleeding with the following finding evident on examination – *see* Figure 67.2. Which statement is true regarding the treatment of this diagnosis?
  A  90% of patients will require surgical management.
  B  Medical therapy includes topical testosterone twice daily.
  C  Prepubertal patients are more likely to fail medical therapy.
  D  Referral to child protective services is mandatory.
  E  If >15–30 mm in size, surgery is more likely.

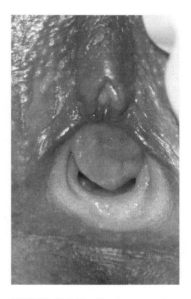

**FIGURE 67.2 Urethral mucosal prolapse**

**A6**  E  Urethral mucosal prolapse has an incidence of 1 : 2880 children; it is more common between the ages of 4 and 8 years, and it varies with ethnicity. The presenting symptom is usually painless bleeding without interference of voiding patterns. Described as an annular, congested or oedematous, anteriorly placed introital mass, it is the protrusion of the urethral mucosa beyond the urethral meatus. Once prolapsed, the muscular tone of the urethral meatus constricts the tissue circumferentially resulting in the oedema, congestion and in some circumstances necrosis of the mucosal tissue.

It is thought that several factors contribute to the prolapse. First, there may be anatomical defects with poor adhesion of the urethral mucosa to the underlying smooth muscles of the urethra. Often there is a precipitating event such as an increase in intra-abdominal pressure from conditions including constipation and straining for bowel movements, or an upper respiratory tract infection and accompanying cough or crying. This precipitating event, when occurring in a susceptible child with prepubertal/unoestrogenised tissue, results in prolapse of the tissue. While the physical findings are often confused for abuse, it is not related to sexual abuse. Medical therapy with topical oestrogen therapy and sitz baths with or without antibiotic treatment will resolve the prolapse in 33%–70% of cases. Surgery, which involves excision of the prolapsed mucosa, is indicated when medical therapy fails, in patients with profuse bleeding, when the mucosa is necrosed, when the prolapse is particularly large (15–30 mm diameter), and in postpubertal patients.

In regard to patients presenting with vaginal bleeding, the differential diagnosis in a prepubertal girl includes vaginitis, foreign body (as discussed in detail for question (3), premature puberty or premature menarche, genital trauma or abuse (*see* questions 4 and 5), skin conditions such as lichen sclerosis with excoriations, urethral mucosal prolapse and vaginal/cervical rhabdomyosarcoma. These diagnoses can be distinguished on history, physical exam and investigations.

 **Q7** A 7-year-old girl presents for consideration of surgical excision of anogenital warts. Which of the following would *not* be appropriate to recommend at the first consultation?

**A** human papilloma virus (HPV) typing to determine mode of transmission

**B** a trial of topical therapy with imiquimod

**C** a trial of topical therapy with 0.5% podophyllotoxin solution

**D** expectant management

**E** referral to child protective services for assessment of potential abuse

 **A7** **A** The mean age of presentation for anogenital warts (AGW) in children varies between 2.8 and 5.6 years. The most common area of involvement is perianal with up to 70% of AGW occurring in that distribution; 23% involve the vulva. The possible modes of transmission for HPV and AGW are: vertical transmission, sexual abuse and non-sexual contact (autoinoculation or heteroinoculation). Studies have documented that HPV types are not predictive of the mode of transmission in children. HPV types are evenly distributed between mucosal, cutaneous and mucocutaneous types in childhood AGW, demonstrating less site specificity than HPV in adults. HPV typing of AGW is therefore not recommended. The proportion of AGW attributed to sexual abuse varies from 3% to 50%. One study of children referred to paediatric surgery for surgical excision of AGW had 47% of their cases attributed to abuse after assessment by a multidisciplinary team. The older the child, the greater the likelihood that abuse is the mechanism of transmission. Compared with a child aged 0–4 years, a child presenting with AGW between 4 and 8 years of age has a 2.9-fold increased likelihood of abuse, and between 8 and 12 years of age this increases to a 12.1-fold increased risk. The American Academy of Pediatrics recommends referral to child protective services for all children with AGW, while other opinions recommend referral if any investigation reveals concerns of abuse, or for children aged over 4–5 years. Given that this child presented at 7 years of age, a referral to child protective services is appropriate on that criterion alone. Prior to considering surgical excision, expectant and medical therapy should be considered. Spontaneous resolution of AGW occurs in up to 75% of children with healthy immune systems within 3–5 years. Multiple treatment modalities may be necessary to effect resolution of AGW. Decisions on the appropriate treatment option should take into account ability to comply with office vs. home treatment, the number of lesions, the cost, the location of lesions, the discomfort associated with treatment and the side effects of treatment. Paediatric studies are available to support topical treatments with podophyllotoxin 0.5% solution/0.15% cream and imiquimod. Regardless of the selected treatment, recurrence rates are similar (20%–30%).

 **8** Which is correct regarding the development of the müllerian ducts *in utero?*

**A** müllerian ducts develop at 9 weeks of gestational age.

**B** müllerian ducts reach the urogenital sinus at 9 weeks of gestational age.

**C** müllerian ducts fuse at 9 weeks of gestational age.

**D** müllerian ducts are of endodermal origin.

**E** müllerian ducts develop in the presence of müllerian inhibiting substance.

 **8** **B** The müllerian ducts are of mesodermal origin. They develop into the structures of the female genital tract (fallopian tubes, uterus, cervix and upper vagina). The lower vagina is of endodermal origin arising from the urogenital sinus. (The ovaries are of a completely separate embryologic origin, migrating from the gonadal ridge.) The elongating müllerian ducts, which develop at 6 weeks of gestational age, lie lateral to the wolffian ducts until they reach the caudal end of the mesonephros. At this point their course shifts medially to reach the midline in the area of the cloaca. At 9 weeks of gestational age, the müllerian ducts elongate caudally to reach the urogenital sinus, inserting at the müllerian tubercle. The müllerian ducts fuse at 12 weeks of gestational age to form a single tube (which will form uterus, cervix and upper vagina). Canalisation of the solid vaginal plate follows, a process that is complete by the fifth month of gestation. The midline septum in the uterus, cervix and upper vagina is resorbed to create a single cavity by 20 weeks of gestational age. The most distal aspect of the sinovaginal bulbs proliferates to form the hymen, which becomes perforate prior to birth. Müllerian anomalies are a result of failure of one of the above processes of embryogenesis and can be summarised as a failure of organogenesis, vertical fusion, lateral fusion or resorption.

**Q9** The most common age for presentation of a completely obstructing outflow tract anomaly of the female genital tract is:

**A** 10 years

**B** 12 years

**C** 15 years

**D** 17 years

**E** 20 years.

**A9** **B** The usual triad of symptoms associated with a completely obstructing outflow tract (imperforate hymen, transverse vaginal septum, partial vaginal agenesis or cervical agenesis) is cyclical abdominal pain, amenorrhoea and a pelvic/abdominal mass. The time of presentation is at the onset of menarche. Symptoms hence usually present around age 12 (average age of menarche), or 2 years after the onset of thelarche (the usual interval between onset of thelarche and onset of menarche). The diagnosis of outflow tract anomalies is often delayed by up to 12 months from onset of symptoms.

**Q10** An adolescent presents with a complete genital outflow tract obstruction. Of the following müllerian anomalies, which diagnosis is most likely?

**A** cervical agenesis

**B** partial vaginal agenesis

**C** transverse vaginal septum

**D** uterine didelphys

**E** unicornuate uterus

**A10** **C** Transverse vaginal septums, partial vaginal agenesis and cervical agenesis are all in the differential diagnosis of a completely obstructed outflow tract. The most common of these is the transverse vaginal septum. Transverse vaginal septums have an incidence of 1 : 21 000 to 1 : 70 000. Cervical agenesis occurs in 1 : 80 000. While both uterine didelphys and unicornuate uteri are more common than a transverse septum, with incidences of 1 : 1828 and 1 : 5400, respectively, neither cause a complete obstruction of the genital outflow tract.

An imperforate hymen is the most common diagnosis resulting in an obstructed outflow tract with an incidence of 0.1%. However, as the hymen is an embryologic septum between the urogenital sinus and the sinovaginal bulbs, it is technically not considered a müllerian anomaly. An imperforate hymen can be easily diagnosed on vaginal exam as, in addition to the symptom triad detailed above, physical exam of the perineum usually reveals a thin, bulging membrane with a bluish hue of obstructed blood behind it. (Imperforate hymens should always be addressed in the operating room.) Complete genital tract obstruction from any müllerian anomaly would present without an obvious bulge on perineal exam.

**Q11** Which of the following anomaly and surgical repair pairings reflects the appropriate management for the genital anomaly listed?

**A** partial vaginal agenesis – hysterectomy

**B** partial vaginal agenesis – mobilisation and pull-through of haematocolpos

**C** uterine didelphys with obstructing hemivaginal septum – hysterectomy

**D** transverse vaginal septum – needle drainage and tract dilatation

**E** cervical agenesis – needle drainage and tract dilatation

**A11** **B** A general guide is that obstructed anomalies with cryptomenorrhoea resulting in haematocolpos or haematometria should not be subject to drainage procedures unless definitive surgical repair is being undertaken, because of the risk of introducing bacteria and subsequent infection of the upper genital tract. Drainage and dilatation of the drainage channel are inadequate means of recreating patent outflow tracts and hence are not advised for management of any müllerian anomaly.

Most transverse vaginal septums are less than 1 cm in thickness, and can be managed either with primary surgical excision and reanastomosis of the upper and lower vaginal mucosal edges or with mobilisation of the upper haematocolpos, pulling the upper mobilised vaginal mucosa inferiorly and reanastomosing this to the lower vaginal mucosa. This mobilisation, pull-through and reanastomosis is applied to thicker vaginal septums and/or partial vaginal agenesis. Stenting the vagina after surgical repair is mandatory to prevent stricture formation at the site of mucosal reanastomosis. Hysterectomy is not required for vaginal obstruction by transverse septum, nor for partial vaginal agenesis where continuity of the outflow tract can be reliably re-established.

Uterine didelphys with an obstructing hemivaginal septum is surgically corrected by resecting the hemivaginal septum.

Surgical management of the rare cervical agenesis case is more controversial. Traditionally, hysterectomy was offered. More recently, successful uterovaginal anastomosis has been reported in several small case series. Referral to centres of excellence is recommended for management of these infrequent anomalies, to optimise outcomes.

In the management of any outflow tract obstruction, menstrual suppression can be prescribed to manage pain symptoms while awaiting definitive surgical management. Menstrual suppression can be achieved with continuous combined hormonal contraceptives, depo-medroxyprogesterone acetate or gonadotropin-releasing hormone agonists with addback combined hormonal replacement.

**Q12** In the investigation of a patient with Mayer–Rokitansky–Küster–Hauser's (MRKH) syndrome, besides the genital abnormalities of absent uterus, cervix and vagina, the investigation most likely to diagnose an associated abnormality is:

**A** audiogram

**B** echocardiogram

**C** karyotype

**D** renal ultrasound

**E** skeletal survey

**A12** **D** MRKH syndrome or müllerian agenesis is the second most common cause of primary amenorrhoea, with an incidence of 1 : 4000. These patients have a normal 46,XX karyotype and normal gonadal function, hence commence puberty with their peers. A blind-ended lower vagina of variable length will be evident on physical examination. Tanner staging for breast and pubic hair will be appropriate for the stage of puberty and congruent with each other.

The diagnosis is confirmed when the anatomical abnormality is demonstrated on imaging. Pelvic ultrasound is often the first modality, but magnetic resonance imaging is considered the gold standard for diagnosis. The major differential diagnosis is androgen insensitivity syndrome (AIS). In AIS, however, women will have an absence of sexual hair, hence there will be a discordance between Tanner staging of pubic hair and breast development. Karyotyping will show a 46,XY configuration and androgens will be in the normal male range.

Sixty-four per cent of women with MRKH syndrome will have a typical presentation with no associated anomalies. The most common anomalies associated with MRKH syndrome are those of the urinary tract. Renal agenesis, pelvic kidney, horseshoe kidney, hydronephrosis, hydroureter and ureteral duplication have all been reported. The overall incidence of renal anomalies is in the range of 36%. Less commonly in MRKH patients, skeletal abnormalities (wedge vertebrae, fused vertebrae, rudimentary vertebral bodies, supernumerary vertebrae, clinodactyly, hypoplastic radius, scaphoid, trapezium) and cardiac anomalies (mitral valve prolapse, mitral regurgitation, ventricular septal defects, truncus arteriosus, patent ductus arteriosus, patent foramen ovale) can be demonstrated in 28% and 16%, respectively. Other less common associations are hernias, unilateral hearing impairment, and unilateral ovarian agenesis. The high incidence of renal anomalies is speculated to be related to the close proximity (during embryogenesis) of the mesonephric and müllerian duct primordiums, and accounts for the fact that, overall, renal anomalies are present in approximately 25% of patients with any müllerian anomaly. Disruption in the development of one system is presumed to lead to maldevelopment or agenesis of the contiguous structures.

Klippel–Feil's syndrome is the association of congenital fusion of the cervical spine, short neck, low posterior hairline and painless limitations of cervical movement associated with uterine and vaginal agenesis. 'MURCS association' refers to müllerian duct aplasia, renal aplasia and cervicothoracic somite dysplasia.

The knowledge of these associated abnormalities guides the investigations when the diagnosis of MRKH is confirmed. Renal imaging and a skeletal survey is recommended. Karyotyping is often performed during the investigations of primary amenorrhoea. Audiogram and echocardiogram can be performed selectively based on the individual medical history and physical examination.

**Q13** An adolescent is brought to the operating room for a diagnostic laparoscopy to investigate persistent dysmenorrhoea despite treatment with anti-inflammatory and oral contraceptive pills over the preceding 3 months. The most likely diagnosis at the time of diagnostic laparoscopy would be:

**A** endometriosis

**B** ovarian torsion

**C** pelvic inflammatory disease

**D** unicornuate uterus with functional rudimentary horn

**E** uterine didelphys with obstructing hemivaginal septum.

**A13** **A** Only 10% of dysmenorrhoea in adolescent is of secondary aetiology. The remainder is defined as primary dysmenorrhoea, related to ovulatory cycles with prostaglandin production leading to myometrial contraction and uterine ischaemia. In adolescents who have pain unresponsive to conservative management with non-steroidal anti-inflammatories (NSAIDs) and/or combined hormonal therapy, up to 69% will be diagnosed with endometriosis at diagnostic laparoscopy. Endometriosis is hence the most common aetiology of secondary dysmenorrhoea. Endometriosis in adolescents is often atypical in appearance, compared with the typical powder-burn lesions seen in adults. Vesicles, flame-like lesions and white lesions predominate. The extent of endometriosis is often restricted to earlier stages; stage I and stage II ASRM (American Society of Reproductive Medicine) disease is found in 61%–92% and 8%–23%, respectively, of laparoscopies in adolescents and young adult women. The stage of visible disease, however, does not necessarily correlate with the degree of symptomatology in patients of any age.

Müllerian anomalies such as the unilaterally obstructed outflow tracts (unicornuate uterus with a functional rudimentary horn and uterine didelphys with obstructing hemivaginal septum), are responsible for only 6%–8% of chronic pain in adolescents. Unicornuate uteri are a result of a failure of organogenesis with absence of development of one müllerian duct. In 74% of cases the arrest is incomplete and a rudimentary horn is evident. These rudimentary horns may or may not have a functional endometrium and may be communicating or not. Horns that contain functional endometrium and are both non-communicating present as secondary dysmenorrhoea due to the cryptomenorrhoea. Twenty-six per cent of horns are in this category and are candidates for surgical excision.

A uterine didelphys is a result of failure of lateral fusion. Longitudinal vaginal septums are commonly associated with didelphic uteri, demonstrable in 75% of these anomalies. When the septum is asymmetrical and obstructs one side, this is known as OHVIRA (obstructed hemivagina, ipsilateral renal anomaly) syndrome. Eighty-nine per cent of didelphic uteri with an obstructing septum have an ipsilateral renal anomaly, most commonly renal agenesis.

Ovarian torsion is an important differential diagnosis of acute pelvic pain, though would not be associated with the persistent dysmenorrhoea in the given case. Complications of sexual activity should always be considered in the adolescent with pelvic pain, i.e. pelvic inflammatory disease, ectopic pregnancies and other early pregnancy complications. Pelvic inflammatory disease can present with new-onset dysmenorrhoea as well as with acute pelvic pain.

**Q14** The imaging modality which will best distinguish between a bicornuate uterus and a septate uterus is:

**A** hysterosalpingogram

**B** hysterosonogram

**C** transabdominal pelvic ultrasound

**D** transvaginal pelvic ultrasound

**E** magnetic resonance imaging.

**A14** **E** A bicornuate uterus is the result of a failure of lateral fusion; a septate uterus is the result of failure of resorption of the central septum once the paired müllerian ducts fuse. Septate uteri have the highest incidence of reproductive complications of all the müllerian anomalies. The poor pregnancy-continuation rates are attributed to the fibrous and avascular septum as well as the defective septal endometrium. Surgical correction of the septate uterus may be accomplished by hysteroscopic division of the septum with subsequent significant improvement in reproductive outcomes. It is important to establish the correct diagnosis – between a septate uterus and a bicornuate uterus – prior to planning surgical repair. No surgical intervention is indicated for the bicornuate uterus. An imaging modality that can accurately assess the external contour of the uterus is essential. While hysterosalpingography and hysterosonography can provide considerable information regarding the interior of the uterine cavity, MRI is superior for determining the external contour. The two anomalies can be distinguished with the following criteria: intercornual distance (4 cm with bicornuate uterus, 2–4 cm with septate uteri), fundal indentation (>1 cm with bicornate uterus) and angle of uterine horns (>105 degrees with bicornuate, <75 degrees with septate uteri). In general, MRI has become the method of choice for assessing anatomical abnormalities of the upper female genital tract.

**Q15** Which of the following statements is true regarding fetal ovarian cysts?
- **A** Between 25% and 70% will develop complexity during the ante-natal period
- **B** Caesarean section should be recommended as the mode of delivery.
- **C** Surgical management is recommended in the neonatal period due to the risk of malignancy in antenatally diagnosed ovarian cysts.
- **D** Complex neonatal ovarian cysts do not resolve with expectant management.
- **E** Simple cysts less than 4 cm in size should be resected.

**A15** **A** The antenatal discovery of a fetal ovarian cyst is infrequent with an incidence of 1 : 2625 pregnancies. The diagnosis is presumptive antenatally, based on the identification of a cystic, non-peristaltic structure in the lower abdomen of a female fetus. Sonographic demonstration of the integrity of the urinary and gastrointestinal tracts separate from the cystic structure supports the diagnosis. While these cysts have been diagnosed as early as 19 weeks of gestational age, the most common gestational age at diagnosis is 33 weeks. Ninety-seven per cent of these cysts are functional, and are speculated to be the result of fol-licular stimulation of the fetal ovary by placental hCG, maternal oestrogens or fetal gonadotropins. There are only rare case reports of ovarian pathology in the neonatal period: cystadenomas, cystic teratomas and granulosa cell tumours. The natural history of these antenatally diagnosed ovarian cysts *in utero* is the development of complexity prior to delivery in 25%–70%. Complex cysts typically represent *in utero* torsion or haemorrhage. While soft tissue dystocia is possible (from abdominal distension related to the ovarian cyst), it is rare and most authors advocate reserving caesarean delivery for obstetrical indications only. Because the vast majority of these ovarian cysts represent functional cysts, management in the neonatal period is not guided by risk of malignancy. Both simple and complex cysts have been demonstrated to resolve spontaneously with observation; 86% of simple cysts may resolve as well as 54% of those that are complex, though com-plex cysts usually take longer to resolve. On follow-up imaging after complex cyst resolution, often no ovary is evident on the ipsilateral side, presumed to reflect an atretic ovary that reabsorbed subsequent to an *in utero* torsion. Neonatal cysts will sometimes be noted on imaging to alternate location in the abdomen, reflecting their mobile nature (some are autoamputated from *in utero* torsion).

For expectant management to be adopted in the neonatal period, the cyst should be confirmed to be ovarian on postnatal imaging, no solid components should be present aside from debris/clot/septation consistent with haemorrhage or *in utero* torsion, the infant should be asymptomatic and tumour markers should be normal for age. The family must also be able to commit to the serial imaging required to monitor cyst resolution. Patients with cysts that are simple and large (over 4–5 cm in size) can be offered postnatal ultrasound-guided needle aspiration in an attempt to reduce the risk of postnatal torsion and to avoid surgical management. Cysts less than this size are most often followed expectantly. If surgery is undertaken, it should be the least invasive, and most conservative, i.e. minimally invasive approaches, with ovarian preservation (ovarian fenestration or cystectomy).

Q16 An otherwise healthy 7-year-old girl presents with fever, a 24-hour history of colicky left lower abdominal pain and synchronous onset of nausea and vomiting. An ultrasound reveals a unilaterally enlarged left ovary (4 cm). There is no focal mass within the left ovary. Multiple peripheral cysts of 8–15 mm containing fluid-debris levels are located within the ovary. Venous flow is absent and arterial flow is decreased to the left ovary. The most appropriate management plan is:

**A** magnetic resonance imaging to confirm or refute diagnosis of ovarian torsion

**B** urgent laparoscopic exploration with plan for detorsion and conservation of the left ovary

**C** urgent laparoscopic exploration with plan for oophorectomy of left ovary given the 24-hour duration of symptoms

**D** elective laparoscopic exploration with plan for oophorectomy of left ovary given the 24-hour duration of symptoms

**E** elective laparotomy after tumour markers and CT scan of the abdomen to assess for malignancy, with plan for staging laparotomy.

A16 **B** Ovarian torsion is a clinical diagnosis. The usual symptoms are colicky lower quadrant pain, often unilateral with radiation to the flank or groin. Nausea and vomiting are present in up to 83% of torsions, and occur with the onset of pain. About 20%–40% of children will have a history of similar episodes of pain within the 4 months preceding presentation, reflecting possible intermittent torsion. Only a third of children will have a palpable mass on examination. Findings of peritoneal signs, fever and leucocytosis occur late in the course of torsion and may be associated with a higher risk of tissue necrosis. Ultrasound imaging assists the diagnosis. The most consistent finding on greyscale ultrasound is ovarian enlargement. An ovary with a volume <20 mL in one series had a 100% negative predictive value for torsion. The presence of peripheral cysts with fluid–debris levels, is thought to be related to transudation of fluid into follicles and intrafollicular haemorrhage as the ovary becomes congested after the interruption of perfusion. The sensitivity of these findings on imaging ranges from 64% to 85%, with a specificity of 97%. While absent or decreased arterial and venous flow on Doppler imaging is suggestive of ovarian torsion, it should be noted that flow may be preserved.

In children, an ovarian mass as a lead point for adnexal torsion is not uniformly present; approximately 20% of torsions in the childhood age group occur in normal adnexae. Excessive mobility of the adnexae due to long ovarian ligaments in the prepubertal patient has been postulated as the aetiology of these normal ovarian torsions. Further, it is rare for malignancies to tort and consequently only <5% of torsions have an underlying malignant aetiology. The more common pathologies associated with adnexal torsion are: dermoid cysts, functional cysts, paratubal or paraovarian cysts and cystadenomas.

While the rate of conservation of ovaries decreases with delayed surgery (from symptom onset), there are numerous paediatric references demonstrating the preservation of function in ovaries judged moderately to severely ischaemic at time of surgery; hence, urgent surgical management, with detorsion and ovarian preservation, is indicated. Rarely, another procedure may be required to remove a necrotic ovary at a later time or follow-up imaging may demonstrate a lack of ovarian function, but more often than not ovarian preservation will result in a functional ovary. Some aspects of surgical management that remain debatable are the role of oophoropexy in the management of normal ovarian torsion, and the timing of ovarian cystectomy in the severely ischaemic ovary. The overall rate of repeat torsion in childhood is increased from 5% to 11% if there is no associated ovarian pathology. However, oophoropexy may interfere with adnexal blood supply and create a risk of mechanical infertility from distorting tubal/ovarian anatomy. One retrospective case series (Oelsner *et al.*, 2003) demonstrated a higher rate of ovarian dysfunction in children and adolescents where an immediate ovarian cystectomy was performed coincident with a detorsion procedure. The authors therefore cautioned that in the severely ischaemic ovary detorsion alone with subsequent cystectomy at a second procedure could be considered.

Q17 Which of the following statements is correct regarding haemorrhagic ovarian cysts?

A The frequency of occurrence is equal in premenarcheal and post-menarcheal populations.

B They do not usually occur in the absence of medical co-morbidities.

C The usual timing of presentation is the luteal phase of the menstrual cycle.

D The symptoms of presentation are indistinguishable from ovarian torsion.

E Surgical management is usually required with possible need for oophorectomy to control haemorrhage.

A17 C Functional ovarian cysts result from failure of the maturing follicle to ovulate and involute, or may reflect persistence of the corpus luteum. These cysts are often simple on ultrasound, with thin walls. They are benign and self-limited, often regressing within 2–3 menstrual cycles. These cysts do not cause pain unless they rupture, haemorrhage or lead to torsion and may be incidental findings on imaging.

Haemorrhagic cysts are complicated functional cysts. Following ovulation, both the luteinised theca cells and the granulosa cell layer of the follicle become vascularised. The vessels are fragile and may rupture leading to haemorrhage. Because they are associated with ovulation, they are rare in the premenarcheal patient. A haemorrhagic ovarian cyst often presents with an abrupt onset of lower abdominal or pelvic pain midcycle or in the luteal phase without fever or leucocytosis. If the cyst wall ruptures, a haemoperitoneum may develop and peritoneal signs or postural hypotension may be evident on examination. Haemorrhagic cysts occur in healthy patients but are predisposed in patients with bleeding diatheses, on anticoagulation therapy or following blunt abdominal or pelvic trauma. The appearance on ultrasonography may be confused with an ectopic pregnancy, an ovarian tumour or an inflammatory process such as a tubo-ovarian abscess. The hallmark of a haemorrhagic ovarian cyst is its evolution over time from acute haemorrhage (anechoic cystic mass), through clot formation (internal echoes, strands and septations), clot retraction (fluid–debris level) to resolution. The average diameter of a haemorrhagic ovarian cyst is 3.0–3.5 cm but they may range in size from 2.5 to 10 cm. While acute pain is often the presentation, the symptoms gradually resolve without intervention. Analgesia, reassurance and serial imaging follow-up are indicated for the stable haemorrhagic cyst. Use of an oral contraceptive pill does not aid regression of the functional ovarian cyst but may prevent new cyst formation.

Q18 What is the overall malignancy rate of surgically managed ovarian masses in childhood and adolescence?

A 0%–5%

B 10%–15%

C 25%–50%

D 70%–75%

E 85%–90%

A18 **B** Of surgically treated ovarian masses in infancy, childhood and adolescence, neoplasms will be responsible for approximately 30%–50%. Mature cystic teratoma is the most common lesion in children and adolescents. Dermoid cysts have characteristic features on imaging, related to the presence of thick sebaceous fluid, hair and calcifications from teeth or bone. The most characteristic feature on ultrasound imaging of a dermoid is the hyperechoic mural nodule known as the 'dermoid plug' or Rokitanksy's protuberance.

Malignancy will be evident on pathological examination in 8%–15% of surgical cases. While the overall incidence of ovarian masses increases with age, the malignancy rate is inversely related to age. In one study of children and adolescents with an overall malignancy rate of 7.9%, the rate of malignancy between 1 and 15 years of age was 11% and for over 15, this rate dropped to 4%. Besides younger age, malignancy is more likely if the mass is associated with endocrine disturbance, i.e. precocious puberty/virilisation or if it is solid or complex on imaging.

Q19 Which of the following is not a correct pairing of histological ovarian tumour type with its corresponding tumour marker?

A $\beta$-hCG : choriocarcinoma

B alpha-fetoprotein : endodermal sinus tumour

C inhibin : granulosa cell tumour

D LDH : immature cystic teratoma

E CA125 : serous cystadenocarcinoma

A19 **D** All histological cell types are evident in ovarian neoplasms in children and adolescents; however, the proportion of each type varies compared with adult populations. Germ cell tumours predominate (73%), followed by epithelial tumours (13%). Stromal tumours comprise a small proportion of ovarian masses at all ages.

The benign germ cell tumour, mature cystic teratoma, is the most common childhood and adolescent ovarian neoplasm. The benign stromal tumour is the fibrothecoma. Malignant germ cell tumours include: dysgerminoma, immature teratoma, endodermal sinus tumour, mixed germ cell tumour, embryonal carcinoma and choriocarcinoma. Malignant sex-cord-stromal tumours are the granulosa cell and Sertoli–Leydig tumours. Epithelial lesions may be benign (cystadenomas), borderline (low malignant potential) or malignant (cystadenocarcinomas).

The ovarian malignancies in children and adolescents and their related tumour markers are indicated in Table 67.1.

| | AFP | β-hCG | Inhibin | Lactate dehydrogenase | CA125 | Testosterone |
|---|---|---|---|---|---|---|
| Dysgerminoma | – | ± | – | + | – | – |
| Endodermal sinus tumour | + | – | – | ± | – | – |
| Immature teratoma | – | – | – | – | – | – |
| Embryonal carcinoma | ± | ± | – | – | – | – |
| Choriocarcinoma | – | + | – | – | – | – |
| Mixed germ cell tumour | ± | ± | – | – | – | – |
| Granulosa cell tumour | – | – | + | – | – | – |
| Sertoli–Leydig tumour | – | – | ± | – | – | + |
| Epithelial LMP or carcinoma (non mucinous) | – | – | – | – | ± | – |

TABLE 67.1 Tumour markers in childhood ovarian malignancies

Q20 Surgical staging guidelines for management of ovarian germ cell tumours in children and adolescents, recommend all of the following procedures *except*:

A collection of ascites or washings on entering the peritoneal cavity

B unilateral oophorectomy of the tumour-containing ovary

C biopsy of any abnormality of the contralateral ovary

D bilateral pelvic lymphadenectomy and para-aortic lymph node sampling

E inspection and palpation of the omentum with removal of adherent or abnormal areas.

A20 D The overall goals of surgery for germ cell tumours in children are to resect the tumour where feasible, to spare uninvolved reproductive organs, and to accurately stage the extent of the disease. The Pediatric Oncology Group surgical guidelines for ovarian germ cell tumours recommend the following.

1 Collection of ascites or washings on entering the peritoneal cavity.

2 Examination of peritoneal surfaces with biopsy or excision of any nodules.

3  Examination and palpation of lymph nodes in the retroperitoneum with sampling of any firm or enlarged lymph nodes.

4  Inspection and palpation of the omentum with removal of adherent or abnormal areas.

5  Inspection and palpation of contralateral ovaries with biopsy of any abnormal areas.

6  Complete resection of tumour-containing ovary.

Lymph nodes that do not appear grossly abnormal have a low risk of positivity and hence routine bilateral pelvic lymphadenectomy is not recommended in the absence of palpable gross abnormalities. Germ cell tumours respond extremely well to chemotherapy (bleomycin, etoposide and cisplatin), resulting in excellent survival rates for these tumours, especially when they present at an early stage of the disease. There does not appear to be any adverse effect of omitting aspects of surgical staging that would be routinely applied in adult populations (sampling bilateral retroperitoneal nodes, omentectomy). Malignant epithelial lesions should be staged according to adult staging recommendations. However, a conservative and fertility-sparing approach is applied to low-malignant-potential tumours of the ovary in reproductive age women, which is especially applicable to children and adolescents.

## Further reading

Breech LL, Laufer MR. Müllerian anomalies. *Obstet Gynecol Clin North Am.* 2009; **36**(1): 47–68.

Dovey S, Sanfilippo J. Endometriosis and the adolescent. *Clin Obstet Gynecol.* 2010; **53**(2): 420–8.

Merritt DF. Genital trauma in the pediatric and adolescent female. *Obstet Gynecol Clin North Am.* 2009; **36**(1): 85–98.

Oelsner G, Cohen, Soriano D, *et al.* Minimal surgery for the twisted ischaemic adnexa can preserve ovarian function. *Human Reproduction.* 2003; **18**(12): 2599–602.

Oltmann SC, Fischer A, Barber R, *et al.* Cannot exclude torsion: a 15-year review. *J Pediatr Surg.* 2009; **44**(6): 1212–16.

Templeman C. Ovarian cysts. *J Pediatr Adolesc Gynecol.* 2004: **17**(4): 297–8.

Van Eyk N, Allen L, Giesbrecht E, *et al.* Pediatric vulvovaginal disorders: a diagnostic approach and review of the literature. *J Obstet Gynaecol Can.* 2009; **31**(9): 850–62.

# SECTION XI

# Oncology

# CHAPTER 68

# Adjuvant therapy in childhood cancer

### JOHANNES VISSER

**From the choices below each question, select the single best answer.**

**Q1** Which of the following is not a characteristic of phase I clinical trials in paediatric oncology?
- **A** They are offered to patients for whom no known curative treatment is available.
- **B** They assess whether a new agent is sufficiently efficacious to warrant further study.
- **C** Small numbers of patients are required.
- **D** They use a dose-escalating design.
- **E** They are conducted in large individual institutions or small consortia of institutions.

**A1** **B** Phase I trials are designed to evaluate the toxicity of new therapeutic agents. They typically use a dose-escalating trial design. Each cohort is monitored for toxicity before the next cohort is given a higher dose. The end point is either the determination of the safety of the agent or the maximum tolerated dose. Phase II trials are designed to determine if a new therapy is sufficiently active in a specific disease to warrant its further study.

**Q2** Which of the following is not a cause of graft vs. host disease?
- **A** umbilical cord blood transplantation
- **B** T-cell-depleted allogeneic haematopoietic stem cell transplantation
- **C** matched unrelated donor haematopoietic stem cell transplantation
- **D** purged autologous haematopoietic stem cell transplantation
- **E** sibling donor haematopoietic stem cell transplantation

**A2** **D** The source of stem cells used in haematopoietic stem cell transplantation is denoted by the descriptions autologous (from the patient themselves) and allogeneic (from someone else). Graft vs. host disease refers to the clinicopathologic process of enteritis, hepatitis and dermatitis. It is mediated by donor T-cells that recognise antigenic disparities between donor and recipient. This is therefore not a problem of autologous haematopoietic stem cell transplants. 'Purged' refers to techniques to remove tumour cells that might be present in the stem cell collection from the patient, before reinfusion.

**Q3** Which of the following is true regarding acute graft vs. host disease?
  **A** It is often the first sign of graft failure.
  **B** It requires lifelong immunosuppression.
  **C** It manifests as lichen planus.
  **D** It manifests as cirrhosis.
  **E** None of the above.

**A3** **E** The appearance of acute graft vs. host disease symptoms often accompanies evidence of successful engraftment (recovering blood counts). It is mediated by donor T-cells and therefore is not a feature of a failing donor haematopoietic stem cell graft.

Acute graft vs. host disease can usually be controlled by a course of immunosuppression which can then be gradually withdrawn completely.

Acute graft vs. host disease develops within the first 100 days after haematopoietic stem cell transplantation and is characterised by enteritis, hepatitis and dermatitis. Lichen planus, ocular sicca, dry mouth and cirrhosis are manifestations of chronic graft vs. host disease.

**Q4** Radiation forms part of multimodal therapy for all of the following *except*:
  **A** large B-cell lymphoma
  **B** Hodgkin's lymphoma
  **C** alveolar rhabdomyosarcoma
  **D** neuroblastoma
  **E** nephroblastoma.

**A4** **A** Large B-cell lymphoma makes up 10% of non-Hodgkin's lymphoma in children. Burkitt's lymphoma makes up 50%, lymphoblastic lymphoma 30% and anaplastic large cell lymphoma 10%. The treatment of non-Hodgkin's lymphoma in children is multidrug chemotherapy.

Large B-cell and Burkitt's non-Hodgkin's lymphoma are treated with intensive pulsed chemotherapy with the most important drugs being cyclophosphamide, high-dose methotrexate and cytarabine. The role of targeted B-cell antibody therapy (anti-CD20, rituximab) has not yet been established in children.

Q5 Which of the following drugs is not a vesicant?
  A doxorubicin
  B cytarabine
  C dactinomycin
  D vincristine
  E daunorubicin

A5 **B** A vesicant is a chemical that, if it escapes from the vein, causes extensive tissue damage with vesicle formation or blistering. The widespread use of central lines reduces the risk of this complication in paediatric oncology. Chemotherapy agents are classified according to their risk of causing tissue damage if extravasated. Vesicants are the highest risk group. Cytarabine is in the lowest risk group (neutrals) and can be given subcutaneously as well as intravenously.

Q6 Adjuvant therapy is based on risk stratification in:
  A localised rhabdomyosarcoma
  B precursor B-cell acute lymphoblastic leukaemia
  C Burkitt's lymphoma
  D childhood medulloblastoma
  E all of the above.

A6 **E** Risk stratification is widely used in paediatric oncology to ensure that patients at lower risk of recurrence receive less intensive treatment and those at higher risk of recurrence receive more intensive treatment. Risk factors were identified and risk-based treatment stratification validated in large multicentre trials for several diseases. Risk stratification varies between different treatment protocols but risk factors include:
  - localised rhabdomyosarcoma – age, size of tumour, presence of spread to local lymph nodes, site of primary, post-surgical stage (Intergroup Rhabdomyosarcoma Study Group), pathology
  - precursor B-cell acute lymphoblastic leukaemia – age, white blood cell count, cytogenetic features, rate of response to induction treatment
  - Burkitt's lymphoma – modified Murphy staging system
  - Childhood medulloblastoma – clinical, pathologic and molecular variables.

**Q7** Which of the following biochemical changes is *not* a manifestation of acute tumour lysis syndrome?

  **A** hypercalcaemia

  **B** hypophosphataemia

  **C** hypokalaemia

  **D** hypocalcaemia

  **E** none of the above

**A7**   **D** Acute tumour lysis syndrome is the result of the rapid release of large quantities of intracellular metabolites (uric acid, potassium and phosphate) from dying cells. This is mainly a feature of rapidly growing tumours that are also very sensitive to chemotherapy (Burkitt's lymphoma, T-cell leukaemia/lymphoma and leukaemia patients with very high white cell counts). It usually occurs during the first 5 days after commencement of chemotherapy but may start even before treatment begins (spontaneous tumour necrosis).

    The serum biochemical features are high uric acid, high potassium, high phosphate and low calcium. The low calcium is secondary to the hyperphosphataemia). Acute renal failure may result. Preventive measures and careful monitoring and management of electrolyte abnormalities are essential.

**Q8** Adjuvant therapy for stage IV neuroblastoma includes all of the following *except*:

  **A** cis-retinoic acid

  **B** allogeneic haematopoietic stem cell transplantation

  **C** myeloablative chemotherapy

  **D** radiotherapy to primary

  **E** anti-GD2 antibody.

**A8**   **B** Allogeneic haematopoietic stem cell transplantation utilises stem cells from a donor and is not an established part of multimodal therapy for neuroblastoma.

    Autologous haematopoietic stem cell transplantation (own stem cells) is used to 'rescue' patients after myeloablative chemotherapy. High-dose chemotherapy is used to treat the neuroblastoma but causes severe or complete depletion of bone marrow cells (myeloablation). Stem cells are collected from the patient before the high-dose chemotherapy and reinfused afterwards.

**Q⁹** First-line chemotherapy for rhabdomyosarcoma includes which of the following?

  **A** cyclophosphamide

  **B** vincristine

  **C** dactinomycin (actinomycin-D)

  **D** ifosfamide

  **E** all of the above

**A⁹** **E** Vincristine and dactinomycin are well established as part of first-line treatment for rhabdomyosarcoma. European groups favour ifosfamide and North American groups favour cyclophosphamide as third agent. The Intergroup Rhabdomyosarcoma Study IV prospective randomised trial compared an ifosfamide-based combination with a cyclophosphamide-based combination and showed no difference in 3-year survival or failure-free survival. Ifosfamide may cause renal toxicity not seen with cyclophosphamide and is not favoured by the North American groups. The European groups favour ifosfamide since data suggests the risk of renal toxicity is low at cumulative doses of <60 g/m² and a higher risk of gonadal toxicity with cyclophosphamide.

**Q10** Which of the following statements regarding haemorrhagic cystitis is *not* true?

  **A** It is a side effect of cyclophosphamide.

  **B** It is a side effect of ifosfamide.

  **C** The risk of this side effect is dose dependent.

  **D** Dactinomycin given in conjunction with pelvic radiation increases the risk of haemorrhagic cystitis.

  **E** Leukovorin (folinic acid) and hyperhydration are used to prevent this side effect of chemotherapy.

**A10** **E** Haemorrhagic cystitis is a potential side effect of ifosfamide and cyclophosphamide. Activated metabolites and biologically active by-products of these agents can cause a chemical cystitis. The incidence of this complication is reduced by hyperhydration, frequent emptying of the bladder and the administration of mesna. Mesna reacts in the urine with urotoxic metabolites of these agents resulting in their detoxification.

    Leukovorin is administered at set times after the administration of the folic acid analogue, methotrexate, to limit the toxicity of this chemotherapy agent.

**Q11** Neo-adjuvant chemotherapy is part of the treatment of which the following conditions?

**A** osteosarcoma

**B** hepatoblastoma

**C** nephroblastoma

**D** nasopharyngeal carcinoma

**E** all of the above

**A11** **E** Neo-adjuvant chemotherapy is administered before definitive surgery in contrast to adjuvant chemotherapy which is administered after surgery.

Neo-adjuvant chemotherapy in osteosarcoma patients allows for the assessment of the chemotherapy responsiveness of the tumour and facilitates limb salvage procedures.

Neo-adjuvant chemotherapy in hepatoblastoma is used in an effort to make unresectable tumours resectable and there is evidence that incomplete resections are less common after preoperative chemotherapy.

The National Wilms' Tumour Study Group based in North America reserves neo-adjuvant chemotherapy for specific groups of patients to facilitate surgical removal. These include bilateral renal tumours, tumour extension into the inferior vena cava above the hepatic veins, and tumours found to be inoperable at surgical exploration. In contrast the Internationale Société d'Oncologie Pédiatrique approach offers neo-adjuvant chemotherapy to all patients. The cure rates of the two approaches appear to be similar and the merits of each remain a matter of debate.

Nasopharyngeal carcinoma is rare in children. Because of the location of nasopharyngeal carcinoma, the tumour usually cannot be totally removed with surgery. When patients are diagnosed early and the tumour is small, the treatment is usually radiation therapy only. Patients with more advanced disease usually get chemotherapy and radiation therapy. These patients commonly have larger tumours, or cancer that has spread to the lymph nodes of the neck.

**Q12** Which of the following is true regarding infants with stage 4S neuroblastoma?

**A** Patients with tumours with N-myc amplification are offered intensive chemotherapy, surgical resection of primary, radiation to site of primary and myeloablative chemotherapy with stem cell rescue.

**B** Carboplatin and etoposide chemotherapy and surgical resection are offered to all patients with tumours without N-myc amplification.

**C** Metastatic disease must be limited to liver, skin and lung.

**D** Limited to age group <18 months.

**E** All of the above.

$A$12 **A** Stage 4S neuroblastoma patients (< 1 year of age) with N-myc amplification have a very poor prognosis and are offered intensive treatment. This is also the case for infants with stage 4 disease.

Stage 4S neuroblastoma patients without N-myc amplification only require treatment in case of life-threatening or organ-threatening symptoms and have an >85% cure rate with this approach. Metastases in stage 4S neuroblastoma must be limited to skin, liver or bone marrow.

$Q$13 Which of the following adjuvant treatments is not potentially cardiotoxic?

   **A** total body irradiation
   **B** anthracyclines
   **C** ifosfamide
   **D** thoracic spine radiotherapy
   **E** left flank radiotherapy

$A$13 **C** Anthracyclines (doxorubicin, daunorubicin, epirubicin, mitozantrone, idarubicin, amsacrine) are potentially cardiotoxic chemotherapy agents.

Radiotherapy to field including thorax, thoracic spine, mediastinum, left flank and total body irradiation is potentially cardiotoxic.

Ifosfamide is not a cardiotoxic agent.

$Q$14 Residual positron emission tomography (PET) scan activity after initial chemotherapy has an established role in risk stratification in:

   **A** osteosarcoma
   **B** rhabdomyosarcoma
   **C** anaplastic large cell lymphoma
   **D** hepatoblastoma
   **E** none of the above.

$A$14 **E** PET is a functional diagnostic imaging modality. The role of PET in identifying Hodgkin's lymphoma patients who need adjuvant radiotherapy (by assessing the PET response after the first two courses of chemotherapy) is under investigation. PET does not yet have an established role in risk stratification in other paediatric malignancies but has been shown to be helpful in selected cases including central nervous system tumours, lymphomas, neuroblastoma, soft tissue tumours, malignant bone tumours and germ cell tumours.

**Q15** Which of the following adjuvant/supportive treatments are *not* complicated by constipation/obstipation?

    **A** tricyclic antidepressants

    **B** pelvic irradiation

    **C** vincristine

    **D** narcotics

    **E** vinblastine

**A15**  **B** Radiation to the pelvis or the lower abdomen may cause acute radiation enteritis. It usually presents with watery diarrhoea, sometimes associated with cramping abdominal pain.

## Further reading

Altman AJ. *Supportive Care of Children with Cancer: current therapy and guidelines from the children's oncology group.* 3rd ed. Baltimore, MD: John Hopkins University Press; 2004.

Pizzo PA, Poplack D. *Principles and Practice of Pediatric Oncology.* 4th ed. Philadelphia, PA: Lippincott Williams & Wilkins; 2002.

Voûte PA, Barrett A, Stevens MCG, *et al.*, editors. *Cancer in Children: clinical management.* 5th ed. New York, NY: Oxford University Press; 2005.

# CHAPTER 69

# Renal tumours

## VICTORIA LANE, MARK POWIS

From the choices below each question, select the single best answer.

 **Q1** Which of the following is *false* with regard to Wilms's tumour?
  **A** Wilms's tumour accounts for 6%–7% of all paediatric malignancies.
  **B** Wilms's tumour is the fourth most common intra-abdominal solid organ tumour in children.
  **C** The annual incidence of Wilms's tumour in North America is 8 per million children.
  **D** 650 new cases are diagnosed a year in North America.
  **E** The 3- to 5-year survival is 85%.

 **A1** **B** Wilms's tumour represents 6%–7% of all paediatric malignancies and is the second most common intra-abdominal solid organ tumour found in children. The annual incidence in North America is 8.1 per million children representing about 650 new cases each year. The 3- to 5-year survival is approaching 85%–90%.

 **Q2** Which of the following is *not* characteristic of WAGR syndrome?
  **A** 30% risk of developing Wilms's tumour
  **B** absence of the iris
  **C** malformations of the genitourinary tract
  **D** mental retardation
  **E** *WT2* gene implicated

**A2** **E** WAGR syndrome comprises **W**ilms's tumour, **a**niridia, **g**enitourinary malformation and mental **r**etardation. The risk of developing Wilms's tumour is more than 30%. Cytogenetic analysis of individuals with this syndrome showed deletions at chromosome 11p13, which has been found to be the locus of the contiguous set of genes including *PAX6* (the gene causing aniridia), and *WT1* (one of the Wilms's tumour genes), rather than *WT2*. *WT1* gene encodes a transcription factor that is crucial for normal kidney and gonadal development.

**Q3** Which of the following syndromes is not associated with Wilms's tumour?

  **A** Beckwith–Wiedemann's syndrome

  **B** Denys–Drash's syndrome

  **C** Perlman's syndrome

  **D** Li–Fraumeni's syndrome

  **E** Down's syndrome

**A3** **E** Down's syndrome (trisomy 21) is not associated with Wilms's tumour.

Beckwith–Wiedemann's syndrome is an overgrowth disorder manifested by large birthweight, macroglossia, organomegaly, hemihypertrophy, neonatal hypoglycaemia, abdominal wall defects, ear abnormalities and a predisposition to Wilms's tumour. About 5% of individuals with this syndrome will develop Wilms's tumour. Beckwith–Wiedemann's syndrome maps to chromosome 11p15, a locus also known as WT2, because loss of heterozygosity at this locus has been detected in Wilms's tumour.

Denys–Drash's syndrome is characterised by pseudohermaphroditism, glomerulopathy, renal failure and a 95% chance of developing Wilms's tumour.

Perlman's syndrome and Li–Fraumeni's syndrome are both associated with Wilms's tumour.

**Q4** Which of the following is not related to Beckwith–Wiedemann's syndrome?

  **A** high birthweight

  **B** macroglossia

  **C** risk of multiple tumours

  **D** hyperglycaemia

  **E** omphalocele

**A4** **D** Beckwith–Wiedemann's syndrome is associated with hypoglycaemia.

**Q5** Of the following statements, which one is true?

  **A** 10% of Wilms's tumours present with stage V disease.

  **B** Mean age at diagnosis for Wilms's tumour is 7 years.

  **C** Renal sparing procedures for patients with Wilms's are only suitable for those with a solitary kidney.

  **D** Chemotherapy agents used in Wilms's include dactinomycin, vincristine and doxorubicin.

  **E** A skeletal survey and bone scan are required for all patients with Wilms's tumour.

**A5**  **D**  The mean age at diagnosis for Wilms's tumour is 3 years. Six per cent of patients with Wilms's tumour present with stage V (bilateral) disease. Partial nephrectomy is indicated in those with a solitary kidney but also in those with bilateral Wilms's tumour. Partial nephrectomy for small polar tumours with no evidence of spread, is practised in some centres, especially in Italy. Chemotherapy agents used include dactinomycin, vincristine and doxorubicin. A skeletal survey and bone scan are not required in all patients with Wilms's tumour but should be routine investigations in those with clear cell sarcoma because of the high metastatic potential of this tumour.

**Q6**  Which of the following is false?

**A**  All patients over 6 months of age in the Société International d'Oncologie Pédiatrique (SIOP) trials undergo prenephrectomy chemotherapy.

**B**  In North America, patients with Wilms's tumour thrombus extending into the right atrium undergo prenephrectomy chemotherapy.

**C**  In North America, children with stage II tumours (favourable histology), treated with vincristine and dactinomycin, also receive radiotherapy.

**D**  In North America, patients with stage V Wilms's tumour should undergo bilateral renal biopsy with staging of each kidney followed by chemotherapy to facilitate renal sparing procedures.

**E**  In North America, all patients with stage V (bilateral) disease undergo prenephrectomy chemotherapy.

**A6**  **C**  In the SIOP studies the therapeutic approach has focused on developing stage specific strategies after prenephrectomy therapy. Stage classification and histopathological diagnosis are delayed until after surgery. It is thought that the use of prenephrectomy chemotherapy facilitates surgical resection and minimises complications. Children under 6 months of age undergo primary nephrectomy unless there is evidence of metastases at presentation. Therefore, patients in the SIOP trial with chemotherapy-induced tumour shrinkage result in a different stage distribution to those patients in the North American National Wilms' Tumour Study Group (NWTSG).

The staging system for the NWTSG is as follows.

- Stage I
  - Tumour confined to the kidney and completely resected; no penetration of the renal capsule or involvement of renal sinus vessels.
- Stage II
  - Tumour extends beyond the kidney but is completely resected

(negative margins and lymph nodes); at least of the following has occurred:

(i) penetration of the renal capsule

(ii) invasion of the renal sinus vessels

(iii) biopsy of the tumour before removal

(iv) spillage of the tumour locally during removal.

- Stage III
  — Gross or microscopic residual tumour remains postoperatively including; inoperable tumour, positive surgical margins, tumour spillage involving peritoneal surfaces, regional lymph node metastases, or transected tumour thrombus.
- Stage IV
  — Haematogenous metastases or lymph node metastases outside the abdomen (e.g. liver, lungs, bone, brain).
- Stage V
  — Bilateral renal Wilms's tumour.

Most Wilms's tumours that appear to involve neighbouring structures usually simply compress rather than invade. This therefore reduces the need for radical en bloc dissection and its associated complications. Tumour extending into the renal vein and proximal IVC can, in most cases, be removed en bloc with the kidney. Tumour extending into the inferior vena cava (IVC) (hepatic level) or into the right atrium should be treated with prenephrectomy chemotherapy to facilitate surgical resection.

At diagnosis, about 6% of children present with bilateral Wilms's tumour. Survival is more than 70%; however, these children are at high risk of renal failure. This risk has led to the recommendation that such children undergo bilateral renal biopsy with staging of each kidney followed by chemotherapy to shrink the tumour and aid renal sparing procedures. Primary excision of the tumour masses is not recommended.

Radiotherapy is an important treatment modality in children with Wilms's tumour. Successive NWTSG trials have refined the indications for radiotherapy. NWTS-2 showed that radiotherapy could be avoided in stage I disease if they received vincristine and dactinomycin. The NWTS-3 study proved that children with stage II disease treated with vincristine and dactinomycin could also avoid radiotherapy.

**Q7** Concerning patients with renal cell carcinoma (RCC), which of the following is false?
   A Between 2% and 5% of paediatric renal tumours are RCCs.
   B M = F.
   C It may be associated with von Hippel–Lindau's disease.
   D Papillary and clear cell subgroups are described.
   E 50% present with lung, liver or brain metastases.

**A7** **E** RCC accounts for 2%–5% of all paediatric renal tumours and 0.5%–2% of all RCCs occur in those under 21 years of age. Patients classically present with frank haematuria, loin pain and a palpable mass. Twenty-five per cent, however, are asymptomatic and are detected on imaging. Twenty per cent of patients will present with metastatic disease (bone, liver, brain). Bilateral presentation can be associated with conditions such as von Hippel–Lindau's disease. Two main morphological subgroups can be identified – namely, papillary and clear cell tumours.

Survival of children with renal call carcinoma is largely affected by stage at presentation and completeness of resection at radical nephrectomy, with overall survival at 64%–87%.

**Five year survival**
Stage I: higher than 90%
Stages II–III: 50%–80%
Stage IV: 9%
Nephrectomy is adequate for stage I–II disease.

**Q8** Regarding clear cell sarcoma of the kidney (CCSK), which of the following is incorrect?
   A Abdominal mass is a common presenting feature.
   B Bilateral cases are well recognised.
   C No familial or syndromic association exists.
   D Peak incidence at 1–4 years.
   E It is more common in boys.

**A8** **B** Clear cell carcinoma occurs with a peak incidence at 1–4 years, boys being more commonly affected (ratio 2 : 1). Classically patients present with an abdominal mass. No patients have been reported with bilateral disease and there is no known syndrome or familial association. Clear cell carcinoma has a high malignant potential; hence it is also known as bone-metastasing renal tumour of childhood. Bone metastases occur in 15%–60% of patients with CCSK and metastases to other organs can also occur. Four per cent will present with distant metastases at presentation.

Standard treatment of clear cell carcinoma is radical nephrectomy followed by aggressive chemotherapy. In the latest NWTSG/COG (Children's Oncology Group) protocols, patients are given four-agent chemotherapy (cyclophosphamide, etoposide, vincristine and doxorubicin) for 6 months along with radiotherapy, regardless of disease stage. The addition of doxorubicin has improved outcome and the National Wilms' Tumour Study III showed a 75%, 4-year survival in 50 patients with clear cell carcinoma.

**Q9** Regarding mesoblastic nephroma, which of the following is false?

   **A** Between 3% and 10% of all paediatric renal tumours are mesoblastic nephromas.

   **B** Mesoblastic nephroma is the most common renal tumour in those under 3 months.

   **C** 90% are diagnosed within the first year of life.

   **D** Mesoblastic nephroma can be divided into classic and papillary types.

   **E** Mesoblastic nephroma is associated with maternal polyhydramnios.

**A9** **D** Mesoblastic nephroma gives rise to 3%–10% of all paediatric renal tumours, and is the most common renal tumour in those under 3 months of age. Ninety per cent are diagnosed within the first year of life and it is twice as common in boys as girls. Two morphological types are recognised and include classic and cellular types and the latter accounts for 42%–63% of cases.

Mesoblastic nephroma classically presents with an abdominal mass and occasional haematuria. Many cases are diagnosed on prenatal ultrasound and give rise to polyhydramnios, hydrops and premature delivery.

Mesoblastic nephroma is treated with radical rather than partial nephrectomy to reduce the risk of local recurrence. Nephrectomy is usually sufficient as the tumour generally follows a benign course. Ninety-five per cent of patients do not relapse, and the 5% who do have the cellular variant of the disease.

**Q10** Regarding malignant renal rhabdoid tumour, which of the following is false?

   **A** It accounts for 2% of all paediatric renal tumours.

   **B** It can present with hypercalcaemia.

   **C** It is more common in females.

   **D** 80% present with metastases.

   **E** 60% occur in those under 1 year of age.

**A10** **C** Malignant renal rhabdoid tumour is a rare but aggressive renal tumour accounting for 2% of all paediatric renal tumours and 80% occur in those under 2 years of age (60% in those under 1 year of age). Male predominance is 1.5 : 1. Haematuria is a common presenting feature, as are symptoms from metastatic spread as metastatic spread occurs in 80% of patients. Patients have also been reported as presenting with hypercalcaemia due to increased parathormone concentrations.

Malignant renal rhabdoid tumour has an 80% overall mortality at 12–18 months follow-up, due to advanced stage at presentation and poor response to traditional chemotherapy and radiotherapy. Completely resected tumours with negative lymph nodes also have a poor prognosis with only 50% survival. NWTS-5 study is using a protocol whereby radical nephrectomy is followed by carboplatin and etoposide alternating with cyclophosphamide for 24 weeks and radiotherapy.

**Q11** Regarding renal medullary carcinoma, which of the following is false?

   **A** It almost exclusively affects carriers of the sickle cell trait.

   **B** The left kidney is more commonly affected.

   **C** The mean age at presentation is 20 years.

   **D** Mortality is near 100%, with death within weeks/months of diagnosis.

   **E** It is more common in boys if diagnosed under 25 years of age.

**A11** **B** Renal medullary carcinoma almost exclusively affects young adults of black ethnicity that have sickle-cell trait and has previously been described as the seventh sickle-cell nephropathy. The age range of presentation is 5–39 years and the mean is 20 years. In those under 25 years, the malignancy mainly affects boys in a 2–3 : 1 ratio; however, above this age the sex distribution is equal. Classically patients present with gross haematuria, abdominal/loin pain, weight loss, fever and a palpable mass. The right kidney is affected more commonly than the left (3 : 1).

Mortality for renal medullary carcinoma is near 100%, with death occurring within weeks or months of diagnosis. This high mortality is because patients usually present with late stage disease (18% with stage III and 81% with stage IV disease). In this setting stage III disease is defined as extension into major veins, adrenal or perinephric invasion, or a single regional lymph node metastasis and stage IV disease is defined as invasion beyond Gerota's fascia, involvement of >1 lymph node or distant metastases.

## Further reading

Ahmed HU, Arya M, Levitt G, *et al*. Part I: primary malignant non-Wilms' renal tumours in children. *Lancet Oncol.* 2007; 8(8): 730–7.

Ahmed HU, Arya M, Levitt G, *et al*. Part II: treatment of primary malignant non-Wilms' renal tumours in children. *Lancet Oncol.* 2007; 8(8): 842–8.

Ehrlich PF. Wilms tumor: progress and considerations for the surgeon. *Surg Oncol.* 2007; 16(3): 157–71.

Kalapurakal JA, Dome JS, Perlman EJ, *et al*. Management of Wilms' tumour: current practice and future goals. *Lancet Oncol.* 2004; 5(1): 37–46.

# CHAPTER 70

# Neuroblastoma

## MADAN SAMUEL

From the choices below each question, select the single best answer.

**Q1** One of the most common solid tumours in infancy and childhood is:
- A neuroblastoma
- B ganglioneuroma
- C Wilms's tumour
- D sarcoma
- E teratoma.

**A1** **A** Neuroblastoma is one of the most common solid tumours in infancy and childhood. It is a neoplasm of the neural crest origin. It commonly arises in the adrenal medulla and along the sympathetic ganglion chain from the neck to the pelvis. This neoplasm exhibits great heterogeneity in its behaviour.

**Q2** Neuroblasts can be identified in the fetal adrenal gland at:
- A 10th to 11th intrauterine week
- B 10th to 12th intrauterine week
- C 10th to 14th intrauterine week
- D 16th to 18th intrauterine week
- E 9th to 10th intrauterine week

**A2** **B** Primitive neuroblasts can be seen in the fetal adrenal gland in the 10th and 12th intrauterine week. They increase in number by the 20th intrauterine week and diminish in number by the third trimester.

**Q3** Which statement is true regarding the autopsy incidence of neuroblastoma *in situ* in the adrenal gland?

    **A** It is found in 1 in 360 neonates who die of congenital heart disease.

    **B** It is found in 1 in 460 neonates who die of congenital heart disease.

    **C** It is found in 1 in 39 infants who die of various causes.

    **D** It is found in 1 in 390 infants who die of various causes.

    **E** It is found in 1 in 16 infants who die of various causes.

**A3**   **C** Neuroblastoma *in situ* occurs in 1 in 260 neonates dying of congenital heart disease and 1 in 39 in neonates who die of other causes.

**Q4** The clinical incidence of neuroblastoma is:

    **A** 1 in 100 000 to 1 in 120 000

    **B** 1 in 7500 to 1 in 10 000

    **C** 1 in 10 000 to 1 in 15 000

    **D** 1 in 10 000 to 1 in 12 000

    **E** 1 in 5000 to 1 in 7500.

**A4**   **B** The clinical incidence of neuroblastoma is 1 in 7500 to 1 in 10000 children.

**Q5** Which of the following correctly lists the primary sites of neuroblastoma in decreasing order of frequency?

    **A** adrenal medulla, paraspinal ganglia, posterior mediastinum and pelvic organ of Zuckerkandl

    **B** adrenal cortex, paraspinal ganglia, posterior mediastinum and pelvic organ of Zuckerkandl

    **C** adrenal medulla, posterior mediastinum, paraspinal ganglia and pelvic organ of Zuckerkandl

    **D** adrenal cortex, posterior mediastinum, paraspinal ganglia and pelvic organ of Zuckerkandl

    **E** adrenal gland, paraspinal ganglia, posterior mediastinum and pelvic organ of Zuckerkandl

**A5**   **A** The primary site that is most commonly afflicted by the tumour is the adrenal medulla (50%). The distributions in the other primary sites are retroperitoneal paraspinal ganglia (25%), posterior mediastinum (20%), pelvic organ of Zuckerkandl (2.5%) and posterior triangle of the neck (2.5%).

Q6  Which of the following statements is true regarding mass screening?

   A  Japan discontinued its programme in April 2004.

   B  Germany discontinued its programme in April 2004.

   C  Quebec discontinued its programme in April 2004.

   D  North America discontinued its programme in April 2004.

   E  Europe discontinued its programme in April 2004.

A6  A  Mass screening programme was discontinued by the Ministry of Health, Japan, in April 2004.

Q7  Mass screening programmes for neuroblastoma were discontinued because of:

   A  overdiagnosis

   B  poor information about the natural history of the tumour

   C  identification of biologically favourable tumours that spontaneously regressed

   D  high false positives

   E  high false negatives.

A7  D  Mass screening provides important information about the natural history of the tumour and about biologically favourable tumours that regress. However, it causes medical and psychological distress to parents because of its high false-positive rates. Overdiagnosis of neuroblastoma has led to unnecessary therapy. Therefore mass screening programmes have been abandoned in Japan, North America, Europe and Canada.

Q8  A 36-month-old presents with localised stage I neuroblastoma with favourable histology and absent N-myc amplification. The best management option for best outcome is:

   A  chemotherapy and total excision

   B  chemotherapy, total excision and radiotherapy

   C  total excision only

   D  chemotherapy only

   E  biopsy, chemotherapy, total excision and chemotherapy.

A8  C  Stage I neuroblastoma is managed by operation only. The cure rate is 100%.

**Q9** What percentage of stage II patients with high-risk prognostic factors require aggressive chemotherapy?

    **A** 5%–10%

    **B** 10%–15%

    **C** 15%–20%

    **D** 20%–25%

    **E** 25%–30%

**A9** **B** Thirteen per cent of stage II cases have high-risk prognostic factors and require aggressive chemotherapy.

**Q10** Neuroblastoma survival rates are better in patients with:

    **A** low levels of proto-oncogene Trk-A

    **B** high levels of proto-oncogene Trk-A

    **C** low levels of proto-oncogene Trk-B

    **D** low levels of proto-oncogene Trk-C

    **E** high levels of proto-oncogene Trk-A and Trk-B.

**A10** **B** High levels of the proto-oncogene Trk-A, a receptor for the neurotrophin nerve growth factor, are associated with excellent survival in infants with neuroblastoma. Trk-A receptor is activated by nerve growth factor and may cause spontaneous regression. Trk-A expression, absence of N-myc amplification, and lower-stage neuroblastoma is usually seen in young patients with good prognosis.

**Q11** Which of the following statements is true about therapeutic outcomes in infants with unresectable neuroblastoma?

    **A** Cellular DNA content is a predictor of good response to chemotherapy.

    **B** Cellular DNA content is a poor predictor of response to chemotherapy.

    **C** Trk-A and Trk-B expression is the only good predictor of response to chemotherapy.

    **D** Favourable histology is a good predictor of response to chemotherapy.

    **E** Unfavourable histology is a poor predictor of response to chemotherapy.

**A11** **A** Flow cytometry studies have shown that hyperdiploidy and triploidy are associated with a favourable outcome.

**Q12** In stage 4S neuroblastoma, complete resolution of the liver size results from:

**A** radiotherapy

**B** chemotherapy

**C** surgery

**D** natural resolution

**E** none of the above.

**A12** **D** Low-dose irradiation may help symptomatic hepatomegaly in infants with stage 4S. Although early reduction in the liver size is observed complete resolution occurs in 6–15 months. Resolution of the liver mass is probably related to the natural course of stage 4S disease rather than to radiotherapy.

**Q13** Which of the following therapeutic combinations may be effective for the treatment of neuroblastoma?

**A** retinoids and IL-2 immunotherapy

**B** retinoids and IL-12 immunotherapy

**C** retinoids and dose-intensive chemotherapy

**D** retinoids and targeted radiotherapy using $^{131}$I-labelled 3F8

**E** retinoids and T-cell-based immunotherapy

**A13** **E** Retinoids and T-cell-based immunotherapy may be an effective combination in treating neuroblastoma. They probably sensitise neuroblastoma cells to cytotoxic lymphocytes.

**Q14** Which biological tumour modulator is experimentally known to promote regression and control progression of neuroblastoma?

**A** cis-retinoic acid

**B** interferon

**C** interleukin-2

**D** interleukin-12

**E** granulocyte colony-stimulating factor

**A14** **A** Cis-retinoic acid may promote regression of the neuroblastoma. It may differentiate the cells to favourable histology and thereby control the progression of the disease. Cis-retinoic acid is known to protect against infections.

Q15 A child with a thoracic posterior-mediastinal neuroblastoma undergoes complete excision. Remnants of tumour extending into the vertebral column are transected at the vertebral foramina. Which of the following statements is true?

   A This would adversely affect the outcome.

   B This does not affect outcome.

   C This would upstage the patient's disease.

   D Spinal deformity is well known in these children.

   E This would lead to paraplegia.

A15 B Remnants of neuroblastoma at the vertebral foramina do not adversely affect the outcome. The excision of spinal extension is controversial.

## Further reading

Brodeur GM, Pritchard J, Berthold F, *et al*. Revisions of the international criteria for neuroblastoma diagnosis, staging, and response to treatment. *J Clin Oncol*. 1993; **11**(8): 1466–77.

Grosfeld JL. Risk-based management: current concepts of treating malignant solid tumors of childhood. *J Am Coll Surg*. 1999; **189**(4): 407–25.

Oue T, Inoue M, Yoneda A, *et al*. Profile of neuroblastoma detected by mass screening, resected after observation without treatment: results of the Wait and See pilot study. *J Pediatr Surg*. 2005; **40**(2): 359–63.

Vertuani S, De Geer A, Levitsky V, *et al*. Retinoids act as multistep modulators of the major histocompatibility class I presentation pathway and sensitize neuroblastomas to cytotoxic lymphocytes. *Cancer Res*. 2003; **63**(22): 8006–13.

## CHAPTER 71

# Hepatic tumours

### N ALEXANDER JONES, ONYEBUCHI UKABIALA

From the choices below each question, select the single best answer.

 **Q1** The most common malignant tumour of the liver in the paediatric population is:

    **A** metastatic lesion

    **B** hepatoblastoma

    **C** hepatocellular carcinoma (HCC)

    **D** infantile haemangioendothelioma

    **E** sarcoma.

**A1**   **A** Metastatic tumours are the most common malignant neoplasms of the liver. These include Wilms's tumour, lymphoma and neuroblastoma. Primary hepatic tumours represent only 1%–4% of all solid tumours in children. Hepatoblastoma is the most common malignant primary hepatic tumour and accounts for almost half of all primary hepatic tumours, both malignant and benign. HCCs and sarcomas account for the second and third most common malignant tumours respectively. Infantile haemangioendothelioma is a benign hepatic neoplasm. It is the most common benign hepatic neoplasm. Infantile haemangioendothelioma is also the most common neoplasm of the liver in the first year of life.

 **Q2** Which one of the following imaging characteristics is diagnostic for focal nodular hyperplasia (FNH)?

    **A** abnormal increase in activity on red blood cell blood-pool scan

    **B** single, hyperattenuating lesion on CT

    **C** solid appearance on ultrasonography, but cystic appearance on CT

    **D** multiseptate, multicystic, anechoic mass at periphery of the liver on CT

    **E** early enhancement on CT with intravenous contrast and a central scar

A2    **E**  FNH presents at a mean age of seven. The majority of these benign neoplasms are found incidentally. FNH characteristically appears on CT as a lesion with early contrast enhancement. Although not always seen, the presence of a central scar is diagnostic. These characteristics can also be seen with HCC, so care must be taken to further workup and differentiate the two neoplasms. Infantile haemangioendothelioma has an abnormal increase in activity on a red blood cell blood-pool scan, which is both specific and sensitive for these benign hepatic neoplasms. Hepatocellular adenoma usually occurs as a single lesion. Because of the presence of fat within the neoplasm it appears as a hyperattenuating lesion on CT. A solid appearance on ultrasound and a cystic appearance on CT or MRI is characteristic of undifferentiated embryonal sarcoma. Mesenchymal hamartoma is usually a multiseptated, multicystic, anechoic mass in the liver periphery on ultrasound or CT.

Q3    Which one of the following is *not* usually associated with multiple infantile haemangioendothelioma?

    **A**  other liver tumours

    **B**  hepatomegaly

    **C**  congestive cardiac failure

    **D**  anaemia

    **E**  cutaneous haemangiomas

A3    **A**  The majority of infantile haemangioendotheliomas will present in the first 2 months of life. These neoplasms commonly occur with hepatomegaly, congestive heart failure (CHF), respiratory distress and anaemia. Some patients will have congenital hypothyroidism. The classic triad of hepatomegaly, CHF and anaemia or other cutaneous haemangiomas occurs in 80% of infants who harbour multiple hepatic haemangiomas. In addition to cutaneous haemangiomas, haemangiomas can occur in the lung, pancreas, lymph nodes and bone. Infantile haemangioendothelioma can be seen in conjunction with FNH, but other liver lesions are not common.

Q4    Which one of the following is the most appropriate initial management for infantile haemangioendothelioma?

    **A**  resection of an asymptomatic lesion due to malignancy risk

    **B**  surgical resection once respiratory compromise or coagulopathy develops

    **C**  initial treatment of a symptomatic lesion with steroids

    **D**  embolisation of asymptomatic lesions to avoid potential associated symptoms

    **E**  thyroidectomy once the diagnosis is made and other systemic symptoms are appropriately managed

**A4** **C** Infantile haemangioendotheliomas tend to grow over the first year of life then regress spontaneously. Asymptomatic haemangioendotheliomas are monitored, but patients should be screened for hypothyroidism. Those with multiple lesions should also be screened for intracranial or pulmonary lesions. Patients presenting with CHF, coagulopathy or respiratory compromise have a significant mortality risk. In addition to treatment focused on the presenting symptoms, steroids are used to treat the haemangioma. Almost half will resolve with a prednisone dose of 2–3 mg/kg/day. If steroids fail after administration for 1–2 weeks, then a trial of alpha-interferon is begun. Alpha-interferon is indicated in patients with Kasabach–Merritt's syndrome.

Surgical resection can be considered for residual lesions (as there is a reported risk of malignant transformation to angiosarcoma), but is not the correct initial management for an asymptomatic or symptomatic haemangioma. Embolisation is being used to treat these lesions more frequently, especially in unstable patients. Embolisation is not indicated in asymptomatic lesions. Thyroidectomy does not have a role in management, but patients should be screened for hypothyroidism since this can complicate management if missed.

**Q5** Historically, the subtype of hepatoblastoma with the worst prognosis is:
 **A** pure fetal
 **B** small cell undifferentiated
 **C** macrotrabecular
 **D** mixed epithelial and mesenchymal pattern
 **E** embryonal.

**A5** **B** Hepatoblastoma has been divided into six different subtypes based on histology. All are listed in the options with mixed epithelial and mesenchymal pattern being further divided into those with or without teratoid features. Historically, the pure fetal type has been associated with the best prognosis. The small cell undifferentiated subtype carries the worst prognosis.

**Q6** Which of the following is *not* true regarding hepatoblastoma?
 **A** Alpha-fetaprotein (AFP) levels are elevated in up to 90%.
 **B** Complete surgical removal at initial presentation is possible in more than 65% of cases.
 **C** It is associated with Budd–Chiari's syndrome, Gardner's syndrome and trisomy 18.
 **D** Complete surgical removal can be improved with chemotherapy.
 **E** It most commonly presents as an asymptomatic right upper quadrant mass.

**B** One of the hallmarks of hepatoblastoma is its association with a variety of clinical conditions, syndromes and malformations. Beckwith–Wiedemann's syndrome has a strong association, and patients must be monitored for its coexistence using ultrasound and AFP levels. A short list of other conditions includes extreme prematurity, Budd–Chiari's syndrome trisomy 18, familial adenomatous polyposis, Gardner's syndrome, and neurofibromatosis. Hepatoblastoma most commonly presents as an asymptomatic right upper quadrant mass. Sexual precocity can be a presenting feature in those producing human chorionic gonadotropin. Up to 90% of hepatoblastoma patients have an elevated AFP level. The levels decrease to normal in 4–8 weeks after a complete surgical resection. AFP levels can be used after resection as a monitoring tool. Complete surgical resection is possible in less than half the cases at initial presentation, but chemotherapy can improve the complete resection rate to greater than 70%. Improved resection rates are seen with both delayed and second-look surgery.

**Q7** A 7-year-old male presents with a right upper quadrant mass associated with some discomfort. Physical examination confirms a large liver mass. Extensive workup reveals a normal laboratory panel. Ultrasound demonstrates a solid 18 cm mass. CT shows a cystic mass within the right lobe of the liver. The child's most likely diagnosis is:

**A** HCC

**B** hepatoblastoma

**C** FNH

**D** mesenchymal hamartoma

**E** undifferentiated embryonal sarcoma.

 **E** Undifferentiated embryonal sarcoma typically presents in children aged 6–10 years of age. It is an extremely malignant lesion associated with a poor outcome. It most commonly presents with right upper quadrant or epigastric pain. A mass may or may not be felt on physical exam. These tumours typically occur in the right lobe of the liver and measure 14–21 cm at the time of diagnosis. Laboratory studies are usually normal. Workup will reveal a solid mass on ultrasound, but a cystic appearance on CT or MRI. Treatment involves a radical surgical resection. Survival rates have improved with chemotherapy.

Q8   Which one of the following is true regarding the lesion diagnosed in question 7?

    **A**   Survival rates are improved to 66% with a combination of surgery and chemotherapy.

    **B**   AFP is an important monitoring tool after resection and adjuvant chemotherapy.

    **C**   Small lesions are managed with chemotherapy alone.

    **D**   Oral contraceptives and exogenous androgens are common aetiologies of this lesion.

    **E**   This malignancy is often associated with Beckwith–Wiedemann's syndrome.

A8   **A**   Undifferentiated embryonal sarcoma, despite historically poor outcomes, is very chemotherapy sensitive. Sarcoma-type protocols have improved survival up to 66%. Survival is around 37% in patients who present with free intraperitoneal rupture. AFP levels are usually normal. Observation is not appropriate for this malignant lesion and aggressive treatment with surgery and chemotherapy is needed to improve survival. Oral contraceptives and exogenous androgens can cause FNH or hepatocellular adenoma. Beckwith–Wiedemann's syndrome is seen in children with Wilms's tumour and hepatoblastoma.

Q9   Which of the following is *not* associated with paediatric HCC?

    **A**   haemochromatosis

    **B**   portal vein thrombosis

    **C**   hepatitis

    **D**   biliary atresia

    **E**   familial adenomatous polyposis

A9   **B**   HCC is the second most common paediatric hepatic tumour, but comprises less than 1% of all paediatric cancers. Cirrhosis is the known predisposing factor in the adult population, but the aetiology is different in children. HCC in the paediatric population follows a variety of metabolic, infectious, congenital and familial disorders. Metabolic disorders include alpha-1 antitrypsin deficiency, haemochromatosis, and type I and III glycogen storage diseases. Hepatitis B and C are infectious disorders associated with the malignancy, especially hepatitis B in areas where this infection is endemic. Congenital abnormalities such as biliary atresia, congenital hepatic fibrosis and Alagille's syndrome have an association with HCC. The association with biliary atresia is strong enough that a screening protocol with hepatic ultrasound and serum AFP levels is recommended. Familial disorders such as familial adenomatous polyposis, Gardner's syndrome and neurofibromatosis have shown an association with HCC.

**Q10** Which of following is *not* a likely complication of mesenchymal hamartoma?

   **A** high-output cardiac failure

   **B** fetal hydrops

   **C** pulmonary hypertension

   **D** rupture

   **E** respiratory distress

**A10** **D** Most of the growth of mesenchymal hamartoma occurs just before or just after birth. Prognosis of neonates with this benign hepatic lesion is often poor. The rapid growth of the neoplasm is felt to be related to the development of fetal hydrops and resulting high mortality. The presentation can also be of high-output cardiac failure with associated pulmonary hypertension. Respiratory distress can occur secondary to mass effect. Tumour rupture is a rare complication. Reports have demonstrated spontaneous involution with observation, while others have shown rare transformation into undifferentiated embryonal sarcoma. When possible, complete surgical excision is curative and is the recommended treatment.

**Q11** Which of the following is *not* a goal of preoperative radiological workup of potentially resectable hepatic neoplasms?

   **A** judging response to neo-adjuvant chemotherapy

   **B** assessing for the presence of metastatic disease

   **C** predicting prognosis and need for adjuvant therapy in resectable cases

   **D** evaluating tumour extension into adjacent organs or vascular structures

   **E** evaluating tumour extent and predicting remnant liver volume

**A11** **C** Preoperative radiological workup is imperative when considering surgical resection of hepatic neoplasms. Assessing for metastatic disease that would preclude resection will help prevent unnecessary exploration. Similarly, tumour extension into adjacent organs or vascular structures that may preclude resection can be evaluated. Neoplasms that may initially appear unresectable on imaging but are known to be responsive to chemotherapy can be monitored radiologically, and their response to chemotherapy and altered potential for resection can be evaluated. When a large portion of functional hepatic tissue needs to be resected for a clear margin, radiological workup can help predict remnant liver volume to ensure adequate postoperative liver function. Prognosis cannot be determined by radiological studies.

**Q12** Which of the following represents correct management of a hepatocellular adenoma?

    **A** cessation of oral contraceptives in a 16-year-old female

    **B** prompt operation in a patient with a ruptured hepatocellular adenoma

    **C** observation of a 7 cm hepatocellular adenoma

    **D** observation of a ruprred hepatocellular adenoma less than 5 cm diameter, after the patient has stabilised

    **E** selective resection of adenomas in a patient with type I glycogen-storage disease (GSD)

**A12** **A** Hepatocellular adenoma is rare in the paediatric population and is most commonly known for its appearance in women in their twenties on oral contraceptives. These lesions in the paediatric population are generally asymptomatic and diagnosed incidentally. There is a risk of spontaneous rupture and symptomatic presentation, albeit the risk is very small. Initial management includes withdrawal of any potential causative medications, and observation. Surgical resection is reserved for lesions that grow during a period of observation, for those with evidence of intralesional haemorrhage, for adenomas larger than 5 cm and those in which the diagnosis is unclear. When operating for tumour rupture, elective resection should follow a period of non-operative monitoring and haemodynamic support if the patient's condition allows. In patients with type I GSD with multiple adenomas, hepatic transplantation should be considered because of the risk of developing HCC in this patient population.

**Q13** Which of the following is *not* true regarding hepatic resection?

    **A** The Pringle manoeuvre should be limited to 20 minutes.

    **B** Extended right hepatic lobectomy includes resection of segments I and IV through VIII.

    **C** Hepatic arterial variations are of no surgical importance.

    **D** Transverse and subcostal incisions are both acceptable approaches to hepatic lobectomy.

    **E** When performing a left hepatic lobectomy, care must be take to identify the variable insertion of the middle hepatic vein.

**A13** **C** When performing a liver resection both transverse and subcostal incisions provide adequate exposure. The surgeon must be familiar with the anatomy and identification of displaced or accessory hepatic arteries. Damage or ligation of these vessels can result in irrreversible ischaemia of the remnant liver tissue and resulting liver failure. Similarly, knowledge of variations of the middle hepatic vein insertion is of utmost importance during left hepatic lobectomy to avoid devastating haemorrhage. This area is extremely difficult to expose and control haemorrhage. The Pringle manoeuvre is an important method of controlling intraoperative haemorrhage. The manoeuvre should be limited to 20 minutes to avoid hepatic ischaemia and postoperative liver failure.

**Q14** A 3-year-old female is being evaluated for new-onset jaundice. On physical exam a mass is palpated in the right upper quadrant. Ultrasound reveals a 9 cm mass within the right hepatic lobe. The mass appears to involve the right hepatic duct and proximal ductal dilatation is seen. The most likely diagnosis is:

   **A** rhabdomyosarcoma

   **B** HCC

   **C** undifferentiated embryonal sarcoma

   **D** infantile haemangioendothelioma

   **E** hepatoblastoma.

**A14** **A** Rhabdomyosarcoma, although the most common sarcoma in children, is a rare liver tumour. The median age at presentation is 3 years of age. The neoplasm arises in the intrahepatic biliary system and then invades the hepatic parenchyma. Because of its origin the most common presenting symptom is jaundice. Elevated direct bilirubin, transaminases and gamma-glutamyl transpeptidases are common laboratory findings.

**Q15** Which one of the following is true regarding the lesion identified in question 14?

   **A** Adequate resection is possible in 69%–81% of patients after a multidisciplinary approach.

   **B** Lymphatic spread is a rare finding.

   **C** Hepatitis B is a common predisposing factor in endemic areas.

   **D** Alpha-fetoprotein is an important monitoring tool after resection.

   **E** Percutaneous transhepatic cholangiography (PTC) can be useful preoperatively.

**A15** **E** Complete resection of rhabdomyosarcoma is possible in only 20%–40% of patients because of tumour spread and invasion into other organs. Surgery, chemotherapy and radiotherapy are needed in a multidisciplinary approach to maximise adequate resection rates. Lymphatic spread is not uncommon due to the aggressive nature of this neoplasm. PTC can aid in evaluating the tumour extent within the biliary system. PTC also provides a means of external drainage to treat the obstructive jaundice. Hepatitis B is a predisposing factor of HCC. AFP is a diagnostic and monitoring tool after resection of hepatoblastoma.

**Q16** Regarding the surgical anatomy of the liver, which of the following is the most accurate statement?

**A** Right hepatic trisegmentectomy includes segment III.

**B** In up to 18% of cases the right hepatic artery arises from the superior mesenteric artery and ascends to the porta hepatis on the *left* side of the common bile duct.

**C** A preduodenal portal vein precludes effective vascular control at the porta hepatis.

**D** The middle hepatic vein usually runs from left to right between segments III and VII to empty into the inferior vena cava.

**E** Left trisegmentectomy may be curative for solitary tumours limited to segments III, IV and V.

**A16** **E** Right hepatic trisegmentectomy (also called extended right lobectomy) includes segments V, VI, VII, VIII, as well as IV on the left side of Cantlie's line. Segment I may or may not be included. An aberrant right hepatic artery, which may be accessory or replacing, does arise from the superior mesenteric artery. It then ascends to the liver on the right side of the common bile duct, *not* the left, where the normal common hepatic artery usually stays. There are fewer than 100 case reports of preduodenal portal vein in the literature. It is usually an incidental finding and has no practical bearing on the surgical anatomy of the liver. The middle hepatic vein runs from right to left and superiorly along, or across segment IV. Left trisegmentectomy (extended left lobectomy) includes everything to the left of Cantlie's line, as well as segments V and VIII – leaving segments VI and VII. Preservation of segment VIII, if uninvolved, may be feasible; however, the operation is technically more difficult.

**Q17** Regarding extensive liver resections, which of the following is not a likely/expected physiological complication?

**A** tendency towards persistent hypoglycaemia

**B** transient encephalopathic features

**C** prolonged hypoalbuminaemia

**D** need for clotting factor replacement

**E** hyperuricaemia

**A17** **E** The liver has a crucial position in intermediary metabolism. It plays a profound role in the maintenance of blood sugar because of its role in gluconeogenesis, glycogenesis and glycolysis. If liver mass is below a critical level, persistent hypoglycaemia is a real danger. Hence, the need to closely monitor blood sugar levels after massive liver resections. Acute liver failure with encephalopathy can be a consequence of acute and massive reduction in liver mass. Almost all serum proteins – including albumin and clotting factors – are synthesised in the liver.

Uric acid is the end-product of organic base catabolism from nucleic acids. Gout and kidney failure can lead to hyperuricaemia. Liver failure does not affect the level. In any case impaired liver function will tend to produce less uric acid.

## Further reading

Ashcraft KW, Holcomb GW, Murphy JP, editors. *Pediatric Surgery*. 4th ed. Philadelphia, PA: Elsevier Saunders; 2005.

Grosfeld JL, O'Neill JA, Fonkalsrud EW, *et al.*, editors. *Pediatric Surgery*. Vol 1. 6th ed. Philadelphia, PA: Mosby Elsevier; 2006.

Herzog CE, Andrassy RJ, Eftekhari F. Childhood cancers: hepatoblastoma. *Oncologist*. 2000; 5(6): 445–53.

Ziegler MM, Azizkhan RG, Weber TR. *Operative Pediatric Surgery*. New York, NY: McGraw-Hill Companies; 2003.

# CHAPTER 72

# Endocrine tumours

## MICHAEL SKINNER, EDUARDO PEREZ

**From the choices below each question, select the single best answer.**

**Q1** A 17-year-old male is being evaluated for a thyroid nodule. During questioning, he admits to recently having headaches and anxiety. After the administration of pentagastrin, his serum calcitonin is 1500 pg/mL. A fine needle aspiration (FNA) of the nodules is performed. What measurement on the FNA sample would aid in making the diagnosis?

- **A** calcitonin
- **B** vanillylmandelic acid (VMA)
- **C** carcinoembryonic antigen
- **D** A and C
- **E** all of the above

**A1** **D** This question describes a typical case of medullary thyroid carcinoma (MTC), with a multinodular thyroid in the setting of an elevated calcitonin level. MTC originates from the parafollicular C cells and is responsible for 5% of all thyroid malignancies. Eighty per cent of medullary carcinomas are sporadic and the remainder are associated with an inherited multiple endocrine neoplasia (MEN) syndrome. Pathological diagnosis can be obtained with FNA. The pathological features of medullary carcinoma include C-cell hyperplasia, presence of amyloid, and specimen staining positive for calcitonin and carcinoembryonic antigen.

**Q2** What is the most important test to consider before any surgical interventions for multiple endocrine neoplasm type 2?

- **A** serum calcium
- **B** serum parathormone (PTH) level
- **C** 24-hour urine catecholamines
- **D** serum thyroid-stimulating hormone (TSH) and T4 levels
- **E** serum phosphorus

A2 **C** This patient presentation with headache and anxiety, should raise the suspicion of a concurrent phaeochromocytoma. Phaeochromocytomas are rare catecholamine-secreting tumours of the adrenal medulla. They affect 40% of patients with MEN2A and similarly with MEN2B, although there is large variability of its penetrance among kindreds. About 10% of phaeochromocytomas in children are familial. Malignant phaeochromocytomas are rare in children (<1%), but there is a higher incidence of bilateral disease. Usually phaeochromocytomas become evident about 10 years after the diagnosis of C-cell hyperplasia or MTC. The symptoms associated with phaeochromocytoma include hypertension, headache, intermittent sweating, pallor and flushing, tachycardia and palpitations, nervousness, weight loss, abdominal or chest pain, and thirst with polyuria. MEN2 patients are characterised by an adrenergic phenotype and show larger elevations of plasma metanephrines and a higher frequency of hypertension and symptoms, particularly of a paroxysmal nature.

Q3 If the CT scan suggests a phaeochromocytoma, what procedure would you perform first?
**A** adrenalectomy
**B** parathyroidectomy
**C** thyroidectomy
**D** A and C
**E** B and C

A3 **A** If a phaeochromocytoma is identified in this patient, it will need to be removed before the thyroid is operated on. The treatment for phaeochromocytoma is surgical removal of the lesion. Phaeochromocytomas can be extraordinarily active for their size, and accurate preoperative localisation of the lesions is essential. In the setting of bilateral disease, partial adrenalectomy should be considered.

Q4 What is the recommended treatment after the possibility of phaeochromocytoma has been definitely excluded?
**A** ipsilateral thyroid lobectomy with ultrasound examination of the contralateral lobe
**B** total thyroidectomy with postoperative iodine-131 treatment
**C** total thyroidectomy with postoperative calcitonin monitoring
**D** total thyroidectomy with postoperative chemoradiation therapy
**E** excisional biopsy with permanent pathology examination

A4 **C** The treatment of choice for sporadic and inherited disease is total thyroidectomy with central lymph node dissection. Ipsilateral modified neck dissection should be performed if there is neck disease, if there are positive findings during central neck dissection, or if tumour size is greater than 1 cm. Postoperatively, patients benefit from thyroid hormone replacement after total thyroidectomy. There is no role for postoperative iodine-131 therapy. Chemotherapy has not been shown to be useful, but radiation therapy has been shown to decrease local recurrence in high-risk patients.

After a period of 8–12 weeks, if serum calcitonin and carcinoembryonic antigen levels are within normal limits, they can be used as sensitive markers for recurrence or metastases. Somatostatin may be used for the treatment of facial flushing and diarrhoea.

**Q5** After an uneventful laparoscopic appendicectomy for acute appendicitis in an 8-year-old, pathology report shows a 2 cm carcinoid in the tip of the appendix. What is the next step in management?

 **A** right hemicolectomy
 **B** chemotherapy
 **C** observation
 **D** caecectomy
 **E** ileocaecectomy

**A5** **C** Carcinoid tumours arise from the amine uptake cells and the carboxylation cells and are classified according to the site of origin as foregut, midgut or hindgut, with midgut tumours accounting for 80%–85% of cases; 46% of these arise from the appendix. Only 10% of patients have symptoms present at time of diagnosis. Sixty per cent of these tumours are detected after an appendicectomy has been performed. As in adults, 2 cm is the threshold between a simple appendicectomy and a right hemicolectomy. Also the proximity to the caecum and mucin production is also taken into account. In this case treatment has been completed, and the patient requires only observation.

**Q6** Which tumour markers can be used to follow this patient?

 **A** serotonin
 **B** chromogranin A
 **C** somatostatin
 **D** inhibin
 **E** CA125

**A6** **A** Carcinoid tumours are derived from chromaffin cells and are able to secrete vasoactive peptides such as serotonin. This makes it a good tumour marker to follow up for recurrence in these patients.

**Q7** A 5-year-old girl who underwent prophylactic total thyroidectomy 24 hours ago now complains of a generalised 'tingling' sensation and muscle cramps. Appropriate treatment would include which of the following?

  **A** intravenous infusion of calcium gluconate

  **B** administration of oxygen by mask

  **C** administration of an anticonvulsant

  **D** administration of a tranquilliser

  **E** neurologic consultation

**A7**  **A** The most common complication of thyroid surgery remains transient hypoparathyroidism, occurring in 0.7%–40% of paediatric patients. The most frequent cause is injury to the blood supply of the parathyroid glands. The manifestations include tingling, muscle cramps, convulsions and a positive Chvostek's sign (contraction of facial muscles after tapping the facial nerve). Mild asymptomatic hypocalcaemia does not require calcium supplementation. In patients with severe disturbances or symptoms of hypocalcaemia, intravenous supplementation should be implemented and patients should be released with an oral calcium regimen until the hypoparathyroidism resolves. In 2% of patients, permanent hypocalcaemia requires permanent calcium and vitamin D supplementation to avoid the long-term complications of hypocalcaemia.

**Q8** A 16-year-old female presents with depression, hypertension, 9 kg weight gain over 6 months and amenorrhoea. On examination, she weighs 75 kg, her height is 152 cms, and she has supraclavicular fullness, abdominal striae, ecchymoses on her arms and facial acne. Which of the following would be the most appropriate next step?

  **A** morning adrenocorticotropic hormone (ACTH) level

  **B** morning cortisol level

  **C** MRI of pituitary

  **D** 24-hour urine free cortisol

  **E** 1 g cosyntropin stimulation test

**A8**  **D** The patient has the clinical features of Cushing's syndrome. Initial screening tests for determining if she has hypercortisolism include dexamethasone suppression testing, midnight cortisol measurement and urinary free cortisol. Of these tests, the urinary free cortisol is most sensitive test. In patients with Cushing's syndrome, the urinary free cortisol level is greater than 100 µg per day.

$Q^9$ After confirming the diagnosis of Cushing's disease, how would you identify pituitary from non-pituitary causes?

A low-dose dexamethasone test

B high-dose dexamethasone test

C morning adrenocorticotropic hormone level

D 24-hour urine free cortisol

E morning cortisol level

$A^9$ **B** After the diagnosis of Cushing's syndrome is established, a specific cause needs to be determined. This can be achieved by using the high-dose dexamethasone test. This test distinguishes between pituitary and non-pituitary causes. An oral dose of dexamethasone is given every 6 hours for 48 hours. Then a 24-hour urine is collected to measure for free cortisol and 17-hydroxysteroids. In patients with an adrenal adenoma or adrenocortical carcinoma, and in most patients with tumours that produce ACTH, the levels are not suppressed. In patients with pituitary neoplasm, the steroid secretion levels are suppressed by 50%.

$Q10$ When a pituitary microadenoma is identified, what is the best option for treatment?

A chemotherapy

B adrenalectomy

C trans-sphenoidal hypophysectomy

D radiation

E none of the above

$A10$ **C** Bilateral adrenalectomy used to be the therapy of choice for Cushing's syndrome due to pituitary tumours. This aggressive treatment took care of the problem, but patients were left with adrenal insufficiency. The treatment of choice is resection of the pituitary tumour, via the trans-sphenoidal route. It is expected that 20% of patients may experience a relapse within 5 years of treatment. If not successful, pituitary irradiation is generally an effective second-line treatment.

**Q11** A 12-year-old male has been diagnosed with asymptomatic primary hyperparathyroidism. Which of the following is *not* a management options?

- **A** sestamibi scan followed by localised parathyroidectomy and frozen section
- **B** observation
- **C** four-gland exploration
- **D** transaxillary parathyroidectomy
- **E** neck ultrasound followed by localised parathyroidectomy and PTH assay

**A11** **B** Primary hyperparathyroidism in childhood most commonly results from a solitary hyperfunctioning adenoma, and more rarely from diffuse hyperplasia of all four glands. Hyperparathyroidism resulting from hyperplasia in all four glands is a feature of MEN1. Furthermore, as stated previously, approximately 30% of patients having MEN2A develop hyperparathyroidism. Once the diagnosis of hyperparathyroidism is established, the offending parathyroid tissue should be resected. There is no place for medical management of primary hyperparathyroidism in children. In the past, bilateral neck exploration with resection of enlarged parathyroid glands was standard treatment for primary hyperparathyroidism. More recent advances in imaging and real-time parathyroid hormone measurements have allowed the use of minimally invasive techniques in adults. Currently, it is recommended that patients with biochemically confirmed primary hyperparathyroidism undergo preoperative localisation with technetium-99m-sestamibi scan. If the scan demonstrates a single parathyroid lesion, a less invasive procedure can be performed. Confirmation that the offending gland has been removed can be obtained by performing a rapid parathyroid hormone analysis while the child remains asleep.

Q12 A 16-year-old female presents with a 4cm nodule of the lower pole of the left lobe of the thyroid gland. It is mildly tender and there are no palpable lymph nodes. Her TSH level is low. She is referred to you with an ultrasonography scan (*see* Figure 72.1a) and nuclear scan (*see* Figure 72.1b). What is the next step in management?

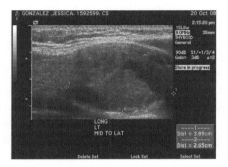

**FIGURE 72.1A** Ultrasonography scan of thyroid gland

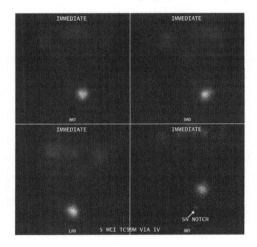

**FIGURE 72.1B** Radionuclide thyroid scan

**A** total thyroidectomy
**B** left lobectomy
**C** thyroid antibody studies
**D** FNA of the nodule
**E** CT of the neck

A12 **D** Although thyroid nodules are uncommon in children, their importance stems from a relatively high likelihood of associated cancer. In more recent paediatric studies, the incidence of malignancy in thyroid nodules has been 20% or less. This is a much lower incidence of cancer than was reported in previous decades and is believed to reflect the decreased number of children who have been exposed to neck radiation for trivial reasons. In a child with a palpable solitary nodule, measurement of free T4, TSH and thyroid antibodies (antithyroglobulin and antithyroid peroxidase) is generally carried out to evaluate thyroid function and screen for autoimmune thyroiditis. When evaluating a sporadic thyroid nodule in a symptomatic paediatric patient, it is critical to determine whether the nodule is malignant or benign. The most important diagnostic test at this point is FNA. The technique is easily accomplished in nodules larger than 1 cm in diameter; smaller lesions may require ultrasound guidance. Interpretations are classified as benign tumour, malignant tumour, indeterminate diagnosis or inadequate specimen. In children, the effectiveness of FNA cytology in the evaluation of thyroid nodules is still being debated. Children are somewhat more difficult to evaluate than adults, owing to the smaller size of the nodules, and the frequent need to sedate the child to allow safe and accurate aspiration. Also, there is a higher incidence of cancer in any thyroid nodule in young children. It is widely accepted to use FNA in adolescent patients because the pattern of thyroid disease is similar to that of adults. CT scan will not reliably separate benign from malignant nodules Total thyroidectomy is not indicated at this time.

**Q13** Her FNA shows this to be a benign follicular lesion. What is the most appropriate treatment?

  **A** total thyroidectomy

  **B** total thyroidectomy with postoperative iodine-131 therapy

  **C** lobectomy

  **D** lobectomy with postoperative iodine-131 therapy

  **F** observation with interval ultrasound examination and thyroglobulin measurement

**A13**  **C**  For a benign follicular lesion, lobectomy should be adequate. If there is any suggestion on the final pathology that this is a malignant lesion then a completion thyroidectomy should be performed. There is controversy about the extent of thyroid resection required for long-term control. Surgeons advocating aggressive thyroid resections argue that total thyroidectomy, with lymph node dissection if the regional nodes are involved, is the most successful method of obtaining local control of the tumour. Moreover, removing the entire thyroid gland makes radioiodine ablative therapy more effective because there is less functioning endocrine tissue to take up the radionuclide. Those who argue that lesser thyroid gland resection is indicated hold that differentiated thyroid carcinoma in children is a relatively indolent disease and that survival is apparently not a function of the extent of gland removal. Further, there is a significant incidence of major surgical complications associated with total thyroidectomy in children.

**Q14** She underwent an uneventful operation, but 6 hours later you get called to the bedside because the patient has breathing difficulties. On examination her condition is stable, her $O_2$ saturation is 94% and the wound is dry, but there seems to be some swelling. What is the next step in management?

**A** intubation

**B** wound exploration

**C** observation

**D** warm compresses

**E** ultrasonography of the neck

**A14** **B** Patient is presenting with possible wound haematoma. This diagnosis should be made at the bedside and warrants immediate treatment. In the setting of respiratory difficulty, even though her $O_2$ saturation is normal, a wound exploration is warranted. Evacuation of the haematoma will result in immediate opening of the airway. Emergency intubation is not indicated as her oxygen saturation is normal. Ultrasonography would delay the diagnosis in the setting of respiratory difficulty. Warm compresses or observation would not correct the problem.

**Q15** An 11-year-old male presents to your clinic complaining of muscle weakness. On exam his BP is 150/90. His serum potassium level is 2.9. He underwent a CT scan of his abdomen (*see* Figures 72.2a and 72.2b) what's the diagnosis?

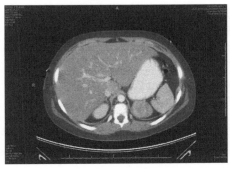

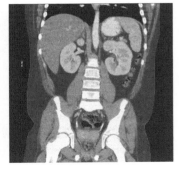

**FIGURE 72.2A** CT scan of abdomen (horizontal section)

**FIGURE 72.2B** CT scan of abdomen (coronal section)

**A** Cushing's syndrome

**B** phaeochromocytoma

**C** adrenal hyperplasia

**D** adrenal adenoma

**E** neuroblastoma

A**15** **D** Signs and symptoms of primary hyperaldosteronism are non-specific. Children usually present with hypertension, muscle weakness, polydipsia and polyuria. Constant high levels of aldosterone causes the total body sodium level to increase, thus increasing the total fluid volume and suppressing renin and angiotensin. When a child presents with hypertension and hypokalaemia, one should consider a diagnosis of primary hyperaldosteronism. Once the diagnosis is confirmed, it is necessary to determine whether it is due to an adenoma or to bilateral adrenal hyperplasia. If a mass greater than 1 cm is identified by CT scan or MRI, adenoma is likely. If no masses are visualised, a selective adrenal vein sampling can differentiate unilateral vs. bilateral adrenocortical hypersecretion.

Q**16** What is the next step in management of the patient in question 15?
  **A** percutaneous biopsy
  **B** radiation
  **C** bilateral adrenalectomy
  **D** unilateral adrenalectomy
  **E** spironolactone

A**16** **D** In patients with adrenal hypercortisolism of unilateral adrenal origin, the treatment is operative removal of the gland. Perioperative exogenous glucocorticoid replacement is required because the contralateral gland is suppressed. The surgical approach to the adrenal gland depends on the size of the lesion, the likelihood of malignant disease, the need for bilateral adrenalectomies, and the surgeon's preference. If adrenocortical carcinoma is suspected, then an open transabdominal approach is necessary to widely excise the tumour and to thoroughly search for metastatic lesions.

Laparoscopic adrenalectomy has emerged as the standard treatment for most patients, including paediatric, when malignancy is not suspected. Laparoscopic approaches can be lateral transabdominal or retroperitoneal.

Q**17** A 12-year-old male presents after fainting in his physical education class. The school nurse found his blood glucose level was 35. He got better after some juice but started feeling light-headed after an hour. His paediatrician obtained the following test results: glucose 30 mg/dL [1.7 mmol/L], insulin 10 µU/mL, C-peptide positive. What is your working diagnosis?
  **A** insulinoma
  **B** diabetes
  **C** vasovagal syncope
  **D** gastrinoma
  **E** carcinoid

**A17** **A** Insulinoma is the most common pancreatic endocrine tumour in children, although it is still quite rare, with an estimated incidence of one case per 250 000 patient-years. Only 10% of insulinomas are malignant, and these metastasise to surrounding tissues. The distinction between benign and malignant tumours of the endocrine pancreas is difficult. It is based on a tumour size greater than 2 cm, and the presence of lymph node or other distant metastases. Presenting symptoms include hypoglycaemia, dizziness, headaches, sweating and seizures. Whipple's triad was originally described in patients with insulinoma, and consists of symptoms of hypoglycaemia with fasting, fasting glucose level less than half of normal, and relief of symptoms with glucose administration. The tumour in insulinoma is usually solitary, except in MEN1 syndrome, which may entail multiple lesions. The diagnosis of insulinoma is made by demonstrating an insulin-to-glucose ratio of more than 0.3 (microunits of insulin per millilitre to milligrams of glucose per decilitre). C-peptide levels should always be measured to rule out the administration of exogenous insulin.

**Q18** Abdominal ultrasonography shows a 2 cm lesion in the body of the pancreas. What is the next step in management?
  **A** enucleation
  **B** distal pancreatectomy
  **C** check the calcium/PTH level
  **D** diazoxide
  **E** pancreatoduodenectomy

**A18** **C** Because pancreatic islet cell tumours can occur as part of MEN type 1 (MEN1), screening for two other diseases – pituitary adenoma and hyperparathyroidism – should be performed. The tumour in insulinoma is usually solitary, except in MEN1 syndrome, which may entail multiple lesions.

**Q19** A 7-year-old male is diagnosed with metastatic MTC. There is no family history of the disease. What is the next step in management?
  **A** total thyroidectomy
  **B** total thyroidectomy with central neck dissection
  **C** genetic screening
  **D** radiation therapy
  **E** chemotherapy

**A19** **C** Genotype–phenotype correlations exist with regard to clinical subtype, age at onset, and aggressiveness of MTC and the presence of other endocrine tumours in MEN2. These relationships are useful when planning the timing of prophylactic thyroidectomy and deciding whether screening for phaeochromocytoma or hyperparathyroidism is necessary. Another important use of these correlations is in patients presenting with apparently sporadic MTC. The presence or absence of *RET* mutations will influence their management. Therefore, genetic testing is recommended before surgical intervention in all paediatric patients diagnosed with MTC.

**Q20** At what age would you perform prophylactic thyroidectomy on a *RET* carrier with a family history of MEN2B?

**A** before the age of 1 year

**B** 2–5 years

**C** 5–10 years

**D** 11–15 years

**E** after the age of 16

**A20** **A** The only effective treatment for MTC is surgical resection, underscoring the importance of early diagnosis and therapy before metastasis occurs. For this reason, current management of MTC in children from families having the MEN2 syndrome relies on the presymptomatic detection of the *RET* proto-oncogene mutation responsible for the disease. Affected children with MEN2A should undergo total thyroidectomy at about the age of 5 years, before the cancer spreads beyond the thyroid gland. Indeed, approximately 80% of children who have thyroidectomy based on the presence of the *RET* mutation will already have foci of MTC within the thyroid gland. Owing to the increased virulence of MTC in children having MEN2B, it may be preferable for them to have their thyroid glands removed in infancy, sometimes before the age of 1 in carriers of some specific *RET* mutations.

## Further reading

Kappy MS, Allen DB, Geffner ME, editors. *Principles and Practice of Pediatric Endocrinology.* 1st ed. Springfield, IL: Charles Thomas Publisher Ltd; 2005.

Holcomb GW, Murphy JP. *Ashcraft's Pediatric Surgery.* 5th ed. Philadelphia, PA: Saunders; 2010.

Oldham KT, Colombani PM, Foglia RP, *et al.*, editors. *Principles and Practice of Pediatric Surgery.* 4th ed. Philadelphia, PA: Lippincott Williams & Wilkins; 2005.

# CHAPTER 73

# Germ cell tumours

## ROSHNI DASGUPTA, RICHARD G AZIZKHAN

**From the choices below each question, select the single best answer.**

**Q1** Primordial germ cells migrate from the yolk sac along the mesentery to the gonads in what week of gestation?

**A** week 1
**B** week 3
**C** week 12
**D** week 5
**E** week 9

**A1** **D** The blastocyst forms primordial cells in week 1 of gestation. At week 3, cells form on the wall of the yolk sac. Actual migration of totipotential primordial germ cells does not occur until weeks 5–6, when cells migrate from the yolk sac along the mesentery to the gonads and then become gonadal or extragonadal. Abnormal migration may give rise to midline tumours, which mainly occur in the cervical, retroperitoneal, sacrococcygeal, mediastinum and pineal gland.

**Q2** What is the most common germ cell tumour in the neonatal age group?

**A** mediastinal teratoma
**B** ovarian neoplasm
**C** cervical teratoma
**D** testicular neoplasm
**E** sacrococcygeal teratoma (SCT).

**A2** **E** SCT is the most common germ cell tumour in the fetal/neonatal age group (50%). Mediastinal teratomas and gonadal neoplasms are seen in children in their second decade of life. The rate of germ cell tumours in the 0–4 age group is 7 per million children. Gonadal tumours are rare in children; they are much more common in girls aged 10–15 years.

**Q3** What malignant germ cell tumours secrete alpha-fetoprotein (AFP)?

   **A** choriocarcinoma

   **B** yolk sac tumours

   **C** germinoma

   **D** testicular tumours

   **E** embryonal carcinoma

 **A3** **B** AFP is produced by yolk sac (endodermal sinus) tumours and has a half-life of 4 days. Embryonal carcinoma, seminoma, dysgerminoma and choriocarcinoma can secrete β-hCG. In addition, lactate dehydrogenase (LDH) and ALP can also be elevated in patients with germinoma tumours.

 **Q4** Klinefelter's syndrome is associated with what type of germ cell tumour?

   **A** mediastinal teratoma

   **B** testicular seminoma

   **C** endodermal sinus tumour

   **D** choriocarcinoma

   **E** embryonal carcinoma

 **A4** **A** Mediastinal teratomas are the most common site of extragonadal germ cell tumours in older children. They are found in the anterior mediastinum and present with airway symptoms. Germ cells make up 20% of all mediastinal tumours. About 80% of mediastinal germ cell tumours are benign; these occur with equal frequency in males and females. However, there is a male predominance (9 : 1) for malignant mediastinal germ cell tumours. Germ cell tumours are associated with Klinefelter's syndrome (47,XXY). In patients with Klinefelter's syndrome, the relative risk of having a malignant mediastinal germ cell tumour is 66.7. At least 8% of male patients with primary mediastinal tumours have Klinefelter's syndrome (50 times the expected frequency).

 **Q5** Which of the following is not generally included in the preoperative workup of an infant with SCT?

   **A** blood screen for tumour markers

   **B** echocardiogram prior to chemotherapy

   **C** MRI of abdomen and pelvis

   **D** chest CT scan

   **E** spinal radiographs

**A5**    **B**   SCTs require extensive preoperative workup that should include an AFP tumour marker. This is generally used as a baseline and to predict recurrence in future follow-up. Spine films should be performed to rule any sacral anomalies. Currarino's triad includes a presacral tumour, anorectal malformation and a scimitar type sacral anomaly. Examination of the chest should be performed to ensure there is no metastatic spread to the lungs. An echocardiogram is not required as 95% of SCTs are benign in the neonatal period.

**Q6**   What is the risk of recurrence of a SCT?

    **A**   10%

    **B**   25%

    **C**   80% if the coccyx is not removed

    **D**   50%

    **E**   70%

**A6**    **B**   The risk of recurrence of SCT is generally thought to be around 25%. Risk factors for recurrence include age greater than one year, immature teratoma on histology, and an elevated AFP. The risk of recurrence is 40% if the coccyx is not removed. Patients should be monitored with serial rectal examinations and serum markers to detect any sign of recurrence. Patients with local recurrence should have resection and be considered for chemotherapy.

**Q7**   What is the current indication for a retroperitoneal lymph node dissection for testicular germ cell tumours in children?

    **A**   enlarged lymph nodes seen on CT scan

    **B**   routine for all children under 10 years of age

    **C**   if a sentinel lymph node test is positive

    **D**   for all germinomas

    **E**   if a patient underwent a trans-scrotal resection for testicular mass

**A7**    **A**   In adults retroperitoneal lymph node dissection (RPLND) may be used as a primary treatment modality for low-volume non-seminomatous germ cell tumours localised to the retroperitoneum as well as a salvage therapy for residual masses following chemotherapy. In children a routine selective lymph node dissection is indicated for patients with enlarged nodes. RPLND may also be used in boys with persistently elevated levels of tumour markers after chemotherapy. In children diagnosed with paratesticular rhabdomyosarcoma over age 10, routine retroperitoneal lymph node dissection is indicated.

**Q8** Which is not part of the staging procedure for a patient with an ovarian teratoma?

**A** palpation of lymph nodes and biopsy of enlarged nodes

**B** examination and biopsy of suspicious lesion in the omentum

**C** peritoneal washings

**D** routine wedge biopsy/bivalving of the contralateral ovary

**E** preoperative tumour markers

**A8**   **D**  The paradigm for staging patients with teratomas includes an examination of the entire peritoneal cavity. The omentum should be examined and suspicious nodules biopsied. Peritoneal washings or ascitic fluid should be taken for cytologic analysis. All suspicious lymph nodes should be biopsied; however, there is no indication for a full retroperitoneal lymph node dissection. Routine wedge biopsy of the contralateral ovary is not indicated; biopsy should be performed only if suspicious lesions are present.

**Q9** Which of the following is false regarding the presentation of cervical teratomas?

**A** They present *in utero* with antenatal polyhydramnios.

**B** They may have respiratory distress due to airway compression and hypoplastic lungs.

**C** They may require an EXIT procedure for management of the airway.

**D** They are usually malignant.

**E** They contain elements from all three germ cell layers.

**A9**   **D**  Cervical teratomas comprise 10% of all teratomas and are most often diagnosed on prenatal ultrasound. They can present with polyhydramnios secondary to obstruction. Many patients also have hypoplastic lungs. The teratomas contain all three germ cell layers and are almost always benign (80%). They are found at the level of the strap muscles and extend posteriorly towards the trachea.

**Q10** What is the standard therapy for a completely resected mature teratoma in a child under age 15?

**A** radiation therapy to primary site

**B** neo-adjuvant chemotherapy if extragonadal

**C** observation

**D** radiation to primary site and six cycles of chemotherapy with cisplatin, etoposide and bleomycin (PEB)

**E** six cycles of chemotherapy with PEB

A10  C  As long as no elements of carcinoma are found, patients with mature germ cell teratomas (regardless of location), may simply be observed at regular interval without the need for any adjuvant therapy. Immature teratomas contain tissue from all three germ cell layers, but predominantly neuroepithelial elements. These are graded from I–III based on the amount of immature tissue. If malignant teratomas are noted the PEB regimen is standard of care.

Q11  Which of the following is true regarding SCTs?

  A  Type I SCT are predominantly external and have the highest incidence of malignancy.
  B  Type IV is completely external.
  C  Type III has a small external component but the majority of the mass is internal.
  D  Type II is the least common type of SCT.
  E  Type IV tumours usually present with congestive heart failure.

A11  C  The Altman classification of SCTs is based on location.
Type I is a predominantly external.
Type II has both an intra-abdominal and an external component.
Type III is predominantly internal with a small external component.
Type IV is exclusively internal with no external component.

   Tumours with an intra-abdominal component are more likely to be malignant, primarily because of the late stage at diagnosis. In neonates the tumour is benign in about 95% of patients, children greater than 1 year of age have a higher rate of malignancy (80%). Congestive heart failure can be secondary to shunting or haemorrhage into the tumour and is most common with the large external SCT.

Q12  Which of the following statements about paediatric testicular seminoma is false?

  A  If discovered at stage I patients are thought to have nearly a 100% survival rate.
  B  Cryptorchidism is not a risk factor for seminoma.
  C  There is an equal incidence in both black and white people.
  D  The treatment for stage I resected seminoma does not include chemotherapy.
  E  Patients diagnosed with testicular seminoma on one side are at increased risk for developing a contralateral seminoma on the other side.

A**12** **C** Cryptorchidism is a risk factor for the development of testicular germ cell tumours. Ten per cent of testis tumours are associated with cryptorchidism. A quarter of the tumours associated with cryptorchidism are actually within the contralateral normally descended testis. The risk of testicular cancer in a boy with cryptorchidism is directly related to the degree of maldescent. The risk is 1 in 20 if the testis is high within the abdomen and decreases to 1 in 80 if the testis is within the inguinal canal. After radical orchidectomy, patients with stage I seminoma are treated only with external beam radiotherapy to retroperitoneal and ipsilateral pelvic lymph nodes, typically 2500 cGy, which gives nearly 100% survival rate, chemotherapy is not required. Although in adults the incidence of testicular cancer is much higher in white people, among paediatric patients the incidence is equal among both black and white people.

Q**13** Which of the following statements is *not* true regarding ovarian germ cell tumours?

   **A** All patients except those with stage I, grade I immature teratoma and stage IA dysgerminoma require postoperative chemotherapy.
   **B** Adjuvant platinum-based chemotherapy for ovarian germ cell tumours is thought to be superior to vincristine, dactinomycin and cyclophosphamide.
   **C** Recurrence rate of immature teratomas is inversely related to the grade of neural elements.
   **D** Second-look laparotomy is not beneficial in patients with initially completely resected tumours who receive cisplatin-based adjuvant treatment.
   **E** Radiation therapy for recurrent germ cell tumours is not effective.

A**13** **C** The recurrence rate of immature teratomas is directly related to the grade of neural elements. Both size and histology are the major factors determining prognosis for patients with immature teratomas. Prognosis is poor for patients with large tumours when more than one-third of the tumour was composed of endodermal sinus elements, choriocarcinoma, or grade III immature teratoma. Tumours greater than 10 cm in size also have a poor prognosis. Studies show treatment with PEB appears to be superior to vacuum-assisted closure (VAC) as there is a 25% recurrence rate in patients treated with 6 months of VAC. In the modern era patients treated with PEB-based chemotherapy have been found not to benefit from second-look surgical procedures because of the effectiveness of the platinum-based chemotherapy.

**Q14** What percentage of patients with SCTs have associated abnormalities?

**A** 5%

**B** 10%

**C** 20%

**D** 40%

**E** 50%

**A14** **C** Twenty per cent of children with SCTs have some sort of associated abnormality. These can include cardiac, genitourinary, musculoskeletal or neurologic abnormalities.

**Q15** Which of the following should not be done to workup a testicular mass?

**A** serum markers including AFP, β-hCG

**B** abdominal CT scan

**C** testicular ultrasound

**D** trans-scrotal biopsy

**E** chest CT scan

**A15** **D** Trans-scrotal biopsy should not be performed; an inguinal approach to testicular lesions should be done. Markers including AFP, β-hCG, ALP and LDH are often helpful in testicular cancer. Chest CT has now replaced chest X-ray as a means of evaluating the chest for spread. Abdominal CT scan is necessary to look at retroperitoneal nodes for staging purposes. Testicular ultrasound also helps differentiate a solid testicular mass from other masses – which may include hydrocele, hernia and varicoceles.

# CHAPTER 74

# Lymphomas

## KEITH J AUGUST, ALAN S GAMIS

From the choices below each question, select the single best answer.

 **1** In Hodgkin's lymphoma, Reed–Sternberg cells are usually derived from:

   **A** granulocytes

   **B** B-lymphocytes

   **C** T-lymphocytes

   **D** plasma cells

   **E** histiocytes.

 **1** **B** Reed–Sternberg cells in classic Hodgkin's lymphoma are large cells that have a characteristic 'owl's eye' nucleus. These cells express CD15 and CD30 and are negative for CD45. Reed–Sternberg cells harbour clonal immunoglobulin rearrangements identifying them as being derived from germinal centre B-lymphocytes. Reed–Sternberg cells make up less than 2% of the cellular content of the tumour and are found among a background of inflammatory cells that typically include B- and T-lymphocytes, granulocytes, histiocytes, plasma cells and eosinophils.

 **2** The most frequent histological subtype of Hodgkin's lymphoma seen in children is:

   **A** nodular sclerosing

   **B** mixed cellularity

   **C** lymphocyte rich

   **D** lymphocyte depleted

   **E** nodular lymphocyte predominant.

 **2** **A** Hodgkin's lymphoma is divided into two main histological types: classic and nodular lymphocyte predominant. Classic Hodgkin's lymphoma is further divided into four subtypes: nodular sclerosing, mixed cellularity, lymphocyte rich and lymphocyte depleted. The nodular-sclerosing subtype comprises 40% of childhood Hodgkin's lymphoma and is more commonly diagnosed in adolescents. The mixed-cellularity subtype is seen in 30% of cases. It occurs more frequently in children less than 10 years of age and often presents with extranodal involvement. The nodular-lymphocyte-predominant subtype is seen in 10%–15% of cases. Lymphocyte-rich and lymphocyte-depleted subtypes are uncommon in children.

**Q3** The most common site of extralymphatic spread for Hodgkin's lymphoma is:

  A  bone marrow

  B  lung

  C  central nervous system (CNS)

  D  liver

  E  skin.

**A3**  **D**  The liver is the most common site for extralymphatic spread in Hodgkin's lymphoma. Central nervous system disease is extremely rare, and sampling of cerebrospinal fluid is not routinely practised. Bone marrow disease is seen in 4%–14% of patients with Hodgkin's disease and should be evaluated in all patients with the exception of those with localised disease and no systemic symptoms.

**Q4** Diagnostic staging of patients with Hodgkin's lymphoma should include all of the following *except*:

  A  complete blood count

  B  CT scan of neck, chest, abdomen and pelvis

  C  chest X-ray

  D  lymph node biopsy

  E  splenectomy.

**A4**  **E**  Although historically, exploratory laparotomy and splenectomy were a routine part of staging for Hodgkin's lymphoma, improved imaging modalities and changes in treatment strategies (with a larger emphasis on chemotherapy) have made these procedures unnecessary. Splenectomy in patients who are treated for Hodgkin's lymphoma results in an increased risk of sepsis during treatment and increases the incidence of secondary leukaemia as a long-term complication. Lymph node biopsy is used to establish a diagnosis and identify the histological subtype of disease. All patients should have a chest X-ray and CT scan of the chest, abdomen and pelvis to assess the extent of disease and number of involved lymph nodes. A complete blood count is used to screen for bone marrow disease and to detect other haematological abnormalities that may be associated with Hodgkin's lymphoma.

**Q5** Important long-term side effects that are caused by chemotherapy for Hodgkin's lymphoma include all of the following *except*:

**A** ototoxicity

**B** infertility

**C** secondary leukaemia

**D** cardiotoxicity

**E** restrictive lung disease.

 **A5** **A** With the current high cure rates seen for patients diagnosed with Hodgkin's lymphoma using intensive, multimodal treatments, the avoidance of long-term side effects has become increasingly important. Chemotherapy is associated with some significant long-term side effects that include cardiomyopathy (following treatment with anthracyclines), restrictive lung disease (bleomycin), infertility (alkylating agents such as nitrogen mustard, procarbazine and cyclophosphamide), and secondary leukaemias (nitrogen mustard, procarbazine, cyclophosphamide and etoposide). Platinum compounds, which can cause high-frequency hearing loss, are not routinely used in Hodgkin's lymphoma treatment protocols.

 **Q6** Important long-term side effects that are caused by radiation therapy in Hodgkin's lymphoma include all of the following *except*:

**A** cosmetic defects

**B** growth retardation

**C** hyperthyroidism

**D** coronary artery disease

**E** secondary malignancies.

**A6** **C** Radiation therapy in Hodgkin's lymphoma has several long-term side effects that often do not manifest until many years following treatment. Cosmetic defects can occur due to decreases in the growth of bone and/or soft tissues exposed to radiation, and this is more common in younger patients. The clavicles and vertebrae are the most commonly affected, due to their presence within the most commonly applied radiation field. Hypothyroidism is commonly diagnosed after radiation to the neck. Secondary malignancies within the radiation field are not uncommon, and the relative risk following radiation is as much as 10 times that seen in the general population. Breast cancer is a particularly common secondary cancer in irradiated females. Mediastinal irradiation increases the risk for coronary artery disease and survivors of Hodgkin's lymphoma have an increased incidence of cardiac death.

**Q7** A translocation involving chromosomes 8 and 14 is characteristic of:

    **A** Burkitt's lymphoma

    **B** Hodgkin's lymphoma

    **C** lymphoblastic lymphoma

    **D** diffuse large B-cell lymphoma

    **E** anaplastic large cell lymphoma.

**A7**   **A** The majority of Burkitt's lymphoma is characterised by a translocation between the *c-Myc* oncogene, found on chromosome 8q24 and the immunoglobulin heavy chain gene found on chromosome 14q32. In a smaller number of cases, the *c-Myc* gene can occur as a part of other translocations involving the immunoglobulin light chain gene. This translocation is thought to mediate tumourogenesis through the dysregulation of *c-Myc* signalling, which normally controls cell cycle progression through $G_1$ into the S phase.

**Q8** Non-Hodgkin's lymphoma in children most commonly presents in which anatomical location?

    **A** mediastinum

    **B** head and neck

    **C** extremities

    **D** abdomen

    **E** skin

**A8**   **D** Although non-Hodgkin's lymphoma can occur anywhere, it is found within the abdomen in approximately one-third of cases. Abdominal presentation is most frequently seen in Burkitt's lymphoma and can range from extensive intra-abdominal disease to a localised tumour that can cause obstruction, bowel perforation, and/or intussusception. Non-Hodgkin's lymphoma is also seen in the mediastinum (27%), head and neck (29%), skin, lymph nodes, bone and CNS.

**Q9** Which of the following is not prognostic in patients with non-Hodgkin's lymphoma?

    **A** stage

    **B** age

    **C** presence of fever

    **D** CNS involvement

    **E** lactate dehydrogenase (LDH)

A⁹  **C**  Advanced-stage disease at diagnosis occurs in the majority of children and is a strong predictor of outcome for all subtypes of non-Hodgkin's lymphoma although more aggressive therapies have significantly improved survival in these patients. Younger patients tend to have better outcomes than older patients, particularly for Burkitt's lymphoma. CNS involvement is more common in Burkitt's lymphoma and lymphoblastic lymphoma and is associated with a poorer prognosis. An elevated LDH is also associated with poorer survival in Burkitt's lymphoma. The presence of fever, considered a B symptom in Hodgkin's lymphoma, is not a known prognostic indictor in non-Hodgkin's lymphoma.

**Q10** For patients that have post-transplant lymphoproliferative disease, initial treatment is:

**A** chemotherapy

**B** resection

**C** reduction of immunosuppression

**D** antivirals

**E** rituximab.

A¹⁰  **C**  Post-transplant lymphoproliferative disease (PTLD) is a clonal disorder that occurs in patients following solid organ or bone marrow transplant. In patients with PTLD, B-lymphocyte proliferation occurs and in almost all cases this process is associated with Epstein–Barr virus infection. The spectrum of disease seen with post-transplant lymphoproliferative disease is diverse. Some patients will respond to a reduction or elimination of immunosuppressive medication, while in others, disease is more aggressive, necessitating treatment with rituximab, a monoclonal antibody against CD20, or more conventional lymphoma chemotherapy.

**Q11** The most common form of non-Hodgkin's lymphoma in children is:

**A** lymphoblastic lymphoma

**B** Burkitt's lymphoma

**C** diffuse large B-cell lymphoma

**D** anaplastic large cell lymphoma

**E** follicular lymphoma.

A¹¹  **B**  Burkitt's lymphoma comprises approximately 40% of non-Hodgkin's lymphoma seen in children. Lymphoblastic lymphoma is seen in another 30% of cases. Diffuse large B-cell lymphoma and anaplastic large cell lymphoma make up 20% and 10% of cases, respectively. Other types of non-Hodgkin's lymphomas that are more indolent and are seen frequently in adults such as follicular lymphoma or peripheral T-cell lymphoma are rare in children.

**Q12** The type of lymphoma most likely to present with respiratory distress from a large mediastinal mass is:

   **A** lymphoblastic lymphoma

   **B** Burkitt's lymphoma

   **C** diffuse large B-cell lymphoma

   **D** anaplastic large cell lymphoma

   **E** Hodgkin's lymphoma.

**A12** **A** Lymphoblastic lymphoma is the most common form of non-Hodgkin's lymphoma to present with mediastinal disease. As opposed to Hodgkin's lymphoma, which also commonly presents with a mediastinal mass, lymphoblastic lymphoma is rapidly progressive and often will present with respiratory distress and/or superior vena cava syndrome due to the obstruction of airways and decreased venous return from the head and neck.

**Q13** Small-bowel intussusception leading to a lymphoma diagnosis is more likely to occur in which type of lymphoma in children?

   **A** lymphoblastic lymphoma

   **B** diffuse large B-cell lymphoma

   **C** anaplastic large cell lymphoma

   **D** Burkitt's lymphoma

   **E** Hodgkin's lymphoma

**A13** **D** Burkitt's lymphoma is frequently seen in the abdomen, and in 25%–30% of cases is diagnosed when it causes small-bowel obstruction or intussusception resulting in acute abdominal pain and a palpable abdominal mass. This presentation is often initially misdiagnosed as acute appendicitis. A diagnosis of intussusception in a child above the age of 5 years should lead to a high index of suspicion that non-Hodgkin's lymphoma may be involved. This is the rare situation where complete resection of the tumour is recommended, and these patients have an excellent prognosis with limited chemotherapy postoperatively.

**Q14** Patients with Burkitt's lymphoma are at high risk of all of the following complications *except*:

   **A** uric acid nephropathy

   **B** hyperphosphataemia

   **C** hyperkalaemia

   **D** hypocalcaemia

   **E** hyponatraemia.

A14 **E** Because of the rapid doubling time of Burkitt's lymphoma, these patients are at risk for the severe electrolyte disturbances seen with tumour lysis syndrome. Rapid turnover of tumour cells results in the release of intracellular contents into the circulation. Metabolic derangements such as hyperuricaemia, hyperkalaemia, hyperphosphataemia and hypocalcaemia are frequently seen. Tumour lysis syndrome can be present at diagnosis or be caused by the rapid destruction of tumour seen immediately after the initiation of chemotherapy. Treatment involves aggressive hydration, allopurinol, and frequent monitoring of serum electrolytes. Rasburicase can be administered when uric acid levels are elevated. Rarely, dialysis may be necessary in extreme cases when renal failure occurs.

Q15 CNS involvement is most likely to occur with which of the following diseases?

  **A** lymphoblastic lymphoma
  **B** diffuse large B-cell lymphoma
  **C** Burkitt's lymphoma
  **D** anaplastic large cell lymphoma
  **E** Hodgkin's lymphoma

A15 **C** Although CNS disease can be found at diagnosis in all forms of non-Hodgkin's lymphoma, it is most commonly seen in Burkitt's lymphoma, and second most frequently with lymphoblastic lymphoma. CNS disease is rarely seen in Hodgkin's lymphoma.

Q16 Radiation therapy is most often used to treat which lymphoma?

  **A** lymphoblastic lymphoma
  **B** Burkitt's lymphoma
  **C** diffuse large B-cell lymphoma
  **D** anaplastic large cell lymphoma
  **E** Hodgkin's lymphoma

A16 **E** Radiation therapy remains an important part of many treatment regimens for Hodgkin's lymphoma. Although some newer protocols are evaluating the possibility of eliminating radiation therapy for patients with low risk disease and a rapid response to chemotherapy, the majority of patients with Hodgkin's lymphoma continue to require radiation therapy to reduce the risk of relapse. Because of the excellent response to chemotherapy and long-term side effects, radiation therapy is not commonly used in childhood non-Hodgkin's lymphoma. It may rarely be used under special circumstances.

**Q17** Which of the following is not considered a B symptom in patients with Hodgkin's lymphoma?

   **A** weight loss of more than 10% in the previous 6 months

   **B** unexplained recurrent fevers greater than 38°C

   **C** drenching night sweats

   **D** pruritus

   **E** all of the above are B symptoms

**A17** **D** B symptoms in Hodgkin's lymphoma are associated with more aggressive disease and worse prognosis. B symptoms include weight loss, recurrent fever, and night sweats. Pruritus can also be seen in patients with Hodgkin's lymphoma, but its presence does not have prognostic significance.

**Q18** Exposure to Epstein–Barr virus is a risk factor for all of the following *except*:

   **A** Hodgkin's lymphoma

   **B** diffuse large B-cell lymphoma

   **C** lymphoblastic lymphoma

   **D** Burkitt's lymphoma

   **E** post-transplant lymphoproliferative disease.

**A18** **C** Patients with a history of infectious mononucleosis or high titres to the Epstein–Barr virus are at increased risk of developing Hodgkin's lymphoma. Exposure to the Epstein–Barr virus is more frequently associated with the mixed cellularity subtype and occurs an average of 4 years after exposure. Epstein–Barr virus exposure increases the risk of developing both Burkitt's and diffuse large B-cell lymphoma. Patients who develop a primary Epstein–Barr virus infection in the months following a transplant are at high risk of developing post-transplant lymphoproliferative disease, and Epstein–Barr viral loads are known to correlate with disease risk.

**Q19** Which of the following is not a potential risk factor for Hodgkin's lymphoma?

   **A** higher socio-economic status

   **B** HIV infection

   **C** exposure to Epstein–Barr virus

   **D** age >15 years

   **E** larger family size

$A$**19 E** Families with a larger number of children have a lower incidence of Hodgkin's lymphoma, presumably due to increased number of infectious exposures at an early age when immunostimulation is less likely to lead to a lymphoid malignancy. This same reasoning is credited for the increased risk of children in families with higher socio-economic status, who tend to have fewer infectious exposures as children. Patients with HIV infection are at increased risk of developing Hodgkin's lymphoma as well as non-Hodgkin's lymphomas such as Burkitt's and diffuse large B-cell lymphoma. Exposure to Epstein–Barr virus is a known risk factor and many patients have evidence of viral proteins within malignant cells. Hodgkin's lymphoma has a bimodal age distribution, and the first peak includes patients that are 15 years of age and older. Hodgkin's lymphoma is the most common cancer diagnosis in children 15–19 years of age.

## Further reading

Holcomb GW, Murphy JP. *Ashcraft's Pediatric Surgery*. Philadelphia, PA: WB Saunders; 2005. pp. 936–53.

Lewing KB, Gamis AS. Lymphoma. In Holcomb GW, Murphy JW (eds). *Ashcraft's Pediatric Surgery*. Philadelphia, PA: WB Saunders; 2009. pp. 936–53.

Pizzo PA, Poplack DG. *Principles and Practice of Pediatric Oncology*. 5th ed. Philadelphia, PA: Lippincott Williams & Williams; 2006.

Weinstein HJ, Hudson MM, Link MP. *Pediatric Lymphomas*. Heidelberg, Germany: Springer; 2007.

# CHAPTER 75

# Teratoma, rhabdomyosarcoma and other tumours

## MADAN SAMUEL

From the choices below each question, select the single best answer.

**Q1** Which of these statements is true regarding the reduction of serum alpha-fetoprotein (AFP) levels during the first 8 months of life?
  A 150 000 ± 50 000 decreases to 25 ± 10 ng/mL.
  B 33 000 ± 15 000 decreases to 75 ± 10 ng/mL.
  C 48 000 ± 35 000 decreases to 8.5 ± 5.5 ng/mL
  D 250 000 ± 50 000 decreases to 15 ± 5.5 ng/mL
  E 500 000 ± 50 000 decreases to 25 ± 5.5 ng/mL

**A1** **C** Serum AFP at birth is high (48 000 ± 35 000 ng/mL), and rapidly declines to normal adult values of (8.5 ± 5.5 ng/mL) by 8 months of age. High levels of serum AFP are suggestive of a malignant mass; milder elevations are seen in hamartoma and teratoma.

**Q2** Kasabach–Merritt's syndrome is characterised by:
  A infantile hepatic haemangioendothelioma, thrombocytopenia, congestive cardiac failure and hypothyroidism
  B infantile hepatic haemangioendothelioma, congestive cardiac failure and thrombocytopenia
  C infantile hepatic haemangioendothelioma, thrombocytopenia, congestive cardiac failure and hyperthyroidism
  D infantile hepatic haemangioendothelioma, congestive cardiac failure and thrombocytosis
  E infantile hepatic haemangioendothelioma, congestive cardiac failure, thrombocytopenia and leucopenia.

**A2**    **B**   Kasabach–Merritt's syndrome presents with congestive cardiac failure, thrombocytopenia and hepatic vascular anomalies such as infantile hepatic haemangioendothelioma.

**Q3**   Stage I hepatoblastoma and HCC is defined as:
- **A** complete surgical resection
- **B** microscopic residual tumour
- **C** macroscopic residual tumour
- **D** distant metastases
- **E** disseminated disease.

**A3**    **A**   Staging of hepatoblastoma and HCC is as follows: stage I – complete resection; stage II – microscopic residual tumour; stage III – macroscopic residual tumour; and stage IV – distant metastases.

**Q4**   The five-year survival rate for gastrointestinal stromal tumours (GISTs) that have been completely resected is:
- **A** 40%–50%
- **B** 50%–65%
- **C** 35%–45%
- **D** 60%–70%
- **E** 80%–90%.

**A4**    **B**   The 5-year survival rate of completely resected GISTs is in the range of 50%–65%.

**Q5**   Which of the following statements about Barrett's oesophagus is true?
- **A** Barrett's is a premalignant lesion leading to adenocarcinoma.
- **B** Barrett's is a premalignant lesion in all cases of oesophageal burns.
- **C** Barrett's is a premalignant lesion that never occurs in the distal oesophageal segment.
- **D** Barrett's is a premalignant lesion not retained in the cervical oesophagus post gastric transposition.
- **E** Barrett's is a premalignant lesion leading to squamous cell carcinoma.

**A5**    **A**   Barrett's oesophagus is a premalignant lesion that predisposes to oesophageal adenocarcinoma. It can occur in the retained cervical oesophagus after gastric transposition. The distal segment of the oesophagus must be removed as chronic inflammation from severe chronic oesophagitis predisposes to Barrett's and adenocarcinoma after oesophageal replacement surgery. There are case reports of adenocarcinoma of the oesophagus after chemical burns of the oesophagus.

**Q6** Which of the following describes the typical location(s) of an appendiceal carcinoid tumour?
- **A** 75% tip of the appendix, 14% body of the appendix, 11% appendicocaecal junction
- **B** 50% tip of the appendix, 25% body of the appendix, 25% appendicocaecal junction
- **C** 100% tip of the appendix
- **D** 50% tip of the appendix, 50% appendicocaecal junction
- **E** 100% appendicocaecal junction

**A6** **A** Paediatric appendicular carcinoid is discovered at operation for appendicitis or incidentally. The carcinoid occurs at the tip of the appendix in 75% of the cases and therefore proximal obstruction of the appendiceal lumen is not seen.

**Q7** Which of the following statements is true?
- **A** Breast cancer in mothers is the major associated malignancy in children with soft tissue sarcomas.
- **B** Breast cancer in mothers is the major associated malignancy in children with Wilms's tumour.
- **C** Breast cancer in mothers is the major associated malignancy in children with yolk sac tumour.
- **D** Breast cancer in mothers is the major associated malignancy in children with hepatocellular cancer.
- **E** Breast cancer in mothers is the major associated malignancy in children with neuroblastoma.

**A7** **A** In mothers of children afflicted with soft tissue sarcoma, the risk of breast cancer is 3–13.5 times greater than that of the normal population.

**Q8** Which statement is true regarding sacrococcygeal teratomas?
- **A** They are isolated and not associated with other anomalies.
- **B** They are associated with anorectal anomalies only.
- **C** They are associated with genitourinary and anorectal anomalies.
- **D** They are associated with spinal anomalies only.
- **E** They are associated with rectal atresia only.

$A^8$    **C**   Teratomas are associated with a spectrum of congenital anomalies. Sacrococcygeal teratomas are associated with genitourinary tract anomalies, rectal atresia and caudal spinal cord.

$Q^9$   Which statement is true regarding teratomas?
- **A**   Nasopharyngeal teratoma is associated with cleft palate.
- **B**   Sacrococcygeal teratomas are always isolated.
- **C**   Cranial teratomas are always isolated.
- **D**   Testicular teratomas are rare.
- **E**   Cranial teratomas are associated with cleft palates.

$A^9$    **A**   Nasopharyngeal teratomas are associated with disfiguring cleft palates.

$Q^{10}$ A 2-year-old girl presents with intractable constipation. On examination the child was not thriving and has a large solid posterior rectal mass. What is the most likely diagnosis?
- **A**   Altman stage IV tumour
- **B**   Altman stage III tumour
- **C**   lipoma
- **D**   myelomeningocele
- **E**   dermoid

$A^{10}$   **A**   Sacrococcygeal teratomas can be classified according to Altman staging. Altman stage IV teratomas are purely intra-abdominal and usually are associated with distant metastases by the time of diagnosis.

$Q^{11}$ Which of these statements regarding fetus *in fetu* is true?
- **A**   Fetus *in fetu* is a mature teratoma.
- **B**   Fetus *in fetu* is an immature teratoma.
- **C**   Fetus *in fetu* is a dermoid tumour with yolk sac components.
- **D**   Fetus *in fetu* is a dermoid tumour with mature cells.
- **E**   Fetus *in fetu* is a rhabdoid.

$A^{11}$   **A**   Fetus *in fetu* is rare and the current World Health Organization categorisation is mature teratoma.

**Q12** Which statement regarding sacrococcygeal teratoma is true?

  **A** 80% of sacrococcygeal teratomas are benign, 10% have familial occurrence and 10% have associated anomalies.

  **B** 70% of sacrococcygeal teratomas are benign, 5% have familial occurrence and 15% have associated anomalies.

  **C** 90% of sacrococcygeal teratomas are benign, 10% have familial occurrence and 10% have associated anomalies.

  **D** 80% of sacrococcygeal teratomas have immature mitotic cells, 15% have familial occurrence and 15% have associated anomalies.

  **E** 70% of sacrococcygeal teratomas have immature mitotic cells, 5% have familial occurrence and 15% have associated anomalies.

**A12** **A**  80% of sacrococcygeal teratomas are benign and 10% have familial predilection. Between 10% and 20% have associated anomalies such as oesophageal fistula with tracheo-oesophageal fistula, anorectal malformation, genitourinary malformations and myelomeningocele.

**Q13** The cardinal step in sacrococcygeal teratoma surgery is:

  **A** ligation of the abdominal aorta prior to excision of tumour

  **B** excision of the coccyx after ligating the common iliacs

  **C** excision of the coccyx and ligation of median sacral artery

  **D** excision of the coccyx and ligation of the superior lateral sacral artery

  **E** excision of the coccyx and ligation of the inferior lateral sacral artery.

**A13** **C**  Median sacral vessels are ligated after the excision of the coccyx to achieve control over majority of the tumour vascularity.

**Q14** Which statement is true regarding the incidence of intracranial tumours?

  **A** Intracranial teratomas account for 50% of all brain tumours in early infancy.

  **B** Gliomas account for 50% of all brain tumours in early infancy.

  **C** Astrocytomas account for 50% of all brain tumours in early infancy.

  **D** Craniopharyngiomas account for 50% of all brain tumours in early infancy.

  **E** Medulloblastomas account for 50% of all brain tumours in early infancy.

**A14** **A** Intracranial teratomas present in a bimodal age pattern and account for 50% of brain tumours in early infancy. The pineal gland is the most common site of origin.

**Q15** Tumours of the testis should be approached by:

   **A** inguinal incision

   **B** inguinoscrotal incision

   **C** scrotal incision

   **D** abdominoperitoneal incision

   **E** laparoscopy.

**A15** **B** An inguinoscrotal incision is used. The testicular vessels are ligated at the level of the internal ring. The tumour is excised with an island of scrotal skin. Ipsilateral hemiscrotectomy may have to be performed. Frozen section is useful for diagnosis and extent of excision.

**Q16** Which of the following statements is true regarding testicular tumours?

   **A** 60% of prepubertal testicular tumours are germ cell with 20% metastases to the lungs and 6% to the retroperitoneal nodes.

   **B** 70% of prepubertal testicular tumours are germ cell with 20% metastases to the lungs and 6% to the retroperitoneal nodes.

   **C** 50% of prepubertal testicular tumours are germ cell with 10% metastases to the lungs and 6% to the retroperitoneal nodes.

   **D** 40% of prepubertal testicular tumours are germ cell with 20% metastases to the lungs and 10% to the retroperitoneal nodes.

   **E** 50% of prepubertal testicular tumours are germ cell with 20% metastases to the lungs and 6% to the retroperitoneal nodes.

**A16** **A** 60% of prepubertal testicular tumours are germ cells. Haematogenous spread to the lungs occurs in 20% and retroperitoneal lymph node metastases occur in 4%–6% of children.

**Q17** The classic triad of presentation in a Leydig cell tumour is:

    **A** 90% unilateral testicular mass, 10% precocious puberty and elevated 17-ketosteroid

    **B** 90% unilateral testicular mass, 20% precocious puberty and elevated 17-ketosteroid and AFP

    **C** 90% unilateral testicular mass, 10% precocious puberty and elevated 17-ketosteroid, AFP and human chorionic gonadotropin (hCG)

    **D** 90% unilateral testicular mass, 20% precocious puberty and elevated 17-ketosteroid, AFP and hCG

    **E** 90% unilateral testicular mass, 5% precocious puberty and elevated 17-ketosteroid.

**A17** **A** Leydig cell tumour is the most common gonadal stromal tumour of adults and children. The classic triad of presentation is precocious puberty in 10%, unilateral testicular mass in 90% and elevated 17-ketosteroid.

**Q18** Which of the following statement is true regarding paediatric phaeochromocytoma?

    **A** Paediatric phaeochromocytoma shows a familial pattern in 10%, occurs in extra-adrenal sites in 30% and paroxysmal hypertension is seen in 70%–90%.

    **B** Paediatric phaeochromocytoma shows a familial pattern in 15%, occurs in extra-adrenal sites in 15% and sustained hypertension is seen in 70%–90%.

    **C** Paediatric phaeochromocytoma shows a familial pattern in 10%, occurs in extra-adrenal sites in 30% and paroxysmal hypertension is seen in 70%–90%.

    **D** Paediatric phaeochromocytoma shows a familial pattern in 10%, occurs in extra-adrenal sites in 30% and sustained hypertension is seen in 70%–90%.

    **E** Paediatric phaeochromocytoma shows a familial pattern in 25%, occurs in extra-adrenal sites in 25% and sustained hypertension is seen in 70%–90%.

**A18** **D** Ten per cent of paediatric phaeochromocytomas occur in families and 30% occur at extra-adrenal sites. Sustained hypertension is seen in 70%–90% of children. Paroxysmal hypertension occurs in adults.

**Q19** Which statement regarding hypercalcaemia is false?
- **A** Hypercalcaemia in younger and older patients presents acutely and is associated with co-morbid conditions.
- **B** Between 10% and 20% of cancer patients develop hypercalcaemia.
- **C** Cancer patients who develop hypercalcaemia have a 50% mortality at 1 month after it appears.
- **D** The longer the duration of hypercalcaemia, the poorer the development of tolerance.
- **E** Two common causes are hyperparathyroidism and malignancy.

**A19** **D** Parathyroid hormone regulates serum calcium levels. Calcium is bound to albumin and the most common cause of hypercalcaemia is hyperparathyroidism and malignancy. Between 10% and 20% of cancer patients develop hypercalcaemia and it is associated with poor prognosis with 50% mortality at 1 month post hypercalcaemia clinical presentation. The longer the duration of hypercalcaemia, the better is the tolerance, and slower the development of co-morbidities.

**Q20** Which statement is false regarding Hodgkin's lymphoma?
- **A** It arises from B-cells.
- **B** It is associated with Epstein–Barr virus.
- **C** Reed–Sternberg cells are not characteristic.
- **D** Positron emission tomography is a useful adjuvant to CT scan.
- **E** Autologous bone marrow transplant is considered following relapse.

**A20** **C** Reed–Sternberg cells are characteristic and are surrounded by a dense inflammatory infiltrate.

**Q21** Which of the following statements is true regarding non-Hodgkin's lymphoma?
- **A** Diffuse large B-cell lymphoma is the most common non-Hodgkin's lymphoma, followed by low-grade follicular lymphoma.
- **B** The incidence of lymphoma is high in young children.
- **C** Cutaneous lymphomas are usually B-cell lymphomas.
- **D** Altered immunity is not a risk factor.
- **E** Antibiotics are contraindicated in gastric lymphoma.

**A21** **A** Diffuse large B-cell lymphoma is the most common non-Hodgkin's lymphoma. The main risk factor is altered immunity. Aggressive B-cell lymphoma is an AIDS defining illness and also can be associated with organ transplant, autoimmune disease and congenital immunodeficiency disorders. It is associated with

Epstein–Barr virus, Hepatitis C and *Helicobacter pylori*. Antibiotics are the first line of treatment for low-grade localised gastric lymphoma followed by radiation as the second line of treatment.

**Q22** A child with mixed gonadal dysgenesis presents for evaluation and further management. What advice would you give regarding gonadal surgery?

**A** bilateral gonadectomy

**B** unilateral gonadectomy of non-palpable gonad

**C** gonadal biopsies and observation

**D** do nothing

**E** annual assessment with pelvic CT scan and postpuberty biopsy

**A22** **B** Unilateral gonadectomy of the non-palpable gonad is recommended. Annual review with ultrasound scan, followed by pre- and postpubertal gonadal biopsy of the gonad in the scrotum is advisable. This is for early detection of testicular carcinoma *in situ*.

**Q23** Which statement is false regarding gonadoblastoma in a child with mixed gonadal dysgenesis (45,X/46,XY)?

**A** Small bilateral tumours occur in 33%, and 10% are malignant.

**B** Early gonadectomy of non-palpable gonad is recommended.

**C** Early bilateral gonadectomy is recommended.

**D** There is a risk of seminoma in the gonad.

**E** These patients have neonatal testosterone imprints.

**A23** **C** Although in the past early bilateral gonadectomy was indicated, this management policy has changed following the development of neonatal testosterone implants in the brain. Because of the risk of seminoma, the non-palpable gonad is excised. The palpable gonad is followed up annually with pre- and postpubertal biopsies to detect testicular carcinoma *in situ*. If carcinoma *in situ* is detected, gonadectomy is advisable.

**Q24** Which statement is false regarding the treatment of adrenocortical tumours?

**A** Surgical resection is the main stay in the treatment of these tumours.

**B** Debulking of unresectable tumours is beneficial.

**C** Chemotherapy is successful.

**D** Medical therapy with mitotane may benefit unresectable tumours.

**E** Chemotherapy is not successful.

$A$24 **C** Complete surgical resection of adrenocortical tumour is the treatment of choice. It ensures good prognosis and long-term survival. Chemotherapy has not been successful in these patients. Debulking of unresectable tumour may be of benefit. Common sites of metastases are lung, liver, lymph nodes, contralateral adrenal gland, bones, kidneys and brain. Mitotane acts as an adrenolytic agent by altering mitochondrial function. It is a useful adjuvant medical therapy in unresectable tumours.

$Q$25 Which is the most common malignant brain tumour of childhood?
  **A** cerebellar astrocytoma
  **B** ependymoma
  **C** medulloblastoma
  **D** brainstem glioma
  **E** craniopharyngioma

$A$25 **C** Medulloblastoma is the most common malignant brain tumour of childhood. Cerebellar astrocytomas are benign and curable by complete surgical excision.

## Further reading

Andrassy RJ. Advances in the surgical management of sarcomas in children. *Am J Surg.* 2002; **184**(6): 484–91.

Andrassy RJ. Rhabdomyosarcoma. *Semin Pediatr Surg.* 1997; **6**(1): 17–23.

Bethel CA, Bhattacharyya N, Hutchinson C, *et al.* Alimentary tract malignancies in children. *J Pediatr Surg.* 1997; **32**(7): 1004–8.

Chen JC, Chen CC, Chen WJ, *et al.* Hepatocellular carcinoma in children: clinical review and comparison with adult cases. *J Pediatr Surg.* 1998; **33**(9): 1350–54.

Darbari A, Sabin KM, Shapiro CN, *et al.* Epidemiology of primary hepatic malignancies in U.S. children. *Hepatology.* 2003; **38**(3): 560–6.

# SECTION XII

# Special areas of paediatric surgery

# CHAPTER 76

# Paediatric radiology

### ASHOK RAGHAVAN, KSHITIJ MANKAD, JEREMY B JONES, NEETU KUMAR

**From the choices below each question, select the single best answer.**

**Q¹** What type of tracheo-oesophageal fistula (TOF) is this likely to be?

A Type A
B Type B
c Type C
D Type D
E Type E

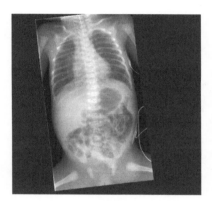

**A¹** C Oesophageal atresia (OA) is a condition in which the proximal and distal portions of the oesophagus do not communicate. The upper segment of the oesophagus is a dilated, blind-ending pouch with a hypertrophied muscular wall that typically extends to the level of the second to fourth

**FIGURE 76.1** X-ray of the chest and abdomen of a newborn with a radio opaque catheter *in situ*

thoracic vertebrae. TOF is an abnormal communication between the trachea and oesophagus. When associated with OA, the fistula most commonly occurs between the distal oesophageal segment and the trachea, just above the carina.

Five types of OA and TOF have been described:

- type A – OA without fistula or so-called pure OA (10%)
- type B – OA with proximal TOF (<1%)
- type C – OA with distal TOF (85%)
- type D – OA with proximal and distal TOFs (<1%)
- type E – TOF without OA or so-called H-type fistula (4%).

The most common abnormality is OA with a distal TOF (85%). Isolated atresia with no fistula is the next most common finding (10%), followed by H-type TOF (no atresia) (4%). OA with proximal and distal fistulas (1%) and OA with a proximal fistula (1%) is less common.

Type A is pure OA without fistula; type B is OA with a fistula between the proximal pouch and the trachea; type C is OA with a fistula from the trachea or the main bronchus to the distal oesophageal segment; type D is OA with both proximal and distal fistulas; type E is an H-shaped TOF without atresia. Of these five types of OA, type C is by far the most common.

 Q2 H-type fistula is a communication between the oesophagus and trachea with the track running in which direction?

    **A** superior to inferior

    **B** inferior to superior

    **C** anterior to posterior

    **D** medial to lateral

    **E** lateral to medial

A2  **B** Congenital TOF without associated atresia is a rare anomaly, representing about 5% of all TOFs. The so-called H-type fistula is in fact N shaped, passing from the oesophagus up to the trachea above the level of the carina, usually between C7 and T2 vertebral levels. Although they can occur at any level between the cricoid cartilage and the carina, TOFs usually course obliquely (with the tracheal end proximal) at or above the level of the second thoracic vertebra

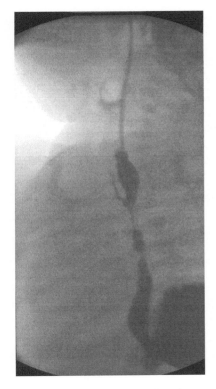

**FIGURE 76.2** Lateral view of a tube oesophagogram

**Q3** Contrast study for the diagnosis of H-type fistula is best done with the baby in:

**A** supine position

**B** prone position

**C** true lateral position

**D** oblique lateral position

**E** sitting position.

 **A3** **C** A contrast study should be done in the true lateral position with attention to the first swallows to exclude aspiration of contrast through the larynx. When fistula is clinically suspected, if it is not demonstrated on a contrast oesophagram, then a tube oesophagram must be performed. The tube oesophagram involves injecting contrast with controlled pressure during withdrawal of a feeding tube through the oesophagus. If the fistula is not demonstrated in the true lateral position it is occasionally useful to inject with the baby in a prone position and perform lateral fluoroscopy.

**Q4** Which of the following is not associated with TOF?

**A** anorectal anomalies

**B** tetralogy of Fallot

**C** renal anomalies

**D** DiGeorge syndrome

**E** Cornelia de Lange syndrome

**A4** **E** Many anomalies are associated with OA; 50%–70% of children with OA have some other defect. The acronym VACTORL (which stands for **V**ertebral, **A**norectal, **C**ardiac, **T**racheal, **O**esophageal, **R**enal and **L**imb) describes the most common combination of defects associated with OA. Cardiac abnormalities are the most common, especially ventricular septal defects and tetralogy of Fallot. Imperforate anus and skeletal malformations might also be found on examination. Congenital diaphragmatic hernia, and not TOF is a recognised finding in Cornelia de Lange syndrome.

 **Q5** X-rays that should be taken in a suspected case of OA/TOF are:

**A** abdomen:

**B** chest anteroposterior view

**C** chest lateral view

**D** both B and C

**E** A, B and C.

A5 **D** In neonates in whom OA and/or TOF is suspected, posteroanterior and lateral plain chest radiographs should be obtained first. Inability to pass a rigid nasogastric tube from the mouth to the stomach is diagnostic of OA and/or TOF, but this finding should be confirmed with a flexible tube and radiographic visualisation of the tube coiled in the proximal pouch. Upper-pouch TOF occurs with OA in less than 1% of all cases of OA/TOF but could be easily missed after birth.

Contrast-enhanced studies are rarely indicated because of the risk of aspiration, but they may be necessary to identify or locate a fistula. Only an experienced radiologist should perform contrast-enhanced studies with fluoroscopic control.

Radiological diagnosis is based on findings at anteroposterior and lateral chest radiography, which reveals a blind pouch of the proximal oesophagus that is distended with air. Radiographic evaluation should always include the abdomen to assess the presence of air in the gastrointestinal (GI) tract (distal fistula). In types A and B, there is complete absence of gas in the stomach and intestinal tract, whereas in types C and D the GI tract commonly appears distended with air.

Q6 On chest X-ray oesophageal duplication is usually:
**A** not seen
**B** seen as a spherical mass in superior mediastinum
**C** seen as a spherical mass in posterior mediastinum
**D** seen as a cylindrical mass in superior mediastinum
**E** seen as a cylindrical mass in posterior mediastinum.

A6 **C** Most oesophageal duplications manifest as spherical cysts located in the right hemithorax; rarely do they communicate with the oesophagus. At chest radiography, they are generally seen as posterior mediastinal masses. Oesophagography shows either the oesophagus displaced to the side opposite the mass or an intramural, extramucosal mass. At CT, the duplication appears sharply marginated, has a homogeneous near-water attenuation, and does not enhance after intravenous administration of contrast material. At MR imaging, most duplications have low signal intensity on T1-weighted images and very high signal intensity on T2-weighted images.

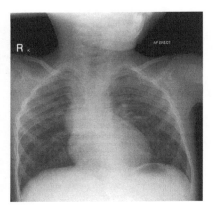

**FIGURE 76.3** X-ray of the chest demonstrating a well-defined mass in the right parahilar region

**Q7** What is the imaging modality of choice in a suspected case of congenital pyloric stenosis?

   **A** plain film

   **B** upper GI contrast study

   **C** ultrasound

   **D** CT scan

   **E** radioisotope study

**A7** **C** Ultrasonography is the imaging modality of choice when evaluating a child for infantile hypertrophic pyloric stenosis. It is both highly sensitive (90%–99%) and specific (97%–100%) in the hands of a qualified sonographer. The pylorus is viewed in longitudinal and transverse planes. The sonographic hallmark of infantile hypertrophic pyloric stenosis is the thickened pyloric muscle. Criteria for making the diagnosis include pyloric muscle thickness greater than 4 mm. The length of the pyloric canal is variable and may range from 14 to 20 mm. The pyloric diameter may range from 10 to 14 mm.

Upper GI imaging (UGI) can help to confirm the diagnosis of infantile hypertrophic pyloric stenosis but is not routinely performed unless ultrasonography is nondiagnostic.

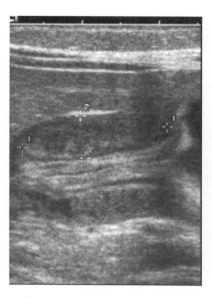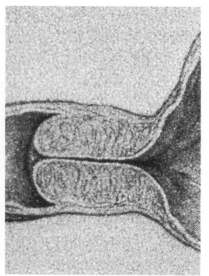

FIGURE 76.4 High-resolution ultrasound scan of the pyloric canal and schematic diagram demonstrating the measurement of a thickened pyloric wall

**Q8** What are the other problems to be considered in a case of congenital pyloric stenosis?

    **A** malrotation

    **B** antral polyp

    **C** gastric duplication

    **D** pylorospasm

    **E** all of the above

**A8** **E**

**Q9** Double track sign is seen on which of the following studies?

    **A** plain film

    **B** ultrasound

    **C** upper GI study

    **D** CT scan

    **E** MRI scan

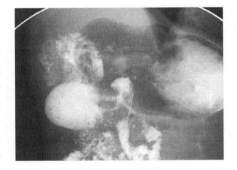

**FIGURE 76.5** Upper GI contrast study showing the shoulder sign

**A9** **C** Barium UGI study is an effective means of diagnosing hypertrophic pyloric stenosis when ultrasonography is not diagnostic. It should demonstrate an elongated pylorus with antral indentation from the hypertrophied muscle. The UGI may demonstrate the 'double track' sign when thin tracks of barium are compressed between thickened pyloric mucosa or the 'shoulder' sign when barium collects in the dilated prepyloric antrum. UGI would demonstrate pyloric obstruction; it is difficult to differentiate accurately between hypertrophic pyloric stenosis and pylorospasm.

**Q10** Regarding development, which one of the following is true?

    **A** The duodenojejunal junction rotates to the left 270 degrees in counterclockwise direction.

    **B** The duodenojejunal junction rotates to the right 270 degrees in counterclockwise direction.

    **C** The duodenojejunal junction rotates to the left 180 degrees in clockwise direction.

    **D** The duodenojejunal junction rotates to the right 270 degrees in clockwise direction.

    **E** The duodenojejunal junction rotates to the right 180 degrees in clockwise direction.

**A10** **A** Conversely, the caecum rotates 270 degrees counterclockwise to the right and resulting in right lower quadrant caecum. The mesentery extends from the duodenojejunal flexure in the left upper quadrant to the caecum in the right lower quadrant.

**Q11** Which of the following is true regarding an abdominal radiograph in a child with obstruction secondary to malrotation?
  **A** Pneumoperitoneum is usually seen at presentation.
  **B** It always shows paucity of gas.
  **C** Multiple dilated loops indicate proximal obstruction.
  **D** A double-bubble sign is commonly seen.
  **E** It may be normal.

**A11** **E** The abdominal radiograph may be normal if the obstruction is recent, intermittent or incomplete. Paucity of bowel gas is an alarming sign in a child with bilious vomiting as seen in the image below. Multiple dilated loops often denote a more distal obstruction from a cause other than midgut volvulus. Duodenum is seldom markedly dilated and the obvious double-bubble sign is not present.

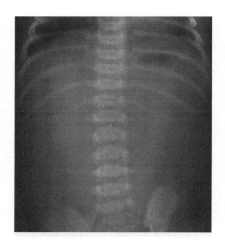

FIGURE 76.6 X-ray of the abdomen showing a gasless abdomen, which is an ominous sign in a child with bilious vomiting

**Q12** The diagnostic procedure of choice in a suspected case of malrotation is:
  **A** ultrasound
  **B** upper GI study
  **C** plain abdominal radiograph
  **D** lower GI study
  **E** lower GI followed by upper GI study.

A12  B  Upper GI study is the test of choice to outline the course and configuration of the duodenum. The normal C loop must cross the midline, and terminate at the same level as the duodenal cap. In case of volvulus the duodenal apex does not reach its normal position as seen in the image below, and a typical corkscrew pattern is seen if the obstruction is not complete.

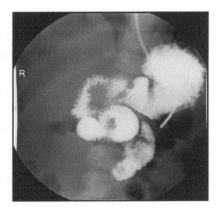

FIGURE 76.7 The duodenojejunal flexure is low in position overlying the spine on an upper GI contrast study

Q13  Which of the following is true about duodenal atresia?
   A  Half occur distal the ampulla of Vater.
   B  A third occur distal to the ampulla of Vater.
   C  Two-thirds occur distal to the ampulla of Vater.
   D  All are distal to the ampulla of Vater.
   E  All are at the ampulla of Vater.

A13  C  Approximately one-third of duodenal atresias occur above the ampulla of Vater and two-thirds below. Figure 76.8 shows the double-bubble sign on the plain film, which is confirmed on the contrast study.

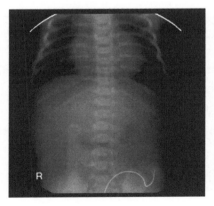
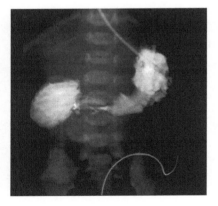

FIGURE 76.8 X-ray of the abdomen and upper GI contrast study demonstrating the classic double-bubble sign

Q14 Which of the following is false about duodenal atresia patients?
  A Multisystem anomalies are present in two-thirds.
  B Half have Down's syndrome.
  C One-quarter have associated cardiac anomalies.
  D One-tenth have associated OA.
  E All of the above.

A14 B One-third of duodenal atresia patients have Down's syndrome.

Q15 Which of the following is not true about jejunal atresia?
  A It is considered to be due to an *in utero* ischaemic insult.
  B It comprises approximately 50% of small-bowel atresia.
  C It can be associated with other jejunal and ileal atresia.
  D Contrast study is seldom required.
  E It is usually associated with multiple anomalies.

A15 D Malformation in other systems, such as cardiovascular, limb and central nervous system anomalies occur in less than 10% of cases. Gender incidence is equal.

Q16 Which of the following is not true about ileal atresia?
  A It is considered to be due to an *in utero* ischaemic insult.
  B It comprises approximately 50% of small-bowel atresia.
  C It can be associated with other jejunal atresia.
  D Intestinal perforation can occur *in utero*.
  E Approximately 75% have a history of polyhydramnios.

A16 E Only 25% have a history of polyhydramnios.

Q17 Which one of the following statements is *false* about meconium ileus?
  A It comprises 20% of cases of neonatal obstruction.
  B Barium enema is the contrast of choice.
  C 15% of patients with cystic fibrosis present in the neonatal period with meconium ileus.
  D Plain film demonstrates distal obstruction with typical air–fluid levels.
  E It is strongly associated with cystic fibrosis.

A17 B Hyperosmolar agents such as undiluted iothalamate meglumine 30% (osmolality approximately 600 mOsm/L) is the contrast of choice in a case of meconium ileus as it helps dissolve the meconium pellets in the ileum and helps in decompression. The hospital stay is significantly reduced compared with patients treated surgically.

**Q18** Which of the following features is most consistent with a diagnosis of the first arch syndrome?

  **A** malformation of the hyoid bone

  **B** absent thymic tissue

  **C** absence of the tonsillar fossa cleft

  **D** absence of the superior parathyroid gland

  **E** malformation of the internal ear ossicles

**A18** **E** The first branchial arch forms the mandible and contributes to the maxillary process of the upper jaw and the tympanic cavity and eustachian tube. Abnormal development of the first branchial arch results in many facial deformities including cleft lip and palate, abnormal shape of the external ear and malformation of the internal ossicles. The second arch forms the hyoid bone and the cleft of the tonsillar fossa. The third cleft migrates lower down to form the thymus and the inferior parathyroid glands. The fourth arch develops into the ultimobranchial body, which contributes to the parafollicular cells of the thyroid gland.

**Q19** A child with a painful neck lump undergoes an ultrasound examination. The scan reveals a homogeneously echogenic thick-walled lesion invested within the strap muscles of the neck, approximately 2 cm lateral to the midline on the left. What is the most likely diagnosis?

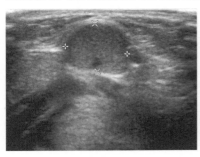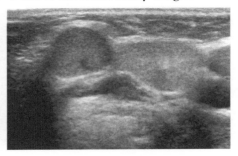

FIGURE 76.9 Longitudinal and transverse ultrasound images of the neck showing a well-capsulated hypoechoic mass

  **A** infected dermoid cyst

  **B** infected thyroglossal duct cyst

  **C** lymph node

  **D** epidermoid

  **E** infected branchial cleft cyst

$A^{19}$  **B**  This is the characteristic location for a thyroglossal duct cyst. The thyroglossal duct is lined by secretory epithelium and connects the foramen caecum at the base of the tongue, to the thyroid, The duct typically involutes between gestational weeks 8 and 10; however, if the involution fails, a cyst may arise anywhere along this course. The cyst wall gets thickened when infected.

The differential diagnosis of a midline neck mass includes epidermoid or dermoid cyst, lymph node and abscess. However, these lesions are typically found in locations superficial to the strap muscles.

$Q^{20}$  A 5-year-old child presents with an enlarging 'doughy' fluctuant lesion overlying the brow. CT scan shows a frontal soft tissue lesion with a subgaleal fluid collection. There is permeative destruction of the underlying frontal bone with opacification of the frontal sinus. What is the most likely diagnosis?

**A**  infected dermoid cyst

**B**  infected frontal epidermoid

**C**  Pott's puffy tumour

**D**  cephalocele

**E**  Langerhans's cell histiocytosis

$A^{20}$  **C**  This is the typical imaging appearance of Pott's puffy tumour. The condition results from frontal sinusitis that leads to thrombophlebitis of the valveless emissary veins, necrosis of the inner and outer tables of the skull and subperiosteal abscess formation. The possible complications of the lesion, which may be evident on imaging, are cavernous sinus thrombosis, subdural/epidural empyema and even parenchymal abscess.

$Q^{21}$  Regarding preoperative imaging to check if a thyroglossal duct cyst contains all of the patient's thyroid tissue, which of the following statements is true?

**A**  An ultrasound of the thyroid is recommended as routine.

**B**  MRI scan of the thyroid should be considered.

**C**  A radioisotope thyroid scan should be regularly requested.

**D**  A preoperative thyroid scan is not generally indicated.

**E**  Surgical planning depends on the amount of thyroid tissue in the cyst.

$A^{21}$  **D**  A preoperative thyroid scan is generally not recommended because excision of the lesion is indicated regardless of the findings on the scan. Should the surgical specimen show significant thyroid tissue, then thyroid function tests should guide the need for replacement therapy.

Q22 A 10-year-old child presents with a cystic lesion. Ultrasound confirms its location as lying anteromedial to the right sternocleidomastoid muscle, anterolateral to the carotid arteries and posterior to the submandibular gland. Which of the following is the most likely diagnosis?

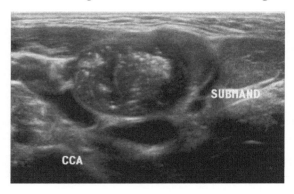

FIGURE 76.10 Well-encapsulated mixed echogenic mass on ultrasound scan of the neck

A first branchial cleft cyst
B second branchial cleft cyst
C third branchial cleft cyst
D fourth branchial cleft cyst
E undetermined branchial cleft cyst

A22 B The above describes the typical location of a second branchial cleft cyst. First branchial cleft cysts are closely related to the parotid gland, typically extending into the external auditory canal. Third and fourth branchial anomalies are rare, more common on the left side and usually associated with a fistulous tract to the pyriform fossa.

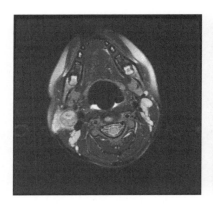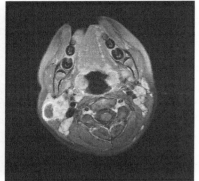

FIGURE 76.11 MRI of the neck: axial T2 fat-saturated and post-contrast axial fat-saturated T1-weighted image showing the location of second branchial cleft cyst

**Q23** Regarding the imaging of cervical lymph nodes, which of the following statements is *untrue*?

   **A** Normal lymph nodes are iso- or hypoattenuating to muscle on CT.

   **B** In comparison with muscle ultrasound, normal nodes appear hypoechoic with a hyperechoic hilum.

   **C** Lymph node measurements are made and stated in their short-axis diameter.

   **D** Normal lymph nodes generally measure less than 10 mm in diameter.

   **E** level IB and IIA nodes are up to 15 mm in diameter.

**A23** **C** Measurements are quoted as long-axis diameters. The other statements are true.

**Q24** An ultrasound was requested for this 1-month-old baby presenting with torticollis. What is the most likely diagnosis?

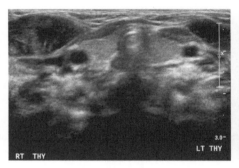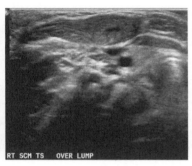

**FIGURE 76.12** Transverse and right longitudinal ultrasound images of the sternocleidomastoid muscle

   **A** normal muscle anatomy

   **B** fibromatosis colli

   **C** tumour of the sternocleidomastoid muscle

   **D** intramuscular lipoma

   **E** intramuscular haematoma

**A24** **B** Fibromatosis colli, or pseudotumour of the sternocleidomastoid is a benign self-limiting condition. It is usually associated with instrumented delivery. Torticollis is seen in an estimated 20% of cases. Ultrasound is the imaging modality of choice and reveals a focal or diffuse enlargement of the muscle with variable echogenicity.

Q25 In Figure 76.13, what is the most likely diagnosis?

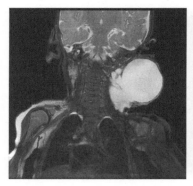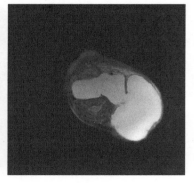

FIGURE 76.13 Coronal and axial fat-saturated T2-weighted images of the neck

  A  laryngocele
  B  branchial cleft cyst
  C  thyroglossal duct cyst
  D  lymphatic malformation
  E  arteriovenous malformation

A25  **D**  Lymphatic malformations (cystic hygroma) are best characterised on MRI. They are typically hypointense on T1- and hyperintense on T2-weighted sequence (as shown). Most of these lesions are detected by the time a patient is 2 years old. The typical location of cervical lymphatic malformation is the posterior cervical space and the oral cavity.

**Q26** A 1-year-old girl presented with progressive dysphagia. There was a week-long history of flu-like symptoms prior to this presentation. A plain film of the neck and CT scan of the neck was performed. What is the most likely diagnosis shown on this axial section?

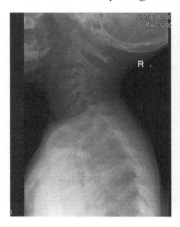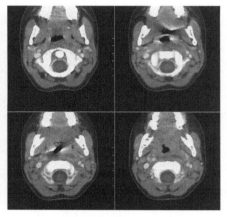

FIGURE 76.14 Lateral X-ray of the neck and post-contrast CT scan of the neck

A infected thyroglossal cyst
B infected branchial cleft cyst
C infected oesophageal duplication cyst
D retropharyngeal abscess
E malignant lymphadenopathy

**A 26** **D** The retropharyngeal space is the second most common location of abscess in children after the peritonsillar space. The typical CT feature is a low-attenuation lesion with a surrounding enhancing rim. The location is not typical for developmental cysts or lymphadenopathy.

**Q27** Regarding pleomorphic adenoma of the parotid gland, which of the following statements is *not* true?

A Pleomorphic adenoma is the most common tumour of the paediatric parotid gland.
B It appears hypoechoic relative to the rest of the gland on ultrasound.
C The tumour matrix may show calcific foci.
D The heterogeneity of the lesion increases with size.
E The tumour may show mild contrast enhancement.

**A 27** **A** Pleomorphic adenoma is the third most common tumour of the paediatric parotid gland after haemangioma and lymphangioma. The other items describe the imaging features of the tumour.

**Q28** A 14-year-old boy presented with weight loss and jaundice. Hepatomegaly was noted on physical examination. CT scan of the liver in arterial and portal venous phases of contrast showed multiple focal lesions demonstrating early arterial enhancement and early washout of contrast in the portal venous phase. What is the most likely diagnosis?

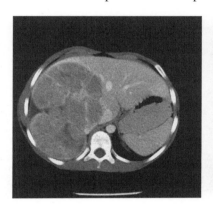 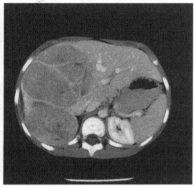

FIGURE 76.15 Axial post-contrast CT scan images of the liver in portal venous phase

**A** focal nodular hyperplasia

**B** multiple capillary haemangiomata

**C** hepatocellular carcinoma

**D** multiple liver metastases

**E** hepatoblastoma

**A28** **C** Hepatoblastoma commonly occurs in children under 3 years of age. The description of the contrast characteristics of the lesions is typical for hepatocellular carcinoma. Focal nodular hyperplasia is usually an incidental finding in adolescents. They usually have central scars and their contrast enhancement is typical for enhancement in the arterial and early portal venous phases, followed by washout in the late portal venous phase.

Q29 A 4-year-old boy presents with an abdominal mass. What is the most likely diagnosis?

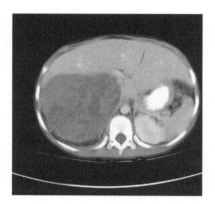

FIGURE 76.16 Post-contrast CT scan of the abdomen at the level of the kidneys

A multilocular cystic renal tumour with liver metastasis

B Wilms's tumour

C hepatic primary with renal metastases

D neuroblastoma

E nephroblastomatosis

A29 B A heterogeneous renal mass displacing the liver. The most likely lesion given the age and CT appearances would be that of a Wilms's tumour.

Q30 Which of the following statements regarding paediatric renal masses is *untrue*?

A 80% of Wilms's tumours present before the age of 5 years.

B Wilms's tumour is associated with cryptorchidism in up to 20% of cases.

C Nephroblastomatosis refers to diffuse or multifocal involvement of the kidneys with nephrogenic rest cells.

D All children with bilateral renal cell carcinoma should be screened for von Hippel–Lindau's syndrome.

E The most common solid renal tumour in the neonate is mesoblastic nephroma.

A30 B Wilms's tumour is associated with cryptorchidism in less than 3% of cases.

**Q31** Regarding the imaging characteristics of paediatric renal tumours, which of the following is *untrue*?

- **A** The assessment of the inferior vena cava for tumour thrombosis is essential in all cases of Wilms's tumour.
- **B** MRI scan of the head is required only for children with clear cell sarcoma or rhabdoid tumour of the kidney.
- **C** The presence of pulmonary nodules on CT chest in cases of Wilms's tumour does not necessitate treatment modification.
- **D** Multilocular cystic renal tumour does not typically show metastatic deposits.
- **E** Imaging can convincingly distinguish clear cell sarcoma from Wilms's tumour.

**A31** **E** Imaging of the inferior vena cava (IVC) is essential in all cases of Wilms's tumour as it has a high propensity to invade the IVC. MRI brain is not recommended in cases of Wilms's tumour. Multilocular cystic renal tumour is not known to metastasise. The imaging features of clear cell sarcoma may be similar to those of Wilms's tumour.

**Q32** A presacral mass lesion is reported as follows on CT: a large heterogeneous lesion with extensive calcification and extension into the sacral neural foramina. Which of the following is most likely to represent the correct diagnosis?

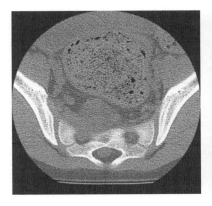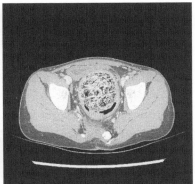

**FIGURE 76.17** Plain CT scan of the pelvis at level of the distal sacrum

- **A** neuroblastoma
- **B** dermoid cyst
- **C** sacrococcygeal teratoma
- **D** anterior sacral meningocele
- **E** pelvic abscess

A**32** **A** All the options form the differential diagnosis of presacral masses in children. Neuroblastoma is a common malignancy in childhood. It can be detected on prenatal ultrasound. CT reveals a heterogeneous lesion (due to haemorrhage, necrosis and calcification).

Q**33** A neonate is reviewed following persistent, fluctuating icterus. His stools are pale and there is a conjugated hyperbilirubinaemia. An ultrasound shows a normal-sized liver with normal architecture. The gallbladder is small and the report finishes saying that the triangular cord sign is present. Technetium-99m ($^{99m}$Tc)-DISIDA scintigraphy shows no tracer in the bowel at 24 hours. What is the likely diagnosis?

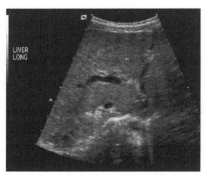 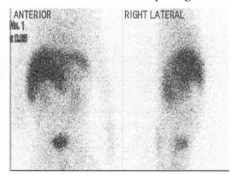

**FIGURE 76.18** Ultrasound of the liver demonstrating the cord sign, and Technetium-99m-DISIDA images

- **A** Alagille's syndrome (biliary hypoplasia)
- **B** physiological jaundice
- **C** biliary atresia
- **D** choledochal cyst
- **E** neonatal hepatitis

A**33** **C** Biliary atresia presents in the neonatal period with persisting and fluctuating icterus, pale stools and conjugated hyperbilirubinaemia. There is a slight female preponderance. The liver is normal initially but with progression becomes large and coarse with periportal fibrotic change. The biliary tree will not be dilated (unlike obstructive jaundice in older children). The presence of the triangular cord sign (obliterated fibrotic biliary tree) and a small or absent gallbladder are high predictors of biliary atresia.

There are three types of biliary atresia.
- Type I: extrahepatic biliary atresia (15%)
  — small gallbladder with visible intrahepatic ducts
- Type II: intrahepatic biliary atresia (10%)
  — small gallbladder with visible extrahepatic ducts

- Type III: complete atresia (75%)
  — atresia of the entire biliary tree.

**Q34** Biliary atresia is associated with a number of developmental abnormalities. Which of the following is *not* associated with biliary atresia?

   **A** preduodenal portal vein

   **B** choledochal cyst

   **C** polysplenia

   **D** hemivertebrae

   **E** Patau's syndrome

**A34** **D** Associated abnormalities occur in about 10% of patients with biliary atresia and include:

- preduodenal portal vein
- choledochal cyst
- azygous continuation of IVC
- polysplenia
- trisomy 13 (Patau's syndrome)
- situs inversus.

Hemivertebrae are associated with Alagille's syndrome (biliary hypoplasia). Other associations that occur with biliary hypoplasia include forehead bossing, pointed chin, butterfly vertebrae, dysplastic kidneys and peripheral pulmonary branch stenosis.

**Q35** A neonate with a prolonged episode of jaundice from birth has a spine radiograph that shows an abnormal segmentation of the vertebral bodies at D8 level. An ultrasound scan shows a collapsed gallbladder and $^{99m}$Tc-DISIDA scintigraphy shows tracer in the bowel at 24 hours. What is the likely diagnosis?

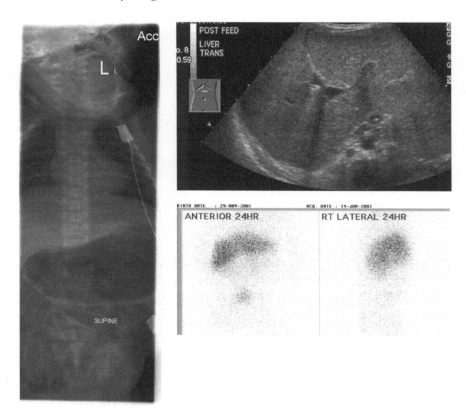

FIGURE 76.19 X-ray of the spine demonstrating segmentation abnormality, ultrasound scan of the abdomen and Technetium-99m-DISIDA scan

- **A** Alagille's syndrome
- **B** biliary atresia (type I)
- **C** neonatal jaundice
- **D** biliary atresia (type III)
- **E** Caroli's disease

**A35** **A** The spine X-ray shows a hemivertebrae at D8 level. The collapsed gallbladder and tracer that makes it into the bowel should suggest Alagille's syndrome (biliary hypoplasia). Biliary atresia would result in no tracer leaving the hepatic system and hence, no tracer would make it into the bowel.

Q36 A 4-year-old girl is admitted with jaundice and on examination has a right upper quadrant mass. An ultrasound confirms an abnormality in the biliary tree. The biliary tree has multiple areas of saccular dilatation that affect the intrahepatic biliary tree as well as the common bile duct. The diagnosis of choledochal cyst is reached. There are five types of choledochal cyst. Which type is described in this case?

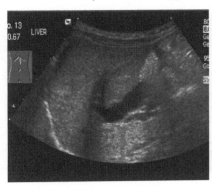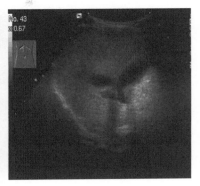

**FIGURE 76.20** Ultrasound scan of the porta hepatis

A Type I
B Type II
C Type III
D Type IV
E Type V

A36 **D** Choledochal cyst is a congenital segmental dilatation of the biliary tree. Presentation in childhood classically occurs with obstructive jaundice, abdominal pain and a right upper quadrant mass. However, these symptoms only occur in 10% of cases. Thirty per cent of cases present in the neonatal period, 50% by age 10 and 80% by young adulthood. There is a 3 : 1 female preponderance.

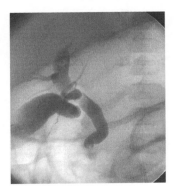

**FIGURE 76.21** Cholangiogram demonstrating the biliary system anatomy

The classification is as follows.

- Type I: most common, accounting for 80%–90%
  - Ia: dilatation of the entire extrahepatic bile duct
  - Ib: focal and segmental dilatation of the extrahepatic biliary tree
  - Ic: dilatation of the common bile duct.
- Type II: rare (2%)
  - true diverticulum of the extrahepatic biliary tree.
- Type III: rare (2%–5%)
  - choledochocele: dilatation of the extrahepatic bile duct within the duodenal wall.
- Type IV: second most common (10%–15%)
  - IVa: multiple dilatations/cysts of the intra- and extrahepatic biliary tree
  - IVb: cysts affecting the extrahepatic biliary tree only.
- Type V (Caroli's disease): rare (1%–6%)
  - multiple dilatations/cysts of the intrahepatic biliary tree only.

**Q37** A 2-month-old boy is admitted following an episode of jaundice. He is the child of an immigrant couple, was born at home and has not been seen at the hospital previously. There have been multiple episodes of jaundice since birth and blood work confirms conjugated hyperbilirubinaemia. The liver is large and has a course echotexture. The gallbladder is not visualised, there was no dilatation of the biliary radicals. The spleen is large and tortuous vessels are evident at the splenic hilum. Given the likely diagnosis, what is the treatment of choice?

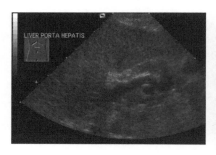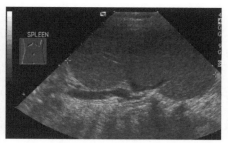

FIGURE 76.22 Ultrasound images of the liver and spleen

**A** liver transplantation

**B** Kasai's procedure

**C** transjugular, intrahepatic, portosystemic shunt

**D** splenectomy

**E** percutaneous drainage

A**37** **B** This child has undiagnosed biliary atresia. Children will often present with fluctuating icterus. The liver is initially normal in size and echotexture when assessed at ultrasound. However, without treatment, the liver increases in size and becomes increasingly coarse. Portal hypertension may occur and with a rise in portal pressure, splenomegaly and shunting through portosystemic anastomoses can occur.

The Kasai procedure (a portoenterostomy) is the treatment of choice in patients who present before 60 days. It allows drainage of bile into a Roux-en-Y jejunal loop and carries a significantly lower morbidity than liver transplantation and also avoids the need for long-term immunosuppression.

Q**38** Which of the following test results is the most sensitive for the diagnosis of biliary atresia?

   **A** $^{99m}$Tc-DISIDA scintigraphy: no tracer in the bowel at 24 hours.
   **B** MRI: multiple cysts at the porta hepatitis.
   **C** Cholangiogram: hypoplastic biliary tree with a collapsed gallbladder.
   **D** Biopsy: bile duct proliferation with fibrosis and cholestasis.
   **E** Ultrasound: triangular cord sign.

A**38** **D** Biliary atresia results in bile duct proliferation, periportal fibrosis and cholestasis, all of which can be seen at biopsy and are characteristic of the condition. The triangular cord sign is seen at the porta on ultrasound and represents fibrosis, characteristic in biliary atresia. No tracer at 24 hours during $^{99m}$Tc-DISIDA scintigraphy is also indicative of biliary atresia. However, of the three findings, the biopsy result is the most sensitive. Multiple cysts at the porta sounds like choledochal cyst and the hypoplastic biliary tree occurs in Alagille's syndrome (biliary hypoplasia).

**Q39** A young child presents with abdominal pain, pale stools and fever. No discriminating features are found on examination; blood test confirms obstructive jaundice and raised inflammatory markers. The liver is normal at ultrasound but there is fusiform dilatation of the common bile duct (CBD). The gallbladder is visualised. Child had a magnetic resonance cholangiography (MRCP) to confirm the diagnosis. What is the likely diagnosis?

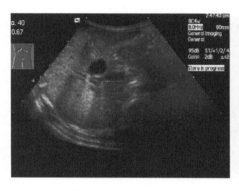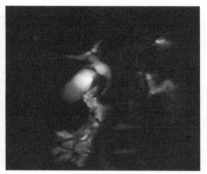

**FIGURE 76.23** Ultrasound and MRCP images

**A** choledochal cyst, type I

**B** sickle-cell crisis

**C** viral hepatitis

**D** Caroli's disease

**E** G6PD (glucose-6-phosphate dehydrogenasee deficiency)

**A39** **A** Choledochal cyst is a congenital segmental dilatation of the biliary tree. Presentation with abdominal pain, obstructive jaundice and fever can mimic hepatitis unless a mass is found. There are five types of choledochal cyst, the commonest being type I.

- Type I: most common, accounting for 80%–90%
  - Ia: dilatation of the entire extrahepatic bile duct
  - Ib: focal and segmental dilatation of the extrahepatic biliary tree
  - Ic: dilatation of the common bile duct.

Caroli's disease is the eponymous name given to choledochal cyst type V and is very rare (only 2% of cases). The other answers would not account for the fusiform dilatation of the CBD, but could cause presentation with jaundice in a young child.

**Q40** Following clinical review the differential diagnosis for a neonate with fluctuating jaundice includes biliary atresia. When considering how to continue the investigative process, which radiological investigation is the best first investigation?

    **A** cholangiogram

    **B** ultrasound abdomen

    **C** MRI cholangiogram

    **D** MRI liver

    **E** $^{99m}$Tc-DISIDA scintigraphy

**A40** **B** The best first investigation in any condition is often not the most sensitive examination. In this situation, the best first test is abdominal ultrasound. It has a relatively high sensitivity, is portable, cheap and is non-invasive. The triangular cord sign may be seen and relates to portal fibrosis, characteristic of biliary atresia.

**Q41** Which GI malformation is associated with Beckwith–Wiedemann's syndrome?

    **A** gastroschisis

    **B** TOF

    **C** omphalocele

    **D** duodenal atresia

    **E** malrotation

**A41** **C** Beckwith–Wiedemann's syndrome is characterised by midline abdominal wall defects (omphalocele, umbilical hernia, diastasis of the recti), macroglossia, macrosomia, ear creases or ear pits and neonatal hypoglycaemia. Many children do not have all these features and may also have other developmental abnormalities including midface hypoplasia, hemihypertrophy, genitourinary anomalies, cardiac anomalies, musculoskeletal abnormalities and hearing loss.

**Q42** A child is born with an anterior abdominal wall defect. The defect is a small, full thickness split in the ventral abdominal wall to the right of the midline. What is the most likely diagnosis?

    **A** umbilical hernia

    **B** omphalocele

    **C** gastroschisis

    **D** cloacal exstrophy

    **E** divarication of the recti

$A^{42}$  **C**  Gastroschisis and omphalocele are both defects that are present in the anterior abdominal wall. Gastroschisis refers to a small, full-thickness defect that is *not* in the midline, classically positioned to the right of the umbilicus. It typically occurs in isolation and its aetiology is postulated to be related to an ischaemic event *in utero*.

$Q^{43}$  A neonate is born with a ventral abdominal wall defect. Which of the following features is *not* associated with the diagnosis of omphalocele?
  **A**  herniation of the liver
  **B**  midline position of the hernia
  **C**  umbilicus at the top of the defect
  **D**  trisomy 13
  **E**  no covering membrane

$A^{43}$  **E**  An omphalocele is a midline ventral abdominal wall defect through which abdominal viscera protrude *in utero*. The liver is often involved, as are other abdominal viscera and the umbilicus inserts at the top of the defect which is covered by a membrane (unlike gastroschisis). There is an association with trisomy 13.

$Q^{44}$  A child is born with a ventral abdominal wall defect to the right of the midline at the level of the umbilicus. There is herniation of bowel that is covered with a thick fibrous substance. There is no membrane covering the bowel. The defect is surgically corrected. The child is subsequently reviewed in clinic. Which of the following is *not* associated with this developmental defect?
  **A**  necrotising enterocolitis (NEC)
  **B**  intestinal atresia
  **C**  dysmotility
  **D**  short bowel syndrome
  **E**  volvulus

$A^{44}$  **E**  The defect that has been described in the stem is gastroschisis, a developmental defect that is likely the result of an *in utero* ischaemic event. Exposure of the bowel to amniotic fluid *in utero* results in damage to the bowel. Postnatally, this results in a thick and fibrous 'peel-covered' coating to the loops of bowel.

Complications include short bowel syndrome and intestinal dysmotility. Other conditions that are associated with gastroschisis include intestinal atresia and stenosis. NEC is reported in 20% of patients.

Q45 A patient who was born with gastroschisis and had a surgical repair in the neonatal period presents to the local surgical service with abdominal pain and altered bowel habit. The concern is that her presentation relates to complications from gastroschisis repair. What is the most helpful radiological investigation?

    **A** abdominal radiograph

    **B** upper GI contrast study

    **C** ultrasound abdomen

    **D** MRI abdomen

    **E** contrast enema

A45 **B** Patients with gastroschisis may present with complications (short bowel syndrome), associated pathology (intestinal atresia and stenoses) or complications related to repair (malrotation). The best radiological investigation is an upper GI contrast study which will help to exclude malrotation and volvulus as the cause for the presentation.

Q46 A child has an abdominal wall defect. On examination, there is a partial thickness defect in the ventral abdominal wall to the right of midline, lateral to the rectus abdominus muscle. What is the diagnosis?

    **A** Bochdalek's hernia

    **B** gastroschisis

    **C** divarication of the recti

    **D** spigelian hernia

    **E** omphalocele

A46 **D** A spigelian hernia is a hernia in the anterior abdominal wall at the linea semilunaris. The linea semilunaris is formed by the aponeurosis of the internal oblique muscle as it meets the rectus abdominus muscle and encloses it. These are partial thickness defects that are quite distinct from gastroschisis and omphalocele. Divarication of the recti is a midline defect and Bochdalek's hernia is a congenital diaphragmatic hernia.

**Q47** A 3-week-old infant presents to the emergency department for the second time with respiratory failure. On the last admission the diagnosis of a chest infection was made clinically, without radiological investigation. On this occasion, the child has a chest radiograph which confirms the reason for the respiratory distress. What is the most likely diagnosis?

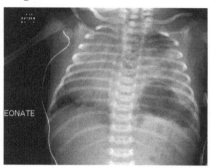

**FIGURE 76.24** X-ray of the chest

**A** diaphragmatic eventration
**B** hiatus hernia
**C** Bochdalek's hernia
**D** Morgagni's hernia
**E** spigelian hernia

**A47** **C** This child has a congenital diaphragmatic hernia with bowel (and possibly other abdominal viscera) in the left hemithorax, which has resulted in compression, and hypoplasia, of the left lung. Bochdalek's hernia is far more common than Morgagni's hernia and tends to occur on the left with features that can be remembered using the 5B mnemonic:

- Bochdalek's
- big
- back
- baby
- bad.

Diaphragmatic eventration would present with a raised hemidiaphragm and hiatus hernia would not produce this appearance and a spigelian hernia is a hernia that involves the anterior abdominal wall.

**Q48** A child with Down's syndrome and cyanotic congenital heart disease is also shown to have a diaphragmatic abnormality. What is this most likely to be?

- **A** diaphragmatic eventration
- **B** Morgagni's hernia
- **C** iatrogenic diaphragmatic rupture
- **D** Bochdalek's hernia
- **E** septum transversum defect

**A48** **B** Morgagni's hernia is a congenital diaphragmatic hernia. It accounts for only <5% of all congenital diaphragmatic hernias, but does have associations with congenital heart disease, intestinal malrotation and chromosomal abnormalities including Down's and Turner's syndromes. It arises from maldevelopment of the septum transversum that is located between the ribs and sternum. It is smaller than Bochdalek's hernia and has features described by the 4Ms:

- Morgagni's
- middle (anterior and central position)
- mature (tend to present in older children)
- minuscule (they are small).

**Q49** A teenager presents to his family doctor with epigastric abdominal pain. He is short, with almond-shaped eyes, a round face and has a single palmar crease. He had a murmur as a child, which was confirmed on ultrasound to be the result of an atrial septal defect (ASD). He had an echocardiogram recently as routine follow-up examination and apart from the ASD, there was no other abnormality. As part of the workup on this occasion, a chest radiograph is performed which shows a soft tissue density in the cardiophrenic angle on the right. Otherwise, the study is normal, with a normal cardiac size, clear lungs and pleural spaces. What is the most likely diagnosis?

- **A** thymoma
- **B** Morgagni's hernia
- **C** pericardial cyst
- **D** germ cell tumour
- **E** hiatus hernia

**A49** **B** This teenager has Down's syndrome and an ASD. Apart from that, his echocardiogram is normal, reducing the likelihood that the diagnosis is of a pericardial cyst. With these associations and epigastric pain, the best answer is Morgagni's hernia.

**Q50** A young child has an abnormal diaphragmatic contour which is lobulated and upwardly displaced to the right anteromedially. Ultrasound of the diaphragm reveals reduced movement on the right, but it is not paradoxical. What is the diagnosis here?

**A** Morgagni's hernia

**B** hiatus hernia

**C** septum transversum defect

**D** diaphragmatic eventration

**E** traumatic diaphragmatic rupture

**A50** **D** Diaphragmatic eventration accounts for about 5% of congenital diaphragmatic abnormalities. There is upward displacement of a congenitally thin and hypoplastic diaphragm. These are often small and just cause a lobulated contour. If unilateral, there are associations with Beckwith–Wiedemann's syndrome and chromosomal abnormalities. When bilateral, there may be a history of cytomegalovirus or toxoplasmosis.

## Further reading

Blumhagen JD, Maclin L, Krauter D, *et al*. Sonographic diagnosis of hypertrophic pyloric stenosis. *Am J Roentgenol*. 1988; **150**(6): 1367–70.

Caniano DA, Beaver BL. Meconium ileus: a fifteen-year experience with forty-two neonates. *Surgery*. 1987; **102**(4): 699–703.

Donoghue V. Neonatal gastrointestinal tract. In: Carty H, Brunelle F, Shaw D, *et al*. *Imaging children*. New York, NY: Churchill Livingstone; 1994. pp. 250–60.

Ng J, Antao B, Bartram J, *et al*. Diagnostic difficulties in the management of H-type tracheoesophageal fistula. *Acta Radiol*. 2006; **47**(8): 801–5.

Nixon HH, Tawes R. Etiology and treatment of small intestinal atresia: analysis of a series of 127 jejunoileal atresias and comparision with 62 duodenal atresias. *Surgery*. 1971; **69**(1): 41–51.

Weiss LM, Fagelman D, Warhit JM. CT demonstration of an esophageal duplication cyst. *J Comput Assist Tomogr*. 1983; **7**(4): 716–18.

# CHAPTER 77

# Paediatric anaesthesia

## NIGEL PEREIRA, ROB E JOHN, LIZ STOREY

**From the choices below each question, select the single best answer.**

**Q1**  Which of the following is true regarding epidural blocks in children?

   **A**  They are rarely indicated in routine paediatric surgery.

   **B**  Epidural blocks can mask the presence of abdominal haemorrhage after laparotomy.

   **C**  They should never be used in day-case surgery.

   **D**  They affect only sensory pathways.

   **E**  Hypotension associated with epidurals in infants is always due to sympathetic blockade.

**A1**  **B**  Epidural blocks include thoracic, lumbar, and sacral or caudal block, the latter being one of the commonest nerve blocks used in paediatric surgery. One of the greatest hazards of after epidural laparotomies is the abolition of pain as a symptom of intra-abdominal haemorrhage. Caudals are frequently used in day-case surgery and are particularly useful in infants undergoing, for example, penile surgery or hernia repairs.

    One of the major problems is that motor block occurs particularly at higher concentrations of local anaesthetic agents. Hypotension during an epidural in a young child is more likely to be due to fluid loss than sympathetic vasodilatation.

**Q2**  Regarding temperature control in the operating theatre, in small infants, which of the following is true?

   **A**  Radiation is not an important cause of heat loss.

   **B**  Anaesthetic agents do not effect temperature regulation

   **C**  Heat loss is due to the relatively small surface-to-volume ratio.

   **D**  Brown fat generates heat.

   **E**  Evaporative heat loss from the respiratory tract cannot be prevented.

**A2**   **D**   Radiation is an extremely important source of heat loss. Since heat is transferred from the warm body to cold surroundings such as walls and equipment, the theatre should be warmed before surgery commences. Anaesthetic agents do effect temperature regulation by a number of mechanisms such as depression of behavioural, hypothalamic and autonomic responses to changes in environmental temperature. Because this can be anticipated, patient warming and temperature monitoring should be instigated for all surgery in these patients. Surface-to-volume ratio is inversely related to the size of the patient. This is a fixed geometric relationship which results in relatively greater heat loss in small infants. Brown fat is more important in small infants as a source of heat generation than in adults. Heat is produced when the normal process of generating adenosine triphosphate in mitochondria is 'uncoupled' and heat is produced instead. Volatile agents inhibit this process. Evaporative losses from the respiratory tract can be prevented by humidification usually using a combined condenser and microbial filter or heated water humidifier.

**Q3**   If a child does not breathe at the end of a 2-hour operation, this is unlikely to be due to:

 **A**   fentanyl
 **B**   vecuronium
 **C**   isoflurane
 **D**   hypocapnia
 **E**   propofol induction.

**A3**   **E**   Fentanyl is a potent opioid with powerful respiratory depressant. The patient will have other signs of opioid depression such as pinpoint pupils. Naloxone will reverse this, but will also reverse the analgesic effects and unless used by infusion the patient could stop breathing later as it has a relatively short half-life. Vecuronium is a non-depolarising muscle relaxant which blocks the motor neurone end plates. A useful test is to use a percutaneous electrical nerve stimulator, usually a 'train of four' pattern and look for 'fade' where the later twitches are absent or much smaller than the first. The relaxant may be reversed by neostigmine and glycopyrrolate, where the neostigmine blocks the breakdown of acetylcholine and the glycopyrrolate blocks the parasympathetic effects of surplus acetylcholine at receptors other than the neuromuscular junction. Isoflurane is a volatile agent and these all have direct respiratory depressant effects. Isoflurane is excreted via the lungs and is removed by switching off the vaporiser and ventilating the patient for a few minutes. Carbon dioxide levels at the respiratory centre control breathing and need to be normal or higher than normal in the face of respiratory depressants to stimulate regular spontaneous breathing. A propofol induction 2 hours before is very unlikely to be the cause and other causes are more likely.

Q4 Regarding postoperative concerns specific to general anaesthesia in ex-premature infants, which of the following is true?

A The risk of postoperative apnoea at 56 weeks' post-conceptual age is 1%.

B Patients less than 60 weeks' post-conceptual age should be monitored 24–48 hours postoperatively.

C Anaemia reduces the incidence of apnoeas.

D Regional anaesthesia should not be used together with general anaesthesia.

E Caffeine and theophylline should not be used to prevent postoperative apnoeas.

A4 A Postoperative apnoea in spontaneously breathing ex-premature infants is common. This can be avoided by using ventilatory support. It may be reduced by delaying surgery, treating anaemia, avoiding respiratory depressant drugs such as morphine, and using respiratory stimulants such as caffeine prophylactically. Spinal or caudal anaesthesia may be used alone, or general anaesthesia combined with a local anaesthetic technique. Use of the shorter-acting volatile agent desflurane may be useful in reducing the incidence of anaesthesia related apnoeas.

Q5 Regarding anaesthetic drugs used in paediatric anaesthesia:

A propofol is contraindicated in children less than 6 months old.

B desflurane is commonly used for inhalational induction in children.

C children are calmer after sevoflurane than other volatile agents.

D Remifentanil is broken down by pseudocholinesterase in children.

E Intralipid is recommended to treat bupivacaine overdose.

A5 E Propofol is indicated for induction and maintenance by infusion from 1 month of age. Because of the risk of fatal side effects (metabolic acidosis, rhabdomyolysis, hyperkalaemia and cardiac failure) of using high-dose infusion over longer periods, propofol is contraindicated for sedation in intensive care below 17 years of age. Desflurane is not recommended for inhalation induction in children as it is irritant and causes cough, breath-holding, apnoea, laryngospasm and increased secretions. Sevoflurane causes emergence delirium in children. Remifentanil is broken down by the ubiquitous tissue cholinesterase, whereas suxamethonium is broken down by pseudocholinesterase. Intralipid is recommended for the treatment of bupivacaine overdose following animal experiments and positive human experience. In addition to oxygen and cardiopulmonary resuscitation, stop injecting the local anaesthetic and treat convulsions. The current recommended dose is: Intralipid 20%: 1.5 mL/kg bolus followed by an infusion of 0.25 mL/kg/min with two repeat boluses at 5-minute intervals if adequate circulation has not been restored. Increase the dose to 0.5 mL/kg if adequate circulation has not been restored.

 **Q⁶** Suxamethonium may be safely used for which of the following?
   A rapid sequence induction for a laparotomy in a 5-year-old with intestinal obstruction
   B intubation in a case of myotonic dystrophy in a 10-year-old
   C intubation in a case of suspected malignant hyperthermia
   D intubation in a 4-year-old, one month after 60% burns
   E intubation in a case of acute tubular necrosis

 **A⁶** **A** Suxamethonium is a depolarising muscle relaxant and is the traditional agent used to facilitate intubation in patients with a suspected full stomach associated with preoxygenation and cricoid pressure, known as rapid sequence induction.

It is contraindicated in myotonic dystrophy as it exacerbates myotonia and this can cause respiratory embarrassment. Suxamethonium is a specific trigger agent for malignant hyperthermia and is absolutely contraindicated in suspected cases. Suxamethonium can cause dangerous hyperkalaemia between 3 and 7 weeks after major burns. The mechanism is thought to be due to both rhabdomyolysis and abnormal increase in acetylcholine receptors in the burn area. Suxamethonium should be avoided in renal failure, because of the potential for dangerous hyperkalaemia.

**Q⁷** Considering prophylaxis against venous thromboembolism in children, which of the following is true?
   A Children have lower levels of α2-macroglobulin than adults.
   B The presence of a central venous catheter poses a high risk.
   C Corticosteroids reduce the risk.
   D Asparaginase reduces the risk.
   E Obesity is unlikely to be relevant.

 **A⁷** **B** Venous thromboembolism is less common in children than adults and occurs in around five per 10 000 children in hospital. Plasma levels of α2-macroglobulin are higher and plasma prothrombin levels are lower and these are thought to be protective. Risks may be congenital such as: factor V Leiden or deficiencies of antithrombin III and protein C and S. Acquired risk factors include the presence of a central venous catheter, puberty, congenital heart disease, inflammatory diseases, burns, trauma, immobility, pregnancy, smoking and obesity. Drugs which increase risk include corticosteroids, asparaginase and oral contraceptives.

**Q8** Regarding paediatric day-case surgery, which of the following is true?

   **A** In general it should account for 10%–20% of elective paediatric surgical workload in a specialist centre.

   **B** It is advantageous because it causes less emotional upset, behavioural problems and parental separation, and releases resources for inpatient care.

   **C** Suitable day-case procedures include: repair of inguinal hernia, circumcision and reversal of ileostomy.

   **D** The only requirements for day-case surgery are the suitability of the case and an ASA 1 or 11 patient.

   **E** It is contraindicated in a term baby who is now 6 weeks old.

**A8**  **B**  The Royal College of Surgeons guidelines suggest that 50%–70% of elective paediatric operations should be done as day cases. The advantages of day care include less emotional upset, parental separation and fewer behavioural problems (such as nightmares and enuresis). Day care also improves parent and child satisfaction, decreases waiting lists and puts less strain on resources for inpatient care.

   Selection for day-case surgery should be based on the following factors.

   • **Health:** children needing specialised perioperative care, e.g. diabetes, metabolic disease, sickle-cell, haemophilia and other bleeding disorders, complex cardiac disorders or projected airway difficulties and sleep apnoea, would all be unsuitable.

   • **Age:** pre-term babies and ex-premature babies are at increased risk of postoperative apnoea and bradycardia and require monitoring; they should not be done as day case until 60 weeks' post-conceptual age. Most specialised units will provide day care to well, term babies over 4 weeks of age.

   • **Complexity of surgery:** prolonged surgery, emergency surgery and surgery associated with significant pain and bleeding are not suitable.

   • **Social:** there must be adequate family support and supervision, suitable home conditions and a telephone readily available.

   • **Geography:** the patient should not have a long distance to travel and there must be adequate transport.

**Q9** With regard to preoperative preparation and anaesthesia for day-case surgery, which of the following is true?

  **A** It is not necessary to have contact with the parents or patient until the day of surgery.

  **B** A sickle screen is not needed in children who may have sickle-cell anaemia.

  **C** Premedication with midazolam is contraindicated because it delays recovery.

  **D** Inhalational induction of anaesthesia with sevoflurane is the method of choice.

  **E** Intravenous opiates may be given if required but addition of opiates to a caudal block is not suitable because of the risk of delayed respiratory depression.

**A9** **E** Effective day care requires streamlined assessment. Preoperative nurse-led clinics which include input from surgeons, anaesthetists and play specialists, are increasingly common and very effective. Protocols for fasting and investigations should be clear, and specific written information given to the parents before the day of admission. Most children require no preoperative investigations. A sickle screen is needed in children who may have sickle-cell anaemia.

Premedication is not contraindicated in day-case surgery and there is no evidence that midazolam 0.5 mg/kg delays recovery. Intravenous or inhalational induction of anaesthesia is appropriate and often depends on the child's choice. Good postoperative analgesia is essential and whenever possible local anaesthetic techniques should be used in combination with general anaesthesia. The addition of paracetamol and non-steroidal anti-inflammatory drugs are the mainstay of analgesia but opiates may be given if required orally or intravenously. The use of opiates as an adjunct in a caudal block is not recommended in day-case surgery because of the risk of delayed respiratory depression.

**Q10** Regarding rapid sequence induction in children, which of the following is true?

  **A** A classic rapid sequence induction technique may need to be modified in paediatric practice.

  **B** Children are not usually at risk of aspiration of gastric contents.

  **C** It is never appropriate to hand ventilate a baby during a rapid sequence induction.

  **D** The child is not at risk of aspiration during emergence from anaesthesia and extubation.

  **E** A cuffed endotracheal tube is required.

A10  A  If a risk of aspiration of gastric contents is foreseen, a rapid sequence induction (RSI) should be performed for induction of anaesthesia. Classically an RSI requires a working cannula, and the patient should be monitored and positioned on a tilting trolley with suction available. Oxygen is administered via a close-fitting face mask for 3 minutes and then anaesthesia is induced with thiopentone 5 mg/kg followed quickly by suxamethonium 2 mg/kg, giving rapid paralysis. As the induction agent takes effect an assistant applies pressure to the cricoid ring and bag-and-mask ventilation is avoided so as not to inflate the stomach. An endotracheal tube is placed in the trachea. A well-fitting uncuffed tube is said to offer protection from airway soiling but there is renewed interest in cuffed tubes in children and in the emergency patient; they offer the advantage that the correct fit should be achieved at the initial intubation. Extubation is the time of highest risk and so awake extubation is recommended.

There are several problems with classic RSI in paediatric practice. Preoxygenation and application of full monitoring can be difficult in an uncooperative child. Oxygen stores in the functional residual capacity in a small child or neonate can easily be exceeded if ventilation is avoided while waiting for suxamethonium to work, leading to hypoxia. It is reasonable to inflate the lungs gently with cricoid pressure in place, even in the context of a RSI.

Q11  Regarding massive blood transfusion, which of the following is true?
  A  It is necessary if 20% of circulating blood volume is lost in a short space of time.
  B  It is focused on maintaining adequate tissue perfusion and oxygenation.
  C  It rarely leads to coagulation defects.
  D  It causes metabolic disturbances, the commonest of which is hyperkalaemia.
  E  It unavoidably causes hypothermia.

A11  B  Massive blood transfusion can be defined as replacement of blood volume with transfused blood within 24 hours or, more usefully in a surgical setting, loss of 50% of the blood volume within 3 hours.

The main considerations are as follows:
  • Maintenance of blood volume and haemoglobin concentration to ensure adequate tissue perfusion and oxygenation.
  • Use of blood components to correct coagulation defects: this may be guided by laboratory measurements but often in the context of massive blood loss they will be out of date by the time the results are available. 5–10 mL/kg platelet infusion is given. Fresh frozen plasma is given as a 10–20 mL/kg infusion to provide coagulation factors.

Cryoprecipitate, rich in factor VIII and fibrinogen, may be needed in disseminated intravascular coagulation or if fibrinogen levels are low.

- The management of metabolic disorders: the commonest problem is reduced ionised calcium due to citrate toxicity. Appropriate treatment is 5–10 mL/kg calcium chloride. Hyperkalaemia, hypomagnesaemia and raised lactic acid levels may also occur.
- Management and avoidance of hypothermia.

**Q12** Which of the following is true with regard to managing an uncooperative child before surgery?

- **A** They are usually uncooperative because they are misbehaving and need to be disciplined.
- **B** The best strategy is to ignore the child's distress and press on – the quicker it's over the better.
- **C** Midazolam has its maximum effect in 20 minutes and is given orally at a dose of 1 mg/kg.
- **D** Distress experienced by a child perioperatively may lead to behavioural problems that can last for weeks.
- **E** Children aged 5–8 years are most at risk of anxiety.

**A12** **D** Children are not usually uncooperative unless they are frightened, distressed or psychologically disturbed. Managing a frightened uncooperative child at induction is distressing for the parents, patients and healthcare workers, but perhaps more worrying is that delayed troublesome *postoperative* behaviour has been recognised as a problem that is related to distress during induction. It can include general anxiety, separation anxiety, poor sleep, temper tantrums and enuresis and can persist for weeks or longer.

With this in mind, the management of uncooperative children should focus on prevention. Identifying the anxious child can be hard, and prediction of children's behaviour is equally difficult. Children between 1 and 5 years are at greatest risk of developing perioperative anxiety. Separation anxiety peaks at 1 year and those over 5 years are more able to deal with unpredictable situations. Shy, withdrawn children and children of anxious parents have higher levels of anxiety. Previous bad experiences with medical services are important and parental prediction of cooperation may be valuable.

Strategies for preventing anxiety can broadly be divided into non-pharmacological and pharmacological interventions. The former may involve preoperative preparation programmes, the preoperative visit, parental presence at induction, play therapy and music. For those children requiring multiple painful procedures, help from a psychologist may be needed. The commonest used pharmacological intervention is midazolam, a short-acting benzodiazepine. The optimum dose is 0.5 mg/kg orally – it causes maximum effect at 30–45 minutes but anxiolysis may be achieved as early as 15 minutes. Ketamine, choral hydrate and triclofos, opioids and clonidine have also been used.

Q13 Which of the following is true of tracheostomy?
  A It is often needed in the treatment of croup.
  B Humidification is a must.
  C Accidental decannulation and plugging of the tube are common postoperative events.
  D It can be life-saving in the presence of a mediastinal mass.
  E When changing the tube, the new one must be introduced as superficially as possible.

A13 C Tracheostomy is performed to relieve airway obstruction and also to provide a means for long-term ventilation and tracheal toilet. It is almost always done under general anaesthesia in children.

It could be part of the management of patients with, e.g. neck tumours or Pierre Robin's syndrome but would hopefully not be needed in supraglottitis or bacterial tracheitis, where short-term endotracheal intubation would be the intention. The hope would be to avoid endotracheal intubation altogether in the treatment of croup. The airway obstruction caused by a mediastinal mass would not be helped by tracheostomy if endotracheal intubation has failed.

Daily management involves cleaning the stoma site, suction of secretions and preventing the accumulation of dried secretions in the cannula and within the tracheobronchial tree. The majority of long-term patients do not need formal humidification.

In the postoperative period patients are prone to accidental decannulation and to blockage of the cannula with blood or secretions. Early on the stoma will not have healed and recannulation could be particularly difficult. Recannulation is performed by inserting the tip of the cannula at right angles to the trachea and then letting the curve of the tube follow the tract into the trachea. This is to prevent accidental superficial placement. Tracheal dilators may help recannulation in the early postoperative period.

Q14 In the management of acute pain, which of the following is true?
  A Non-steroidal anti-inflammatory drugs (NSAIDs) should be prescribed to all patients to reduce the need for opiates.
  B It is unnecessary to give regular paracetamol while a patient is still on an opiate infusion.
  C Giving intravenous opiates on demand is ultimately safer and more effective than an infusion or patient-controlled analgesia (PCA).
  D Oral codeine is a reliable and effective alternative to morphine.
  E Pain scoring is central to the control of postoperative pain.

$A$14 **E** The use of pain-scoring tools appropriate for age and ability combined with a multimodal approach (including non-pharmacological interventions) usually results in strategies that relieve postoperative pain.

Regular prescriptions of paracetamol and NSAIDs can reduce the need for, and the dose of, opiates and improve pain scores. They should be given before the effect of local or regional analgesia wears off. NSAIDs are safe in the majority of patients but they are now used so commonly that it is easy to forget that they could cause problems with bleeding in major surgery or trauma and could be contraindicated in some patients with severe asthma, renal impairment or a history of GI bleeding.

Morphine is the most commonly used parenteral opiate. The use of morphine infusions or PCA helps smooth out the peaks and troughs that result from intermittent bolus injections, making it more effective and potentially reducing side effects. PCA can be used from the age of about 5 years but a small background infusion will help the younger child to sleep without rousing in pain. Strict standards of observation need to be in place for opiates to be used safely, especially in neonates, infants, and those with co-morbidities that make them more susceptible to respiratory depression, e.g. obstructive sleep apnoea.

Codeine is used very commonly as the oral opiate of choice but about 10% of children lack the enzymes needed to convert codeine to morphine, so it could fail to produce analgesia.

## Further reading

*Continuing Education in Anaesthesia, Critical Care & Pain.* Oxford University Press [Journal].

Doyle E. *Paediatric Anaesthesia.* Oxford: Oxford University Press; 2007.

Lerman J, Steward D, Cote CJ. *Manual of Pediatric Anesthesia: with an index of pediatric syndromes.* Philadelphia, PA: Elsevier; 2010.

Gregory GA. *Pediatric Anesthesia.* 4th ed. Philadelphia, PA: Churchill Livingstone; 2002.

*Pediatric Anesthesia.* Wiley-Blackwell [Journal].

# CHAPTER 78

# Solid organ transplantation

## ERIK B FINGER

From the choices below each question, select the single best answer.

**Q1** Which of the following is *not* true regarding post-transplant lympho-proliferative disease (PTLD)?

    **A** The incidence of PTLD is approximately 50% in transplant recipients.

    **B** PTLD is associated with Epstein–Barr virus (EBV) infection.

    **C** The incidence of PTLD is greater in children than adults.

    **D** PTLD is more common in small-bowel transplant recipients than for other organs.

    **E** Initial treatment for PTLD is reduction in immunosuppression.

**A1**   **A** PTLD is a lymphoma affecting transplant recipients. It occurs in ~1% of transplant recipients, but ranges of 1%–10% have been reported. It is associated with EBV infection and the incidence is higher in children who are more likely to be seronegative for EBV exposure at the time of transplant, and who have a longer post-transplant lifespan for development of disease. PTLD is most common in small-bowel transplantation (up to ~20% incidence), presumably due to the large lymphoid mass that accompanies the organ and increased levels of immunosuppression needed for these transplants. Initial treatment is reduction of immunosuppression. Additional treatment options include surgery, radiation, chemotherapy, antibody therapy directed at B-cells, and therapy to reduce EBV load. Prognosis depends on location of disease (central nervous system, disseminated, localised), clonality (monoclonal vs. polyclonal), and subset of cells involved (T-cells, B-cells, lymphocyte subsets).

**Q2** Which of the following is *not* an indication for pancreas transplantation?
  **A** hypoglycaemic unawareness
  **B** desire to avoid insulin injections
  **C** progressive secondary complications of diabetes (nephropathy, retinopathy, neuropathy)
  **D** co-transplant of a non-pancreas organ
  **E** difficulty in controlling blood sugar despite intensive regimen of insulin administration

**A2**  **B**  Desire to avoid insulin injection is not considered an indication for pancreas transplantation. While recipient selection is not uniform, the other options listed are all factors that favour transplant in the risk/benefit evaluation. Patients with hypoglycaemic unawareness can have life-threatening episodes of low blood sugar that can be prevented with transplant. Progressive secondary complications of diabetes include retinopathy, neuropathy and nephropathy. The progression of these complications slows with transplant and may even improve in some. Need for co-transplant of another organ lessens the additional risk of immunosuppression for treatment of diabetes. This is most often a simultaneous kidney and pancreas transplant (SPK), but others can be considered as well. This can either be performed simultaneously as for SPK transplants, or serially. Difficulty managing blood sugars despite an intensive regimen of insulin therapy is also considered an indication for transplant. These are patients that have large fluctuations in blood sugar despite insulin pump or frequent insulin dosing.

**Q3** Which of the following is not true regarding organ donors?
  **A** Declaration of brain death requires an EEG or brain perfusion scan.
  **B** Brain death is associated with cardiovascular, autonomic and hormonal lability.
  **C** Diabetes insipidus is frequent in organ donors and electrolyte abnormalities need to be corrected in order to prevent organ dysfunction following transplant.
  **D** Under some circumstances patients with unrecoverable brain injury can be used as organ donors even if not declared brain dead.
  **E** Brain death is determined by absence of brainstem reflexes and spontaneous breathing.

**A3**  **B**  Determination of brain death is based on clinical exam. Brain perfusion scans or EEGs are often used for the confirmation of brain death but are not an essential component of its determination; however, many institutions require such a confirmatory test before proceeding with organ harvesting. The clinical determination is based on the absence of brainstem reflexes and spontaneous breathing. Breathing is often assessed by performing an apnoea test. The patient is disconnected from the ventilator for 10 minutes and a blood-gas measurement is made. A diagnostic apnoea test requires a $CO_2$ elevation to $\geq 60$ mmHg or $\geq 20$ mmHg over baseline normal $PCO_2$ and no evidence of spontaneous breathing. Some potential donors are too unstable for such a test to be feasible and in these cases the secondary methods are used (EEG or brain perfusion scan). In some cases patients who are not brain dead can be used as organ donors. In this process, called *donation after cardiac death*, the patient has irreversible brain injury. If the family wishes and consents, medical care is withdrawn (usually by extubation). If the heart stops and cardiac death is declared, a rapid procurement of organs can be performed. The exact details of this procedure vary by region or institution. Usually a waiting period of 5 minutes is observed after cardiac death is declared.

 **Q4** Which of the following is *not* true regarding opportunistic infections in transplant patients?

**A** Infections in the first month following transplant are similar to those in other patients undergoing surgery for similar non-transplant indications.

**B** Due to extensive screening of donors, transmission of infection from donor to recipient does not occur.

**C** Reactivation of chronic infection in the recipient (i.e. hepatitis C), is an important cause of infection in transplant recipients.

**D** Appropriate antimicrobial prophylaxis against cytomegalovirus (CMV) and mycobacterial infection has lessened the incidence of these diseases and has improved patient survival.

**E** Invasive fungal infections have significant risk of morbidity and mortality in transplant patients.

**A4** **B** Infections in transplant patients come in three main phases. Initially these patients are susceptible to donor- or recipient-related nosocomial or technical infections. Later in the first year these patients see reactivation of latent infections. After the first year transplant patients face community-acquired infections

During the first month following transplant, patients are susceptible to similar infections as those affecting non-transplant patients (line, wound, catheter infections). Disease transmission from donor to recipient does occur despite screening. Transmission of hepatitis, HIV, West Nile virus and other exotic infection such as rabies has occurred, but fortunately is quite rare. Prophylaxis against CMV with aciclovir or valganciclovir has decreased CMV disease in recipients. CMV-negative recipients receiving organs from CMV-positive donors are at the most risk for development of clinically significant disease. Antibiotic prophylaxis with trimethoprim-sulfamethaxazole or equivalent in sulfa allergic patients is used to reduce the risk of pneumocystis pneumonia, which is caused by *Pneumocystis jiroveci* (formerly carinii). Invasive fungal infections carry a ~30% mortality in transplant patients.

**Q5** Which of the following causes of end-stage renal disease (ESRD) in children is most likely to recur following kidney transplant?

A congenital obstructive uropathy

B hypertension

C focal segmental glomerulosclerosis

D glomerulonephritis

E polycystic kidney disease

**A5** **B** There are many causes of renal failure in children, including each of the causes listed. Focal segmental glomerulosclerosis is one of the causes of renal failure that can recur following transplant, and it does so in up to 50% of transplant recipients. Recurrence is diagnosed after the development of proteinuria or graft dysfunction and is confirmed by biopsy. In many children, native nephrectomy is performed prior to transplant so that postoperative proteinuria can be correctly attributed to the allograft rather than native kidneys. Recurrent disease can be corrected in many patients with plasmapheresis, but rapid diagnosis and initiation of treatment are essential. Other causes of ESRD such as diabetes and hypertension also recur, and corrective measures can be taken to lessen their impact following transplant.

**Q6** Which of the following is not true about early postoperative complications following renal transplant?

A Graft thrombosis does not occur if the kidney reperfused well after transplant.

B Delay in graft function leading to dialysis in the first week following transplant is associated with longer cold-ischaemia times, older-aged donors and technically difficult transplants.

C Anastomotic leak of the ureteral anastomosis often occurs several days following transplant and presents with pain (often severe) and a peri-transplant fluid collection.

D Rising serum creatinine following transplant can be attributed to supratherapeutic levels of immunosuppression.

E Ultrasound and biopsy are useful tools for diagnosing the cause of graft dysfunction following transplant.

**A6** **A** Graft thrombosis can occur following kidney transplant, even in technically straightforward cases. Indicators of graft dysfunction such as drop in urine output, rising serum creatinine, new development of haematuria and pain over the graft can be seen with thrombosis. Diagnosis is made by urgent ultrasound and operative attempt at graft salvage ensues urgently. Other causes of graft dysfunction can be donor related (long cold time, older-age donor), technical (difficult transplant operation with longer warm-ischaemia time) or patient related (postoperative hypotension, recurrent disease, dehydration). Elevated serum creatinine is seen with thrombosis, vascular narrowing, urinary obstruction, rejection and supratherapeutic levels of cyclosporine or tacrolimus. Ultrasound and biopsy are helpful at identifying the cause of graft dysfunction if drug levels are within the accepted range.

**Q7** Which of the following is not a benefit attributable to living kidney donation compared with deceased renal transplant?

A reduced transplant wait time

B less delayed graft function

C longer graft and patient survival

D less number of patients who receive transplants

E fewer postoperative complications

**A7** D Living donor transplant is superior to deceased donor kidney transplantation in most regards. The use of living donors shortens wait times and increases the number of patients receiving transplants. In addition, there are fewer postoperative complications such as delayed graft function and there is an increase in both graft and patient survival following transplant.

**Q8** Which of the following factors is not included in the allocation algorithm for deceased donor liver organs?

A age of recipient

B geographic proximity of donor to recipient institution

C laboratory indicators of severity of hepatic dysfunction including bilirubin, INR, and creatinine (Cr)

D donor and recipient human leukocyte antigen (HLA) matching

E liver dysfunction in patient in an ICU

**A8** E Organ allocation policy for livers follows a complex algorithm. Attempts are made to base decisions on severity of disease and proximity between donor hospital and recipient institution. In the United States patients are ranked on the bases of their MELD (model of end-stage liver disease) or PELD (paediatric end-stage liver disease) scores, which are calculated with a formula based on serum bilirubin, INR, and Cr. Serum albumin is also included in children under 12. Priority is given to patients in an ICU who have a significant risk of mortality from 7 days without transplant (Status I). Paediatric patients have priority for paediatric donors. HLA matching, as is done for kidney allocation, is not considered for liver allocation. Allocation in Europe is similar, but other factors such as serum sodium values are considered in disease severity scales.

**Q9** Which of the following statements regarding paediatric heart transplant is not true?

   **A** The most common indications for paediatric heart transplant are the presence of congenital defects and dilated cardiomyopathy.

   **B** Presence of renal disease requiring dialysis at the time of transplant is a contraindication for isolated heart transplant.

   **C** Fixed elevated pulmonary vascular resistance is a contraindication for heart transplant.

   **D** The most common techniques for implant of the donor heart are bicaval and biatrial, both including anastomoses of the aorta and pulmonary artery.

   **E** Paediatric heart transplant cannot be performed under cold circulatory arrest.

**A9** **E** Congenital defect is the most common indication for paediatric heart transplant in infants less than 1 year old. In older children the most common indication is dilated cardiomyopathy. Contraindications to heart transplant include irreversible pulmonary hypertension, severe renal or liver disease, active systemic infection, current malignancy, and severe central nervous system disease. Dialysis is a contraindication for isolated heart transplant unless simultaneous heart-kidney transplant is planned. Fixed pulmonary hypertension of 4–5 Wood units/m$^2$ is considered an absolute contraindication unless a simultaneous heart–lung transplant is performed. Bicaval or biatrial approaches are both used for the implantation of the heart. The bicaval technique has fewer short-term complications such as the reduced need for postoperative pacemaker insertion, but both techniques have similar long-term patient survival. Paediatric heart transplants are often performed with deep cold circulatory arrest.

**Q10** Which of the following approximate overall 5-year transplant patient survival rates is incorrect?

   **A** living-donor kidney, 90%

   **B** deceased-donor kidney, 80%

   **C** heart, 75%

   **D** liver, 73%

   **E** lung, 75%

**A10** **E** The overall (all ages) 5-year patient survival rates for each organ recipient category listed are correct, except for lung transplant where the actual 5-year patient survival is ~54%. Intestine (55%) and heart-lung transplants (49%) are similar.

**Q11** Which of the following are classic side effects of the indicated immunosuppression medications?

   **A** cyclosporine A: nephrotoxicity, hypertension, gingival hyperplasia

   **B** tacrolimus: nephrotoxicity, hypertension, diabetes mellitus

   **C** steroids: hypertension, hyperlipidaemia, hyperglycaemia, osteoporosis

   **D** mycophenolate mofetil: diarrhoea, leucopenia

   **E** all of the above

**A11** **E** Immunosuppressant medications are associated with a wide range of side effects. In addition to increased risk of cancer and infection, there are a number of nuisance side effects. The above pairings are all classic side effects of the listed medications.

**Q12** Which of the following medication is not associated with significant alteration of the blood levels of both cyclosporine A (CsA) and tacrolimus?

   **A** erythromycin

   **B** fluconazole

   **C** rifampin

   **D** verapamil

   **E** atorvastatin

**A12** **E** There are many interactions between immunosuppressive mediations and other pharmaceuticals. Classic medications that cause the increase in drug levels of cyclosporine and tacrolimus include azole antifungals (ketoconazole and fluconazole), calcium-channel blockers (verapamil), and antibiotics (erythromycin). Rifampin is an example of a medication that induces the cytochrome p450 system, increases metabolism of hepatically cleared mediations, and results in significant decreased blood levels of tacrolimus and CsA. Drug dosing must be monitored and adjusted for any of these drugs. Atorvastatins do not alter the blood levels of CsA and tacrolimus. However, there is an increase risk of myopathy, seen with combination therapy of CsA and atorvastatin, but not with tacrolimus.

**Q13** Which of the following is not an agent used for induction immunosuppression?

   **A** polyclonal anti-T-cell or anti-thymocyte antibody.

   **B** monoclonal anti-T-cell receptor antibody (OKT3)

   **C** monoclonal anti-IL2 receptor antibody

   **D** high-dose steroid

   **E** cyclosporine

**A13** **E** Many centres use an induction immunosuppression protocol. This often includes a short course of high-dose steroid and an antibody treatment. This is usually a polyclonal anti-lymphocyte preparation, OKT3, or monoclonal anti-IL2 receptor antibody. Cyclosporine is used for maintenance immunosuppression.

**Q14** Which of the following donor factors are *not* associated with worse outcomes following liver transplant?

**A** donor age >60 years

**B** donation after cardiac death

**C** partial-liver or split-liver transplant

**D** organ preservation time <8 hours

**E** hypernatraemia (Na >165) in donor at time of procurement

**A14** **D** Several donor factors have been identified as having increased risk following liver transplant. Such factors include donor age >60, split- or partial-liver transplants, donation after cardiac death, long organ preservation time, hypernatraemia, and high levels of intracellular macrovesicular fat deposits. These can be assembled into a 'Donor Risk Index' to rate the quality of donors.

**Q15** Which of the following organs has the greatest ability to recover from an episode of acute rejection?

**A** kidney

**B** liver

**C** pancreas

**D** heart

**E** lung

**A15** **B** The liver's ability to regenerate following injury and its lower incidence of acute rejection episodes make it more resilient and tolerant of rejection episodes. Because of this difference, immunosuppression levels are typically lower than for other organs.

## Further reading

*2009 Annual Report of the U.S. Organ Procurement and Transplantation Network and the Scientific Registry of Transplant Recipients: transplant data 1999–2008*. Rockville, MD: U.S. Department of Health and Human Services, Health Resources and Services Administration, Healthcare Systems Bureau, Division of Transplantation; 2009.

Canter CE, Shaddy RE, Bernstein D, *et al*. Indications for heart transplantation in pediatric heart disease: a scientific statement from the American Heart Association Council on Cardiovascular Disease in the Young; the Councils on clinical cardiology, cardiovascular nursing, and cardiovascular surgery and anesthesia; and the Quality of Care and Outcomes Research Interdisciplinary Working Group. *Circulation*. 2007; **115**(5): 658–76.

Feng S, Goodrich NP, Bragg-Gresham JL, *et al*. Characteristics associated with liver graft failure: the concept of a donor risk index. *Am J Transplant*. 2006; **6**(4): 783–90.

Gottschalk S, Rooney CM, Heslop HE. Post-transplant lymphoproliferative disorders. *Annu Rev Med*. 2005; **56**: 29–44.

Jacob S, Sellke F. Is bicaval orthotopic heart transplantation superior to the biatrial technique? *Interact Cardiovasc Thorac Surg*. 2009; **9**(2): 333–42.

Tjang YS, Stenlund H, Tenderich G, *et al*. Pediatric heart transplantation: current clinical review. *J Card Surg*. 2008; **23**(1): 87–91.

# CHAPTER 79

# Neonatology

## ELIZABETH PILLING

From the choices below each question, select the single best answer.

 **Q1** Infants born to mothers with diabetes have the following problems *except*:
- **A** hypoglycaemia
- **B** hyperglycaemia
- **C** hyperinsulinism
- **D** macrosomia
- **E** small for gestational age.

**A1** **B** Infants born to mothers with diabetes mellitus have a number of medical problems, principally related to their exposure to a hyperglycaemic environment before birth. Maternal hyperglycaemia leads to fetal hyperinsulinism, which acts as a growth factor producing fetal macrosomia. Hyperinsulinism also causes inactivation of the surfactant system increasing the incidence of respiratory distress syndrome. The fetal hyperinsulinism after birth leads to neonatal hypoglycaemia. Maternal microvascular disease can produce infants small for gestational age.

 **Q2** Which of the following is not a cause of early (first 24 hours) jaundice?
- **A** ABO incompatibility
- **B** hypothyroidism
- **C** rhesus disease
- **D** G6PD deficiency
- **E** spherocytosis

**A2** **B** Hypothyroidism is a cause for late and conjugated hyperbilirubinaemia. Early jaundice is caused by sepsis or haemolytic disease of the newborn until proved otherwise.

Q3 Regarding intraventricular haemorrhage (IVH), which of the following is true?

A Incidence of IVH in infants <750 g is 45%.

B The germinal matrix regresses in the first 2 months post term.

C Periventricular infarction is a common complication of a severe IVH.

D Porencephalic cyst is caused by extension of intraventricular haemorrhage.

E Maintaining normal coagulation is critical to preventing IVH.

 A3 **A** Germinal matrix haemorrhage-intraventricular haemorrhage is the commonest cause of neonatal intracranial haemorrhage. The majority of these lesions occur in pre-term infants, with 45% of infants born less than 750 g having a haemorrhage.

The area of initial haemorrhage is from the germinal matrix – a fragile capillary bed in the subependymal region. This matrix regresses over the last 16 weeks of gestation and is almost completely involuted by 36 weeks' gestation.

Following haemorrhage, the blood can enter the lateral ventricles and cause ventricular dilatation. This is due to the blood inciting an arachnoiditis, causing obstruction to cerebrospinal fluid drainage or by direct obstruction to flow by the clot.

Fifteen per cent of infants with IVH also demonstrate haemorrhagic necrosis in the periventricular white matter. This is not due to 'extension' of the haemorrhage (as is frequently thought), but haemorrhagic venous infarction due to obstruction in venous drainage following large intraventricular haemorrhage. This area of infarction may break down to form a porencephalic cyst.

 Q4 Which of the following is *not* a risk factor for respiratory distress syndrome?

A male sex

B African race

C being small for gestational age

D haemolytic disease of the newborn

E second twin

 A4 **B** Respiratory distress syndrome is caused by immaturity of the lungs, especially the surfactant synthetic systems. The principal risk factor is prematurity – 50% of infants less than 30 weeks have respiratory distress syndrome compared with 2% of those born at 35–36 weeks. Other predisposing factors are male sex (male-to-female 1.7 : 1), race – African infants have a reduced incidence, birth depression, maternal diabetes (because of insulin delaying maturation of the surfactant synthetic pathways), second twins, hypothermia and haemolytic disease of the newborn (probably due to hyperinsulinism as in maternal diabetes). Infants born small for gestational age have a reduced incidence compared with their appropriate-for-gestational-age contemporaries.

 **Q5** Evidence-based treatments for bronchopulmonary dysplasia (BPD) include which one of the following?

- **A** oral corticosteroids
- **B** inhaled corticosteroids
- **C** oxygen saturations about 95%
- **D** regular diuretic therapy
- **E** nebulised bronchodilators

**A5** **A** BPD is defined as oxygen requirement at 36 weeks' corrected gestation. Development of BPD is inversely related to gestational age. Risk factors include oxygen toxicity, barotrauma and volutrauma caused by ventilation. High fluid intake and the presence of patent ductus arteriosus also increase the incidence, possibly due to abnormal handling of fluid in infants who go on to develop BPD. Infection, including antenatal chorioamnionitis and postnatal cytomegalovirus also is associated with the development of BPD.

 **Q6** Which of the following is *not* a risk factor for the development of BPD?

- **A** hypercarbia
- **B** patent ductus arteriosus
- **C** high fluid intake
- **D** high tidal volume ventilation
- **E** antenatal steroid use

**A6** **E** Treatment of BPD begins with prevention of lung damage, minimising oxygen toxicity, barotrauma and volutrauma. Permissive hypercarbia, maintaining pH>7.25 should be used. Oral corticosteroids have been proven to facilitate extubation; however, this also increases the risk of cerebral palsy. Inhaled steroids demonstrated no statistically significant effects on BPD on a review of randomised controlled trials. Diuretic therapy is commonly used and has been shown to have very short-term effects on lung function; however, it has no long-term benefits.

Q7 With respect to this chest X-ray of a 4-hour-old 28-week-gestation infant, management should include:

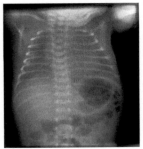

FIGURE 79.1 X-ray of the chest of a 4-hour-old neonate in respiratory distress

A diuretic therapy
B physiotherapy
C oral corticosteroids
D inhaled bronchodilators
E intravenous antibiotics.

A7 E The chest X-ray demonstrates classic respiratory distress syndrome with the 'ground glass' appearance of the lung fields. Appropriate management would include respiratory support as indicated by clinical signs, blood gases and oxygen saturation levels, surfactant therapy and antibiotics (CXR findings of infection and RDS are identical).

Q8 Which of the following is not a risk factor for developing hypoglycaemia after birth?
A maternal beta-blocker usage
B maternal hyperglycaemia
C low apgar score at birth
D birthweight 2.8 kg
E maternal metformin

A8 D Maternal beta blockers increase the risk of hypoglycaemia because of stimulation of insulin secretion. Maternal hyperglycaemia would suggest gestational diabetes and therefore is a risk of hypoglycaemia. Infants born with low apgars may have used their glucose stores and are at risk. Infants of 2.8 kg are appropriately grown, and therefore are not at increased risk.

**Q9** Which of the following conveys a survival advantage after pre-term birth?

   **A** Asian race vs. Caucasian race

   **B** male sex vs. female sex

   **C** second twin vs. first twin

   **D** multiple pregnancy vs. singleton pregnancy

   **E** normal delivery vs. caesarean section

**A9**  **C** Second twins have an increased mortality and morbidity.

**Q10** Which one of the following factors contributes to early onset sepsis?

   **A** antenatal corticosteroids

   **B** multiple intravenous access

   **C** skin abrasions

   **D** prolonged rupture of membranes

   **E** coagulase-negative staphylococcus

**A10**  **D** Early onset sepsis – within the first 48 hours. This is infection acquired before or during birth. The common causative organisms are group B streptococcus, *Escherichia coli*, *Haemophilus influenzae* and *Listeria monocytogenes*.

# CHAPTER 80

# Paediatric orthopaedic disorders

## GLEESON REBELLO

**From the choices below each question, select the single best answer.**

**Q1** Regarding osteomyelitis in children which of the following statements is untrue?

    **A** Acute haematogenous osteomyelitis (AHO) is the most commonly occurring form of osteomyelitis in children.

    **B** It is caused by deposition of blood-borne organisms in the metaphysis of the bone.

    **C** In the absence of purulence in the metaphysis in the early phases of the disease, antibiotic treatment alone may control infection.

    **D** Once purulence develops it remains within the confines of the metaphysis and does not extend into the subperiosteal space.

    **E** Septic arthritis can be caused by osteomyelitis in regions where the metaphysis is intra-articular.

**A1**   **D** Purulence forms in the proximal metaphysis in untreated situations. It then extends laterally through the porous metaphyseal cortex into the subperiosteal space, elevating the periosteum. As a result, the bone looses its intramedullary as well as its periosteal blood supply leading to bone necrosis and sequestrum (dead bone) formation. New bone laid down by the osteogenic layer of the periosteum is called involucrum. Antibiotic accessibility is poor in this region hence chronic osteomyelitis may result which leads to chronic sinus formation and expulsion of dead, infected bone. If left untreated the pus can also track down the entire length of bone leading to its ischaemia.

    AHO is the most commonly occurring form of osteomyelitis in children and affects 1 in 5000 children younger than 13 years of age. Males are 2.5 times more commonly affected than females. It is caused by deposition of blood-borne organisms in the metaphysis of the bone where the capillary system has a relatively slow flow and few available reticuloendothelial cells for phagocytosis.

**Q2**   Regarding presentation of AHO, which of the following is true?

  **A**  Neonates with AHO may have poor feeding and display irritability or present with florid sepsis.

  **B**  Lower extremity involvement may lead to limping or refusal to walk.

  **C**  Between 30% and 50% of patients will have had a recent non-orthopaedic bacterial infection.

  **D**  The differential diagnosis of AHO includes fracture, toxic synovitis, cellulitis, arthritis, thrombophlebitis and malignancies that include Ewing's sarcoma and leukaemia.

  **E**  All of the above.

**A2**   **E**  AHO covers a broad spectrum in terms of presenting signs and symptoms. Presentation modes range from malaise and low-grade fevers to florid sepsis. Neonates may display poor feeding and irritability. In ambulating children there will be a refusal to crawl or walk. There might be loss of spontaneous movement in the affected upper extremity which is referred to as pseudoparalysis. There might be a recent history of bacterial or viral infections. The differential diagnosis of AHO can include Gaucher's disease, sickle-cell crisis and the others stated in option D. Malignancies that can present like osteomyelitis include Ewing's sarcoma and leukaemia. Bone pain is the chief complaint in 18% of patients presenting with acute lymphocytic leukaemia.

**Q3**   Regarding diagnosis of AHO, which of the following statements is false?

  **A**  Erythrocyte sedimentation rate (ESR) is a non-specific marker of inflammation and is elevated in 90% of patients with AHO.

  **B**  C-reactive protein (CRP) levels increase markedly within the first 24–48 hours of the onset of infection and decline within 6–8 hours of the initiation of antibiotic therapy.

  **C**  Blood culture results are positive in all patients with AHO.

  **D**  Cultures taken from bone are positive in 50% of patients and guide the antimicrobial therapy.

  **E**  Plain radiographs on presentation may appear normal but show changes 7–14 days after onset of infection.

**A3**   **C**  Blood cultures are positive in only 30% of patients with AHO. ESR is a non-specific marker of inflammation and takes 1–2 weeks to decline once antibiotic therapy is initiated, unlike the CRP which begins to trend downwards within a few hours of appropriate antibiotic therapy. Plain radiographs can detect obvious changes like periosteal elevation 7–14 days after onset of infection. Bone scanning may be useful for localising early infection in the presence of an inconclusive physical examination. It will also help in ruling out multifocal osteomyelitis. MRI is useful in detecting osteomyelitis as early as 3–5 days after disease onset and can also help localise an abscess that will merit surgical drainage. Ultrasound may be useful in differentiating a septic hip from osteomyelitis of the proximal femur.

 **Q4** Regarding the management of AHO, which of the following statements is untrue?

  **A** After localising a bone infection a bone aspiration should be performed and aspiration of pus indicates need for surgical drainage.

  **B** *Haemophilus influenzae* is the most common pathogen in AHO.

  **C** Parenteral antibiotics are necessary to prevent spread of disease and optimise bactericidal levels in the affected bone.

  **D** Intravenous antibiotics until normalisation of CRP levels, and ongoing oral treatment until normalisation of ESR, will result in a low rate of recurrence.

  **E** Chronic osteomyelitis, pathological fractures and growth disturbance with subsequent angular deformities/limb length discrepancy, are complications AHO.

 **A4** **B** *Staphylococcus aureus* is the most common pathogen in AHO, representing 60%–90% of all instances. Group B beta haemolytic streptococcus is commonly associated with neonatal osteomyelitis. In children with underlying diseases like sickle-cell anaemia, more atypical organism like salmonella may be considered. The preferred antibiotics for empiric staphylococcus coverage are oxacillin and cefazolin. Vancomycin and clindamycin are often used for treatment of methicillin-resistant *S. aureus* infections. A positive response to parenteral antibiotic treatment includes a return to normal temperature, local improvement and a decline in the CRP. Chronic osteomyelitis, pathological fractures and growth disturbance with subsequent angular deformities/limb length discrepancy are complications of AHO. Chronic osteomyelitis is characterised by sequestrum formation and usually occurs if AHO is unrecognised or left untreated. The risk of pathological fractures occurs as a result of deossification, and a protective cast may be necessary to prevent such an occurrence. Growth plates that lie adjacent to the metaphysis may be damaged by initial infection or surgical procedure leading to angular deformity or shortening of limb.

**Q5** Regarding septic arthritis in a child, which of the following statements is untrue?

  **A** The best treatment for a proven case of septic arthritis is close observation with regular follow-up.

  **B** Septic arthritis most commonly involves the large joints (hip 35%, knee 35%, ankle 10%).

  **C** Fever, limp, refusal to bear weight, limited and painful range of motion, erythema, warmth, tenderness and swelling are common physical findings in septic arthritis.

  **D** The most commonly identified infecting organisms are *S. aureus* (56%), Gr A streptococci (22%), *Streptococcus pneumoniae* (6%).

  **E** Ultrasonography (USG)-guided joint fluid aspiration (especially in the hip) is necessary to confirm diagnosis of sepsis when clinical, laboratory and imaging findings suggest septic arthritis.

**A5** **A** Proven septic arthritis in a child constitutes a surgical emergency. Prompt diagnosis and treatment which includes arthrotomy and surgical drainage are essential. The release of proteolytic enzymes by polymorphonuclear cells and bacteria in addition to increased intrarticular pressure can result in rapid and irreversible hyaline cartilage damage in few hours as demonstrated on animal models. If unrecognised or left untreated this can result in joint destruction with subsequent deformity and lifelong disability. If treated in a timely fashion with surgery and appropriate antimicrobial therapy, a good outcome with minimal sequelae can be expected. Fever, limp, refusal to bear weight, limited and painful range of motion, erythema, warmth, tenderness and swelling are common physical findings in septic arthritis. Four clinical predictors have been used to help differentiate septic arthritis of the hip from transient synovitis. History of fever greater than 38.5°C, inability to bear weight, ESR greater than 40 mm/hr and white blood cell count greater than 12 × 10⁹/L. In one study the presence of three out of four factors was 93.1% predictive of septic arthritis and presence of all four factors was 99.6% predictive. The most commonly identified infecting organisms are *S. aureus* (56%), Gr A streptococci (22%) and *S. pneumoniae* (6%). In the neonate, group B beta haemolytic strep are common infecting agents. USG-guided joint fluid aspiration (especially in the hip) is necessary to confirm diagnosis of sepsis when clinical, laboratory and imaging findings suggest septic arthritis. A white blood cell count of greater than 50 × 10⁹/L or a positive Gram stain suggests the presence of septic arthritis. Aspirate cultures are positive in 50%–70% of patients with septic arthritis and Gram stain may be positive in 30%–50% of patients.

**Q6** Regarding paediatric orthopaedic disorders in general, which of the following statements is untrue?

**A** A congenital disorder differs from a developmental disorder.

**B** A congenital disorder is the same as a genetic disorder.

**C** Malformations are structural disorders that result from an interruption of normal organogenesis during the second month of gestation.

**D** Deformations differ from dysplasias.

**E** Disruptions are structural disorders that result from extrinsic interference with normal growth and development.

**A6** **B** A congenital disorder is one that is present at birth. A genetic disorder is one that results from alteration of DNA sequence of the individual's genome. Theoretically, all genetic disorders are congenital. In conditions like Duchenne's muscular dystrophy, which is a genetic disorder, the children are phenotypically normal till 4 years of age and hence appear normal at birth. If the phenotype is evident at birth such as clubfeet, it is referred to as congenital talipes equinovarus. A congenital disorder differs from a developmental disorder. A congenital condition like clubfeet exists at birth and is acquired during the embryonic or fetal part of intrauterine gestation. A developmental disorder refers to disorder that appears after birth such as Scheuermann's kyphosis is a developmental disorder of the spine. Deformations are structural disorders resulting from either mechanical pressure or muscular activity. Examples of deformations include calcaneovalgus of an infant's foot, posteromedial bowing of the tibia, metatarsus adductus. Dysplasias are structural disorders caused by genetic or cellular abnormalities and include conditions like achondroplasia and spondyloepiphyseal dysplasia. Deformations are easier to treat by eliminating the deforming force or countering with a corrective force like casting or bracing. Dysplasias are not amenable to correction by simple mechanical measures and may need complex medical and surgical management. Disruptions are structural disorders like a congenital constriction band that result from extrinsic interference with normal growth and development.

**7** In developmental dysplasia of the hip (DDH), which of the following statements is untrue?

   **A** Treatment of dislocated hips in neonates with a positive Ortolani's test should be initiated immediately and not delayed.

   **B** From the neonatal period till 6 months of age radiographs are the best imaging modality to detect hip dysplasia.

   **C** Treating with a Pavlik harness is effective in achieving reduction of a reducible dislocation in more than 85% of patients.

   **D** Closed reduction and spica casting of the hip is the preferred method of treatment in children up to 18 months of age provided reduction is stable and can be achieved without undue force.

   **E** Open reduction is performed in all hips where closed reduction cannot be achieved and at times needs a concomitant femoral shortening procedure ± acetabular osteotomy especially in children older than 2 years of age.

 **7**  **B**  In the first 4–6 months of life, pelvic radiographs are of little benefit in the evaluation of an infant with DDH because of the cartilaginous structure of the acetabulum and femoral head. Ossification of the femoral epiphysis that begins at roughly 4–6 months permits better radiographic evaluation using a combination of various lines and angles that are well described in standard orthopaedic texts. Hip USG is used to evaluate the hip in children prior to appearance of the femoral epiphysis. USG interpretation usually combines anatomical evaluation of acetabular socket development and assessment of instability by measuring the displacement of the femoral head from the acetabulum while simultaneously performing stress manoeuvres.

Treatment of dislocated hips in neonates with a positive Ortolani's test should be initiated immediately and not delayed. Treatment with a Pavlik harness is effective in achieving reduction of a reducible dislocation in more than 85% of cases. After successful treatment with a Pavlik harness, less than 5% of hips will show evidence of persistent severe late dysplasia. An Ortolani-negative dislocation (inability to reduce the hip) may be briefly treated with a Pavlik harness but the harness must be abandoned if reduction is not achieved and confirmed by USG in 2–3 weeks. Hips that are unremarkable on clinical examination but reveal sonographic dysplasia without sonographic instability, do not warrant abduction splinting because they will improve within the first 3 months of life in up to 97% of infants.

Closed reduction is the preferred method of treatment in children younger than 18 months provided it can be achieved without undue force but can lead to prolonged treatment and secondary femoral or acetabular procedures to address residual deformity. In children older than 2 years of age a femoral shortening osteotomy is warranted during open reduction to diminish the pressure on the reduced femoral head and lessen the chance for avascular necrosis of the femoral head.

**8** Regarding idiopathic clubfeet (congenital talipes equinovarus), which of the following statements is untrue?

    **A** Clubfoot is the most common birth defect with an incidence ranging from 1 : 250 to 1 : 1000 live births depending on the population.

    **B** Prenatal diagnosis of this condition using ultrasound is highly effective with a true positive predictive rate of 83%.

    **C** Clubfoot may be also present in neurological conditions like spina bifida

    **D** The treatment for idiopathic clubfoot is primarily surgical.

    **E** Surgical correction of idiopathic clubfoot is usually performed in older children with residual deformity or relapse following manipulative treatment.

**8**   **D** The treatment for idiopathic clubfeet is primarily conservative and was first described by Ponsetti. It involves gentle manipulations beginning in the neonatal period followed by serial cast applications to hold the correction. The cast is an above-knee cast with the knee in 90 degrees of flexion, and through serial manipulation the foot is gradually externally rotated. Depending on severity of clubfeet the period of treatment goes on for 4–8 weeks with weekly cast changes. An Achilles tenotomy is performed in 90% of cases after this period of casting in order to correct the hindfoot equinus. After correction is achieved the child is placed in a foot abduction orthosis full time for the first 3 months and night-time and nap time for 2–4 years. Early relapse may be treated with repeat casting but approximately 10%–20% of patients need anterior tibialis tendon transfer at 2–4 years of age for recurrent deformity. Clubfoot may also be present in children with neurological disorders and arthrogryposis multiplex congenital. The treatment of clubfeet when associated with these conditions is much more complex with a greater chance for recurrence and multiple surgeries.

**Q**9 As regards other congenital paediatric foot conditions, which of the following statements is false?

    **A** Calcaneovalgus deformity that is characterised by dorsiflexion of the entire foot at the ankle joint is caused by intrauterine positioning and usually resolves over time.

    **B** Metatarsus adductus is a congenital foot deformity in which there is medial deviation of the forefoot with a normal hindfoot.

    **C** Congenital vertical talus is a rigid rocker-bottom flatfoot deformity in which the talus is vertically orientated with fixed dorsal displacement of the navicular.

    **D** Polydactyly is a common congenital toe deformity that most commonly manifests as duplication of the fifth toe and is treated surgically.

    **E** Tarsal coalition is a condition that leads to union between various tarsal bones and is easily diagnosed at birth.

**A**9   **E** The two most common types of tarsal coalition are calcaneonavicular coalition and talocalcaneal coalition. Calcaneonavicular coalition becomes symptomatic between 8 and 12 years of age and talocalcaneal coalitions between 12 and 14 years of age. Coalitions usually present as a rigid flatfoot with a history of repeated episodes of pain in the ankle and foot. The first line of approach is usually conservative with immobilisation of the foot in a cast for 4–6 weeks and surgery is reserved for cases with persistent pain that fail conservative treatment. The results of surgical treatment are better with calcaneonavicular coalitions than with talocalcaneal coalitions.

    Calcaneovalgus deformities in the neonate are caused by intrauterine positioning and usually improve over time. The hindfoot in metatarsus adductus is usually normal looking with good range of motion which differentiates it from the clubfoot which has hindfoot varus and equinus. Most cases of metatarsus adductus resolve over time before 4 years of age. Surgery is only indicated in more severe rigid deformities that persist and interfere with shoewear. Correction is usually achieved with soft tissue release and multiple tarsal/metatarsal osteotomies. Congenital vertical talus is a rare condition in which the foot is shaped like a Persian slipper. There is a fixed dorsal dislocation of the navicular on a vertically orientated talus with tight heel cords and a calcaneus in equinus. Treatment for this condition is always surgical. Polydactyly is a common congenital toe deformity that most commonly manifests as duplication of the fifth toe and is treated surgically. Duplication of the fifth toe is called post-axial polydactyly. Pre-axial polydactyly is rarer and involves duplication of the great toe. Surgery is usually performed at 1 year of age to improve cosmesis and shoe fitting. In some instances there is duplication of the metatarsal which then needs to be removed with the extra digit.

Q10 Regarding scoliosis, which of the following statements is untrue?

   A  Idiopathic scoliosis is the most common spinal deformity that develops in otherwise healthy children and most often affects females.

   B  The typical curve pattern in adolescent idiopathic scoliosis (AIS) is left thoracic and right lumbar.

   C  Patients with AIS usually do not have neurologic complaints.

   D  In patients with AIS, curve progression is related to growth remaining and curve magnitude.

   E  Curves greater than 45–50 degrees are usually treated with surgical instrumentation and fusion.

A10  B  The typical curve pattern in AIS is right thoracic and left lumbar. Left thoracic curve patterns are distinctly unusual and occasionally associated with underlying syndromes or syringomyelia. A left thoracic curve is an indication for an MRI which is otherwise not routinely indicated in AIS.

Idiopathic scoliosis is the most common spinal deformity that develops in otherwise healthy children. Infantile scoliosis occurs between birth and 3 years, juvenile scoliosis between 3 and 10 years and AIS occurs after 10 years of age. AIS is defined as a curve greater than 10 degrees and its diagnosis is made after excluding all other causes which could include congenital scoliosis, neuromuscular scoliosis and scoliosis associated with conditions like neurofibromatosis and Marfan's syndrome. Typical standing radiographs are obtained in the PA projection on large cassettes to asses the Cobb angles and the radiograph is repeated every 6 months in growing children to assess curve progression. Patients with AIS usually do not have neurologic findings; if present, other diagnoses must be considered. Curve progression is related to growth remaining and curve magnitude at the time of initial diagnosis. Therefore, assessment of physical maturity is critical for planning treatment either by bracing or surgery. In girls, growth remaining and maturity are assessed by considering the age of menarche, Tanner stage, Risser sign (degree of ossification of iliac apophysis) and the presence of an open tri-radiate cartilage. Bracing is commonly prescribed for growing adolescents if the curve is 25–40 degrees at presentation. Bracing is discontinued at cessation of growth and onset of skeletal maturity or when the curve reaches dimensions that warrant surgery (45–50 degrees). Surgical treatment usually consists of instrumentation and fusion of the spine, either by anterior or posterior approaches, to attain correction and arrest progression.

Q11 Regarding paediatric spine conditions, which of the following statements is false?

A Spondylolysis is a stress fracture of the pars interarticularis (part of vertebra located between the inferior and superior articular processes of the facet joint) caused by repetitive hyperextension.

B Spondylolisthesis is the forward slippage of one vertebra on another and most commonly occurs at L5–S1 in the paediatric population.

C Significant progression of spondylolisthesis is common in adulthood.

D Symptomatic patients with spondylolysis usually do well with non-surgical measures that include activity restriction, physical therapy and bracing.

E Scheuermann's kyphosis is a self-limiting condition characterised by wedge-shaped deformation of the thoracic vertebrae accompanied by increased kyphosis.

A11 C Significant progression of spondylolisthesis is uncommon in adulthood and is usually associated with adolescent growth spurt, lumbosacral kyphosis, magnitude of initial slippage on presentation, younger age with immature skeleton, female gender and certain local anatomical predispositions like a dome-shaped sacrum and dysplastic lumbosacral junction. Patients with spondylolysis and spondylolisthesis most often present with mechanical back pain that is activity related. Plain radiographs are helpful to identify the lesions and bone scanning is often positive in patients with new lesions. SPECT (single-photon emission CT) is highly sensitive for demonstrating a pars defect.

Most of the patients are managed conservatively with a combination of bracing, activity restriction and physical therapy. Indications for surgery include uncontrolled pain, slippage greater than 50% on initial presentation or progressive slippage from 25% to 50% and the presence of neurological symptoms.

Scheuermann's kyphosis is a self-limiting condition characterised by wedge-shaped deformation of the thoracic vertebrae accompanied by increased kyphosis. Bracing helps assist its progress though it does not produce correction. Indications for surgery are individualised and based on the amount of deformity, existence of accompanying pain and presence of spinal cord compression with neurological deficit which is extremely rare in this condition.

Q12 Regarding limb length discrepancy and deformity in the lower limb, which of the following statements is false?

A Proximal focal femoral deficiency (PFFD) is a congenital shortening and abnormal development of the femur in which the hip joint may or may not be present.

B Congenital pseudarthrosis of the tibia is a condition whose aetiology is unknown, which manifests as anterolateral bowing of the tibia with or without bony continuity and is extremely difficult to treat.

C Legg–Calvé–Perthes's disease is a disease of unknown aetiology that results in osteonecrosis of the immature femoral capital epiphysis and occurs in children between the ages of 4–9 years.

D Slipped capital femoral epiphysis (SCFE) is displacement between the proximal femoral epiphysis and femoral neck and is usually seen in children less than 5 years of age.

E Blount's disease is caused by growth retardation of the medial and posterior part of the proximal tibial physis and epiphysis leading to progressive genu varum and internal tibial torsion in children.

A12 D SCFE usually occurs in the adolescent age group. The peak age for boys is 13 years and for girls is 11 years with a range from middle childhood to maturity. It occurs most commonly in obese individuals. Endocrine disorders such as hypothyroidism, hypopituitarism and hypogonadism, metabolic disorders such as rickets, and treatment with chemotherapy and radiation may contribute. It is clinically classified into two types of slips. Patients who can bear weight and walk with discomfort are known to have stable slips and unstable slip occurs in patients who cannot bear weight on the affected limb even with crutches. A chronic stable slip can suddenly turn into an unstable slip. Unstable slips have a much higher incidence of complications that include osteonecrosis of the femoral head and chondrolysis.

The absence of a hip joint in PFFD severely limits reconstruction. The main problems associated with this condition are instability because of absence of joint or poor joint formation and limb length discrepancy, which can be profound in certain instances.

Congenital pseudarthrosis of the tibia is a condition of unknown aetiology which manifests as anterolateral bowing of the tibia with or without bony continuity and is extremely hard to treat. Current surgical techniques utilised include intramedullary fixation and bone grafting, vascularised fibular grafts and resection coupled with bone transport.

Legg–Calvé–Perthes's disease is a disease of unknown aetiology that results in osteonecrosis of the immature femoral capital epiphysis and occurs in children between the ages of 4 and 9 years. Though it is self-limiting, it can result in loss of sphericity of the femoral head causing incongruency of the joint and leading to early osteoarthrosis in adulthood. Treatment depends largely on age at presentation and degree and site of involvement of the capital epiphysis. It ranges from observation to containment of the femoral head either by prolonged casting of lower extremities in abduction or proximal femoral/acetabular osteotomies.

Blount's disease is caused by growth retardation of the medial and posterior part of the proximal tibial physis and epiphysis leading to progressive genu varum and internal tibial torsion in children. Infantile Blount's develops shortly after ambulation and needs to be differentiated from physiological genu varum. It can be treated with bracing in the very young (<3 years) and corrective osteotomies in older children with more advanced disease. Adolescent Blount's disease which occurs in older, usually obese, children needs surgical treatment either with hemiepiphysiodesis or corrective osteotomies.

**Q13** Regarding malignant bone tumours, which of the following statements is false?

  **A** The most common symptom for bone tumours is pain.

  **B** Incisional biopsies in bone tumours are generally straightforward procedures that do not require too much planning or meticulous execution.

  **C** In imaging bone tumours MRI is the imaging modality of choice to determine soft tissue extent, bone marrow, neurovascular structure and response to chemotherapy, while CT is useful to evaluate the extent of osseous destruction.

  **D** Osteosarcoma is the most common primary malignant bone tumour in children and histologically has a malignant spindle cell stroma that produces osteoid.

  **E** Ewing's sarcoma is a malignant neoplasm of primitive mesenchymal cell origin and belongs to the family of small round blue cell tumours.

**A13** **B** Incisional biopsies should be performed by the orthopaedic oncologist that will perform the definitive surgery on the bone tumour. A biopsy is fraught with potential complications that can significantly impact the patient's prognosis and treatment. The incision for biopsy should be along the line of potential incision for definitive resection of tumour. Tourniquet should be inflated without exsanguination using Esmarch's bandage. The incision should avoid multiple compartments and internervous planes. Meticulous haemostasis should be performed at the end of the procedure.

Pain in a teenager for longer than 6 weeks following an injury should be carefully evaluated and followed up with more sophisticated imaging if necessary.

Pain at rest is a generally more ominous symptom and may indicate significant bone destruction.

The peak diagnosis of osteosarcoma occurs at 15 years of age. The most common locations are the distal femur, proximal tibia and proximal humerus.

Ewing's sarcoma is the second most common malignant tumour of bone in children and is more common in Caucasian children with a peak incidence in the second decade of life.

**Q14** Regarding benign bone tumours, which of the following is false?

**A** The clinical features of osteoid osteoma include constant pain that is more conspicuous in the night and is relieved by NSAIDs.

**B** Osteochondromas are benign intramedullary cartilage tumours that appear as lytic lesions within the bone.

**C** Non-ossifying fibroma is a benign fibrous lesion that occurs in the metaphysis, is eccentrically located and usually cortically based.

**D** A unicameral bone cyst is an intraosseous fluid-filled lesion that is centrally located in the metaphysis of the bone and usually occurs in the proximal humerus and proximal femur.

**E** Aneurysmal bone cyst is a benign but aggressive tumour that causes expansile, eccentrically located lesions in bone with mixed blood-filled cavities and fibroconnective tissue.

**A14** **B** Osteochondromas are benign bony protuberances with cartilage caps that grow on the surface of bone and are relatively common. Locations include the distal femur, proximal tibia and proximal humerus. Growth usually stops with skeletal maturity. If the lesion continues to grow in adulthood (which is extremely rare) a malignant transformation into a chondrosarcoma should be ruled out.

Osteoid osteoma is a benign but painful tumour that produces fibrovascular tissue and immature osteoid. It can be treated with NSAIDs, surgical resection or radiofrequency ablation. NSAID therapy must be continued until the lesion regresses or burns out with respect to its effect on hepatic and renal function. Surgical resection is effective but intraoperative localisation of lesion can be troublesome. CT-guided radiofrequency ablation that is performed percutaneously is rapidly becoming the treatment of choice for osteoid osteoma.

Non-ossifying fibroma is a benign lesion that is most often an incidental finding on radiographs. Small lesions are usually followed up with serial radiographs. Lesions that cause pain, pathological fracture or are of significant size may be considered for surgical treatment.

A unicameral bone cyst is an intraosseous fluid-filled lesion that is centrally located. Treatments of the cysts include aspiration of the cyst fluid followed by injection with either steroid, bone marrow or bone substitutes as no single technique demonstrates complete efficacy.

Aneurysmal bone cyst (ABC) is a benign but aggressive tumour that causes expansile, eccentrically located lesions in bone with mixed blood-filled cavities and fibroconnective tissue. MRI is useful in demonstrating the presence of a double-density fluid level and multiple septations within the lesion. Treatment of an ABC consists of open curettage and bone grafting using allograft or bone substitutes. Adjuvant liquid nitrogen or phenol is commonly used. Recurrence rates average 20% and can be higher.

## Further reading

Kim HJ, Blanco JS, Widmann RF. Update on the management of idiopathic scoliosis. *Curr Opin Pediatr*. 2009; **21**(1): 55–64.

Loder T, Torode I, Joseph B, *et al. Paediatric Orthopaedics: a system of decision making.* 1st ed. London: Hodder Arnold; 2009.

Weinstein SL, Mubarak SJ, Wenger DR. Developmental hip dysplasia and dislocation. *Instr Course Lect*. 2004; **53**: 523–42.

# CHAPTER 81

# Paediatric neurosurgical disorders

## DESIDERIO RODRIGUES

From the choices below each question, select the single best answer.

**Q1** Which of the following signs is not commonly encountered in infants with hydrocephalus?
   A accelerated head circumference
   B bulging fontanelle
   C tonic–clonic seizures
   D sunset sign
   E dilated scalp veins

**A1** **C** Infants with hydrocephalus will have increasing head circumference with bulging fontanelle and widely separated sutures. They may be drowsy or irritable. The scalp veins may be dilated and they can have a downward gaze known as 'sunset sign'. Infants with hydrocephalus rarely present with tonic–clonic seizures but occasionally may have an episode where they are stiff or even opisthotonic – a 'hydrocephalic fit'.

**Q2** All the following could be the causes of hydrocephalus in children *except*:
   A intraventricular haemorrhage
   B third ventriculostomy
   C colloid cyst of the third ventricle
   D posterior fossa tumours
   E myelomeningocele.

**A2** **B** All except third ventriculostomy are causes of hydrocephalus. Third ventriculostomy is used as a mode of treating hydrocephalus.

**Q3** All of the following procedures have been used to treat hydrocephalus *except*:

    **A** ventriculoatrial shunt

    **B** ventriculoperitoneal shunt

    **C** ventriculopleural shunt

    **D** ventriculocolonic shunt

    **E** lumboperitoneal shunt.

**A3**   **D** All the mentioned procedures can be used to treat hydrocephalus except ventriculocolonic shunt because of the risk of infection.

**Q4** Which of the following is the commonest single-suture synostosis?

    **A** metopic synostosis

    **B** bicoronal synostosis

    **C** lambdoid synostosis

    **D** sagittal synostosis

    **E** unicoronal synostosis

**A4**   **D** The incidence of craniosynostosis is approximately 0.6/1000 live births. Sagittal synostosis accounts for 40%–60% of all cases. The coronal suture is involved in 20%–30% patients; unilateral coronal synostosis is twice as common as bilateral involvement. Metopic synostosis accounts for <10% followed by lambdoid suture synostosis, which is the least common type.

**Q5** Which of the following is *not* a known cause of craniosynostosis?

    **A** familial

    **B** rickets

    **C** valproic acid

    **D** thalassaemia

    **E** head trauma

**A5**   **E** All except head trauma are known causes of craniosynostosis.

**Q6** Which of the following statements about myelomeningocele is *not* true?

    **A** Myelomeningocele is a result of defective caudal neurulation.

    **B** Open myelomeningocele is associated with Chiari malformation.

    **C** Patients often have hydrocephalus that needs treatment.

    **D** Open myelomeningocele should be treated electively when the baby is 3 months or older.

    **E** Patients may have congenital dislocation of hip.

**A6** **D** Myelomeningocele is a result of failure of caudal neurulation. Failure of cranial neurulation leads to anencephaly. Myelomeningocele patients usually have hydrocephalus, which may need to be treated at the same time as the repair of the myelomeningocele. These patients commonly also have Chiari II malformation. The other anomalies which can be present are congenital talipes deformity and congenital dislocation of the hip, in addition to neuropathic sphincters. All cases with an open myelomeningocele should be treated urgently to prevent central nervous system infection and prevent further damage to the placode that is exposed.

**Q7** Regarding tethered cord, which of the following statements is not true?
  **A** Fat may be seen in the filum terminale on MRI scan.
  **B** The child can present with back or leg pain.
  **C** The child can present with bowel or bladder function decline.
  **D** Deterioration in gait is an extremely rare presentation.
  **E** The conus is usually below the L1/L2 level.

**A7** **D** Signs and symptoms of spinal cord tethering can be divided into six broad categories: (1) pain either in the back or legs; (2) motor deterioration, manifested as a decrease in muscle strength and/or an increase in tone; (3) sensory decline; (4) a decline in bowel or bladder function; (5) a deterioration in gait; and (6) progressive orthopaedic deformities of the lower extremities or spine (scoliosis). The MRI findings are usually thickened filum terminale with or without fat within it. A low-lying conus below L1/L2 level with the other symptoms and signs is very often seen on MRI scan of the spine.

**Q8** Which of these statements regarding Currarino's syndrome is incorrect?
  **A** It is an inherited autosomal recessive disorder.
  **B** There is malformation of the sacrum.
  **C** A mass is present in the presacral space.
  **D** Anal and rectal malformations are present.
  **E** There can also be an anterior meningocele.

**A8** **A** Currarino's syndrome (also Currarino's triad) is an inherited autosomal dominant congenital disorder where (1) the sacrum is not formed properly, (2) there is a mass in the presacral space in front of the sacrum and (3) there are malformations of the anus or rectum. It can also cause an anterior meningocele or a presacral teratoma.

$Q^9$ The characteristic feature of Chiari malformation is:
  A hypoplasia of the vermis
  B retrocerebellar cyst
  C cerebellar tonsillar descent of more than 5 mm
  D hypoplasia of the odontoid peg
  E absence of the posterior arc of the atlas.

$A^9$ **C** Chiari malformation is a malformation of the brain. It consists of a downward displacement of the cerebellar tonsils through the foramen magnum. To be called a Chiari malformation the tonsils have to be at least 5 mm below the foramen magnum. Sometimes there can be an obstruction to cerebrospinal fluid outflow causing hydrocephalus.

$Q^{10}$ Which of the following is *not* part of the management of a child with Chiari malformation?
  A analgesics
  B observation
  C foramen magnum decompression
  D ventriculoperitoneal shunt
  E lumboperitoneal shunt

$A^{10}$ **E** Children with Chiari malformation who are asymptomatic can be kept under observation. Those with mild headaches that are not strain induced can be managed with simple analgesics. If the malformation is secondary to tumour or hydrocephalus it is important to treat the primary problem first. Foramen magnum decompression is the most frequently performed procedure. In presence of a Chairi malformation lumboperitoneal shunt is contraindicated, as it can aggravate the tonsillar descent.

## Further reading

Albright AL, Pollack IF, Adelson PD. *Operative Techniques in Pediatric Neurosurgery.* Stuttgart: Thieme; 2000.

Albright AL, Pollack IF, Adelson PD. *Principles and Practice of Pediatric Neurosurgery.* 2nd ed. Stuttgart: Thieme; 2007.

Greenberg MS. *Handbook of Neurosurgery.* 6th ed. Stuttgart: Thieme; 2005.

# CHAPTER 82

# Fetal surgery

## ASHWIN PIMPALWAR

From the choices below each question, select the single best answer.

**Q1** Alfa-fetoprotein (AFP) in the amniotic fluid may be elevated in:
   **A** neural tube defects
   **B** gastroschisis
   **C** omphalocele
   **D** sacrococcygeal teratoma (SCT)
   **E** all the above.

**A1** **E** AFP is a plasma protein produced by the fetal yolk sac and liver. Its level in the newborn gradually decreases after birth. AFP in the fetus reaches a peak level of 3 mg/mL at 13–15 menstrual weeks. AFP concentrations in the fetal serum and the amniotic fluid follow the same curve but at 150-fold dilution. Conditions in the fetus that increase the transudation of fetal serum into the amniotic fluid result in an increased level of AFP in the amniotic fluid. Elevated AFP in maternal serum and the amniotic fluid is therefore a reliable indicator of fetal abnormality. All the conditions mentioned above increase the transudation of the serum in the amniotic fluid and hence have an increased level of AFP in amniotic fluid.

**Q2** Which of the following statements is not true?
   **A** Chorionic venous sampling allows diagnosis of chromosomal abnormalities in the first trimester.
   **B** Amniocentesis allows diagnosis of chromosomal abnormalities in the second trimester.
   **C** Fetal blood can be obtained by percutaneous ultrasonography (US) guidance as early as 14 weeks' gestation.
   **D** Culture of fetal blood cells allows more rapid karyotyping then amniocentesis.
   **E** Fetal loss from sampling techniques is about 10%.

**A2** **E** Fetal loss from sampling techniques is 1%–5%. Cell samples can be obtained for karyotyping and DNA analysis for diagnosis of genetic and inherited metabolic disorders. Chorionic venous sampling allows diagnosis in the first trimester while amniocentesis is performed in the second trimester. The most common indications are advanced maternal age, genetic disease and a previous child with genetic disorder. Fetal blood can be obtained by percutaneous US guidance as early as 14 weeks' gestation. Culture of fetal blood cells allows more rapid karyotyping than amniocentesis. Recently it has been possible to isolate fetal cells from the maternal circulation for genetic testing.

**Q3** EXIT procedure stands for:

   **A** *ex utero in situ* treatment

   **B** extrauterine *in vivo* treatment

   **C** *ex utero* intrapartum treatment

   **D** extrauterine *in situ* treatment

   **E** none of the above.

**A3** **C** EXIT procedure stands for *ex utero* intrapartum treatment. The principle of EXIT procedure is to maintain a state of controlled uterine hypotonia to preserve uteroplacental circulation. The EXIT procedure was first described for reversal of tracheal occlusion in fetuses with severe congenital diaphragmatic hernia (CDH). These patients required removal of tracheal clips applied for blocking the trachea to prevent egress of the lung fluid. The EXIT procedure helped in maintaining the uteroplacental circulation until the fetal airway was secured by endotracheal intubation. Experience with this technique has shown that it can be performed with safety in the mother and the fetus, hence its applications have expanded. It can be used for treatment of giant neck masses causing airway obstruction, large lung masses (congenital cystic adenomatoid malformation (CCAM)) causing mediastinal compression, CHAOS (congenital high airway obstruction syndrome) and bad prognosis CDH.

**Q4** In which of the following is an EXIT procedure *not* used?

   **A** congenital high airway obstruction

   **B** large cervical teratoma or lymphatic malformation

   **C** large omphalocele

   **D** chest mass preventing lung expansion

   **E** CDH requiring immediate extracorporeal membrane oxygenation (ECMO) cannulation

**A**4 **C** EXIT procedure is used for treatment of giant neck masses causing airway obstruction, CCAM causing mediastinal compression, CHAOS and bad prognosis CDH. All types of omphaloceles can be managed postnatally without problems and hence do not need an EXIT procedure.

**Q**5 Which of the following statements is true?

**A** Hysterotomy for open fetal surgery is the same as that for classic caesarean section.

**B** All subsequent deliveries after fetal surgery should be normal vaginal deliveries whenever possible.

**C** Chorion–amnion membrane separation occurs more often after fetal endoscopic surgery as compared with open fetal surgery.

**D** Tocolysis is contraindicated after fetal surgery.

**E** Exogenous nitric oxide may increase the risk of pre-term labour after fetal surgery.

**A**5 **C** Open fetal surgery is performed in mid-gestation. The hysterotomy cannot be performed in the lower segment of the uterus, but may be placed at the fundus of the uterus or based on the position of the placenta. All subsequent deliveries after open fetal surgery should be done by caesarean section because of an increased risk of uterine rupture during labour.

During fetal endoscopic surgery the amniotic membrane gets tented and pushed away from the chorion and the amniotic fluid leaks in between the membranes thus allowing separation of the membranes. During open fetal surgery absorbable staples are used for the hysterotomy and all layers are stapled across hence the separation rate is very low.

There is high uterine irritability after open fetal surgery which leads to a high incidence of premature delivery hence long-term tocolysis is essential for prevention of this complication. Exogenous nitric oxide is a potent tocolytic agent and has been shown to decrease the risk of pre-term labour after fetal surgery.

**Q**6 Which of the following is *not* a fetal treatment for posterior urethral valves (PUVs)?

**A** vesicoamniotic shunt

**B** fetal vesicostomy

**C** fetal cystoscopic valve ablation

**D** fetal bilateral ureterostomy

**E** restoration of fetal amniotic volume to prevent pulmonary hypoplasia

A⁶ **D** PUVs cause obstruction to the antegrade flow of urine. The urinary bladder gets enlarged and thick walled and the posterior urethra becomes dilated. This is seen on US as the 'keyhole' sign. The backpressure on the ureters and kidneys results in hydroureteronephrosis. Obstruction to the kidneys in fetal life causes irreversible dysplasia, which may be prevented by early intervention. This is the goal of fetal intervention in fetuses with PUVs. US-guided percutaneous placement of vesicoamniotic shunts has been used with good results in fetuses with PUVs. Fetal vesicostomy and fetal cystoscopic valve ablation are more invasive procedures and have been performed less commonly. Fetal bilateral ureterostomy is not done in fetal life but can be done postnatally if required. Restoration of amniotic fluid volume is an essential component of treatment if there is associated oligohydramnios to prevent pulmonary hypoplasia in the fetus. It is used in conjunction with the other interventions mentioned above.

Q⁷ Regarding CCAM, which of the following is *not* true?
  **A** Most lesions can be treated after birth.
  **B** Only large lesions that develop fetal hydrops before 26 weeks of gestation may be candidates for fetal surgery.
  **C** Macrocystic lesions may be treated by thoracoamniotic shunting.
  **D** Regression of large lesions and hydrops may occur after treatment with steroids.
  **E** Spontaneous resolution in very unusual.

A⁷ **E** CCAM of the lung is a part of the spectrum of bronchopulmonary foregut malformation. It can be classified as macrocystic, microcystic or mixed. Most lesions are slow growing and can be treated after birth. Several show spontaneous regression and resolution in fetal life and also postnatally. This resolution may be partial or complete. Some lesions, however, grow faster during fetal life and cause substantial pulmonary compromise. Large lesions can cause mediastinal compression and reduce the venous inflow to the heart causing hydrops in the fetus and placentomegaly in the mother. Such large lesions causing cardiopulmonary compromise may benefit from open fetal resection (pulmonary lobectomy) if they are seen during mid-gestation. Fetuses with large lesions near term may benefit from an EXIT to resection policy. Large macrocystic lesions may also be treated initially with thoracoamniotic shunting. Shunts do have a problem of migrating and blockage and hence some people have used serial aspiration of macrocystic CCAM with similar results. Some authors have shown regression of large CCAM after treatment with steroids.

**Q8** Regarding CDH, which of the following is true?

    **A** Lung-area to head-circumference ratio (LHR) is one of the prognostic indicators.

    **B** Liver herniation does not alter the prognosis.

    **C** Repair of CDH on ECMO is contraindicated.

    **D** It needs emergency repair after birth.

    **E** Pulmonary hypertension is usually treated after repair of the diaphragm.

**A8**   **A** CDH is comprises a defect in the diaphragm with herniation of abdominal contents into the chest. One of the contents may be liver. The left side is more common than the right side. LHR is defined as the two-dimensional right lung area measured at the level of the four-chamber view of the heart, divided by the head circumference normalised for gestational age. The LHR measured at 24–26 weeks' gestation has been assessed retrospectively and prospectively and is a useful predictor of postnatal outcome. Patients with an LHR of less than 1.0 have a very bad prognosis whereas all patients with an LHR greater than 1.4 are considered to have good prognosis. LHR values between 1.0 and 1.4 are associated with a 38% survival rate and have a moderate prognosis. The LHR has predicted the severity of lung hypoplasia in left CDH based on ultrasound appearance before 26 weeks. The absence of liver herniation indicates a good prognosis with a survival of 93%, whereas liver herniation is associated with a 43% survival rate. Ultrafast fetal MRI using rapid HASTE (Half-Fourier Acquisition Single-shot Turbo Spin Echo) technique is a powerful tool to accurately show liver herniation.

Abnormal blood vessels with pulmonary hypertension is a major problem with CDH. Pulmonary hypertension needs to be treated before attempting CDH repair. A period of stabilisation is essential before repair.

High-risk CDH (LHR less than 1.0 and liver herniation) with pulmonary hypertension may have severe pulmonary and cardiac compromise. In such fetuses separation from the uteroplacental circulation may lead to immediate instability in the newborn. An EXIT-to-ECMO procedure allows endotracheal intubation and the insertion of venous and/or arterial cannulae for ECMO while on placental support and avoids hypoxia or acidosis during neonatal resuscitation.

**Q9** Regarding CDH, which of the following is true?

    **A** Fetal diaphragm repair has not been shown to improve the prognosis.

    **B** Tracheal occlusion performed via open fetal surgery has not improved prognosis.

    **C** Isolated CDH, LHR >1.4, and no liver herniation, has a good prognosis.

    **D** Fetal tracheal occlusion with percutaneous balloon placement has shown some promise.

    **E** All of the above are correct.

**A9** **E** *In utero* repair does not improve survival rate over standard postnatal treatment in CDH fetuses without liver herniation, primarily because survival in this group is very favourable without prenatal intervention. The original approach of complete *in utero* CDH repair proved technically impossible when liver herniation was present because acute reduction of the liver compromised umbilical venous flow resulting in fetal bradycardia and cardiac arrest. Most patients with CDH who may benefit from prenatal repair are the ones with bad prognosis, i.e. with liver herniation. Since open fetal repair was not successful in this group of patients, *in utero* repair did not improve survival in CDH patients.

    It has been recognised for many years that the dynamics of fetal lung fluid affects lung growth: increased fetal lung fluid egress results in pulmonary hypoplasia, whereas decreased fetal lung fluid egress results in large fluid-filled lungs. This concept was used to improve lung growth and prevent hypoplasia in patients with CDH but tracheal occlusion performed via open fetal surgery has not improved prognosis. However, fetal tracheal occlusion with percutaneous balloon placement has shown some promise.

    Isolated CDH, LHR >1.4, and no liver herniation has good prognosis (*see* question 8).

**Q10** Regarding, fetal myelomeningocele, which of the following is *not* true?

    **A** It can be treated by open fetal surgery.

    **B** It is usually operated before 18 weeks of gestation.

    **C** It is under investigation by the MOMS (management of myelomeningocele study) randomised trial.

    **D** There is recent evidence to suggest that the damage to the spinal cord may be due to exposure to the *in utero* environment.

    **E** It is a cause of fetal hydrops.

**A10** **B** Myelomeningocele is a birth defect with disastrous sequelae that affect both the central and peripheral nervous systems. Leakage of cerebrospinal fluid (CSF) leads to Chiari II malformation. Hydrocephalus develops due to obstruction to CSF flow by the Chiari II malformation. Damage to the spinal cord from fetal exposure leads to neurological impairment of the extremities, sexual dysfunction, urinary and stool incontinence and skeletal deformities. This can be treated by open fetal surgery done beyond 18 weeks of gestation and is under investigation under the MOMS randomised trial.

**Q11** CHAOS stands for:

   **A** congenital hip and airway obstruction syndrome

   **B** congenital high airway obstruction syndrome

   **C** congenital heart and airway obstruction syndrome

   **D** coloboma, heart anomalies, airway anomalies, orbital anomaly syndrome

   **E** coloboma, heart anomalies, airway anomalies, oesophageal anomaly syndrome.

**A11** **B** CHAOS (congenital high airway obstruction syndrome) is a prenatally diagnosed clinical condition associated with hydrops in which near-complete or complete intrinsic obstruction of the fetal airway prevents the egress of lung fluid from the tracheobronchial tree. CHAOS is a rare condition with only 50–60 cases reported so far. The true incidence may be higher because many of the cases die *in utero* or are stillborn. There are multiple aetiologies for the intrinsic obstruction of the airway in CHAOS such as laryngeal atresia, laryngeal web, tracheal atresia and laryngeal cyst. The clinical features and presentation of CHAOS are bilaterally enlarged echogenic lungs, dilated airways and flattened or inverted diaphragms with associated fetal ascites and non-immune hydrops.

**Q12** Regarding fetal SCT, which of the following is *not* true?

   **A** Prenatally diagnosed SCT has a good prognosis.

   **B** Malignant invasion is unusual.

   **C** Fetal heart failure may develop.

   **D** Maternal mirror syndrome may occur.

   **E** Open fetal surgery may be beneficial.

**A12** **A** A fetus with a prenatally diagnosed large mass displacing the anus and with high-output heart failure usually has an SCT. Prenatally diagnosed SCT has a bad prognosis. The SCT may enlarge and develop wide arteriovenous connections with low-resistance channels. This leads to a high-output state and subsequently to hydrops, placentomegaly, maternal mirror syndrome and heart failure. If these changes are seen before 28 weeks of gestation then open fetal surgery should be considered. Radiofrequency ablation is another option but causes unacceptable damage to surrounding structures.

**Q13** Regarding twin–twin transfusion syndrome (TTS), which of the following is *not* true?

**A** It is a complication of monochorionic multiple gestation.

**B** It is a complication of dichorionic multiple gestation.

**C** It accounts for 17%–20% of the mortality associated with twin gestation.

**D** It may be treated with serial amnioreduction.

**E** Selective laser photocoagulation may be used for treatment.

**A13** **B** TTTS is a complication of monochorionic multiple gestation. There are multiple vascular communications between the two fetuses such that one is compromised and the other one is favoured. It affects 4%–35% of all monochorionic twin gestations and accounts for 17%–20% of the mortality associated with twin gestation. Serial amnioreduction and laser photocoagulation has been used for treatment. Serial amnioreduction is associated with 18%–25% incidence of neurologic and cardiac complications. Laser photocoagulation of the abnormal vascular communications has proven to be a comparable alternative.

**Q14** Regarding CCAM of the lung, which of the following is *not* true?

**A** It may involve multiple lobes of the lung.

**B** It does not have separate blood supply from the aorta.

**C** It may resolve spontaneously.

**D** It may be confused with intralobar sequestration.

**E** It has a different aetiology compared with the other bronchopulmonary foregut malformations.

**A14** **E** CCAM of the lung is a part of the bronchopulmonary foregut malformation. It can be classified as macrocystic or microcystic. Mixed type also exists. Most are usually located in one lobe of the lung but lesions may involve multiple lobes. Most lesions are slow growing and can be treated after birth. Many of them show spontaneous regression and resolution in fetal life and also postnatally. This resolution may be partial or complete. Some intralobar sequestrations may be confused with CCAM. Sequestrations have a separate blood supply from the aorta and this differentiates them from CCAM. Lesions that persist in the postnatal period are removed by either open surgical thoracotomy and lobectomy or by thoracoscopic lobectomy/resection depending upon the surgeon's choice.

**Q15** Which of the following is not true of epignathus (oropharyngeal teratoma)?

   **A** It may lead to fetal demise.

   **B** It may cause airway obstruction in fetal life.

   **C** It may severely deviate and deform the trachea.

   **D** Tracheostomy on placental support may be life-saving.

   **E** Early surgery is important to prevent malignant degeneration.

**A15** **E** Giant masses like epignathus, cervical teratoma and cervical cystic lymphangioma cause significant tracheal deviation and distortion leading to airway obstruction. It is extremely difficult to secure the airway of these patients immediately after birth and the mortality of these conditions is high. Hence a fetus with a large epignathus may need an EXIT procedure. The EXIT procedure allows the time needed to secure the airway of these patients by laryngotracheobronchoscopy, endotracheal intubation or tracheotomy. In this way these fetuses that are otherwise normal can be saved. These masses are well seen on US and MRI. While early surgery is important to prevent respiratory distress, most of these lesions are benign. Malignant degeneration can occur in incompletely resected lesions.

**Q16** Regarding hydrocephalus due to aqueductal stenosis, which of the following is true?

   **A** In severe cases, decompressing the ventricles may ameliorate the adverse effects on the developing brain.

   **B** Ventriculoamniotic shunts have improved the outcome greatly.

   **C** Shunt malfunction and complication rate is low.

   **D** Fourth ventriculostomy is a treatment of choice in refractory cases.

   **E** All of the above are correct.

**A16** **A** Aqueductal stenosis causes obstruction to the flow of CSF and dilates the ventricles. This compresses the developing brain and leads to neurological sequelae. In fetuses with severe hydrocephalus, decompressing the ventricles may ameliorate the adverse effects on the developing brain. Percutaneously placed ventriculoamniotic shunts have been used but have not improved the outcome greatly. High malfunction rate and complication rate are the major reasons for this problem. A multicentre randomised trial regarding this is currently in progress to determine the real benefits of this technique. Third ventriculostomy and not fourth is an alternative treatment option for hydrocephalus due to aqueductal stenosis.

Q17 Regarding twin reversed arterial perfusion (TRAP) sequence, which of the following is *not* true?

A It occurs with monochorionic twins.

B The pump twin perfuses the acardiac twin.

C The pump twin is susceptible to heart failure

D Ligation, division or cauterisation of the umbilical cord may be required.

E Percutaneous radiofrequency ablation of the umbilical cord of pump twin is essential.

A17 E TRAP sequence occurs with monochorionic twins. TRAP sequence results from a pump twin perfusing an acardiac twin. In the acardiac monochorionic twin gestation this compromises the viability of the normal pump twin. Although the pump twin is structurally normal, polyhydramnios and high-output cardiac failure can occur. The acardiac twin needs to be destroyed in order to save the pump twin. This can be achieved by a percutaneous US-guided selective radiofrequency ablation of the umbilical cord of the acardiac fetus. This can also be achieved by fetectomy, cauterisation of the cord or obliteration of circulation in the acardiac twin by alcohol injection.

Q18 Regarding gastroschisis, which of the following is *not* true?

A It is a defect on the right side of the umbilical cord.

B It has been treated with amniotic fluid exchange to reduce the toxic effects of amniotic fluid on the fetal bowel.

C It may be associated with midgut volvulus.

D It has a 30–40% risk of associated bowel atresia.

E Chromosomal anomalies are rarely seen.

A18 D Gastroschisis is a defect on the right side of the umbilical cord. Vascular insult to the abdominal wall early in gestation may be a possible aetiology for this condition. This condition is treated after birth and does not need open fetal surgery. Some authors have used prenatal amniotic fluid exchange on the assumption that exposure of the fetal bowel to the amniotic fluid causes the changes that are seen with gastroschisis bowel (matting and thick peel with motility disorder in neonatal period), and that dilution of the toxins in the amniotic fluid may improve the motility problems in these patients. Gastroschisis is not usually associated with chromosomal anomaly and is an isolated anomaly but has a 10%–15% risk of associated bowel atresia. Gastroschisis also has a risk of midgut volvulus of the extruded bowel and sometimes with complete bowel loss leading to short gut syndrome.

**Q19** Regarding 'mirror' syndrome, which of the following statement is not true?

   **A** It is a severe pre-eclamptic state with hypertension, proteinuria, ankle and pedal oedema or even generalised fluid retention.

   **B** It is associated with fetal hydrops.

   **C** Small molecules, present in the fetoplacental unit cross the placenta to cause this syndrome in the mother.

   **D** It is associated with TTTS.

   **E** Usually associated with elevated liver enzymes and thrombocytopenia.

**A19** **E** Hydrops in a fetus can occur with any condition that compresses the main veins and thereby reduces the venous return to the heart. It may also occur in a high-output state where the venous return is more than the heart can take. The fetus develops anasarca, which can lead to fetal demise. Similar changes may be seen in the mother and this condition is called the maternal mirror syndrome. Maternal mirror syndrome or Ballantyne's syndrome is defined as a severe pre-eclamptic state with hypertension, proteinuria, ankle and pedal oedema or even generalised fluid retention. Platelet count, aspartate transaminase, alanine transaminase and haptoglobulin are usually not affected in this syndrome and this may be used to distinguish it from the HELLP (haemolytic anaemia, elevated liver enzyme and low platelet count) syndrome. Common conditions that may lead to hydrops are CCAM, CDH, SCT and large mediastinal masses. One of the possible etiologic mechanisms could be that small molecules present in the fetoplacental unit cross the placenta to cause this syndrome in the mother.

**Q20** Which of the following is correct?

   **A** Erythroblastosis fetalis can be treated by intraperitoneal or intravenous red blood cell (RBC) transfusion to the fetus.

   **B** Fetal hypothyroidism can be treated with transamniotic thyroid abstracts.

   **C** Fetal adrenal hyperplasia can be treated with transplacental corticosteroids.

   **D** Pulmonary immaturity can be treated with transplacental glucocorticoids.

   **E** All of the above are correct.

**A20** **E** Some fetal deficiency states may be alleviated by prenatal medical treatment. Blood can be transfused into the fetal peritoneal cavity or directly into the umbilical artery. When the placental route cannot be used the drug may be delivered into the amniotic fluid where the fetus can swallow it to get the desired effects. Thus, erythroblastosis fetalis can be treated by intraperitoneal or intravenous

RBC transfusion to the fetus, fetal hypothyroidism can be treated with transamniotic thyroid abstracts, adrenal hyperplasia can be treated with transplacental corticosteroids and pulmonary immaturity can be treated with transplacental glucocorticoids.

## Further reading

Adzick NS, Kitano Y. Fetal surgery for lung lesions, congenital diaphragmatic hernia, and sacrococcygeal teratoma. *Semin Pediatr Surg.* 2003; **12**(3): 154–67.

Harrison MR, Evans M, Adzick NS, *et al. The Unborn Patient: the art and science of fetal therapy.* 3rd ed. Philadelphia, PA: WB Saunders; 2001.

Marwan A, Crombleholme TM. The EXIT procedure: principles, pitfalls, and progress. *Semin Pediatr Surg.* 2006; **15**(2): 107–15.

# CHAPTER 83

# Bariatric surgery in children

## HARIHARAN THANGARAJAH, SANJEEV DUTTA

From the choices below each question, select the single best answer.

**Q1** What is the most widely accepted definition of overweight and obesity in the paediatric population?
  **A** Body mass index (BMI) ≥30 (overweight) or ≥35 (obese)
  **B** BMI ≥35 (overweight) or ≥40 (obese)
  **C** BMI ≥40 (overweight) or ≥40 with associated co-morbidities (obese)
  **D** BMI >85th percentile (overweight) or >95th percentile (obese)
  **E** BMI >95th percentile (overweight) or >99th percentile (obese)

**A1** **D** An adult with a BMI ≥35 is considered obese. In children and adolescents who are still growing and have changing body shapes, BMI can be less accurate, particularly as it fails to distinguish between fat and fat-free mass. Thus, the application of growth charts and multiple percentiles is necessary to determine overweight and obesity for age and sex in this group. The United States Centers for Disease Control and Prevention now define paediatric *obesity* as a BMI greater than the 95th percentile, and *overweight* as a BMI greater than the 85th percentile. Exceeding the 99th percentile is referred to as extreme paediatric obesity.

**Q2** Which of the following is not considered a risk factor for childhood obesity?
  **A** maternal obesity
  **B** gestational diabetes
  **C** higher birthweight
  **D** lower birthweight
  **E** paternal prematurity

**A2** **E** Evidence exists to support an association between higher birthweight and higher attained BMI in childhood and early adulthood. Lower birthweight has also been associated with an increased risk of developing central obesity later, insulin resistance, and the metabolic syndrome. Maternal obesity and gestational diabetes have been shown to be strong predictors of childhood and adolescent obesity. No convincing evidence currently exists to support an association between paternal prematurity and childhood obesity.

**Q3** Adolescent obesity is associated with innumerable health consequences, including the metabolic syndrome. Which of the following is not a criterion for the metabolic syndrome?
- **A** elevated fasting glucose
- **B** hypertension
- **C** reduced high-density lipoprotein cholesterol
- **D** fatty liver
- **E** elevated triglycerides

**A3** **D** The metabolic syndrome is a cluster of risk factors that links elevated fasting glucose levels, dyslipidaemia, hypertension, and central obesity with an increased risk of later cardiovascular disease. Recent evidence suggests that metabolic syndrome may occur in nearly 50% of overweight children and adolescents, and that its prevalence increases directly with age. Fatty liver, while associated with metabolic syndrome, is not a criterion.

**Q4** Regarding the psychosocial impact of childhood obesity, which of the following is not true?
- **A** Obese young women are less likely to marry than their non-obese counterparts, though the same disparity has not been identified for obese young men.
- **B** Obesity as a young adult has a lasting impact on life satisfaction and aspirations.
- **C** Extreme obesity in adolescents is associated with an increased risk of suicide and suicidal ideation.
- **D** Relative to average-weight peers, obese adolescents are socially marginalised and less likely to be nominated by their peers as a friend.
- **E** Obese young women have lower incomes.

**A4** **A** Obesity is one of the most stigmatising and least socially acceptable conditions of childhood. Studies have demonstrated that obese young women are less likely to marry, have lower incomes, and have completed less schooling than non-obese women, and that obese young men are less likely to marry than their non-obese counterparts. Options B through D are true.

**Q5** Which of the following is an incorrect criterion for bariatric surgery in adolescents, according to the consensus guidelines established in 2004 and endorsed by the American Academy of Pediatrics?

**A** Attainment of physiologic maturity

**B** Failure of ≥18 months of organised weight loss attempts

**C** BMI ≥40 with serious obesity-related co-morbidities such as type 2 diabetes mellitus, obstructive sleep apnoea or pseudotumour cerebri

**D** BMI ≥50 with less-serious obesity-related co-morbidities such as dyslipidaemias, gastro-oesophageal reflux disease or psychosocial distress

**E** Failed multiple non-surgical weight loss efforts

**A5** **B** Adolescents who have failed multiple non-surgical weight loss efforts may be considered candidates for surgical intervention; however, failure of ≥6 months of organised weight loss attempts is sufficient. Attainment of physiologic maturity is necessary prior to undergoing bariatric surgery as stunted growth can accompany the potential dietary and nutritional perturbations that result from such intervention. In general, bariatric surgery may be considered appropriate in adolescents with very severe obesity (BMI ≥40) with the presence of serious obesity-related co-morbidities, in addition to those with higher BMI values (≥50) with less-serious co-morbid conditions.

**Q6** Which of the following obese adolescents represents the best candidate for bariatric surgery according to consensus guidelines established in 2004?

**A** A 15-year-old boy with a BMI of 38 and hypertension, who has failed several organised weight loss attempts and comes from a very supportive family environment.

**B** A 16-year-old girl with a BMI of 46 and type 2 diabetes mellitus, who has yet to undergo any attempt at non-surgical weight loss but appears committed to the postoperative medical and nutritional requirements that accompany bariatric surgery.

**C** A 16-year-old boy with a BMI of 59 and hypertension attributable to his obesity but no other serious co-morbid conditions who has failed several organised weight loss attempts

**D** A 15-year-old girl with a BMI of 47, type 2 diabetes and obstructive sleep apnoea. Her parents, who will be providing informed consent for the procedure, are quite keen on having the operation performed but she appears reluctant.

**E** None of the above individuals represent good candidates for bariatric surgery.

**A6** **C** Bariatric surgery may be considered appropriate in adolescents with very severe obesity (BMI ≥40) with the presence of serious obesity-related co-morbidities (type 2 diabetes mellitus, obstructive sleep apnoea, pseudotumour cerebri), or in those with higher BMI values (≥50) with less-serious co-morbid conditions (hypertension, dyslipidaemias, non-alcoholic steatohepatitis, venous-stasis disease, gastro-oesophageal reflux disease, weight-related arthropathies that impair physical activity, and psychosocial distress, among others). Prior attempts at non-surgical weight loss are generally considered a requisite before proceeding with operative intervention. While informed consent for the procedure must be obtained from the parents, the decisional capacity of the adolescent and his or her ability to provide assent for the procedure are also central factors that must be clarified prior to proceeding with surgery.

**Q7** Which of the following is not a contraindication for bariatric surgery in adolescents?
   **A** presence of a medically correctable cause of obesity
   **B** recent substance abuse problems
   **C** current pregnancy or lactation
   **D** depression
   **E** Tanner stage 1

**A7** **D** Medically correctable causes of obesity should be addressed before consider-ing bariatric surgery. Substance abuse problems within the preceding year and concerns about adherence to postoperative recommendations are also contrain-dications given the compliance with close post-surgical surveillance required to ensure proper outcomes. The rapid weight loss and potential consequent nutri-tional perturbations that accompany bariatric surgery make current lactation or pregnancy (or planned pregnancy within 2 years after surgery) contraindications to the procedure. Physiologic maturation, which should be established prior to consideration of bariatric surgery, usually occurs along with sexual maturation (Tanner stage 3 or 4). A significant proportion of overweight and obese adoles-cents seeking bariatric surgery demonstrate signs of clinical depression. Existing evidence suggests that preoperative depression does not adversely affect short-term outcome after bariatric surgery. As such, the presence of depression does not preclude surgery (though appropriate treatment should be instituted).

Q8    Which of the following is not a component of the preoperative evaluation of an adolescent being considered for bariatric surgery?

     **A**   assessment by a psychiatrist

     **B**   abdominal ultrasound

     **C**   polysomnography

     **D**   upper and lower endoscopy

     **E**   assessment by a dietician

A8    **D**   Psychologic evaluation of the candidate adolescent and his/her parents serves to define potential supports and barriers to patient adherence as well as patient and family preparedness for surgery and the required postoperative lifestyle changes. Preoperative ultrasound can characterise the presence of steatohepatitis and cholelithiasis; patients with symptomatic gallstones should be considered for cholecystectomy before or during the bariatric procedure. Polysomnography may be obtained to evaluate obstructive sleep apnoea (OSA) if suggested by clinical history – up to 55% of adolescents presenting for weight loss surgery have OSA. Upper endoscopy can delineate lesions that may no longer be accessible following certain bariatric surgical procedures (e.g. Roux-en-Y gastric bypass). Evaluation by a dietician is necessary to ensure that the patient understands the dietary changes that will be required postoperatively in order to avert nutritional deficiencies. There is no present role for routine lower endoscopy in the evaluation of adolescents undergoing bariatric surgery.

Q9    Of the following bariatric procedures, which is most likely to produce adverse malabsorptive nutritional sequelae?

     **A**   laparoscopic adjustable gastric banding (LAGB)

     **B**   vertical banded gastroplasty (VBG)

     **C**   Roux-en-Y gastric bypass (RYGB)

     **D**   laparoscopic sleeve gastrectomy (LSG)

     **E**   biliopancreatic diversion with duodenal switch (BPDS)

A9    **E**   Being a primarily malabsorptive procedure, biliopancreatic diversion with duodenal switch has the capacity to engender significant nutritional perturbations including deficiencies in vitamins A, $B_{12}$, D, E and K, iron and protein. RYGB may produce similar effects, though not typically to the same degree as BPDS. LAGB, VBG and LSG are primarily restrictive procedures that harbour a lower risk of producing malabsorptive sequelae.

**Q10** In comparing surgical and non-surgical therapies to address adolescent obesity, which of the following is not true?

**A** Non-surgical options such as dietary and behavioural modification have produced generally unsatisfactory results with poor weight loss, high attrition rates and high probability of weight regain.

**B** Medications that serve to promote weight loss through appetite suppression or malabsorption have shown limited efficacy as benefits tend to be short-lived and side effects poorly tolerated.

**C** Bariatric surgery has demonstrated successful long-lasting (>1 year) effects on body weight in severely obese adolescents.

**D** There is an abundance of long-term outcomes literature suggesting bariatric surgery is safe and efficacious in the treatment of adolescent obesity.

**E** Non-surgical options for the treatment of adolescent obesity are associated with poor compliance.

**A10** **D** Non-surgical therapies for the treatment of adolescent obesity have generally yielded poor results because of problems with compliance and modest/short-term weight loss. While bariatric surgery has been shown to have beneficial extended effects on weight loss for adolescents, long-term outcomes data in this population is lacking. Studies are underway to define the long-term consequences of weight loss surgery in adolescents.

Q11 Which of the following adolescents is likely to have the most favourable outcome following bariatric surgery?

A A 12-year-old boy, Tanner stage 2, with a BMI of 52 and a history of gastro-oesophageal reflux disease but no serious co-morbid conditions. Surgery is performed at a tertiary care facility by a paediatric surgeon who recently finished her surgical training, in concert with an adult bariatric surgery specialist.

B A 14-year-old boy, Tanner stage 4, with a BMI of 44 and a history of pseudotumour cerebri. Surgery is performed at a tertiary care facility by a paediatric surgeon with limited bariatric surgical experience but >20 years of general operative experience.

C A 14-year-old boy, Tanner stage 4, with a BMI of 55 and a history of intertriginous soft tissue infections, but no serious co-morbid conditions. Surgery is performed at a tertiary care facility by a paediatric surgeon who recently finished her surgical training, in concert with an adult bariatric surgery specialist.

D A 16-year-old girl, Tanner stage 5, with a BMI of 48 and a history of type 2 diabetes mellitus. Surgery is performed at a tertiary care facility by a paediatric surgeon with limited bariatric surgery experience but >20 years of general operative experience.

E A 16-year-old boy, Tanner stage 5, with a BMI of 34 and a history of obstructive sleep apnoea. Surgery is performed at a tertiary care facility by a paediatric surgeon who recently finished her surgical training, in concert with an adult bariatric surgery specialist.

A11 **C** Physiologic maturity must be established prior to consideration of bariatric surgery in adolescents, as the dietary complexities and potential nutritional consequences following surgery can stunt completion of growth. Physiologic maturation usually occurs along with sexual maturation (Tanner stage 3 or 4). It is also important that surgery be performed by practitioners who have specialised training in bariatric procedures. Abundant evidence exists to show that minimally invasive bariatric surgery is one of the more technically difficult operations to perform, with a steep learning curve and demonstrated differences in outcome depending on training background of the surgeons. Paediatric surgeons involved in bariatric surgery should pursue advanced training in bariatric procedures and their early experience should be done in partnership with an experienced bariatric surgical specialist. The adolescent described in option E is not a qualified candidate as his BMI falls below generally accepted guidelines.

**Q12** Regarding potential nutritional consequences of bariatric surgical procedures in adolescents, which of the following is *not* true?

    **A** Malabsorption can lead to deficiencies in vitamins A, $B_{12}$, C, D and E.

    **B** Malabsorption can produce anaemia through deficiencies in folate and iron.

    **C** Gastric restrictive procedures can produce a hypochloraemic metabolic alkalosis resulting from the decreased number of parietal cells available for HCl secretion.

    **D** Malabsorption can produce protein–calorie malnutrition.

    **E** Malabsorption can produce metabolic bone disease.

**A12** **C** Hypochloraemic metabolic alkalosis deriving from a decreased number of parietal cells is not a typical nutritional consequence of restrictive bariatric procedures. The deficiencies described in the remaining answer choices all represent potential nutritional sequelae of weight loss surgery – vitamin/mineral supplementation and appropriate dietary modifications are required to avoid these consequences in growing adolescents.

**Q13** Which of the following is not true regarding bariatric surgery in adolescents?

    **A** Compliance with postoperative multivitamin and nutrient supplementation is generally low.

    **B** Adolescent females who undergo bariatric surgery may engage in more sexually promiscuous behaviour after weight loss.

    **C** Even after the period of rapid weight loss, there is a slightly elevated risk of miscarriage in adolescent females who undergo bariatric surgery.

    **D** Adolescents <18 years old constitute <1% of all bariatric surgery patients.

    **E** Childhood obesity is associated with left ventricular hypertrophy during young adulthood.

**A13** **C** Compliance with postoperative healthcare recommendations in adolescents undergoing bariatric surgery is generally poor, with one study documenting a <15% compliance rate with postoperative dietary multivitamin and nutrient supplementation. Girls undergoing bariatric surgery also have an increased risk of pregnancy, a result that may be attributable to more sexually promiscuous behaviour after weight loss, or to increased fertility. Surgery does not appear to affect the outcome of subsequent pregnancies as long as the period of rapid weight loss has passed (hence, pregnancy is contraindicated for 2 years after surgery). Cardiovascular disease risk is elevated with childhood obesity. Presently, adolescents comprise a small minority of patients undergoing bariatric surgery.

**Q14** Towards the conclusion of a laparoscopic RYGB, the gastrojejunal anastomosis is assessed by way of saline immersion of the anastomosis and insufflation of the gastric pouch with air. Marked bubbling of the saline irrigant is noted. The most appropriate next step(s) in management is(are):

**A** Aspiration of the irrigant, placement of a closed suction drain adjacent to the anastomotic site, and closure of the trocar sites.

**B** Immediate conversion to an open operation.

**C** Aspiration of the irrigant, closure of the trocar sites, and a water-soluble upper gastrointestinal contrast study on postoperative day 1.

**D** Aspiration of the irrigant, closure of the trocar sites, and a water-soluble upper gastrointestinal contrast study on postoperative day 1.

**E** Attempt at laparoscopic suture closure of a likely anastomotic leak.

**A14** **E** This scenario describes intraoperative identification of an anastomotic leak. These should be repaired at the time of their intraoperative identification by placing reinforcing sutures at the suspected site of leakage (laparoscopically, if technically feasible). Subsequent adjunctive measures that may be considered include placement of a closed-suction drain adjacent to the anastomotic site, and obtaining a postoperative water-soluble upper gastrointestinal contrast study to further evaluate the anastomosis.

**Q15** A 15-year-old boy with a BMI of 45 and a history of type 2 diabetes mellitus undergoes laparoscopic RYGB. On postoperative day 1, he is noted to be febrile, mildly tachypnoeic and tachycardic. A water-soluble upper gastrointestinal contrast study is obtained which demonstrates free extravasation of contrast in the left upper abdomen. The most appropriate next step(s) in management is(are):

  **A** CT imaging of the abdomen for further characterisation

  **B** administering intravenous antibiotics, keeping the patient nil per mouth through postoperative day seven, and subsequently initiating a diet

  **C** administering intravenous antibiotics, keeping the patient nil per mouth through postoperative day seven, and subsequently obtaining a repeat contrast study

  **D** immediate operative exploration

  **E** percutaneous placement of a drain adjacent to the gastrojejunal anastomotic site and administration of intravenous antibiotics.

**A15** **D** This scenario describes postoperative identification of an anastomotic leak. In this case, the leak is not contained and the patient is demonstrating signs of systemic toxicity. Immediate operative exploration is warranted with an attempt at repair of the leak.

## Further reading

Chandra V, Dutta S. Bariatric surgery in adolescents. In: Alvarez AO, Brodsky JB, Alpert MA, *et al.*, editors. *Morbid Obesity: peri-operative management.* 2nd ed. Cambridge: Cambridge University Press; 2010. pp. 223–33.

Inge TH, Krebs NF, Garcia VF, *et al.* Bariatric surgery for severely overweight adolescents: concerns and recommendations. *Pediatrics.* 2004; **114**(1): 217–23.

Pratt JS, Lenders CM, Dionne EA, *et al.* Best practice updates for pediatric/adolescent weight loss surgery. *Obesity (Silver Spring).* 2009; **17**(5): 901–10.

Treadwell JR, Sun F, Schoelles K. Systematic review and meta-analysis of bariatric surgery for pediatric obesity. *Ann Surg.* 2008; **248**(5): 763–76.

# CHAPTER 84

# Medical statistics and hospital management

## MADAN SAMUEL

**From the choices below each question, select the single best answer.**

**Q1** Two hundred and twenty-eight of 1320 patients with moderate to severe congestive cardiac failure who received placebo treatment died, as did 156 of 1327 who received bisoprolol. What was the *relative risk* of dying?

   **A** 17%

   **B** 12%

   **C** 68%

   **D** 53%

   **E** 22%

**A1**   **C** In clinical trials subjects with different characteristics are followed up to see whether an outcome of interest occurs. The proportions having the outcomes in each group is calculated and so the ratio of these two proportions is a measure of the *raised risk* in one group compared with the other. This ratio is termed the *relative risk*. Under the null hypothesis the expected value of **RR** is 1. In the above example, the risk of death in the placebo group is 0.1727272 (228/1320) and the risk in the treated group is 0.1175584 (156/1327) making the RR of dying (if untreated) 0.1727272/0.1175584 or 68.06%.

**Q2** The true treatment effect of bisoprolol on congestive cardiac failure will not be known because of:

   **A** chance

   **B** poor design

   **C** non-randomisation

   **D** poor methodology

   **E** probability.

$A^2$  **A**  However powerful and well designed an experiment, there will always be considerable uncertainty about the magnitude of the treatment effect.

$Q^3$  Which one of the following correctly describes the general sequence of steps in a research project?

    **A**  study design, data collection, data processing, data analysis, presentation, interpretation

    **B**  planning, design, data collection, data processing, data analysis

    **C**  planning, design, data collection, data processing, data analysis, presentation

    **D**  planning, design, data collection, data processing, data analysis, presentation, interpretation, publication

    **E**  study design, data collection, data analysis, presentation, interpretation

$A^3$  **D**  Self-explanatory.

$Q^4$  Height, weight, blood pressure and serum cholesterol values are examples of what type of data?

    **A**  ranks

    **B**  continuous

    **C**  percentages

    **D**  rates and ratios

    **E**  scores

$A^4$  **B**  Continuous data is the type of data obtained from some sort of measurement (in contrast to counting discrete objects). The accuracy of the data is limited by the accuracy of the measuring instrument.

$Q^5$  The Apgar system of evaluating the well-being of a newborn baby is a:

    **A**  score

    **B**  rank

    **C**  rate

    **D**  percentage

    **E**  analogue scale.

$A^5$  **A**  Patients' symptoms and signs can be given numerical values and the various values added up to give a total score. This score is then an observation.

**Q6** Standard deviation is the:

    **A** average of the squared differences

    **B** average distance from the median

    **C** average distance from the mean

    **D** average distance from the sum of all mean values

    **E** average distance of all observations from a set of observations.

**A6**   **C**  Standard deviation is the average distance each value is from the mean.

**Q7** Surveys and epidemiological studies are examples of:

    **A** observational study

    **B** experimental study

    **C** prospective study

    **D** retrospective study

    **E** cross-sectional study.

**A7**   **A**  In an observational study, information is collected on attributes or measurements of interest without influencing events. A good example is prevalence of sickle disease in the Middle East. Observational studies include surveys and most epidemiological studies.

**Q8** Studies to derive cross-sectional growth charts for children are best described as:

    **A** pseudo-longitudinal study

    **B** observational longitudinal study

    **C** observational cross-sectional study

    **D** experimental cross-sectional study

    **E** experimental longitudinal study.

**A8**   **A**  In pseudo-longitudinal study each subject is seen at only one time, but the data is used to describe changes over time. Hormone levels during the menstrual cycle are another example of pseudo-longitudinal study.

**Q9** Sensitivity is defined as:

    **A** the proportion of negatives that are correctly identified by the test

    **B** the proportion of patients with negative test results who are correctly diagnosed

    **C** the proportion of patients with positive test results who are correctly diagnosed

    **D** the proportion of near positives that are correctly identified by the test

    **E** the proportion of positives that are correctly identified by the test.

**A⁹ E** Sensitivity is the proportion of positives that are correctly identified by the test.

**Q10** Negative predictive value is defined as:
- **A** the proportion of patients with positive test results who are correctly diagnosed
- **B** the proportion of patients with negative test results who are correctly diagnosed
- **C** the proportion of positives that are correctly identified by the test
- **D** the proportion of negatives that are correctly identified by the test
- **E** none of the above.

**A10 B** Negative predictive value is the proportion of patients with negative test results who are correctly diagnosed.

**Q11** Which of the following is not a feature of Pocock study protocol?
- **A** study objective
- **B** treatment schedules
- **C** grants
- **D** trial design
- **E** patient consent

**A11 C** The main features of a study protocol are: background and study objectives, specific objectives, patient-selection criteria, treatment schedules, methods of patient evaluation, trial design, registration and randomisation of patients, patient consent, required size of study, monitoring of trial progress, forms and data handling, protocol deviation, statistical analysis, administrative responsibilities.

**Q12** Semigraphical summarisation of data using centile is best represented by:
- **A** histograms
- **B** scatter plots
- **C** cumulative relative frequency graph
- **D** cumulative distribution
- **E** box and whisker plot.

**A12 E** Self-explanatory.

**Q13** Stem and leaf diagrams represent:
  **A** actual observations
  **B** relative observations
  **C** cumulative frequencies
  **D** distribution frequencies
  **E** cumulative relative frequency.

**A13** **A** Actual observations can be visualised in a stem and leaf diagram.

**Q14** An example of stratified randomisation is:
  **A** stratification by tumour size in testicular cancer
  **B** stratification by age for neuroblastoma outcome
  **C** stratification by menopausal status when comparing two alternative treatments for breast cancer
  **D** stratification by tumour size for resectability in Wilms's tumour
  **E** prognostic stratification by sex.

**A14** **C** Self-explanatory.

**Q15** Treatment outcome in two groups with 10 individuals in each group is best evaluated by:
  **A** Student's $t$-test
  **B** Chi-square test
  **C** Fisher's exact test
  **D** Wilcoxon test
  **E** Stuart–Maxwell test.

**A15** **C** Fisher's exact test consists of evaluating the probability associated with all possible 2 × 2 tables which have the same row and column totals as the observed data, making the assumption that the null hypothesis is true.

## Further reading

CIBIS-II Investigators and Committees. The Cardiac Insufficiency Bisoprolol Study II (CIBIS-II): a randomised trial. *Lancet.* 1999; **353**(9146): 9–13.

Pocock SJ. Current issues in the design and interpretation of clinical trials. *Br Med J (Clin Res Ed).* 1985; **290**(6461): 39–42.

# Index

11β-hydroxylase deficiency 602
17-hydroxyprogesterone 144, 602
21-hydroxylase deficiency 601–2
5α-reductase deficiency 606

AAST Organ Injury Grading Scale 73, 87
ABC (aneurysmal bone cyst) 773–4
abdominal compartment syndrome 76, 270
abdominal distension
    and jejunoileal atresia 304–5
    and meconium ileus 322
    and trauma 53
abdominal pain
    and ATDs 340
    and CDH 735
    and choledochal cyst 437, 727, 730
    colicky 390, 393
    differential diagnosis of 374, 394
    and genital tract obstruction 622
    and GOR 231
    and intussusception 344–5, 390
    investigations of 488
    and ovarian torsion 628
    and radiation enteritis 643
abdominal radiograph
    and caustic ingestion 220
    and intussusception 346
    and malrotation 712
    and meconium ileus 327
abdominal trauma
    blunt, see blunt abdominal trauma
    evaluation of 80
    indicators of 121
    organs injured in 71
abdominal wall contusion 76–7
abdominal wall defects
    embryogenesis of 278
    and GORD 228
    and inguinal hernia 284
    and intestinal atresia 303
abdominal wall hernias 288–9
abdominal X-ray (AXR), and foreign bodies 206
accessory nerve 131–2
ACE (antegrade continence enema) 416, 552, 560
acid burn 113
acid ingestion 218–19, 223
aciduria, paradoxical 297
ACL (anterior cruciate ligament) injuries 98–9
acupuncture 540–1
Addison's disease 137–8
adenocarcinoma
    and Barrett's oesophagus 696–7
    hilar 441
adenomas
    adrenal 671, 675–6

and hyperaldosteronism 136–7
    and malignancy 387
    pleomorphic 720
    sporadic 140
adenomatous polyps 386–7
adenotonsillectomy 493
adenovirus 344–5
adjuvant therapy
    and breast cancer 153
    and neuroblastoma 639
    and risk stratification 638
adnexal torsion 629
ADPKD (autosomal dominant polycystic kidney disease) 459, 502–3, 505–6
adrenal dysfunction 136
adrenal gland, and neuroblastoma 651–2
adrenal hyperplasia 675, 790
    bilateral 137, 676
    congenital, see congenital adrenal hyperplasia (CAH)
adrenal insufficiency, relative 26–7
adrenalectomy 668, 671, 676
adrenalin, racemic 205–6
adrenocortical tumours 136, 671, 676, 703–4
aganglionosis 397–404
AHO (acute haematogenous osteomyelitis) 761–3
AIDS 584, 702
air embolism 38–40, 324
airway
    assessment of 494
    differences in paediatric 49
airway obstruction
    acute 166
    causes of 48
    symptoms of 166, 193
AIS (adolescent idiopathic scoliosis), see scoliosis
AIS (androgen insensitivity syndrome) 573, 576, 624
    complete 285–6, 570, 572, 601, 605
    partial 573, 588, 601
Alagille's syndrome 428, 661, 724–6, 728–9
alarm therapy 538–40
albumin, and nutritional status 8
alimentary tract duplications (ATDs) 338, 340–3
alkali burns 113
alkali ingestion 218–19
alkalosis 13, 297, 798
all-terrain vehicles (ATV) 85
alpha–fetoprotein (AFP)
    and Beckwith–Wiedemann's syndrome 660
    during first 8 months 695

elevation of 779
    and germ cell tumours 680
amenorrhoea 151, 383, 622, 670
    primary 605, 624–5
amino acids 9, 11, 15
amniocentesis 320, 779–80
Amyand's hernia 285
anaemia
    chronic 454
    and GOR 231
    and haemangioendothelioma 658
    haemolytic 431, 789
    iron deficiency 140, 309, 392
    megaloblastic 366
    pernicious 138
    and SGA infants 3
    sickle cell 481, 742, 763; see also sickle cell disease
anaesthesia
    caudal 737, 739, 742
    for day-case surgery 742
    drugs used in 739–40
    general 739
    and temperature regulation 737–8
anal dilatations 425–6
analgesia
    patient-controlled (PCA) 745–6
    postoperative 742
anastomosis
    and FAP 385
    gastrojejunal 799
    and gastroschisis 280
    and Hirschsprung's disease 403
    and jejunoileal atresia 308
    lymphaticovenous 265–6
    and Meckel's diverticulum 335
    and meconium ileus 325
    and NEC 357
    and pyloric atresia 293
anastomotic leak 212–13, 309, 750, 799–800
androgen insensitivity syndrome, see AIS
androgens, exogenous 661
angle of His 228, 235
aniridia 322, 572, 644
ankle fractures 99
anogenital warts 620–1
anoplasty 420–1, 426
anorectal defects, most frequent 417
anorectal malformation
    associations of 424
    and colostomy 419
    and faecal incontinence 413, 416
    and neurogenic bladder 555–6
    radiological studies of 418
    and sacrococcygeal teratomas 699
    surgical treatment of 407–8
    in VACTERL 210
    without fistula 420

anthracyclines 642, 688
antibiotic prophylaxis
  and asplenia 74
  and open fractures 96
  and organ transplant 749
  and PUV 491
  and splenectomy 486
  urinary tract 517, 525, 542, 550
  and VUR 522
antibiotics
  and appendicitis 375
  and bacterial overgrowth 364
  and bactericides 19
  and breast infection 148
  and caustic ingestion 222
  and colitis 382
  and empyema 68, 183
  intravenous, see intravenous
    antibiotics
  and lymphoma 703
  and respiratory distress 759
anticholinergics
  and bladder dysfunction 542–3
  and Hinman's syndrome 544
  and sacral agenesis 554
  and spina bifida 550–1
  and urinary incontinence 528,
    532–3, 559
antidiuretic therapy 539
antimuscarinics, see oxybutynin
antireflux barrier 227
antireflux procedures 228, 238
antireflux surgery
  and circumcision 585
  complications of 231, 234, 237, 239
  and neuropathic bladder 550
antispasmodics 542, 544
antivenins 103–5, 115
antral polyps 711
anxiety, preventing 744–5
aorta
  coarctation of 492–3
  and D-transposition of arteries 247
aortic aneurysms 497
aortic arch
  and ECHO 212
  and PDA 257
  segments of 246–7
aortic coarctation 246, 248
aortic dissections 65, 246, 261
aortic valves, bicuspid 245–6, 248
Apgar system 802
aphthoid ulcers 378–9, 381
apnoea
  postoperative 285, 739, 741
  sleep, see sleep apnoea
appendicectomy
  complications of 374–5
  and Ladd's procedure 315, 375–6
  laparoscopic 375
  and Meckel's diverticulum 335
  and meconium ileus 318, 325
appendicitis
  acute 373, 669, 691
  intrauterine 302–3
  investigations for 373–4
  perforated 374–6
appendicostomy 318, 325, 409
  continent, see Malone procedure
appendix, tumours in 669, 697
appendix testis 593
apple-peel deformity 303–4, 306

aPTT (activated partial thromboplastin
    time) 17, 118, 268, 273–4
aquaporin 536, 541
aqueductal stenosis 787
AR (androgen receptor) 572–4, 576
ARDS (acute respiratory distress
    syndrome) 25, 62, 67
Arnold–Chiari's malformation 548–9
ARPKD (autosomal recessive polycystic
    kidney disease) 504
arrhythmia
  atrial 254–5
  and commotio cordis 65
  ventricular 64
arteriovenous malformations
  genetic associations of 265
  and puberty 269
  treatment for 260
arthralgia 394, 489
arthritis 58, 394, 489, 761–2, 764
arthrogryposis 301
ascites
  and biliary atresia 433
  chylous 457
  and hydrops 178
  and inguinal hernia 284
  and liver disease 456
  and portal hypertension 430, 454,
    456, 462
  urinary 565
asparaginase 740
ASPEN syndrome 590
asplenia 255–6, 294–5, 478–80, 483;
  see also Ivemark's syndrome
asthma, and GORD 229–30
asymmetrical neck reflex 4
athelia 147–8
atorvastatin 753
atretic bowel, proximal segment of
    307–8
atrial septal defect (ASD) 243–5,
    249–52, 735
atropine 49–50
AUS (artificial urinary sphincters) 555,
    558–9
autoimmune disease 137–8, 702
AVP (arginine vasopressin) 540
azathioprine 381–2
azoospermia 321, 601

bacterial overgrowth
  and enterocolitis 401
  and microgastria 294
  and SBS 362–4
bacteriuria
  asymptomatic 517, 520–1
  symptomatic 518
balanitis 587
Bardet–Biedl's syndrome 509
bariatric surgery
  in adolescents 798–9
  criteria for 793–5
  outcomes of 795, 797–8
barium enema, see contrast enema
barium study 232
Barrett's oesophagus 223, 230, 233,
    696–7
Bartter's syndrome 136
Bassini's repair 288
battery ingestions 200, 202, 206–7
Battle's sign 55
Beck's triad 63

Beckwith–Wiedemann's syndrome
  associations of 645, 731, 736
  and hypoglycaemia 468
  and umbilical hernia 288
bedwetting, see PNE
behavioural therapy 532, 540, 544
beta blockers
  and haemangiomas 266
  and Marfan's syndrome 261
  maternal 759
  and variceal bleeding 461
Bianchi procedure 369, 371–2
bicycle accidents 77, 85, 473, 493–4,
    618
bile duct, common, see common bile
    duct
bile duct stenosis 431
bile duct strictures 428, 443, 450
bile lake infection 433–4
bile leak 81–2, 450
biliary atresia
  associations of 725
  characteristics of 429, 432–3,
    724–5
  and choledochal cyst 438
  diagnosis of 428, 432–3, 441, 726,
    729
  and HCC 661
  imaging for 731
  and jaundice 431
  and jejunoileal atresia 301
  outcome of 431, 435
  viral agents of 429
biliary cirrhosis 438–9, 441, 443
biliary dyskinesia 445, 448
biliary hypoplasia, see Alagille's
    syndrome
biliary sepsis 434, 440
biliary tree, diverticulum of 447
biliopancreatic diversion 795
bilious vomiting
  and annular pancreas 466
  and intussusception 345
  and jejunoileal atresia 304
  and malrotation 712
biofeedback 532–3, 542–4
biopsy, incisional 772
Bishop–Koop's procedure 322, 325–6,
    328
bladder
  function in infants 527
  hostile 551, 556, 558
  neurogenic, see neurogenic
    bladder
  in PBS 608
  small capacity 542, 547
bladder augmentation 512, 551, 558–9
bladder contractions
  involuntary 540
  uninhibited 528, 557
bladder distension 536, 608–9
bladder dysfunction
  assessment of 546–7
  causes of 548–9
  neuropathic causes of 537, 546,
    550, 554
  and PUV 567
  types of 547
bladder enlargement 512
bladder exstrophy 608–14
bladder instability 529, 531
bladder neck surgery 558–9

bladder outlet obstruction
  causes of 562
  conditions associated with 510–11
  fetal 564
  management of 558
  and PBS 609
bladder pressure, increased 522
bladder rupture
  extraperitoneal 90
  intraperitoneal 90–1
Blalock–Taussig shunt 253
blisters, sucking 118
blood, cord 12
blood cultures 12–13, 488, 762
blood loss
  in children 51
  clinical signs of 29
blood sugars 9, 665, 748
blood transfusion
  and fluid resuscitation 51
  and haemophiliacs 18
  massive 743–4
  risks of 14
blood volume 22, 743
Blount's disease 771–2
blunt abdominal trauma
  and CT scan 80, 86
  and haemorrhagic cysts 630
  and kidney injury 84
  non-operative management of 72–3
  organs injured in 71
  and pancreatic pseudocysts 474
  and renovascular injury 89
BMI (body mass index) 791, 793–4,
  797, 800
Boari flap 89–90
Bochdalek's hernia 733–5
Boerema's repair 238
Boix–Ochoa's repair 238
bone cysts 773–4
bone marrow disease 687
bone tumours
  benign 773
  malignant 642, 772–3
Bougienage method 202
bowel duplications 345
bowel dysfunction 528, 546
BPD (bronchiopulmonary dysplasia)
  758, 795
bradycardia, postoperative 741
brain death 748–9
brain injury, traumatic, see TBI
brain tumours 699–700, 704
branchial arch
  embryology 129
  removal of remnants 131–2
branchial cleft cysts 717
breast, anatomy of 146–7
breast abscesses 148, 150
breast cancer
  common malignancies 154
  genetics of 153–4
  primary 153
  and PTEN mutation 271
  risk factors for 152
  secondary to radiotherapy 688
  and soft tissue sarcoma 697
breast deformities, congenital 147–8
breast development, asymmetric 148–9
breast discharge 146, 151
breast milk
  and lactobezoars 209

and NEC 351
nutritional content of 9
and SBS 368–9
bronchial artery embolisation 185
bronchiectasis 184–5, 230
bronchodilators 113, 203, 759
bronchogenic cysts 131, 195–6
bronchopulmonary sequestrations
  (BPS) 176, 180–1, 243
bronchoscopy
  OA and TOF 212, 215–16
  and foreign bodies 203, 205
bruising
  causes of 117
  unexplained 118
buckle fractures 97
Buck's fascia 587
Budd–Chiari's syndrome 453, 457, 463,
  659–60
Burkitt's lymphoma 594, 637–9,
  689–93
burn dressings 110
burn injuries 10, 106, 108
burns
  chemical 113–14, 697
  depth of 106–7, 107
  electrical 114–15
  fluid management in 10
  hyper-metabolic response to 111–12
  oral 220
  pharyngeal 221
  topical agents for 109
BXO (balanitis xerotica obliterans)
  511, 578, 583–4

C-cell hyperplasia 667–8
café-au-lait macules 117–18
caffeine
  and anaesthesia 739
  and incontinence 524, 532
  and jejunoileal atresia 301
CAIS, see AIS (androgen insensitivity
  syndrome), complete
calcaneovalgus 765, 768
calcium, absorption of 309, 367
Calot's triangle 437
calyces 496–8
canal of Nuck 284
cannabis 151, 155
cannulation 37, 43, 449, 453
capillary haemangiomas 117–18
caput medusae 453
caput succedaneum 121
carbon dioxide ($CO_2$) 32–3, 173, 738
carbon monoxide 112–13
carboplatin 641, 650
carcinoid syndrome 333–4
carcinoid tumours 333, 669, 697
cardiac anomalies
  congenital 245–6, 248, 250
  and ECHO 212
  and ECMO 34
  fetal 172
  and malrotation 316
cardiac contusion 65, 69
cardiac injury
  blunt 244
  and guide wires 40
  and OR equipment 157
  and pectus bars 157, 160
cardiac lesions 28

congenital 251
cardiac output
  and abdominal compartment
    syndrome 76
  changes in 27
cardiac tamponade
  and central venous catheters 38, 42
  and shock 23
  signs of 63–4
  and TPN 14
cardiac transplantation, see heart
  transplant
cardiac tumours 242–3
cardiogenic shock 24, 28
cardiomyopathy 251, 688, 752
cardiothoracic surgery, equipment for
  157
cardiovascular collapse 22
Caroli's disease 726, 728, 730
catecholamines 26–8, 30, 111, 667–8
catheterisable channels 533, 560
catheters
  Hickman and Broviac 40
  migration of tip 42–3
  peripheral IV 52
caudal block, see anaesthesia, caudal
caustic agents
  burns 113
  ingestion 218–23
cavitary disease 189
CCAM (congenital cystic adenomatoid
  malformation of the lung) 176,
  780–2, 786, 789
CDH (congenital diaphragmatic hernia)
  and Cornelia de Lange syndrome
    708
  and CPAP 34
  and ECMO 33–4
  and EXIT treatment 780
  and GORD 228
  long-term complications of 173
  and malrotation 315
  and Meckel's diverticulum 332
  and MIRROR syndrome 789
  multiple children with 174
  presentation of 170–1
  prognosis for 172, 783
  and pulmonary development 170
  repair of 171, 173
  and respiratory distress 734
cellulitis 150, 762
central venous catheters
  and cardiac tamponade 14, 38
  and complications 39–40
  and haemophilia 39
  infection rate of 36
  percutaneous 38–9
  peripheral, see PICCs
  positioning of 41–2
  and thromboembolism 740
  and TPN 12, 14
cephalhaematoma 57, 121
cerebellar astrocytomas 704
cerebral palsy
  and bladder dysfunction 547, 557
  and corticosteroids 758
  and cryptorchidism 595
  and neglect 120
cervical agenesis 622–3
cervical spine 49, 54, 102, 274, 625
cervical teratoma 679, 682, 787
CFTR gene 319–22, 329

CHAOS (congenital high airway obstruction syndrome) 780–1, 785
chemotherapy
  and acute tumour lysis syndrome 639
  and CCSK 649
  and embryonal sarcoma 661
  and germ cell tumours 633
  and lymphoma 637, 690
  myeloablative 639, 641
  neo-adjuvant 641
  and neoplasms 662
  and neuroblastoma 654
  prenephrectomy 646–7
  and PTLD 747
  and rhabdomyosarcoma 640, 664
  and SCFE 771
  side effects of 688
  and tumour lysis syndrome 692
chest injury
  and cardiac contusion 69
  and cardiac tamponade 64
  and oesophageal perforation 68
  and pneumothorax 63
chest tube placement 66
chest wall deformities 157, 173
chest X-ray
  and foreign bodies 203, 204
  and fractures 119
  and respiratory distress 759
Chiari malformation 776–8, 785
child abuse
  and bruising 117–18
  and burn injuries 106
  conditions mistaken for 117–18
  fractures associated with 119
  risk of 116
  types of 47
  and vaginal lacerations 93
child protective services, referral to 616, 619–21
cholangiocarcinoma 439, 443, 447
cholangiography 727
  operative 440, 442, 446
cholangitis
  causes of 443
  postoperative 430
  recurrent 430, 434–5, 442
  sclerosing 438–9
  uncontrolled 442
cholecystectomy
  endangered structures in 437, 450
  and gallstones 483
  indications for 441–2, 446, 448–9
  laparoscopic 446–7, 449–50
  and mesenteric adenitis 445
  and SCD 18
cholecystitis 81–2, 444–7
  acalculous 446
choledochal cyst
  and biliary atresia 725
  complications of 438–9
  diagnosis of 441, 447, 727–30
  fetal 441
  investigations for 440
  and jaundice 431
  in liver biopsy 428
  presentation of 436–9
  surgery of 442
  type I 436, 440–1
  viral agents of 429
choledochoduodenoscopy 450

choledochojejunostomy 440, 450
choledocholithiasis 446
cholelithiasis
  and bariatric surgery 795
  and choledochal cysts 439
  and gallbladder disease 444
  incidence of 444–5
  and jaundice 431
  and jejunectomy 363
  and spherocytosis 448
cholestasis 362, 428, 443, 729
chordee
  in epispadias 614
  and hypospadias 576–7
  and penile torsion 591
  recurrent 579
choriocarcinoma 197–8, 631–2, 680, 684
chorionic venous sampling 779–80
Chvostek's sign 670
chylothorax 188–90, 257–8
chylous cysts 312
CIC (clean intermittent catheterisation)
  and diurnal incontinence 532
  and neurogenic bladder 512, 558–9
  and PUV 567
  and spina bifida 551
  and spinal injury 558
  and VUR/UTI 525
cimetidine 155, 235
circumcision
  and BXO 583
  complications from 585–6
  and concealed penis 587
  incidence of 582
  indications for 584
  and penis injury 92
  and urethritis 511
  and UTIs 524, 566
cirrhosis
  childhood 428
  compensated 455–6, 458, 462
  and graft vs. host disease 637
  and gynaecomastia 155
  and HCC 661
  and Kasai's procedure 434–5
  and variceal bleeding 461
cis-retinoic acid 639, 655
cisapride 235–6
clear cell carcinoma 648–9
clindamycin 188, 763
clinical trials, relative risk in 801
cloaca
  and hydrocolpos 422–3
  and neurogenic bladder 555–6
  and rectovaginal fistula 425
  rectum in 423–4
  short-channel 413
cloacal exstrophy
  and cryptorchidism 595
  and neurogenic bladder 556
  presentation of 614
  theory for development of 610
clotting factors, activation of 17
clotting tests 17
CLOVES syndrome 274
clubfeet 765, 767–8
CNS (central nervous system), and bladder dysfunction 547–8
coagulation, inhibition of 16
coagulation necrosis 113, 219
coagulopathy

consumptive 457
  and haemangioendothelioma 659
  and snakebite 104
cobblestone pattern 379–81
codeine 368, 746
Cohen technique 523
coin ingestions 201–2, 205
colectomy 382
colitis
  acute severe 382
  infectious 380, 394
  symptoms of 394
  ulcerative 381
colloid goitre 137
colloids 10, 25, 30, 51
colocystoplasty, seromuscular 560
colon injuries 79
colonic atresia 301, 304
colonic duplication 339
colonic polyps 384, 386–7
colorectal cancer 385, 392
colostogram, high-pressure distal 419–21, 420–1, 423
colostomy 79, 402–3, 407–8, 418–19, 423
  diverting descending 419
common bile duct
  dilated 446
  perforation of 431
  repair of 450
  retained terminal 443
commotio cordis 65
compartment syndrome 53, 97, 103
condylar fractures 97
congenital adrenal hyperplasia (CAH) 143–4, 492, 601–2, 604–5
congenital anomalies, and kidney injury 85
congenital haemangioma 263, 273
congenital heart disease
  and aortic arch anomalies 246
  and atrial morphology 248
  and Blalock–Taussig shunt 254
  and CDH 735
  and ELS 182
  and malrotation 313
  radiography of 251
  and septal defects 245
  and thromboembolism 740
congestive heart failure (CHF)
  and embolisation 267
  and haemangioendothelioma 658–9
  and Kasabach–Merritt's syndrome 696
  and sacrococcygeal teratomas 683
constipation
  and adjuvant therapy 643
  and Crohn's disease 383
  idiopathic 397, 401, 403–5, 412
  and LUTS 529
  and overflow incontinence 408
  and sexual abuse 119
  and teratomas 698
  and UTI management 524
continence protocol 524
contrast enema
  agents for 319
  and Crohn's disease 378–9
  and Hirschsprung's disease 398
  and idiopathic constipation 404
  and incontinence 414–15
  and Meckel's diverticulum 335

contrast enema (*continued*)
and meconium ileus 318–19, 323, 326–8
of rectosigmoid 415
contrast oesophagram 220, 708
Convention on the Rights of the Child 123
Cooper's ligaments 147
coronal synostosis 776
corticosteroids
and BPD 758
and foreign bodies 206
and haemangioma 266–7
and hyperplasia 790
and thromboembolism 740
and vascular tumours 264–5
coughing
chronic 232
and foreign bodies 205
Cowden's syndrome 271, 387
cow's milk protein allergy 392, 395–6
CPAM (congenital pulmonary adenomatoid malformation) 175–82
CPAP (continuous positive airway pressure) 34
craniosynostosis 776
craniotomy 58
creatinine 492, 506, 609, 750–1
cremasteric reflex 592, 596
Crohn's disease (CD)
genetic features of 377
investigations for 378–80
and Meckel's diverticulum 332, 334
presentation of 380–1, 383
in remission 381–2
and SBS 359
treatment for 383–4
croup 164, 745
CRP (C-reactive protein) 158, 353, 762–3
cryptorchidism
associations of 595
and gastroschisis 281–2
and hypospadias 570, 572, 575
and inguinal hernia 284
and PUV 568
and TDS 575
and testicular tumours 684
and Wilms's tumour 722
CSF (cerebrospinal fluid) 55, 687, 757, 778, 785, 787
CT (computed-tomography)
and abdominal trauma 80, 473
and alimentary tract duplications 341
and ankle fractures 99
and bone tumours 772
and bruising 118
and choledochal cysts 440
and gallbladder dysmotility 445
and hepatoblastoma 721
and investigation of haematuria 86–7
and oesophageal duplication 709
pelvic 723–4
and retropharyngeal abscess 720
single photon emission, *see* SPECT
CT-angiography 61, 65, 459
Currarino's syndrome 549, 554, 681, 777
Curreri formula 112
Cushing's syndrome 138, 142, 670–1

cutaneous haemangiomas 167, 169, 272, 658
cutaneous necrosis 104
cyanide toxicity 112–13
cyclophosphamide
and CCSK 649
and haemangioma 266
and lymphoma 637
and renal rhabdoid tumour 650
and rhabdomyosarcoma 640
cyclosporine 191, 382, 751, 753–4
cyst rupture 439, 442
cystadenocarcinomas 632
cystadenomas 627, 629, 632
cysteine 9, 15
cystic duct diverticulum 448–9
cystic fibrosis
genetic testing for 320–1
and haemoptysis 185
and inguinal hernia 284
and liver biopsy 428
and meconium ileus 318–22, 328–9
and pancreas 467
and pathogens 184
and pneumothorax 187
and *Pseudomonas* 190
surgical indications 190
cystic hygroma, *see* lymphatic malformations, macrocystic
cystic lung lesions, *see* lung lesions, cystic
cystitis, haemorrhagic 640
cystogram 86–7, 90, 511, 531
cystosarcoma phyllodes 150, 152
cytarabine 637–8
cytomegalovirus (CMV) 3, 123, 429, 736, 749, 758
cytoscopic valve ablation, fetal 781–2

dactinomycin 638, 640, 645–7, 684
data
continuous 802
semigraphical summarisation of 804
daunorubicin 642
day-case surgery 285, 737, 741–2
DCMO (diffuse capillary malformation with overgrowth) 274
DDAVP, *see* desmopressin
DDH (developmental dysplasia of the hip) 766
death, causes of 46–7
decannulation, accidental 745
defibrillation, and pectus bars 158
Deflux 524–5, 559
dehydration, and urinary incontinence 530
Denver Developmental Screening test 7
Denys–Drash's syndrome 645
depression, clinical 794
dermoid cysts 132, 629, 631, 716
desflurane 739
desmopressin 536, 539–41
detrusor hyperreflexia 550, 553–4, 558
detrusor hypertonicity 550–1
detrusor instability 528, 531, 536, 567
detrusor irritability 542
detrusor overactivity 528, 536, 540–3, 547–8
detrusor sphincter dyssynergia 548, 550–1, 553, 567
detrusorectomy 560
developmental assessment 7, 123

developmental delay 123, 294
dexamethasone 181, 670–1
dextrocardia 243
diabetes
complications of 748
gestational 759, 791–2
and hypovolaemia 23
maternal 571, 756–8
and priapism 589
and renal failure 750
and surgery 741
diabetes insipidus 537, 566, 748
diabetes mellitus
and bariatric surgery 794, 800
genetics of 321
and Graves's disease 138
and urinary incontinence 537
diagnostic laparoscopy
and diaphragmatic injuries 70
and dysmenorrhoea 625
and stab wounds 82
dialysis
and acquired cystic renal disease 503
and heart transplant 752
diaphragmatic eventration 734–6
diaphragmatic injuries 70
diaphyseal fractures 101–2, 119
diarrhoea
controlling 368
and cow's milk exclusion diet 392
and hypovolaemia 23
and microgastria 294
and NEC 395–6
and SBS 364, 372
secretory 401
diazoxide 143, 468, 677
Dieulafoy lesion 395
dihydrotestosterone (DHT)
and genital development 572
and hypospadias 573, 576
and micropenis 588
and testosterone 606
DIOS (distal intestinal obstruction syndrome) 467
distal atresia 280, 308
distal radius 97, 101
diurnal incontinence
beginning of symptoms 527–8
and constipation 529
and LUTS 530
and PUV 564, 566–7
and stress activity 541
treatment of 532–3
and urodynamics 541
diverticulectomy 335
DMSA scan
and pyelonephritis 491, 526
and renal investigations 500, 507, 513
and UTIs 517, 520, 522
dobutamine 24–5
dog bites 105–6
domperidone 235–6
Donation after Cardiac Death (DCD) 749, 754
dorsal midline albuginea plication 576
dorsal tunica albuginea plication 577, 579
double bubble sign 311, 712, 713
double track sign 711
Down's syndrome
and annular pancreas 465

associations of 645
and CDH 735
and duodenal atresia 301, 714
and exomphalos 279
and imperforate anus 424
and intestinal pseudo-obstruction 405
and Meckel's diverticulum 332
and umbilical hernia 288
doxorubicin
cardiotoxicity of 642
and CCSK 649
teratogeny of 302
as vesicant 638
and Wilms's tumour 645–6
DPL (diagnostic peritoneal lavage) 53, 70, 80–2
drowning 46–7
DSD (disorders of sexual differentiation), and hypospadias 580, 604
Duchenne's muscular dystrophy 405, 765
Duhamel procedure 403
duodenal atresia
aetiology of 302
and annular pancreas 465
associations of 214, 714
and distant gas 313
and jejunoileal atresia 301
location of 713
and malrotation 315
with OA and TOF 214
and pyloric atresia 293
duodenal duplications 340, 447
duodenal injury 77–9
duodenal lesions 385
duodenal stenosis 313, 466
duodenal ulcers 296, 334
duodenoduodenostomy 466
duodenojejunal junction 306, 308, 310–12, 711–12
duodenojejunal loop 310
dysfunctional elimination syndrome 528–30, 537, 546
dysgerminoma 631–2, 680
dysmenorrhoea 625–6
dysphagia
and alimentary tract duplications 340
and GOR 213, 230–1, 233
progressive 720
dysplasias, definition of 765
dyspnoea
and airway obstruction 193
exertional 455
dysuria, and circumcision 584

EBL (estimated blood loss) 29, 51
ecchymoses 55, 618, 670
ECG (electrocardiogram) 69, 114–15, 212
echocardiogram, and sacrococcygeal teratoma 680
ECMO (extracorporeal membrane oxygenation) 33–4, 173–4, 780, 783
eczema 392
EGF (epidermal growth factor) 360, 574
Ehlers–Danlos's syndrome 117, 284, 286
elbow dislocations 100–1
elbow fractures 100–1
electrical injuries 114–15

embolisation
and arteriovenous malformations 260, 265, 267
bronchial artery 185
embryonal carcinoma 197, 631–2, 680
emesis, see vomiting
EMLA cream, and cannulation 37
empyema
and haemothorax 67–8
organisms causing 190
primary therapy for 183
treatment for 186–7
encephalopathy
hypoxic ischaemic 122
and portal hypertension 455
encopresis 119, 403–4, 529, 544
EndoCinch procedure 239
endodermal sinus tumour, see yolk sac tumour
endometriosis 376, 625
endopyelotomy 513–14
endoscopic surgery, fetal 781
endoscopic variceal ligator (EVL) 393
endoscopy
capsule 379–80
and caustic ingestion 221, 225
and foreign body removal 202
and GOR 233
grading of injury 221
upper GI 378, 390, 458
wireless capsule, see WCE
endothelial cells 16
endotracheal intubation
and epignathus 787
and EXIT procedure 780, 783
frequency of 49
and resuscitation 108
and RSI 743
and TOF 216
and tracheostomy 745
enemas
administering 410–11
bowel management with 412–15
checking colon after 408
and constipation 412
contrast, see contrast enema
and enterocolitis 401
and incontinence 412–16, 552, 560
and laxatives 410
and Malone procedure 409
and voiding disorders 545
enteral feeding
and Crohn's disease 381–2
and duodenal haematoma 78
and lactobezoar 209
and SBS 364–6
enterectomy 363, 368
enteric duplications 338, 341, 391
enterocolitis
and Hirschsprung's disease 400–2, 404
necrotising, see NEC
enterocystoplasty 559–60
enteroplasty
serial transverse, see STEP
tapering 309, 370
enteroscopy, intraoperative 394–5
enterostomy 319, 324–7
enuresis risoria 528
environmental disrupting chemicals (EDC) 574
epicondylar fractures 101

epidermoid cysts 384–5
epidermolysis bullosa 293
epididymo-orchitis 593–4
epidural blocks 737
epiglottitis 162, 164–5
epignathus 787
epilepsy, post-traumatic 60
epispadias 537, 610, 613–14
epithelial metaplasia 386, 437
epithelial plugging 302
Epstein–Barr virus 429, 690, 693–4, 702, 747
Erb's palsy 121–2
ERCP (endoscopic retrograde cholangiopancreatography)
and bile leak 82
and choledochal cyst 439–40
complications of 449
and gallbladder disease 445, 447
and PD 466
ergotamine tartrate 300–1
erythroblastosis fetalis 789
erythromycin 19, 753
Escherichia coli 148, 515, 760
ESR (erythrocyte sedimentation rate) 762–4
etoposide 633, 649–50, 688
Ewing's sarcoma 762, 772–3
EXIT procedure
and CCAM 782
and CDH 783
and hydrops 181
and teratoma 682, 787
uses of 780–1
exomphalos 34, 278–82
exstrophy; see also bladder extrophy; cloacal extrophy
classic 611–12
closure 612–13
embryonic development of 610
male genital defects in 611
external fixation 96, 98
extrahepatic biliary system 437
extraintestinal anomalies 301
extralobar sequestrations (ELSs) 176, 180, 182
extraperitoneal haematoma 90

facial haemangiomas 168
facial nerve 131–2, 670
factor VII 17, 461
factor VIII 39
faecal disimpaction 412
faecal incontinence 403, 407–16, 551–2, 555, 558
falls 52, 56–7
FAP (familial adenomatous polyposis) 384–5, 387, 660–1
FAST exam 53, 64, 69, 80–1
fat, brown 737–8
fat malabsorption 309, 363–4, 366
femoral fractures
open 51, 98
proximal 97
shaft 98
femoral hernia 287–8
fentanyl 49, 738
fetal circulation 35–6, 244, 441
fetal deficiency states 789
fetal loss 280, 563–4, 779–80
fetal surgery, open 182, 781, 784–5, 788
fetus, fluid compartments in 11

fetus in fetu 698
fever
    and lymphoma 690
    unexplained 68, 516
FGF (fibroblast growth factor) 435, 574
fibrinolytic therapy 67
fibroadenomas 149–50, 152
fibroma 242
    non-ossifying 773
fibromatosis colli 718
fibromuscular dysplasia 493
fibrosing colonopathy (FC) 467
fine needle aspiration (FNA) 131, 667, 673–4
first-arch syndrome 715
Fisher's exact test 805
fistula
    enterocutaneous 326
    enteroenteric 205
    locations of 420
    perineal 413, 417, 420, 422, 424
    recto-bladder neck 413, 421, 424
    rectobulbar 417, 421
    rectourethral 417
    rectovaginal 425
    rectovestibular 413, 417, 425
    tracheo-oesophageal, see TOF
        (tracheo-oesophageal fistula)
    tracheocutaneous 161
    urethral cutaneous 578
    vestibular 413, 417, 422
fluconazole 753
fluid compartments 11
fluid management
    in premature infants 11
    in severe burns 10
fluid overload 14, 25
fluid resuscitation
    and ARDS 25
    colloid 30–1
    steps in 51
FNH (focal nodular hyperplasia)
    657–8, 661, 721
Fogarty catheter 207–8, 212, 214
folate 366–7, 798
Foley catheter
    and bladder rupture 90–1
    and enemas 410
    and foreign body removal 202
    and intra-abdominal pressure 76
    and urethral injury 86
follicular lesions 674
follicular lymphoma 690
Fontan procedure 254–5
food bolus 208, 227
foot conditions, congenital 768
foramen magnum decompression 778
forearm fractures 101–2
foregut cysts 192–3, 196
foreign bodies
    aspiration of 203–5, 208
    impaction of 201, 205–6, 208
    and intussusception 390
    and Meckel's diverticulum 333
    removal of 201–2, 205–8
    vaginal 617
Fournier's gangrene 585–6
fracture fixation 96
fracture remodelling 94–5
fractures
    Chance 77

and child abuse 119
    with high complication rates 96–7
    open 51, 90, 96
    pathological 763, 773
functional bladder capacity (FBC) 535–7
functional bladder disorder 541
fungal infections 750
furosemide 141, 507

gallbladder
    duplication of 447
    hydrops of 445
gallbladder disease, aetiology of 444
gallbladder dysmotility 445
gallstones
    and bariatric surgery 795
    and cholelithiasis 444
    and SBS 309
    and SCD 18
    and splenectomy 483
    types of 448
ganglioneuromas 192–3, 195, 197, 387
Gardner's syndrome 385, 659–61
gastric acid 235, 342
gastric atresia 301
gastric duplications 293–4, 341–3, 711
gastric hypersecretion 362–3, 366–8
gastric juice 227, 235
gastric lesions 385
gastric mucosa
    ectopic 333–5, 340–2, 391
    heterotopic 331–4, 336, 391
    and rectal bleeding 391
gastric outlet obstruction 223, 295
gastric perforation
    and antibiotics 222
    and lactobezoars 209
    in newborn 296
    and TOF 216
gastric volvulus, see volvulus, gastric
gastrinomas 470–2
gastritis 389, 441, 443, 458
gastro-oesophageal reflux (GOR)
    and caustic ingestion 225
    and CDH 173
    diagnosis of 231, 233
    and exomphalos 282
    features of 226
    and gastric duplications 293
    and gastrostomy 234–5
    and microgastria 294–5
    natural barriers to 227
    and neurological impairment 234
    and OA/TOF 213, 217
    symptoms of 231–2
    treatment for 235–6, 239–40
gastro-oesophageal reflux disease
    (GORD)
    definition of 226
    and bariatric surgery 794
    complications of surgery 239
    damage caused by 227
    incidence of 228–31
    presentation of 374
gastroenteritis 344, 405
gastrografin 318–19, 322–4, 327, 467
gastrointestinal anastomosis (GIA)
    371–2
gastrointestinal bleeding
    acute 82
    causes of 396
    lower 393

and Meckel's diverticulum 332
    obscure 393–5
    and portal hypertension 454
gastrointestinal stromal tumours (GIST)
    389, 696
gastrointestinal tract, upper 221,
    232–3, 236
gastrojejunostomy 79
gastroschisis
    associations of 279, 732
    complications of repair 733
    and CPAP 34
    diagnosis of 731–2
    fetal 788
    and GORD 228
    and malrotation 282
    management of 280
    outcome of 281–2
    and SBS 359
gastrostomy
    and caustic ingestion 221
    and GOR 230, 234–5
    percutaneous endoscopic, see PEG
    and TOF 214, 216
    tubes 365
GCS (Glasgow Coma Score) 53–4,
    54–5, 60, 62, 81, 473
gender reassignment 587–8
genital anomalies 496, 570
genital defects, male 611
genital tract, outflow obstruction
    622–4, 626
genital trauma 618–20
genitalia, ambiguous 601–3, 605–6
genu recurvatum 98–9
germ cell tumours
    associations of 680
    mature 683
    most common 679
    ovarian 632–3, 684
    and PET scan 642
    secretions of 680
    testicular 681, 684
germ cells, primordial 679
germinoma tumours 680
Gerota's fascia 85, 650
GH (growth hormone) 142, 360, 588
giggle incontinence 528
Gilbert's disease 431
glans, amputation of 585
glans dehiscence 577, 579
Glenn shunt 254
glomerulosclerosis, focal segmental
    499, 750
GLP-2 360
glucagon 334, 360, 468
glucocorticoids 143–4, 468, 604–5,
    789–90
glue ear 232
glutamine 360, 365
glycogen storage disease 141, 468, 661
glycopyrrolate 544, 738
glycosuria 10, 531
goitres 137
gonadal dysgenesis 573
    mixed 572, 601–2, 703
gonadal neoplasms 679
gonadoblastoma 594, 602, 703
Gorham–Stout's disease 274
gout 589, 666
graft thrombosis 750
graft vs. host disease 636–7

granulomas 263, 380
granulosa cell tumour 632
grasp reflex 4–5, 121–2
Graves's disease 134, 137–8
great vessels, transposition of 478
greenstick fractures 101–2
Grisel's syndrome 58
growth charts 124, 125
growth failure 138, 383
growth plates 94–6, 98–9, 763
GTN (nitroglycerine) 37
guide wire 39–40, 80, 212, 215
gunshot wounds 29
gut development 314
gynaecomastia 154–5, 601

haemangioendothelioma, infantile
    657–9, 664, 696
haematemesis
    evaluating 389–90, 395
    and GOR 231
    in neonates 396
    and portal hypertension 454–5
haematochezia 391, 454–5
haematoceles 92, 598
haematopoiesis, primary organ of 477
haematuria
    and graft dysfunction 750
    and HSP 489
    investigation of 86
    macroscopic 493–4
    and renal rhabdoid tumour 649
haemobilia 81–2
haemodynamic instability 72, 79,
    87–8, 185
haemofiltration 33, 477
haemopericardium 64, 69
haemophilia 18, 39, 118, 741
Haemophilus influenzae
    and early onset sepsis 760
    and empyema 190
    and splenectomy 74, 485
    type B 19
    and vaginitis 617
haemoptysis 185, 189–90
haemorrhage
    and ECMO 33
    intralesional 272, 663
    and skull fracture 56
haemorrhagic cysts 630
haemorrhagic shock 51, 81
haemostatic response 16
haemothorax 61–2, 66–7
Hagen–Poiseuille formula 35
hamartoma
    and intussusception 345
    lipovascular 271, 274
    mesenchymal 658, 662
hamartomatous polyps 384–5, 387,
    595
handlebar contusion 473
HBS, see scintigraphy, hepatobiliary
HCC, see hepatocellular carcinoma
head trauma 46, 58, 121
hearing impairment, and language
    development 6
hearing loss, and platinum 688
heart block 135
heart disease, cyanotic 478
heart failure
    and Fontan procedure 254–5
    high output 270, 662, 788

low output 178
    and thyrotoxicosis 135, 247
heart–lung transplants 752
heart transplant 34, 255, 752
heartburn 230–1, 374
Hegar dilator 425–6
Heimlich's manoeuvre 203
Heliobacter pylori 232–3, 333, 703
HELLP syndrome 789
hemihypertrophy 271, 468, 645, 731
hemivaginas 423–4, 423
hemivertebrae 555–6, 725–6
Henoch–Schönlein's purpura (HSP)
    117, 349, 390, 393, 488–9
hepatic dysfunction, and TPN 362
hepatic encephalopathy 430, 462
hepatic fibrosis 437, 439, 441
    congenital 456, 459, 661
hepatic haemangioma 270, 658
hepatic neoplasms, surgical resection
    of 662
hepatic trisegmentectomy 665
hepatic tumours, most common 657
hepatic venography, transjugular 458–9
hepaticoduodenostomy 441, 443
hepaticoenterostomy 441
hepaticojejunostomy 440–3
hepatitis
    differential diagnosis of 730
    and HCC 661
    idiopathic neonatal 431–2
    and lymphoma 703
    and organ transplant 749
hepatoblastoma
    associations of 659–61
    and chemotherapy 641
    diagnosis of 721
    incidence of 657
    and PET scan 642
    staging of 696
    subtypes of 659
hepatocellular adenoma 658, 661,
    663
hepatocellular carcinoma (HCC)
    associations of 661
    diagnosis of 721
    and hepatitis 664
    incidence of 657
    signs of 658
    staging of 696
    and type I GSD 663
hepatocellular diseases 456–7, 460
hepatomegaly 270, 456, 658
hepatopulmonary syndrome 440, 455
hepatorrhaphy 75
hernias
    incarcerated 284–6
    internal 302–3
    sliding 285–6
heterotaxy syndrome 249, 255, 313
HIDA scan 82, 445–7
Hill's repair 238
hindgut duplications 341–2
Hinman's syndrome 542, 544, 547
hip dislocation, congenital 284
hip dysplasia, developmental, see DDH
hip fractures 97
Hirschsprung's disease
    and aganglionosis 399–400
    diagnosis of 398–9, 404–5
    and enterocolitis 401
    familial involvement in 397–8

and idiopathic constipation 404
incidence of 397
and IND 406
and jejunoileal atresia 301
and Meckel's diverticulum 332
pathology of 400
and SBS 359
and small bowel obstruction 317
treatment of 402–3
histamine H1-receptor antagonists 236
histamine H2-receptor antagonists 235
HIT procedure 525
HIV infection 130, 584, 693–4, 749
hoarseness 66, 166, 232, 257–8
Hodgkin's lymphoma
    B symptoms of 693
    and chemotherapy 688
    diagnosis of 687
    in the mediastinum 193
    and PET scan 642
    presentation of 691
    and radiotherapy 688, 692
    risk factors for 693–4
    sites of extralymphatic spread 687
    and splenectomy 481
    types of 686–7
HOSE (Hypospadias Objective Scoring
    Evaluation) 580
human papilloma virus (HPV) 166,
    429, 620
humerus fractures 100
humoral immunity 19
Hunter–Hurler's syndrome 284, 286,
    288
hydrocephalus
    and aqueductal stenosis 787
    associations of 775, 777
    causes of 775, 778
    and myelomeningocele 785
    post-traumatic 58
    and puberty 552
    treatment for 776
hydrocele 286–7, 489
hydrocolpos 422–3
hydrocortisone 30, 382
hydrofluoric acid 114
hydrogen peroxide 20, 324
hydronephrosis
    bilateral 511, 565
    and dysfunctional voiding 531
    and hydrocolpos 423
    and kidney injury 85, 88
    and MRKH 624
    and PBS 607
    and stone disease 498
    unilateral 508
    and VUR 522
hydrops
    and CPAM 177–8
    fetal 789
    of the gallbladder 445
    and nephroma 649
    treatment for 181
hydrostatic reduction 344, 347–8
hydroureter 424, 499, 624
hydroureteronephrosis
    bilateral 490, 563, 565
    in PBS 609
    and PUV 567, 782
    and spina bifida 550
    and spinal injuries 558
hymen, imperforate 622–3

hyperaldosteronism
  primary 136–7, 675–6
  secondary 297
hyperammonaemia 454–5, 457
hyperbilirubinaemia 431, 433
  conjugated 724, 728, 756
hypercalcaemia
  in cancer patients 650, 702
  familial hypocalciuric 135–6
  and HPT 141
hypercalciuria, absorptive 541
hypercortisolism 138, 670, 676
hyperglycaemia
  and burns 112
  maternal 756, 759
  and tissue perfusion 26
  TPN-induced 10
hyperinsulinism
  congenital, see PHHI
  fetal 756
hyperkalaemia
  and anaesthesia 739–40
  and blood transfusions 14, 744
  and Burkitt's lymphoma 692
  and CAH 143
hyperparathyroidism 140–1, 672, 677, 702
hyperphosphataemia 639, 691–2
hyperprolactinaemia 151
hypersplenism 18, 455, 457, 461
hypertension
  and ADPKD 505
  and adrenal dysfunction 136
  and artery stenosis 259
  and bariatric surgery 794
  and herniotomy 492
  and hyperaldosteronism 676
  intracranial 60
  and kidney injury 88
  and metabolic syndrome 792
  and MIRROR syndrome 789
  and phaeochromocytoma 668
  pulmonary, see pulmonary
    hypertension
  and renal failure 750
  renovascular 492–3
  and SGA infants 3
hyperthyroidism
  and breast discharge 151
  causes of 134, 137–8
  and gynaecomastia 155
hypertrophic pyloric stenosis
  associations of 711
  and gastric duplication 294
  and GI bleeding 396
  imaging for 710–11
  incidence of 297
  management of 298
  and metabolic derangement 297–8
hyperuricaemia 665–6, 692
hypoalbuminaemia 455, 489, 665
hypocalcaemia 14, 639, 670, 692
hypochloraemia 13, 297
hypoganglionosis 318, 399, 404, 406
hypoglycaemia; see also PHHI
  and adrenal insufficiency 140
  and Beckwith–Wiedemann's
    syndrome 645
  and diabetes 759
  and insulinoma 471
  and liver resections 665
  neonatal 645, 731, 756, 759
  and propranolol 266

hypoglycaemic unawareness 748
hypogonadism 771
hypokalaemia
  and adrenal dysfunction 136
  and hyperaldosteronism 676
hyponatraemia
  and adrenal insufficiency 140
  and burn ointments 109
  and CAH 143
  and ileostomy 358
hypoparathyroidism 670
hypoperfusion, secondary brain 81
hypopituitarism 605, 771
hypospadias
  distal 575–6, 604
  and DSD 604
  and ectopic kidney 496
  endocrine causes of 573
  environmental factors in 574
  evaluation of 575–6
  examination for 537
  genetics of 572
  idiopathic 571
  incidence of 570–1
  and penile torsion 591
  posterior 575–7, 580
  and proteins 574
  and TDS 575
hypospadias repair 509, 576–81
hypotension
  and air embolism 40
  and cardiac tamponade 63
  delayed 22
  and epidurals 737
  and intussusception 347
  and propranolol 266
  and shock 27, 31, 51
  and snakebite 103
  and spider bites 104
hypothermia
  and blood transfusion 744
  controlled 122
  and respiratory distress 758
hypothyroidism
  acquired 139
  and breast discharge 151
  in children 133–4
  congenital 270, 288, 658
  fetal 789–90
  and gynaecomastia 155
  and haemangioendothelioma
    659
  and hyperbilirubinaemia 756
  and radiotherapy 688
  and SCFE 771
hypovolaemia
  and blood loss 29
  and enterocolitis 401
  and meconium ileus 323
  and peritonitis 322, 324
hypovolaemic shock 22–4, 26, 28,
    51, 327
hypoxaemia
  and inhalation injury 112
  persistent 455
  and priapism 590
  secondary 67
hypoxia
  and ATD 338
  and RSI 743
  and SCD 589
hysterotomy 781

icterus, fluctuating 724, 729
ifosfamide 640, 642
ileal atresia, see small bowel atresia
ileal disease 381
ileocaecal junction 310–11
ileocaecal valve 331, 361–4, 367, 560
ileostomy
  complications of 358
  and faecal incontinence 416
  and Hirschsprung's disease 402
  and meconium ileus 328
  and NEC 357
  T-tube 325
ileum
  endoscopy of 378
  resection of 363, 366, 444, 448
immunodeficiency 303
immunosuppression
  and graft vs. host disease 637
  induction 753–4
  side effects of 753
immunotherapy 655
imperforate anus
  and anal dilatations 425–6
  and Down's syndrome 424
  and faecal incontinence 414–15
  in neonates 418–19
  and OA/TOF 708
  and rectovaginal fistula 425
indomethacin 28, 247, 296, 356
infantile haemangioma 169, 263–4,
    266–73
infections, factors in occurrence 19
inferior vena cava
  compression of 270
  and portal vein 452
  and right atrium 248–9
infertility
  and CF 467
  and chemotherapy 688
  and PUV 568
inflammatory bowel disease (IBD)
  diagnosis of 394
  and SBS 359
infliximab 381–4
inguinal canal, anatomy of 283–4
inguinal hernia
  clinical manifestation of 284–5
  complications of 286
  female 285–6
  incidence of 284
  management of 285
inguinal herniotomy 492
inguinal pouch 595
inhalation injury 108, 112–13
inotropes, mechanism of action 25
inspissated bile plug syndrome 439
insulin, and hyperglycaemia 10
insulinoma 470–1, 676–7
intercostal nerve 289
intercostal vessels 50, 66, 248
interferon 198, 264–6
international normalised ratio (INR) 457
intersex disorders 581, 594
intestinal adaptation 360–1, 367
intestinal atresia
  and alimentary tract duplications
    339
  and gastroschisis 279, 281–2, 732–3
  genetic aspects of 304
  and late intrauterine insults 302–3
  mechanism of 302

morbidity of 309
and SBS 359
and ultrasound 305
intestinal continuity 369–70
intestinal loops, recirculating 370
intestinal neuronal dysplasia (IND) 406
intestinal obstruction
adhesive 309, 324, 376, 405
and ingested magnets 205
and intestinal atresia 309
and Meckel's diverticulum 332–3
intestinal perforation
and abdominal trauma 71
and meconium ileus 324
and NEC 355–6
and seat-belt syndrome 77
intestinal pseudo-obstruction, chronic
405–6
intestinal segments, reversed 369, 372
intestinal walls 307, 330, 381
intestine transplants 752
intra-abdominal abscess 375
intra-abdominal bleeding 81
intra-abdominal injury
and bladder rupture 90
diagnosis of 53, 82
and kidney injuries 84
missed 73–4
and TBI 81
intra-abdominal pressure, indirect
measurement of 76
intracranial bleeding 51, 455, 757
intracranial pressure monitoring 60
intracranial tumours 699
intralipid 739
intralobar sequestrations (ILSs) 176,
180, 786
intramedullary fixation 96, 102, 771
intraosseous access 37, 41, 52
intraperitoneal lavage 20
intraperitoneal sepsis 328
intrathoracic injury 66
intrauterine growth retardation (IUGR)
3
intravenous antibiotics
and empyema 183
and meconium ileus 327
and renal disease 488
and UTIs 518, 521
intravenous hyperalimentation 111–12
intravenous urogram (IVU) 509–10
intubation
and aspiration pneumonia 62
and brain injury 60
and burn injuries 108
endotracheal, see endotracheal
intubation
rapid-sequence 49–50
intussusception
aetiology of 344–5
age-related correlation 349
and alimentary tract duplications
340
and appendicectomy 375
bowel segments associated with 345
and Burkitt's lymphoma 689
idiopathic 344, 390
and intestinal atresia 303
investigations of 346–7
management of 347–9
and Meckel's diverticulum 333, 335
postoperative 316, 348, 350

and rectal prolapse 346
recurrent 349
small-bowel 345, 691
invertograms 418–19
Iowa procedure 371–2
IQ testing 7
iron, absorption of 366–7
isoflurane 738
ITP (idiopathic thrombocytopenic
purpura) 117–18, 481, 489
Ivemark's syndrome 295, 478
IVH (intraventricular haemorrhage) 15,
34, 757, 775

jaundice
and bile leak 82
and cholangitis 430
and choledochal cyst 436–7
differential diagnosis of 431, 721,
726–7, 731
early 432, 726, 756
and jejunoileal atresia 304
obstructive 437, 439, 664, 724,
727, 730
and portal hypertension 456
and thyrotoxicosis 135
jejunal atresia 301, 304, 714
jejunoileal atresia 300–9
jejunum
removal of 367
resection of 362–3
jugular veins 38, 41, 62–4, 188
juvenile polyposis 384, 386–7, 391–2

kaposiform haemangioendothelioma
(KHE) 263, 265, 268, 273
karyotyping
and hypospadias 576
and inguinal hernia 286
Kasabach–Merritt's phenomenon 263,
268, 273, 659, 695–6
Kasai's procedure 428–35, 728–9
Kawasaki's disease 445, 589
ketoconazole 753
keyhole sign 563, 565, 782
kidney disease
chronic 493
polycystic 85, 459, 496; see also
ADPKD; ARPKD
kidney injury
frequency of 84
non-operative management of 87–8
progressive 523
and sports 85
vulnerability of children to 85
kidney transplant 750–1
kidneys
absent 424
bright 508, 511
clear cell sarcoma of (CCSK) 648–9
cysts of, see renal cysts
dysplastic 608, 725
echogenic 563
ectopic, see renal ectopia
horseshoe 85, 496–8, 624
multicystic dysplastic 502–3
solitary 89, 499, 646
upper moiety of 510, 513
Klinefelter's syndrome
and cryptorchidism 595
and gynaecomastia 155
and hypospadias 572

karyotype of 601
and micropenis 588
and tumours 680
Klippel–Feil's syndrome 625
Klippel–Trénaunay's syndrome 261–2,
274
knee injuries 98, 129

labia majora 2, 284
labia minora 2, 615
labial adhesions 537, 615–16
lactic acid levels, increased 113, 744
lactobezoar 209
Ladd's bands 311, 315
Ladd's procedure 313, 315, 375
LAGB (laparoscopic adjustable gastric
banding) 795
lambdoid suture synostosis 776
Langerhans's cells 274, 584
laparoscopy, diagnostic, see diagnostic
laparoscopy
laparotomy
diagnostic, see diagnostic
laparotomy
emergency 81
epidural 737
exploratory 81, 137, 687
and intraperitoneal lavage 20
and intussusception 350
and lactobezoars 209
and NEC 357
laryngeal cleft 162–3
laryngomalacia 34, 163
laryngospasm 48, 205, 232, 739
laryngotracheo-oesphageal cleft
(LTOC) 217
laxatives
and constipation 119, 407
and enemas 410, 412
lazy-bladder syndrome 541–3, 547
Legg–Calvé–Perthes's disease 771–2
leucocyte esterase 516, 518
leucocytosis 12, 629–30
leucopenia 109, 454–5, 457, 753
leukaemia
and acute tumour lysis syndrome
639
and AHO 762
and cardiac tumours 242
precursor B-cell 638
and priapism 589
secondary 688
leukovorin 640
Leydig cell tumours 701
Leydig cells
hypoplasia 573
and hypospadias 572
LHR (lung–head ratio) 783–4
Li–Fraumeni's syndrome 271, 645
lichen amyloidosis 139
lichen planus 637
lichen sclerosis 583–4, 617, 620
ligament of Treitz, see duodenojejunal
junction
limb length discrepancy 95, 771–2
lipids, in parenteral nutrition 9
lipomas
and Cowden's syndrome 387
and intussusception 345
liposuction 265–6, 587
liquefaction necrosis 113, 207, 219
Littre's hernia 284–5, 333

liver
anatomy of 665
neonatal 17
tumours of, *see* hepatic tumours
liver biopsies 428–9, 432–3, 459
liver decompensation 430, 457
liver disease
advanced 12, 454–8, 462
hepatocellular 460
progressive 428, 433
TPN-induced 11
liver injuries
non-operative management of 72–3,
73, 81–2
operative management of 75
and physical abuse 121
liver resection 75, 82, 454, 663–5
liver transplantation
allocation of donor organs 751
and cholestasis 443
donor factors in 754
and Kasai's procedure 428, 434–5
and portal hypertension 460
rejection episodes 754
thrombosis after 454
lobar emphysema, congenital 175–6,
180
lobectomy
and cystic fibrosis 185
of liver 665
and lung disease 179, 191
of thyroid 674–5
loperamide 368, 412, 415
lower oesophageal sphincter (LOS)
as anti-reflux barrier 227
and foreign bodies 201–2
LSG (laparoscopic sleeve gastrectomy)
795
lumbar nerves 289
lumbar puncture 488
lumbosacral spine 188, 272, 473, 547,
549
Lund and Browder chart 106–7, 109
lung abscesses 187–8, 205
lung development 170, 176, 180, 508
lung disease
chronic interstitial 191
restrictive 270, 688
lung lesions, cystic 177–81, 502, 717
lung masses, large, *see* CCAM
lung transplant 190, 752
lungs, hypoplastic 682
LUTS (lower urinary tract symptoms)
528–33
lymph nodes
biopsy 687
cervical 716, 718
dissection 179, 668, 674, 681
lymphadenitis 20, 130, 164
lymphangioma 130, 193, 720, 787
lymphatic malformation
macrocystic 130, 198–9, 198, 266,
272, 719
microcystic 266–7, 274
progression over time 263
lymphatic obstruction, cystic 130
lymphatic spread 664
lymphoedema 265–6, 273
lymphoma; *see also* Hodgkin's
lymphoma; non-Hodgkin's
lymphoma
anaplastic large cell 637, 642

and intussusception 345, 349, 390,
691
large B-cell 637, 690, 693–4, 702
of the liver 657
lymphoblastic 637, 690–2
and PET scan 642
and respiratory distress 691
lymphoproliferative disease, post-
transplant 690, 693, 747

MACE, *see* Malone procedure
macroglossia 468, 645, 731
macrosomia 731, 756
MAG3 renogram 507–10, 513
magnesium 114, 309
magnets, ingestion of 200, 205
malabsorption 205, 309, 364, 370,
796, 798
male phenotypic differentiation 574, 600
Mallory–Weiss's tear 389
malnutrition
assessing 8
and biliary atresia 433
and chylothorax 189–90
and microgastria 294
and NEC 358
protein-calorie 111, 311, 798
and SGA infants 3
Malone procedure 409, 411
malposition 310, 315
malrotation
and alimentary tract duplications
339
and annular pancreas 465
associated anomalies 315–16
diagnosis of 312, 712–13
and gastroschisis 733
intestinal 316, 735
and intestinal atresia 303, 306
management of 313, 315
and Meckel's diverticulum 332
and microgastria 294
and pyloric atresia 293
and pyloric stenosis 711
radiography of 712
and small bowel gas 313
and umbilical cord hernia 280
Marfan's syndrome 160, 260–1, 286, 769
marijuana, *see* cannabis
Martin's procedure 402–3
Mayer–Rokitansky–Küster–Hauser's
syndrome 339, 601, 605, 624–5
MCIH (metachronous contralateral
inguinal hernia) 284–5
meatal stenosis 529–30, 577–9, 585–6
meatal ulceration 585–6
meatus, abnormal 537
Meckel's diverticulum
association of 332
asymptomatic 335–6
complications of 334–5
development of 330
and hernia 285
incidence of 331
incidental 336
and intussusception 348–9, 390
investigations for 334–5
presentation of 332–4, 391
and rectal bleeding 391
meconium
failure of passage 398
irrigating 324–5

meconium aspiration syndrome 33–4
meconium ileus
causes of 320–2
diagnosis of 317–18, 320
imaging for 714–15
and intestinal failure 328
management of 322–3, 326–8
morbidity and mortality 329
surgery for 325–6
meconium peritonitis 305, 321–2, 324
meconium plug syndrome 317
median nerve 100–1
mediastinal compartments 192–3, 192
mediastinal compression 780–2
mediastinal masses 193–5, 194–5, 691,
745, 789
mediastinal tumours 193, 679–80
mediastinitis 202, 220–2, 462
mediastinum, widened 14, 61, 63–4
medulloblastoma 638, 704
megameatus intact prepuce (MIP) 584
megaoesophagus 294–5
megaprepuce 577
megarectosigmoid 405, 412, 415, 419
megaureters 423, 513
melanomas 154, 345
meningitis 123, 343, 485
meningococcal sepsis 117
meningocele
anterior sacral 723, 777
anterior thoracic 195
and neurogenic bladder 556
upper lumbar 549
menstrual cycle, and ovarian cysts 630
mesenteric adenitis 445, 617
mesentery
base of 310–11
cysts in 312
mesna 640
metabolic acidosis
and burn injuries 108–9, 113
and midgut volvulus 311
and NEC 353–4
and propofol 739
and shock 31
and TAPVR 256
metabolic disorders 589, 661, 744,
771, 780
metabolic syndrome 792
metal allergies 158–9
metaplastic polyps 386–7
metastatic disease 242, 641–2, 648, 662
metastatic lesions 154, 657, 676
metatarsus adductus 765, 768
methotrexate 191, 381–2, 637, 640
metoclopramide 235–6
metopic synostosis 776
metronidazole 188, 382, 401
microcephaly, causes of 123
microcolon 318, 323, 329
microcystic lesions 179–80
microgastria, congenital 294–5
micropenis 570, 572–3, 584, 587–8
micturating cystourethrogram (MCUG)
490
and bladder dysfunction 547
and renal dilatation 508–9
and spina bifida 550
and urethral valves 565, 567–8
and UTIs 517, 522
and UVJ obstruction 513
and voiding dysfunction 531, 542–3

midazolam 742, 744
midgut volvulus
    acute 311
    and cholecystitis 446
    chronic 311–12
    and gastroschisis 788
    and malrotation 316
    and SBS 359
midline cysts 131–2
milk-back phenomena 542–3
MIRROR syndrome 785, 789
mitozantrone 642
mixed germ cell tumour 631–2
Mongolian blue spots 118
Morgagni's hernia 734–6
moro reflex 4, 121
morphine 739, 745–6
motor development
    fine 5, 7
    gross 5
motor neurone lesions
    lower 553–5
    upper 553–4, 557
motor vehicle collisions
    and cardiac trauma 244
    as cause of death 47
    evaluating abdomen in 473
    and fluid resuscitation 51
    and genital trauma 619
    and infants 557
    and seat-belt sign 76
    and tension pneumothorax 50
    and thoracic injury 69
    Waddell's triad 48
MR angiography 459
MR urogram 509–10
MRCP (magnetic resonance
    cholangiography) 432, 439, 730
MRI (magnetic resonance imaging)
    and bone tumours 772, 774
    and CDH 783
    and oesophageal duplication 709
    and osteomyelitis 763
    and spinal cord injuries 102
    and spinal cord tethering 777
    and uterine anomalies 626–7
    and Wilms's tumour 723
MRSA infections 763
MTC (medullary thyroid carcinoma)
    139, 667–8, 677–8
mucosal rosette 227–8
müllerian anomalies 622–3, 625–6
müllerian duct syndrome, persistent 601
müllerian ducts
    degeneration of 600
    development of 621–2
müllerian inhibiting substance (MIS)
    573, 595, 600
multimodal therapy 637, 639, 746
multiple atresias 303–4, 306–8
multiple endocrine neoplasia
    and HPT 140
    type 1 139–40, 470–1, 672, 677
    type 2 133, 138–9, 667–8, 672, 677–8
muscle weakness 136, 675–6
mycobacteria, atypical 130
Mycobacterium fortuitum 151
mycophenolate mofetil 753
myelomeningocele
    and anorectal malformations 555
    and cryptorchidism 595
    and faecal incontinence 411–12

fetal 784–5
    and inguinal hernia 284
    and sacrococcygeal teratomas 699
    and spina bifida 549
    treatment of 776–7
    and urinary tract dynamics 551
myxoma 242

naloxone 738
narcotics 406, 643
nasal tip haemangiomas 272
nasogastric decompression 78, 295,
    327
nasogastric tube
    and bowel injuries 78–9
    and caustic ingestion 223
    contraindications to 55
    and meconium ileus 322, 324, 328
nasopharyngeal carcinoma 641
nasopharyngeal teratomas 698
nasopharynx, obstruction of 163
neck cysts
    bronchogenic 131
    midline 132
neck fractures
    femoral 97
    radial 100–1
neck masses 134, 715
    giant 780–1
necrotising enterocolitis (NEC)
    Bell's criteria for 354
    complications of 358
    diagnosis of 352–5, 357
    and ex-prems 396
    and gastric perforation 296
    and gastroschisis 282, 732
    occurrence of 351
    pathogenic mechanisms for 352
    and SBS 359
    surgical treatment of 355–7
necrotising fasciitis 91, 375, 585–6
needle decompression 50
neglect 47, 116, 120, 122, 383
Neisseria meningitidis 19, 74, 485
neonates, see newborns
neostigmine 738
neovascularisation 184, 371
nephrectomy
    and kidney injury 88
    and kidney transplant 750
    partial 88, 646, 649
    radical 648–50
    and renovascular injury 89
nephroblastoma 641
nephroma, mesoblastic 649, 722
nephropathy
    and diabetes 748
    reflux 501, 520, 522
    sickle cell 650
nephrostomy, percutaneous 514
nephrotic syndrome 489, 589
nesidioblastosis, see PHHI
neuroblastoma
    and bone lesions 274
    imaging for 642, 724
    incidence of 651–2
    of the liver 655, 657
    management of 653–4
    mass screening for 653
    in the mediastinum 193, 195
    metastasing 154, 274
    outcomes of 654

primary sites of 652
    stage 4 639, 641–2
    thoracic 196–7
    treatment of 655–6
neuroenteric cysts 195, 343
neurofibromatosis 389, 405, 660–1, 769
neurogenic bladder
    and anorectal malformation 555–6
    associations of 512
    causes for 547–8
    and circumcision 585
    high-pressure 512
    surgery for 558–60
neurological impairment 234, 237–8,
    785
newborns
    fluid compartments in 11
    gestational age and weight 2–3
    normal growth for 3
    PICC placement in 43
    renal function in 12
    shock in 28
NICH (non-involuting congenital
    haemangioma) 273
nipple piercing 151
Nissen fundoplication 213, 230–1, 237–9
nitric oxide 173–4, 256, 400, 589
nocturia 533–4, 539, 542–3
non-Hodgkin's lymphoma
    in the mediastinum 193–4
    metastasing 154
    prognosis of 689–90
    sites of 689
    treatment of 637
    types of 690, 702
non-rotation 316
non-selective shunts 463
Norwood procedure 254
NSAIDs (non-steroidal anti-
    inflammatory drugs)
    and acute pain 746
    and bone tumours 773
    and PDA 247
    and pectal bars 160
    postoperative 742
Nuss's procedure 156, 159
nutrition, parenteral, see parenteral
    nutrition
nutritional status, measuring changes
    in 8
NWTSG (North American National
    Wilms' Tumour Study Group) 641,
    646–7, 649–50

obesity
    definition of 791
    and cardiovascular disease 799
    and cholelithiasis 444–5
    and concealed penis 587
    and gallstones 448
    non-surgical treatment of 796
    psychosocial impact of 792
    risk factors for 791–2
    and SGA infants 3
    and venous thromboembolism 740
observational studies 803
obstructive shock 24, 28
octreotide
    and chylothorax 188–9
    and PHHI 143, 468
    and portal hypertension 461
    and variceal bleed 393

oedema, postoperative 350, 578
oesophageal atresia (OA)
  associations of 708
  clinical signs of 211
  and CPAP 34
  and duodenal atresia 214
  and GOR 213, 230
  investigations for 212, 708–9
  and LTOC 217
  prenatal diagnosis of 211
  surgical repair of 215
  and tracheomalacia 213–14
  types of 210, 706
oesophageal cancer 223, 225
oesophageal dilatation 224–5
oesophageal duplication 339, 341, 709
oesophageal duplication cysts 195–6
oesophageal injury 68, 207, 218, 220, 222
oesophageal manometry 233
oesophageal monitoring 233
oesophageal pathology 201, 208
oesophageal perforation, and antibiotics 222
oesophageal peristalsis 227–8, 232
oesophageal strictures
  after OA repair 212–13
  and caustic ingestion 223
  management of 224
oesophageal ulceration 224, 462
oesophageal varices 430, 433, 463
oesophagitis 229, 233, 235, 441
oesophagus
  congenital stenosis of 216
  foreign objects in 200–2, 207
  intra-abdominal 227–8
oestrogen therapy, topical 616, 620
OGD (oesophagogastroduodenoscopy) 230, 472
OHVIRA (obstructed hemivagina, ipsilateral renal anomaly) syndrome 626
oligohydramnios
  and PBS 609
  and PUV 511, 563–4, 782
  and renal dilatation 508
omphalocele
  associations of 732
  and Beckwith–Wiedemann's syndrome 731
  embryogenesis of 278
  and GORD 228
  and malrotation 315
  management of 781
  and Meckel's diverticulum 332
  and small bowel atresia 303
  and treatment options 281
omphalomesenteric duct anomalies 330–2
operating theatres 280, 738
opiates 742, 745–6
opioids 368, 738, 745
OPSI (overwhelming post-splenectomy infection) 73–4, 482, 484–6
oral contraceptives
  and breast discharge 151
  and cholelithiasis 445
  and hepatocellular adenoma 661, 663
  and thromboembolism 740
orchidopexy 480, 568, 595, 597–8
organ donation 748–9, 751

organ transplants
  acute rejection 754
  opportunistic infections in 749–50
  survival rates 752
oropharyngeal injury 219–20
oropharyngeal teratomas, see epignathus
oropharynx, obstruction of 163
orthopaedic disorders 765
Ortolani's test 766
osteochondromas 773
osteolysis, progressive 274
osteomas 384–5, 773
osteomyelitis 18, 37, 53, 761–3
osteonecrosis 97, 101, 771
osteopontin 435
osteosarcoma 641–2, 772–3
osteotomy, femoral shortening 766–7
ostial lesions 259
ovarian cysts 438, 627–8, 630
ovarian masses 629, 631
ovarian teratoma 682
ovarian torsion 376, 625–6, 628–9
ovarian tumours 631–3
  markers of 632
overflow incontinence 408, 548, 566–7
overweight 139, 791
oxybutynin
  and neuropathic bladder 512
  and PNE 539–40, 543–4, 550, 577
oxygen, and shock 27

packed red blood cells (PRBCs) 51, 72, 81, 482
pain, acute 630, 745–6
PAIS, see AIS (androgen insensitivity syndrome), partial
pancreas
  annular 465–6
  cysts of 469
  ectopic 439
pancreas divisum (PD) 466
pancreas transplantation 748
pancreatectomy
  95% 468–9
  distal 471, 473, 677
  near-total 143
  total 474–5
pancreatic ductal stenosis 320
pancreatic duplications 340
pancreatic embryology 465
pancreatic injuries 71, 77, 473
pancreatic insufficiency 320–1, 467
pancreatic islet cell tumours 470–1, 677
pancreatic pseudocysts 474
pancreatic resection 143, 469
pancreaticobiliary malunion 438–9
pancreaticoblastoma 469
pancreatitis
  acute 439–40, 474
  chronic 474–5
  and ERCP 449
  iatrogenic 440
  and splenectomy 483
panhypopituitarism 143, 587
papillomatosis
  juvenile 152
  recurrent respiratory, see RRP
paracetamol 742, 745–6
parachute reflex 4–5
parenchymal laceration 72, 87
parental responsibility 116–17

parenteral nutrition, lipids in 9
parotid gland 717, 720
patent vitelline duct 333
Pavlik harness 98, 766
PBND (primary bladder-neck dysfunction) 530–1
PDA (patent ductus arteriosus)
  characteristics of 247
  complications of closure 257, 356
  and ligation 166
  and MRKH 624
  nerve damage and 166–7
  and shock 28
PEB 682–4
pectus bar 156–60
pectus excavatum, repairing 156–7
PEEP (positive end-expiratory pressure) 32–3
PEG (percutaneous endoscopic gastrotomy) 120, 125, 778
pelvic floor muscle retraining 532–3
pelvic fracture
  and bladder rupture 90
  as cause of bleeding 80
  and child abuse 47
pelvic inflammatory disease 625–6
pelvic irradiation 643
pelvic osteotomies 612
pelvic trauma 630
penicillin 74, 187, 190, 486
penile cancer 584
penile lymphoedema 585–6
penile torsion 591
penis
  concealed 584, 586–7
  injury to 92
pentalogy of Cantrell 279, 281
peptic ulceration 235, 294
pericardial effusions
  and cardiac trauma 244
  and central venous catheters 14, 38
  and hydrops 178
  and hypothyroidism 140
pericardiocentesis 38, 42–3, 64
perineal trauma 588–90, 618
perineum
  abnormal female 537
  burns to 106
  examination 422
periportal fibrosis 439, 729
peristalsis, ineffective 307, 370
peritoneal dialysis 284, 288, 503
peritoneal drainage 296, 355–6
peritoneal lavage 20
  diagnostic, see DPL
peritoneal sepsis 20
peritonitis
  and antibiotics 222
  diffuse 74–5, 82
  and gastric duplications 294
  and hypervolaemia 324
  and hypovolaemia 322
  and intussusception 347
Perlman's syndrome 645
PET scan 481, 642, 702
Peutz–Jeghers's syndrome (PJS) 345, 349, 385–6, 392, 595
Peyer's patches 344
Peyronie's disease 91
PFFD (proximal focal femoral deficiency) 771
phaeochromocytoma 668–9, 677, 701

phase I clinical trials 636
PHHI (persistent hyperinsulinaemic hypoglycaemia of infancy) 141–3, 468–9
phimosis
  pathological 583
  recurrent 586
phrenic nerve paresis 39–40
phyllodes tumours 150, 152
physeal injury, *see* growth plates
physical abuse 47, 121
PI (pneumatosis intestinalis) 352–5
PICCs (peripherally inserted central catheters) 36, 38, 42–3
pinchcock action 228
pineal gland 679, 700
PIP (positive inspiratory pressure) 32–3
pituitary adenoma 671, 677
pituitary neoplasm 671
platelet counts, range for 17
platelet function defects 118
platelet transfusion 18, 268, 273
platelets, agents released by 17
platinum, and chemotherapy 151, 684, 688
PNE (primary nocturnal enuresis) 533–40
pneumatic reduction 333, 346–8
pneumatoceles 186
pneumomediastinum 66, 68, 161, 202
pneumonia
  aspiration 62, 231, 294
  and ATDs 340
  and empyema 186
  and GOR 230, 234
  and laryngeal cleft 163
  management of 183
  pneumocystis 749–50
  post-obstructive 203, 205
  and splenic trauma 74
pneumothorax
  and fractures 61
  open 63
  spontaneous 187
  tension 23, 28, 50, 62–3
  and tracheocutaneous fistula 161
  and vascular access 40
Politano–Leadbetter technique 523
polydactyly 768
polydipsia 136, 676
polyhydramnios
  antenatal 294
  and cervical teratomas 682
  and CPAM 178
  maternal 211, 304–5, 649
  and nephroma 649
  and small bowel atresia 714
polymastia 147–8
polysorbate 319, 323, 327
polysplenia 255–6, 434–5, 478, 725
polyuria
  and adrenal dysfunction 136
  nocturnal 535–7, 539
  and phaeochromocytoma 668
  and PUV 567
porta hepatis 447, 665, 727
portal fibrosis 731
portal hypertension
  and biliary atresia 433, 729
  and choledochal cysts 439
  investigations for 457–9
  and portal venous system 452–3

posthepatic 453–4, 463
presentation of 435, 454–6
symptomatic 430
treatment of 460
and variceal bleeding 461–2
portal vein
  development of 451–2
  preduodenal 478, 665, 725
portal vein thrombosis
  associations of 453
  extrahepatic 453, 455–6, 458–9
  and venous catheters 303
portal venous gas 317, 353–5
portal venous system 452–3, 459
portosystemic shunts 393, 459, 462
Pott's puffy tumour 716
potty training 6
PPV (patent processus vaginalis) 283–4, 287, 489, 597
Prader–Willi's syndrome 587–8
pre-eclampsia 3, 524, 571, 789
pre-term infants, *see* premature infants
predictive value, negative 804
pregnancy 120, 794, 798
premature infants
  definition of 2
  and bowel perforation 296
  and ECMO 34
  fluid management for 11, 15
  and general anaesthesia 739
  and lactobezoars 209
  and NEC 351
  nutritional requirements of 8–9
  PDA in 247
  and pyloric stenosis 297
  and shock 28
  and surgery 18, 741
  survival advantages for 760
  and umbilical hernia 288
prematurity, extreme 660
prenatal ultrasound, and CDH 172
prepuce 574, 577, 583–4
presacral masses 554, 724
presacral teratoma 777
*Prevotella melaninogenica* 151
priapism 588–90
primitive gut 314
Pringle manoeuvre 75, 663
procoagulants 17–18, 457
projectile vomiting 297
propanolol 393, 461
propofol 738–9
propranolol 169, 266, 272
prostacyclin 16
prostatic hypoplasia 607–8
prostatic urethra, dilated 563, 565–6, 607
protein-losing enteropathy 254–5
proteins, and nutrition 8–9
proteinuria
  and HSP 489
  and MIRROR syndrome 789
  and nephrotic syndrome 489
  postoperative 750
prothrombin time (PT) 17, 118, 268, 457, 459
proton pump inhibitors 235, 368
prune belly syndrome (PBS)
  classic triad in 607
  and cryptorchidism 595
  features of 563, 608
  and GORD 228

incidence of 607–8
management of 609
and neurogenic bladder 512
prenatal intervention for 608
testes in 611
pruritus 139, 693
pseudo-longitudinal study 803
pseudoephedrine 300–1
pseudokidney sign 346–7
*Pseudomonas* 109, 148, 184, 190
pseudopapillary tumour 469–70
pseudotumour cerebri 793–4, 797
psoas hitch 89
PTC (percutaneous transhepatic cholangiography) 440, 664
PTEN mutations 265, 271
PTLD, *see* lymphoproliferative disease, post-transplant
puberty, delayed 139, 383
pubic diastasis 611, 613–14
pubic symphysis 284, 612
pubourethral ligament 603
PUJO (pelviureteric junction impaired drainage) 498
pulmonary branch stenosis 725
pulmonary hypertension
  and CDH 171–4, 783
  and heart transplant 752
  in newborns 28
  and portal hypertension 455
pulmonary hypoplasia
  and CDH 171–2
  and ECMO 33–4
  and exomphalos 279, 282
  and PBS 609
  preventing 564, 782
  and PUV 564
pulmonary immaturity 789–90
pulmonary sepsis 328
pulmonary sequestrations, extralobar 173, 176
pulmonary stenosis 250, 253
pulmonary venous drainage, anomalous 250, 256
putty sign 322
PUV (posterior urethral valves)
  and circumcision 585
  and cryptorchidism 595
  diagnosis of 490, 511, 563–5
  fetal intervention in 563–4
  incidence of 562
  long-term outcome of 568
  presentation of 564–5
  treatment of 491, 566–7, 781–2
  and upper tract dilatation 508
pyelonephritis
  acute 491
  incidence of 515
  indications of 518
  and kidney injury 88
  pseudomonas 491
  unilateral 526
pyelopexy 513–14
pyeloplasty 498, 514
pyelostomy, cutaneous 566
pyloric atresia 293, 296, 304
pyloric stenosis 13, 297–8
pylorospasm 219, 711

rabies 105–6, 749
raccoon eyes 55
radial nerve injuries 100

radiation enteritis, acute 643
radiofrequency ablation (RFA) 773, 786, 788
radiography
  and AHO 762
  cross-table lateral 418
  and fractures 56
  and OA/TOF 708
radioiodine ablative therapy 674
radiological workup, preoperative 662
radionuclide scanning 391, 673
radiotherapy
  cardiotoxicity of 642
  and lymphoma 637, 692
  and phaeochromocytoma 669
  and PTLD 747
  and renal rhabdoid tumour 650
  and rhabdomyosarcoma 664
  and SCFE 771
  side effects of 688
  and Wilms's tumour 647
randomisation, stratified 805
rapid sequence induction (RSI) 740, 742–3
RCC (renal cell carcinoma) 501, 648, 722
reactive airway disease 173, 203, 232–3
receptor/action associations 24–5
rectal atresia 425, 698
rectal biopsy 319, 398–9, 404
rectal bleeding
  and cow's milk exclusion diet 392
  investigation of 390–1, 394
  and portal hypertension 454
rectal injuries 79
rectal prolapse 119, 346, 391, 467
rectosigmoid, dilated 416
recurrent laryngeal nerve 131–2, 166–7, 215, 217
recurrent respiratory papillomatosis (RRP) 166
recurrent UTIs
  and detrusor irritability 542
  investigation of 522
  risk factors for 500
  and sexual abuse 119
  and spina bifida 550, 553
  and voiding disorders 541, 544
Reed–Sternberg cells 686, 702
reflexes, primitive 4
remifentanil 739
renal agenesis 499, 601, 624, 626
renal artery fibrodysplasia 259
renal artery stenosis, bilateral 259
renal cysts 502–3, 563
renal dilatation, antenatal 508–9
renal disease, end-stage (ESRD) 501, 505, 567–8, 750
renal dysplasia 491, 563, 607–9
renal ectopia 495–6, 498
renal enlargement, massive 505
renal failure
  chronic 568
  and spider bites 104
renal function, in newborns 12
renal masses 722
renal medullary carcinoma 650
renal parenchyma 89, 499, 563
renal rhabdoid tumour, malignant 649–50
renal scarring
  and antibiotic prophylaxis 501, 517, 525

risk factors for 500
  and VUR treatment 525
renal trauma, see kidney injury
renal tumours, imaging of 723
renal ultrasound 509–10
  and antenatal dilatation 508
  and hydroureteronephrosis 490
renorraphy 88
renovascular injuries 89
reovirus 429
research projects, sequence of steps in 802
resection
  and haemangioma 267
  and KHE 265
  and lymphatic malformation 266
  and venous malformation 264–5
respiratory compromise
  and ARPKD 504
  and cystic hygroma 199
  and haemangioendotheliomas 658
  and hepatic haemangioma 270
  and lung haemorrhage 455
  and scorpion sting 105
respiratory depression, delayed 742
respiratory distress
  and ATDs 340
  and cardiac tumour 242
  and haemangioendothelioma 658
  and hamartoma 662
  and OA 211
  and PUV 564
  and tracheobronchial tree injuries 66
respiratory distress syndrome 34, 756–9
  acute, see ARDS
respiratory failure 76, 504, 734
respiratory insufficiency 167, 282
resuscitation
  and burn injuries 108
  fluid, see fluid resuscitation
  and intravenous access 22
  neonatal 783
retinal haemorrhages 47
retinoids 655
retinol binding protein 8
retroperitoneal haematoma 88
retroperitoneal lymph node dissection 681–2
retropharyngeal abscess 164–5, 720
retrosternal pain 220, 230–1
revascularisation 89
rhabdomyolysis 104, 739–40
rhabdomyomas 242
rhabdomyosarcoma
  and chemotherapy 640
  localised 638
  metastasis of 154
  paratesticular 681
  presentation of 640
  prevalence of 242
  and risk stratification 642
rib fractures 47, 61–2, 119
RICH (rapidly involuting congenital haemangioma) 273
rickets 139–40, 771, 776
rifampin 753
right atrium, morphology of 248
risk stratification 638, 642
rituximab 637, 690
rooting reflex 4
rotary subluxation, atlanto-axial 58

rotavirus 344–5, 429
Roux-en-Y procedures
  and bariatric surgery 795, 799–800
  and cysts 440–1, 443
  and Kasai procedure 729
  and pancreas injury 473
rubella 3, 123

sacral agenesis 530, 554
sacral anomalies 555, 681
sacral cord injury 557
sacral nerve stimulation 533
sacral vertebrae 413, 415, 556
sacrococcygeal teratoma
  Altman classification of 683
  associations of 685, 697–9
  fetal 785
  incidence of 679
  and MIRROR syndrome 789
  preoperative workup for 680–1
  risk of recurrence 681
  staging of 698
  surgery for 699
sacrum, absent 411–12
sagittal synostosis 776
salmonella 381, 394, 763
salt wasting 601–2
Salter–Harris type fractures 95, 99, 101
Sandifer's syndrome 232
Sano shunt 254
sarcoma
  clear cell 646, 648, 723
  soft-tissue 697
  undifferentiated embryonal 658, 660–2, 664
SBS (short bowel syndrome)
  acquired 328
  algorithm for management 371
  causes of 359, 361–2
  combination therapy for 360
  and gastroschisis 732–3, 788
  and jejunal atresia 308–9
  and malrotation 313, 316
  and nutrition 368–9
  operative intervention for 364, 369, 371–2
  and TPN 362
Scarpa's fascia 283, 587
SCFE (slipped capital femoral epiphysis) 771
Scheuermann's kyphosis 765, 770
Schilling's test 294
scimitar syndrome 243, 250
scintigraphy 232–3
  hepatobiliary 432, 440
  renal 500, 565
SCIWORA (spinal cord injury without radiographic abnormality) 53–4, 102, 557
sclerotherapy
  endoscopic 393, 462
  and haemangiomas 264
  and lymphatic malformation 266, 272
  and varicoceles 599
  and venous malformations 260, 264–5, 267
scoliosis 234, 274, 557, 769, 777
scorpion stings 105, 115
scrotal haematoma 84, 86, 92, 598
scrotal injuries 92
scrotal oedema, idiopathic 593